Clinical Pediatric Ophthalmology and Strabismus

Clinical Pediatric Ophthalmology and Strabismus

Editors

Yogesh Shukla MS (Ophth)
Professor and Advisor
Department of Ophthalmology
National Institute of Medical Sciences
Jaipur, Rajasthan, India

Rohit Saxena MD (Ophth) PhD
Professor
Head Strabismus Service
RP Centre for Ophthalmic Sciences
All India Institute of Medical Sciences
New Delhi, India

Foreword

David L Guyton

JAYPEE

JAYPEE BROTHERS MEDICAL PUBLISHERS
The Health Sciences Publisher
New Delhi | London

Jaypee Brothers Medical Publishers (P) Ltd.

Headquarters
EMCA House, 23/23-B
Ansari Road, Daryaganj
New Delhi 110 002, India
Landline: +91-11-23272143, +91-11-23272703
+91-11-23282021, +91-11-23245672
e-mail: jaypee@jaypeebrothers.com

Corporate Office
4838/24, Ansari Road, Daryaganj
New Delhi 110 002, India
Phone: +91-11-43574357
Fax: +91-11-43574314
e-mail: jaypee@jaypeebrothers.com

Overseas Office
JP Medical Ltd.
83, Victoria Street, London
SW1H 0HW (UK)
Phone: +44-20 3170 8910
e-mail: info@jpmedpub.com

EU GPSR Authorised Representative
Logos Europe, 9 rue Nicolas Poussin
17000, La Rochelle, France
Phone: +33 (0) 6 67 93 73 78
e-mail: contact@logoseurope.eu

Website: www.jaypeebrothers.com
Website: www.jaypeedigital.com

Inquiries for bulk sales may be solicited at: jaypee@jaypeebrothers.com

Clinical Pediatric Ophthalmology and Strabismus

First Edition: 2023, *Reprint*: **2025**

ISBN: 978-93-5465-353-7

Printed at: Samrat Offset Pvt. Ltd.

Dedicated to

Our parents and our families

Contributors

Abhay R Vasavada MS FRCS
Director
Raghudeep Eye Hospital
Ahmedabad, Gujarat, India

Adrianna Jensen MD
Ophthalmology Resident
Zanvyl Krieger Children's Eye Center
Wilmer Eye Institute
Johns Hopkins Medical Center
Baltimore, Maryland, USA

Ahmad Kheirkhah MD
Assistant Professor
Eye Department
UT Texas University College of Medicine
San Antonio, Texas, USA

Aniruddha Agarwal MS (Ophth)
Consultant
Eye Institute, Cleveland Clinic
Abu Dhabi, UAE

Ankita Aishwarya MD
Consultant
Department of Ocular Oncology
Centre for Sight
Hyderabad, Telangana, India

Birsen Gökyiğit MD
Associate Professor
Department of Ophthalmology
University of Health Sciences
Istanbul, Turkey

Courtney L Kraus MD
Faculty
Zanvyl Krieger Children's Eye Center
Wilmer Eye Institute
Johns Hopkins Medical Center
Baltimore, Maryland, USA

Dhikshitha Balaji MD
Faculty
Case Western Reserve University
School of Medicine
Cleveland, Ohio, USA

Edward Kuwera MD
Assistant Professor
Pediatric Ophthalmology and Strabismus
Wilmer Eye Institute
Johns Hopkins Medical Center
Baltimore, Maryland, USA

Emmanuel Y Chang MD
Retina Specialist
University of Texas Medical School
Houston, Texas, USA

Fatema Ghasia MD
Associate Professor
Department of Ophthalmology
Cleveland Clinic
Cleveland, Ohio, USA

Fatma Yülek MD
Professor
Department of Ophthalmology
Ankara University Medical College
Ankara, Turkey

Jordan Murray PhD
Faculty
Visual Neurosciences and
Ocular Motility Laboratory
Cole Eye Institute, Cleveland Clinic
Cleveland, Ohio, USA

Joseph Conway MD
Resident
Department of Neurology
Cleveland Clinic
Cleveland, Ohio, USA

Karthikeyan Mahalingam MD
Senior Resident
RP Centre for Ophthalmic Sciences
All India Institute of Medical Sciences
New Delhi, India

Kim Jiramongkolchai MD
Assistant Professor
Retina Unit, Wilmer Eye Institute
Johns Hopkins Medical Centre
Baltimore, Maryland, USA

Leela V Raju MD
Faculty
Cornea and Refractive Surgery Unit
NYU Langone Health Tisch Hospital
Brooklyn, New York City, USA

Marina Roizenblatt MD
Retina Specialist
Department of Ophthalmology
Federal University of Sao Paulo
São Paulo, Brazil

Mehmet C Mocan MD
Associate Professor
Department of Ophthalmology
University of Illinois
Chicago, Illinois, USA

Michael O'Rourke
MB FRCS (Ophth) PhD
Consultant
Orbit and Lacrimal Unit
Royal Victorian Eye and Ear Hospital
Melbourne, Australia

Miho Sato MD PhD
Professor
Department of Ophthalmology
Hamamatsu University
School of Medicine
Tokyo, Japan

Mireille Jabroun MD
Assistant Professor
Department of Ophthalmology
University of Arizona College of Medicine
Tucson, Arizona, USA

Mohamad Ibrahime Asif MD
Senior Resident
RP Centre for Ophthalmic Sciences
All India Institute of Medical Sciences
New Delhi, India

Monika Yadav MD
Senior Resident
RP Centre for Ophthalmic Sciences
All India Institute of Medical Sciences
New Delhi, India

Namrata Sharma MD
Professor
Cornea Unit
RP Centre for Ophthalmic Sciences
All India Institute of Medical Sciences
New Delhi, India

Nils Mungan MD
Professor
Department of Ophthalmology
University of Mississippi
Medical College
Jackson, Mississippi, USA

Nitin Kumar Menia MS (Ophth)
Assistant Professor
Department of Ophthalmology
All India Institute of Medical Sciences
Bilaspur, Himachal Pradesh, India

Oded Lagstein MD
Faculty
Department of Ophthalmology
The Bnai Zion Medical Center
Technion—Israel Institute of Technology
Haifa, Israel

Prateek Nishant MD
Senior Resident
Department of Ophthalmology
All India Institute of Medical Sciences
Patna, Bihar, India

Priyadarshini KM MD
Resident
RP Centre for Ophthalmic Sciences
All India Institute of Medical Sciences
New Delhi, India

Rajvardhan Azad MD FRCS
Professor Emeritus
Eye Institute
Indira Gandhi Institute of Medical Sciences, Patna, Bihar, India

Raksha Rao MD
Consultant
Narayana Nethralaya
Bengaluru, Karnataka, India

Rasik Vajpayee MD
Professor
Department of Ophthalmology
Royal Victorian Eye and Ear Hospital
Melbourne, Australia

Rebika Dhiman MD
Assistant Professor
RP Centre for Ophthalmic Sciences
All India Institute of Medical Sciences
New Delhi, India

Rinky Agarwal MD
Faculty
Department of Ophthalmology
Lady Hardinge Medical College
New Delhi, India

Rohit Saxena MD (Ophth) PhD
Professor
Head Strabismus Service
RP Centre for Ophthalmic Sciences
All India Institute of Medical Sciences
New Delhi, India

Samiksha Fouzdar Jain MD
Assistant Professor
Department of Ophthalmology and Visual Sciences, Truhelsen Eye Institute
University of Nebraska Medical Center
Omaha, Nebraska, USA

Sangeeta Khanna MD
Associate Professor
Department of Neuro-Ophthalmology
St Louis University
St Louis, Missouri, USA

Santosh G Honavar MD
Director
National Retinoblastoma Foundation
Ocular Oncology Service, Centre for Sight
Hyderabad, Telangana, India

Sarika Gopalakrishnan
BS (Optom) FAAO PhD
Head
Low Vision Unit
Shankara Netralaya
Chennai, Tamil Nadu, India

Satya S Yalla DO MS
Faculty
Goutami Eye Institute
Rajamahendravaram
Andhra Pradesh, India

Shivanand J Sheth MS FICO
Consultant Ophthalmologist
Royal Victorian Eye and Ear Hospital
Melbourne, Australia

Sony Sinha MS
Associate Professor
Department of Ophthalmology
Patna Medical College
Patna, Bihar, India

Srijana Adhikari MS (Ophth)
Professor
Department of Ophthalmology
University of Nepal Medical College
Kathmandu, Nepal

Srinivas Reddy MS
Director and Vitreo-Retinal Surgeon
Goutami Eye Institute
Rajamahendravaram
Andhra Pradesh, India

Srinivasa R Nambula DNB
Consultant
Department of Pediatric Ophthalmology
Goutamy Eye Institute
Rajamahendravaram
Andhra Pradesh, India

Swati Phuljhele MD
Associate Professor
Strabismus Unit
RP Centre for Ophthalmic Sciences
All India Institute for Medical Sciences
New Delhi, India

Syed Faraaz Hussain MS
Assistant Professor
MGM Medical College
Consultant
Fazal Eye Clinic
Navi Mumbai, Maharashtra, India

Thomas Hardy MBBS FRANZCO
Director
Oculoplasty Unit
Royal Victoria Eye and Ear Hospital
Melbourne, Australia

TS Surendran DO MPhil FRCS (ED)
Vice-Chairman and Director
Department of Pediatric Ophthalmology
Sankara Nethralaya
Chennai, Tamil Nadu, India

Vadrevu K Raju MS FRCS
Clinical Professor
West Virginia University
Director
Eye Foundation of America
Morgantown, West Virginia, USA

Vaishali Rakheja MD
Senior Resident
RP Centre for Ophthalmic Sciences
All India Institute of Medical Sciences
New Delhi, India

Vaishali Vasavada MS (Ophth)
Consultant
Raghudeep Eye Hospital
Ahmedabad, Gujarat, India

Vishali Gupta MS
Professor
Department of Ophthalmology
Advanced Eye Centre
Postgraduate Institute of Medical Education and Research
Chandigarh, India

Yogesh Shukla MS (Ophth)
Professor and Advisor
Department of Ophthalmology
National Institute of Medical Sciences
Jaipur, Rajasthan, India

Foreword

The exponential increase in new studies and exciting discoveries in the field of pediatric ophthalmology and strabismus is out-stripping the abilities of practitioners to keep up. The internet returns hundreds or thousands of articles pertinent to each topic that is searched, but many of the materials are in publications of subspecialty societies that are not open access. Unless one is associated with a university that subscribes to each of these journals, the newest information, however tantalizing, is simply not available or affordable. There is thus a definite need for this book, *Clinical Pediatric Ophthalmology and Strabismus*, by editors/authors Professors Yogesh Shukla and Rohit Saxena. They have solicited chapters from an impressive array of international authors who are best able to condense the past, present, and developing knowledge in their fields to readable and affordable text for the practicing pediatric ophthalmologist/strabismus surgeon.

In reviewing many of the chapters, and in picking up new pearls of knowledge on every page, I was pleased to find mention of some of my own favorite contributions. But others were not to be found, such as my teachings regarding sensory exotropia, divergence insufficiency, and the etiology of dissociated vertical deviation (DVD). So the book is serving another purpose as well stimulating more and better teaching regarding subjects not widely known or appreciated!

Ideally this book, which can function as a valuable conduit between the flood of new knowledge and the needs of the individual practitioner, will continue to grow and prosper through subsequent editions. The editors and the contributors are to be heartily congratulated for a job well conceived and well done!

David L Guyton MD
The Zanvyl Krieger Professor of Pediatric Ophthalmology
Krieger Children's Eye Center, Wilmer Eye Institute
Johns Hopkins University School of Medicine
Baltimore, Maryland, USA

Introduction of Authors-cum-Editors

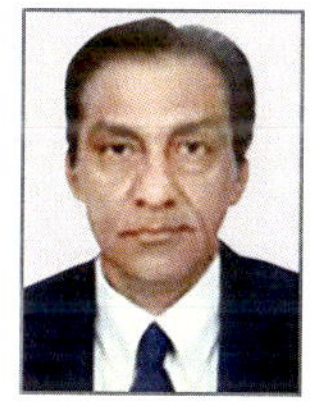

Yogesh Shukla is Professor and Head (Retd.) and currently Professor and Advisor, Department of Ophthalmology at National Institute of Medical Sciences, Jaipur, Rajasthan, India. He has more than 35 years of clinical and teaching experience. He has done Fellowship in Comprehensive Ophthalmology from Eye Foundation of America, West Virginia University, USA in 1997 and Fellowship in Pediatric Ophthalmology and Strabismus from Wilmer Eye Institute, Johns Hopkins Medical Center, USA in 2000. He has chapters in number of books in Ophthalmology, Author of 2 books on Pediatric Ophthalmology; delivered guest lectures/talks on various aspects of Pediatric Ophthalmology and Strabismus in All India Conferences (AIOS); held Instruction courses in AIOS Conferences, SAARC International conferences, Asia-Pacific Society of Pediatric Ophthalmology and Strabismus Conferences. Organizer of World Ocular Trauma Conference in 2012 and International Conference on Pediatric Ophthalmology and Strabismus in Association with AAPOS in 2016. Awarded numerous awards including "Life-Time Achievement Award" by State Society in 2021; "Life-Time Achievement Award" by National Society SPOSI in 2016; and "Times of India National Achievers Award" in 2018. He has served as Secretary, Strabismus and Pediatric Ophthalmology Society of India (SPOSI).

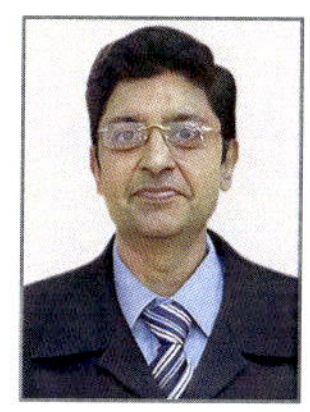

Rohit Saxena is currently Professor and Head of Strabismus Services at Dr RP Centre for Ophthalmic Sciences, All India Institute of Medical Sciences, New Delhi, India. He has more than 22 years of clinical and teaching experience at this prestigious institution. He has 230 indexed publications, 50 chapters in national and international books and has been editor of 3 books on strabismus surgery including a video atlas. He has attended and presented talks in 25 International conferences; routinely presented and conducted Instruction courses at All India conferences and as invited speaker at various national conferences and meetings on Strabismus. He has received more than 30 awards including the Hari Mohan Oration by DOS 2020; Excellence in Strabismology Award by SPOSI 2020; Best of Show Video for AAO (2011) and APAO (2013); AAO 2019, Best video presentation at SPOSI 2019, Best Indexed publication by SPOSI 2016; Best Paper Award in Asia ARVO 2013; AAO (2011) and APAO (2013) Achievement Award and AIIMS Excellence Award in 2018 and 2019.

Preface

Pediatric ophthalmology is one of the fastest growing subspecialties in ophthalmology, but it is still the most understudied and underdeveloped branch. Not too long back, a small child standing in line at a busy hospital outdoor was looked upon with discomfort. But it should not be forgotten that the majority of eye diseases and disorders, stem as congenital or present in childhood or school-age, and if not addressed, remain a distressing stigma for whole life. Practicing pediatric ophthalmology requires skill, patience and some talent. To acquire this, you must have the pearls of text, a fountain of knowledge, from which you gather the proficiency.

Unfortunately, a comprehensive book on this subject is seldom written. An acronym that "don't put all your eggs in one basket", is redundant in the present context. We have gathered eggs from all over the world, the best of them, and presented in one basket for your convenience and understanding. The book is laced with chapters from experts in their respective fields, who are the faculty in renowned institutions of the world, and who have so painstakingly and meticulously written each chapter. It was an expedition in choosing the best, and what they have delivered, is for you to see.

This book is passion and labor of dedication, of commitment and a pledge to deliver the best possible clinical knowledge to the readers. The book stands unique in the sense that information regarding some disorders in children which have never been addressed or given in completeness, is presented here. For example, accommodation in children is supposed to be flawless and has never been questioned. But surprisingly, many ocular problems arising from near work in children are due to accommodative anomalies. Similarly, refractive errors are a different cup of tea when addressed in children and their management requires a different perspective. Vision evaluation in infants and children has been made to understand in a simplified way; Retinitis of prematurity (ROP) has been extensively explained and so is genetics in ophthalmology; to name a few. Strabismus, which in most part, is a pediatric problem, has been dealt as a whole section. It also encompasses strabismic disorders in adults as well.

We the authors-cum-editors, are ourselves experts in various fields of pediatric ophthalmology and have a long clinical experience. The growth of pediatric ophthalmology and strabismus, has inspired us to come out with a comprehensive and simplified textbook and which is affordable. Making of this book has been a journey, a long journey both in time and space. But our greatest solace will be when this book will serve the purpose both to the learner and the learned.

We are also greatly indebted and grateful to all contributing authors of this book, who have given their time and effort in writing each chapter so judiciously.

Though surgical procedures have been briefly described, but details of surgery is outside the scope of this book and for that the reader will have to refer a surgical atlas.

Yogesh Shukla
Rohit Saxena

Contents

SECTION 1

Pediatric Ophthalmology

CHAPTER 1

Pediatric Eye Examination

Yogesh Shukla

"The only thing worse than being blind is to have sight but no vision."

—Hellen Keller

INTRODUCTION

In a general patients outdoor, the presence of a small child as patient is viewed with some distaste, as most of clinicians are not conversant with the techniques of eye examination of a small child. In essence, ocular examination of a small child requires patience, skill, and some talent. If one has to become proficient as a pediatric ophthalmologist, the person has to train himself to learn the techniques for a smooth and efficient examination in children. We will focus most of our attention on learning examination of infants and preschool children where the examination is difficult and requires special skills.

Sophisticated technological advances in medicine have proved to be remarkably useful in the diagnostic process, yet the well-observed history and physical examination remain a clinicians most important tools. They are venerated elements of the art of medicine, the best series of tests we have. Numerous medical anecdotes relate instances in which the examination revealed findings unrelated and unexpected from the patients complaints and concerns.

Timely eye examination and visual assessment are critical for detection of conditions that may result in irreversible visual impairment and in some cases threaten a child's life.

There is a difference in your approach when taking history/examining a small child's eyes than an older child with only vague complaints by parents. Many a times parents will bring children for just routine examination as their other sibling already has an eye problem. The approach to examination will depend upon the age, level of development, and level of understanding of the child. Inspection and observation are probably the most important part of examination.

To architect a pediatric clinic, one has to make certain changes in the environment of the clinic. For example, the waiting area should be different than a general patients area with comfortable sitting and some toys, big and small which makes the child feel at home rather than a hostile hospital atmosphere. Some institutions arrange a "play area" where the child can play during the waiting period. The waiting period should not be too long, as the child may become sleepy or hungry and would be uncooperative during examination. It is imperative that the child must be accompanied by the parents, preferably mother. The examination room should be well lighted at the beginning so that the child is not apprehensive to enter. This has an additional benefit, i.e., the clinician can "observe" the child as he/she comes to the doctor.

THE PROCESS OF EXAMINATION

Observation

Immense amount of information can be had during simple observation of a child. Do not rush to examine the child. Let the child sit comfortably on parents lap for sometime. This will give time for the child to adjust to the new surroundings and more importantly, gives time to the clinician to observe the child. Simple observation will reveal a lot of information, viz. the fixation of eyes, any obvious misalignment, nystagmus, etc. The child's behavior can also be ascertained at this juncture. An irritable child would not cooperate, may not even open eyes, and therefore the examination may be deferred for some other time, or the child may be recalled once he/she has settled. It must be remembered that a sleepy or hungry child will not cooperate and therefore it is prudent to let the child have its timely feed and then recalled after an hour or so.

History

This is most crucial and should be listened carefully from the parents, since, no information can be had from a small child. A very detailed history is not needed as you may loose precious time till the child is cooperative. Relevant and "focused" history is the key and unnecessary questions should be avoided. An old adage that "the patient is always right" does not necessarily apply here. Many a times the mother/parent are ignorant and may not understand the illness; the social circle around them may not perceive subtle strabismus or nystagmus as a threat to vision. The general thinking that such problems occur frequently in infants and small children and will gradually outgrow with time is deeply prevalent and the parents may not record the time when it was noticed. Sometimes, the parent will casually declare that this problem is present since "beginning", even it may have arisen just a couple of weeks back.

History relating to perinatal birth trauma, hypoxia, febrile illness, or any such birth problem should be specifically asked. At times, it is a good idea to ask direct questions if unnecessarily time is being wasted. A slightly older child may himself narrate certain symptoms and this should be carefully noted. Many children may not complain of blurry vision—as they have learned to live with it and appropriate visual test is mandatory. In an older child, the head posture can be observed while he/she is speaking and other facial anomalies can also be observed at this time. Any rubbing of eyes and photophobia should be enquired.

The problem for which the child has been brought for should be asked from the parent or the older child himself (a child of 4–6 years is verbal and should be well communicative), and further queries in that direction should be focused. Whether the ailment is congenital or acquired should be asked and if acquired, then the age of onset. This has a bearing on the prognosis of treatment. If strabismus or nystagmus is observed, the time of onset and frequency should be asked; but if vision defect is the chief complaint, then parents need to specify whether the baby can see lights, respond to gestures, catches small toys, or very small objects. In small child with strabismus, most of times, a vague answer that strabismus is present from beginning is given. As a rule, the parents should be asked to show photographs of child since birth which will reveal the time of onset. This will greatly help in deciding management and prognosis of vision.

In older children, the child's behavior in school should be asked, especially for fatigues, headaches, vertigo, sleepiness, and regarding any specific complaint which has come from school management. Any neurological deficit should be enquired and the referring physicians notes be seen. Whether the child is on any medication, should be specifically asked and the type of medication enquired into. Many medications for any neurologic problem or gastrointestinal (GI) problem contain salts that may cause drowsiness and create unattentiveness which may be perceived as vision defect. Sudden occurrence of strabismus, diminution of vision, or diplopia needs a thorough neurologic checkup and appropriate referral should be done.

The sequence of developmental milestones should be asked and any discrepancy noted.

It is important to remember that all general and visual milestones in a premature infant are delayed and thus all parameters of visual functions are extended.

Lastly, the family history is also important. Enquiry should be done of any similar problem in other sibling, or parents or other direct relatives. Previous miscarriages should be enquired.

In short, as much of history possible should be collected in the shortest time possible; as the child may not cooperate for longer period and the actual physical examination would become difficult.

Older children are better to deal with. They can answer regarding their problems and whatever they narrate should be taken note of it. It is again prudent to develop some kind of friendship by asking about their hobbies, their school program, and about their likes and dislikes before commencing the physical exam.

Physical Examination

Children can be unpredictable, uncooperative, and noncommunicative.

Children between 1 and 2 years are most difficult to examine. In later ages they become more playful and communicative. They start knowing toys and listen to your requests.

For infants, the only source of information is their parents and examination during feeding with a bottle makes things easier. Larger and brightly colored toys are usually used to attract their attention. Noise making toys are not recommended, as movement of eyes due to "sound" gives false information.

Infants and small children should always be examined when seated on mothers lap, where they feel most comfortable and secure. There should be no hurry to finish the examination and it is advisable to keep as much distance away as possible.

Examination should be done with subdued light, as bright light can be intimidating and irritate the child and may close the lids making examination difficult.

Children over 2 years are more responsive, and therefore, calling by their name or nickname, makes them feel better. A friendly rapport should be first established with the child before embarking on any maneuver. Always begin with "noncontact" things: cover test, fixation pattern, red glow, pupillary examination, etc. Many small children get afraid by touch of a stranger, and once they get upset, it is the end of the examination. Allow the parent to show them toys of "appropriate size", while you watch the eye movements for fixation. Appropriate size means the size of an object recommended for that particular age for testing purpose.

External Examination

The child's overall appearance and level of alertness can be judged during history taking from parents or child himself. Ocular alignment and position of head should be the first thing noted. The history will guide in which direction the physical examination should proceed including any specific tests required. The position of lids and lid aperture can be evaluated at this time.

VISUAL ACUITY ASSESSMENT: INFANTS

After a general idea, the first and foremost step is to assess their visual acuity.

Gross visual acuity in infants is mostly tested for fixation and following movements, monocularly. The examiner must know the appropriate size to which the infant may hold attention. For a 1–3 months old, the "human face" is the best target while a toy of size of "thumb" suffices for 1 year infant. Objects (toys) of variable sizes fall in between these two ages. Usually in infants, slow pursuit movement arises around 4–6 months but saccadic pursuit is even present before this age. Therefore, during evaluation this has to be kept in mind **(Figs. 1 and 2)**.

Preverbal children above 1 year of age, respond to different varieties of vision testing which has been described in chapter on vision evaluation.

FIXATION

Fixation is tested monocularly and binocularly. In monocular fixation one assesses whether the patient fixes with the fovea (central) and the quality of fixation. Each eye should be occluded in turn and the smallest possible target, appropriate for that age, that elicits the response should be used. Fixation is assessed for three different functions: (1) location (central versus (eccentric); (2) quality (good versus poor); and (3) duration (maintaining fixation). In day-to-day practice the dictum CSM is used which denotes "central, steady and maintained". "Central" denotes "foveal fixation"; "steady" denotes "quality" (no nystagmus or any unsteady movements); and "maintained" proves that the fixation is maintained when the patient "follows" the movement of light across from one side to another.

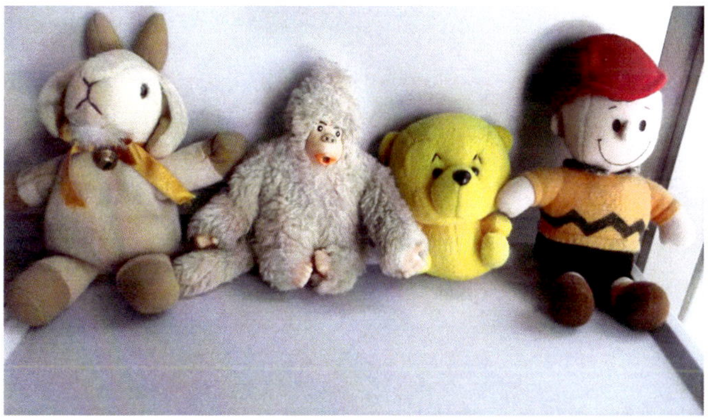

Fig. 1: Recommended toy photos for infants around 6 months.

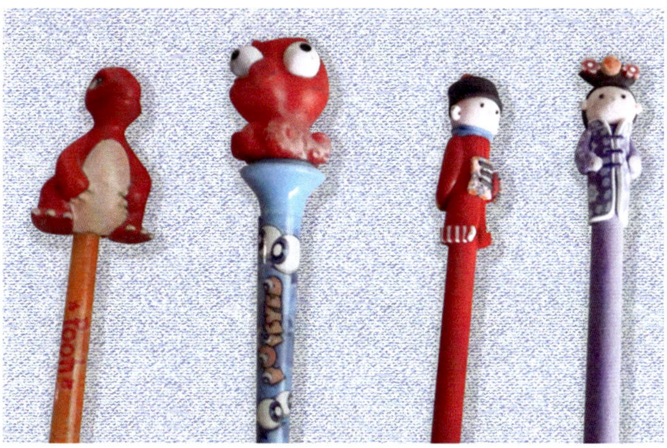

Fig. 2: Fixation toys for infants around 1 year.

Sometimes, the word FF is also used for quality maintenance which means "fix and follow". Steady, central fixation is a good sign and the vision for that age seems to be normal. Eccentric fixation is an ominous sign and the vision is assumed to be 20/200 or less on Snellen chart. The target should be moved slowly across the visual field to assess the "quality" of fixation. The target size and distance should be documented. The "fix and follow" movements will also simultaneously show the range of both monocular and binocular eye movements. The examiner should be aware of visual milestones in an infant. Newborns have only "sporadic saccadic" movements with very poor fix and follow pattern. By 6 weeks, infants show some smooth pursuit movements with central fixation and by 8 weeks they have well-developed central and steady fixation with good fix and follow movements. It should be remembered that up to 3–4 months the smooth pursuit movement (as demonstrated by Optokinetic testing) is predominantly temporal to nasal, and this has to be kept in mind when testing for fix and follow movements. One should remember that there is a small subset of patients who have delayed maturation and may not comply to the normal testing; in these cases, it is better to recall after some months but should show definite CSM by 1 year of age.

Binocular testing compares the vision of one eye to the other. This test shows "fixation preference" of one eye and predicts diminished vision or amblyopia in the nonpreferred eye. This test has the advantage over monocular testing as even small deficiency of vision can be brought forth as the nonpreferred eye may deviate or may not follow coordinated movement along with preferred eye during "maintenance" of fixation testing. Binocular testing also has the advantage that the vision of one eye may be very low, still the eye may fix monocularly, if the target is very attractive; but the discrepancy will be elicited in binocular testing.

It is important to do monocular testing prior to binocular testing to rule out possibility of bilateral symmetric visual loss. In patients with straight eyes or microtropia (strabismus <10 pd), the fixation preference can be tested using the vertical prism test. In straight eyes, it is impossible to say which eye is fixing. The vertical prism test induces a vertical deviation and therefore allows us to examine fixation pattern. Fixation preference testing is a quick and accurate way of knowing fixation preference in cases of amblyopia due to anisometropia, unilateral ptosis, postoperative residual tropias, and other conditions that could cause unilateral amblyopia.

Children who demonstrate poor fixation to above mentioned techniques, can be assessed by optokinetic nystagmus (OKN) drum or the Catford drum. OKN is an involuntary pursuit response to a moving target of high contrast. Since, the OKN drum consists of stripes of high contrast, the child is attracted to them even who are disinterested in other targets. The standard response is equivalent to finger counting of 3–6 ft. This is a good test to evaluate fixation as well as vision in infants and younger children.

Other ways of assessing visual function are the preferential looking tests and the pattern visual evoked potentials (PVEP). These have been already described in chapter on visual acuity.

In preverbal children, Allen's figures, Lea symbols, and HOTV charts are the standard means of evaluating the visual acuity.

Corneal reflection test: Evaluation of misalignment of eyes (strabismus) is extremely important in infants and young children. Congenital esotropias or exotropias, both have their importance with regard to vision, amblyopia, or any ominous sign. Faint leukocoria may not be evident to the parents but an obvious tropia may bring them for examination. As of strabismus per se, cover, cover-uncover testing can reveal qualitatively the type of strabismus. Though sixth nerve palsy is rare, but the author has seen cases being referred as sixth nerve palsy in infants, but actually having infantile esotropia with contracture of medial rectus. Some of these may be accommodative in nature, therefore, the author emphasizes on cycloplegic refraction under atropine and a full fundus examination. Some infants or a child may resist the cover tests; in such circumstances, the Hirschberg's corneal reflection test may be helpful. Since, this is done from a distance, the child may not be alarmed and a gross idea of strabismus can be achieved. Remember, this is a corneal "reflection" of a point light from the front surface of cornea (first Purkinjee image) and its position on both cornea will give assessment of the tropia and to some extent, quantitatively also.

PUPILLARY RESPONSES

Newborns have small, miotic pupils which increase in size to about 6–7 mm by teenage and then gradually decrease in size throughout life. It is difficult to elicit direct pupillary response due to extreme miosis and uncontrolled near reflex. Bright light should be avoided as the infant may close the lids; also effort should be made to have the baby fix at a distance toy target to avoid the near reflex. Older child can control their near reflex but still it is wise to let them look at distance. It is important to identify any "afferent pupillary defect", especially in unilateral amblyopias and vision loss due to macular or optic nerve disease. The "swinging light test" is a good way of knowing the afferent pupillary defects as the "paradoxical" dilatation to light is an ominous sign of macular or optic nerve disease.

THE RED REFLEX

With the induction of high power bimicroscopy and other technologically advanced evaluation methods, the simple evaluation modules have taken a back seat. Nevertheless, in very young children who would be uncooperative, the "red reflex" from the fundus, has its own place to begin with. It would instantly show any media opacities and gross refractive errors and subtle misalignment.

Bruckner described a very useful test to determine these anomalies. He used a direct ophthalmoscope in a darkened room and examined the "red reflex" from the pupil simultaneously in both eyes **(Fig. 3)**. In case of strabismus, the affected eye would show a brighter reflex with a slightly larger pupil. It has been demonstrated that as small as 5 pd of deviations can be ascertained by this method. An eye with refractive error will show a darker reflex. Amblyopia too can be detected, as when the slit beam is focused on the affected eye, nonfixation means that the eye is amblyopic. Other information like media opacities showing a dark spot or fundus anomaly showing a "pale" reflex can be obtained from Bruckner's test.

PHOTO SCREENING

This instrument-based testing for visual anomalies has gained lot of importance in recent times. This is used for large scale evaluation in general population to screen children for various visual problems. This has become a standard practice pattern for testing of ocular anomalies in developed countries, where a normal protocol is that the first testing should be done at 6 months of age, then at 3 years and finally at 5–6 years of age before the child starts formal schooling.

Purpose of early vision screening and ocular examination is to identify children who may have eye disorders which may contribute to development of severe visual impairment, amblyopia, and lack of cognitive development of a child, at

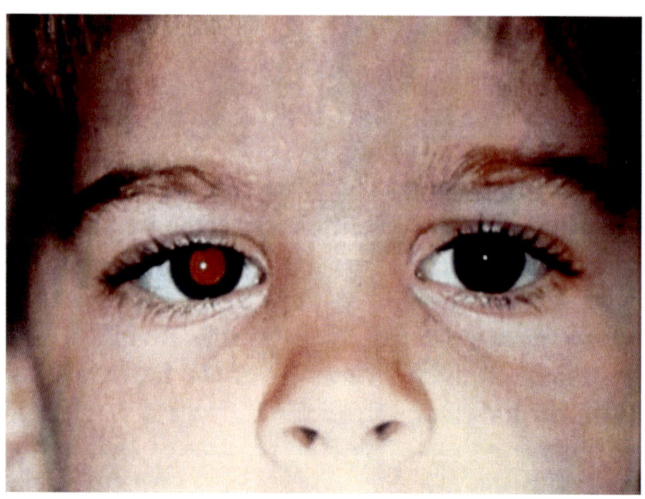

Fig. 3: Bruckner's red reflex: The brighter reflex in right eye shows small esotropia.

an early age, so that effective treatment may be initiated. Although there is limited direct evidence demonstrating the effectiveness of "preschool vision screening" in reducing the prevalence of amblyopia or improving other milestones, a convincing indirect evidence supports this practice. Early detection of vision threatening refractive errors and amblyopia, helps in better chances of visual recovery.

Photo screening uses off-axis photography and photo-refraction of the eye's red-reflex to evaluate refractive errors and small angle strabismus and thus identify risk factors in both eye simultaneously. A multicentric study revealed that photo screening was superior to optotype-based screening for children between ages 3 and 6 years and children who underwent their first photo screening at 2 years of age had superior eventual outcomes of treatment. Instrument-based vision screening techniques are more useful alternatives to visual acuity testing using optotype charts for very young children and children with developmental delays. But, they are not superior to quantitative vision testing with charts in children who can participate in those tests. Instrument-based vision screening detects the presence of risk factors for amblyopia, strabismus, media opacities, retinoblastoma, and retinal diseases.

REFRACTION

Determination of refractive errors is most important in all examinations. It is mandatory for not only knowing refractive error in cases of strabismus and vision impairment, but for a host of other complaints.

The clinician may be surprised to detect refractive errors in so many vague complaints by children. It should be remembered that the adequacy of cycloplegia, not dilatation, is important.

Also, the type of cycloplegic agent used according to age, the presence of any comorbidity, and color of iris should be kept in mind. The details of these drugs are listed in **Table 1**.

In infants: Objective refraction (retinoscopy) is indicated in all infants with defective fixation, preferential fixation, tropias, nystagmus, premature births, or any abnormality noted. The choice of cycloplegic agent is 1.0% atropine sulfate ointment, instilled twice or thrice daily for 3 days. Some infants may not show full dilatation even after this period, particularly premature or dark iris infants. In these cases, a diluted 2.5% phenylephrine can be instilled half an hour prior to examination, whence sufficient pupillary dilatation would occur. Normally sedation with phenergan (promethazine), chloral hydrate, or atarax (hydroxyzine) is sufficient in an infant for retinoscopy and fundus examination.

Toddlers do not sedate well with the above medications and where proper evaluation is necessary, general anesthesia should be used. We have now very safe agents for short-time anesthesia. Loose lenses or a lens-rack are recommended for retinoscopy. In infants, where atropine is contraindicated or previous use showed allergic reaction, a mixture of 0.5% tropicamide and 2.5% phenylephrine serves good purpose for fundoscopy and reasonably accurate retinoscopy. In preschool children, homatropine 2% is a good alternative; and in children 5 years and above, cyclopentolate 1% can be used. In author's clinical view, cyclopentolate is normally used above 5 years of age, except in Down's syndrome, cerebral palsy, or any neurological disorder, or if child showed "abnormal behavior" on previous use of this drug. In such situations, homatropine 1% or even tropicamide 1% is recommended. Children of school going age, who come with complaints of ocular asthenopia or headaches or tropias, usually esotropia, tropicamide may not be effective to unleash the full hyperopia, and a stronger cycloplegic drug is required.

For information purpose, following types of refraction techniques are available:

- Static retinoscopy, noncycloplegic, using a distant fixation target, followed by subjective correction.
- Noncycloplegic refraction using an auto-refraction equipment.
- Cycloplegic refraction using retinoscope or an Autoref.
- Mohindra near noncycloplegic retinoscopy.

TABLE 1: Characteristics and dosages of cycloplegic agents.

Cycloplegic drug	*Concentration*	*Age range*	*Dose*	*Onset of effect*	*Mydriasis*	*Cycloplegia*
Atropine sulfate ointment	1%	Below 1 year	TDS-3 days	2–3 days	10–12 days	15 days
Atropine sulfate solution	0.5–1.0%	1–5 years	1 drop-3 days	2–3 days	10–12 days	15 days
Homatropine hydro-bromide solution	2%	3–18 years	1 drop-10 mins apart 3 times	60 mins	3 days	7 days
Cyclopentolate drop	0.5%–1%	5–21 years	1 drop-10 mins apart	45 mins	24 hours	24 hours
Tropicamide drop	0.5%, 1.0%, 2%	12 years above	2 drop-10 mins apart	30 mins	6–12 hours	6–12 hos
Scopolamine solution and ointment	1–2%	3–12 years	2 drop-10 mins apart	60 mins	3 days	3–5 days

In infants, alternatively, a "mixture of 0.5% tropicamide and 2.5% phenylephrine" can be used.

Mohindra near-retinoscopy, without use of any cycloplegia, is another objective method of estimating refractive error in infants and small children. The technique involves performing retinoscopy at near, about 50 cm, in an otherwise dark room, as the patient fixates at the retinoscope light with one eye, while the other eye is occluded. However, it is not very reliable for quantification of refractive error and the gross refractive error is usually 1.0–1.5 D on myopic side. Near-retinoscopy may be useful in the following situations:

- When frequent follow-up is required.
- When the child extremely anxious for instillation of any drops.
- When the child showed any adverse reaction to any of the above agents.

Cycloplegic retinoscopy: As a rule, "cycloplegic" retinoscopy is mandatory in all infants, preschool, and school going children, as the full and proper error can only then be established. The author uses cycloplegia till age 21 years. A common mistake is using auto-refractor in older children without cycloplegia. It should be mentally noted that children, particularly hyperopic, automatically accommodate more on autorefractor; which gives a false reading of myopia. Thus, a myopic prescription now, would exaggerate their asthenopic symptoms and a vicious circle ensues. Even in "static noncycloplegic retinoscopy", a child may not be able to relax accommodation at distance, particularly a hyperopic child. Therefore, there is no substitute for a "cycloplegic refraction" using a proper cycloplegic agent.

Dynamic retinoscopy: Dynamic retinoscopy is a type of near retinoscopy where the child first focuses on a distant target and then at a handheld near target. The change in retinoscopic findings gives an idea of the accommodative amplitude. It is useful in determining the "accommodative lag" (insufficiency of accommodation) where the required amount of accommodation is not available for near work. The technique helps to gauge the accommodation in preverbal and school going children who cannot comply with the Royal Air Force (RAF) ruler, and who have a plethora of vague complaints. Associated with hyperopia, accommodative lag can have serious effect on a child's reading and writing capabilities.

Visual Fields

As soon as the child begins to fix steadily, say around 2 years, visual fields should be routinely tested. The easiest and quickest way is by "confrontation method" using an interesting target. Both uniocular and binocular fields should be assessed. If the child resists patching, binocular testing will also yield homonymous defects. Even in an infant, a fixation target may be used to fixate centrally and then a different attractive target may be brought in the peripheral field. Owing to good saccadic reflex, the infant may suddenly look at the peripheral target, once it is brought in the child's field of vision.

Color Vision

Although color vision is not routinely done in children but may be helpful in decreased vision of uncertain etiology and constant monitoring in progressive macular disease and optic neuropathies. More often than not, a parent may bring the child to the clinician claiming that he/she confuses between red and green pencil while during drawing for homework. Congenital red-green color defects are prevalent in about 8–10% of male population and earlier it is diagnosed, it will be better for future of the patient.

The easiest way to determine color defects are the color plates. There are two popular types of plates which are helpful in specific situations. The "Ishihara pseudoisochromatic color plates" work on the principle of "color confusion" and are useful for detection of red-green defects. Most acquired color defects show in the blue-yellow range, and will be missed on Ishihara plates, unless the defect has extended to red-green range. The advantage of this test is it can be done on illiterate patients as well as children of preverbal age, as only fingers have to be moved on the color lines.

The other test called "Richmond pseudoisochromatic plates", previously known as "Hardy-Rand-Rittler" plates works on the principle of "color saturation" and can detect both red-green and blue-yellow defects. Unfortunately, these do not come in illiterate plates and is difficult for young children. In general, optic nerve disease will more likely show red-green defects, while retinal disease will show blue-yellow defects.

Slit-lamp Examination

Slit lamp in young children is difficult due to obvious reasons. Infants would not open eyes and bright light is not appreciated by infants and young children. Handheld slit lamps are available which are useful in a cooperative child. In infants and small children, examination under general anesthesia is the best way for microscopic, indirect ophthalmoscopic examination, and retinoscopy.

Fundus Examination

Last but not the least, an adequate fundus examination is imperative for children. For most patients, visualization of posterior pole (optic disc and macula) usually suffices. For detailed peripheral examination, general anesthesia is usually required. Infants below 1 year can be sedated and examination can be performed with slightly dim light. Young children around 2 years may not get sedated and general anesthesia may be required. Children who are older than 3 years are more cooperative and periphery can be examined in sitting position by explaining them the procedure which is more acceptable to the child.

SUMMARY

- In all pediatric examinations, a subdued, nonscary light should be used. A small "pen-light" or a direct ophthalmoscope may suffice.
- The child should be alert and cooperative, well fed, and comfortable.
- Examination of child on parents or any known relatives lap is an ideal position.
- "Focused" history is the key prior to any physical examination. No time should be wasted as children loose interest very quickly. If necessary, direct questions should be asked relevant to the complaints.
- Observation of the child while the brief history is taken, gives enormous amount of information.
- Try to establish some sort of rapport with the child by doing a handshake or calling by nicknames are helpful and drives out the fear from the child. Toddlers and preschool children will be more cooperative with this kind of gesture.
- Always use the "age appropriate" toy target for examinations of fixation, motility testing, cover-testing, etc.
- Visual acuity, even qualitative, is important to assess.
- Examine under anesthesia, whenever necessary.
- Call the child some other time, if examination is improper due to any reason. Enquire the time of day when the child is most cheerful and try examination at that time.
- Insist on photographs—current and previous—as they are valuable in knowing the time onset of the disorder.
- Fundus examination is mandatory in cases of suspicious red-reflex, strabismus, leukocoria, etc.
- Do not alarm the parents, if some sight-threatening or life-threatening disorder is detected.
- Never spell out disaster at first meeting. And refer to a higher center, if further evaluation facilities do not exist at your center.
- There is no set protocol in the routine of examination of child. The examiner should understand the gravity of situation and mold the physical examination accordingly. The examiner should also be innovative and adaptive to attract the child's attention during examination.

SUGGESTED READING

1. Adams RJ et al: Non-cycloplegic auto refraction in infants and young children. Inves. Ophthalmol. Vis. Sci. 2001, 42.
2. American Academy of Ophthalmology. Pediatric ophthalmology/strabismus panel. Preferred Practice Pattern Guidelines. San Francisco; 2012.
3. American foundation for vision awareness. Children's vision and literacy campaign position paper. St. Louis: AFVA; 1993.
4. Archer SM, Sondhi N, Helveston EM. Strabismus in infancy. Ophthalmology. 1989;96(1):133-7.
5. Bell AL, Rodes ME, Collier Kellar L. Childhood eye examination. Am Fam Physician. 2013;88(4):241-8.
6. Hoyt CS, Nickel BL, Billson FA. Ophthalmological examination of the infant. Surv Ophthalmol. 1982;26(4):177-89.
7. Improving early childhood eyecare. Am Public Health Assoc. 2011.
8. Komar B. How to successfully perform a pediatric eye exam. Optometry Times. 2017.
9. Mohindra I. A non-cycloplegic refraction technique for infants and young children. J Am Optom Assoc. 1977;48(4):518-23.
10. Ottar WL, Scott WE, Holgado SI. Photoscreening for amblyogenic factors. J Pediatr Ophthalmol Strabismus. 1995;32(5):289-95.
11. Simon JW, Kaw P. Commonly missed diagnoses in the childhood eye examination. Am Fam Physician. 2001;64(4):623-8.
12. Tingley DH. Vision screening essentials: screening today for eye disorders in the pediatric patients. Pediatr Rev. 2007;28(2):54-61.

2

CHAPTER

Vision Assessment in Infants and Children

Rohit Saxena, Vaishali Rakheja

INTRODUCTION

Vision is the ability of the eye to see and is a combination of the light sense, form sense, contrast sense, and color sense. Visual acuity is defined as the spatial limit of visual discrimination and is the most common measure of visual function in clinical practice. It involves the measurement of the visual threshold which is estimated as the reciprocal of the visual angle. The visual angle is the angle subtended by the object at the nodal point of the eye and denotes the spatial extent of elements in the visual field.

The organic basis of the visual acuity depends on the size and separation of the foveal cones. It is known that two adjacent points of an object appear separate only if they cause stimulation of two cones separated by an unstimulated cone.

Visual acuity can be measured in a number of ways:

- Test of whether a target is present or absent (*detection acuity*)
- Evidence that the spatial detail contained within the target have been fully resolved (*resolution acuity*) or
- Identification of the target using the cognitive ability and communication skills (*recognition acuity*).

Tests of visual acuity can provide valuable information regarding the refractive status of the eye and the pathologies of the visual pathway **(Flowchart 1)**.

VISUAL DEVELOPMENT

It is clear that a neonate cannot see as well as an adult and the visual system undergoes rapid development during the first year of life followed by a slow phase of visual maturation until 8–9 years of age.

Anatomical factors that contribute to this process of development are:

- Muscle insertions and their relationship to the limbus and equator changes markedly in the first year of life.
- Foveal differentiation is not complete until at least 4–8 months of age and the foveal cone density and size increases with age.

Flowchart 1: Tests for assessment of visual acuity.

Visual acuity

Detection acuity tests: Measure the ability to detect the smallest stimulus
- Dot visual acuity test
- Catford drum test
- Boek candy bead test
- STYCAR graded-balls test

Recognition acuity tests: Measure the ability to recognize and distinguish a stimulus from surrounding stimuli
- Direction identification tests like Snellen's E-chart test, Landolt's C-chart test, and Sjögren's test
- Letter identification tests such as Snellen's letter chart test, Sheridan's letter test, and Lipman's HOTV test
- Picture identification tests like Allen picture cards test and miniature toy test
- Tests combining picture identification and behavioral responses such as Cardiff acuity card test

Resolution acuity tests: Measure the ability to discern the details of various elements in the same target
- Optokinetic nystagmus test
- Preferential looking tests such as two-alternative forced choice tests (2-AFC) and Teller acuity card tests
- Visually evoked response (VER)

- The peripheral rods and cones attain adult dimensions by 4 months and the maturation of retinal vascularization occurs by 3 months from birth.
- Myelination of the optic nerve and visual pathway continues to occur until 2 years of age.
- The neuronal circuits in the visual cortex continue to strengthen till 2 years of life.

Other visual attributes such as accommodation and fusional convergence develop by 5-6 months of age. Initially, infants superimpose the images formed by the two eyes and start developing binocular fusion by the third month of life. Stereopsis develops rapidly from 3-6 months of age and adult levels are achieved by 5-7 years **(Table 1)**. This is the period during which the visual system can be influenced by environmental manipulations and is known as the critical period. Any interference during this critical phase can have life-long effects like amblyopia leading to irreversible visual impairment and loss of binocularity. It is therefore essential to identify the children who have disturbed visual development and so can benefit from early interventions.

TABLE 1: The vision milestones.

Age	*Visual milestones*
29–30 weeks of intrauterine life	• Pupil reacts to light • Closes eyelids in response to bright light
Birth	• Infant blinks in response to bright light or touching eye. Eyes are sometimes uncoordinated, may look crosseyed • Able to stare at objects, if held 8–10 inches away • Initially fixes eyes on a face or lighted objects then begins to follow a moving object • Visual acuity is equivalent to 6/120 on acuity card tests
4 weeks	• Maintains stable eye contact when awake and alert and initiated by parent or caregiver • Follows objects with both head and eyes moving together up to 90°
8 weeks	• Fuses to view the object as a single image • Attentive to objects such as toys held till 6 inches from face • Follows vertical movement better than horizontal movements • Starts becoming aware of the colors primarily red and yellow • Doll's head eye movements can be elicited • Intently watches mother's face
3 months	• Coordinated ocular movements most of the time • Pays attention to both black-white and colored targets • Starts reaching out to interesting objects • Visual attention to objects as small as 1 inch • Begins to associate a visual stimulus to an event (bottle and feeding)
4 months	• Hand regard-marked interest in one's hand movements • Reacts with a smile to familiar faces • Able to follow a visual target past midline and can track horizontally, vertically, and in a circle • Foveal differentiation is largely complete
5 months	• Menace reflex present • Eye-hand coordination is achieved and the infant gazes at the objects held in his own hands • Stereopsis develops
6 months	• Fusional convergence well developed and the child can shift gaze from near to far easily • Reaches out and grasps the visual targets • Interested in falling objects and fixates as to where the objects disappear • VEP acuity of the adult level achieved (6/6), card acuity equivalent to 6/36
6–9 months	• Picks and transfers small objects from hand to hand • Explores the environment visually • Interested in geometric patterns
9–12 months	• Visually alert to new people and objects in the surroundings • Judges distance fairly well and throw objects with precision
1 year	• Can differentiate simple geometric patterns • Scribbles with crayons and interested in pictures
2 years	• Optic nerve myelination complete • Can match objects by single property like shape or color • Visual acuity on acuity cards equivalent to 6/6
3 years	Recognition acuity 6/9–6/6
5–7 years	Stereopsis matures to the adult level

(VEP: visual evoked potentials)

Visual Acuity Measurement in Different Age Groups

Pediatric vision assessment can be a daunting task due to the lack of patient cooperation and poor reliability of the assessment techniques. The measurement of visual acuity in children needs ample patience and experience to interpret the specific tests.

There are certain special considerations for vision assessment in infants and toddlers.

- A feed or short nap provides a good window of opportunity and can improve the child's cooperation.
- Watch the child as soon as he/she enters the room and be observant of what the child looks at and the head posture.
- The child should be seated comfortably on the parent's lap with the head supported and the body cradled by the parent's arms.
- Clean and attractive toys should be available to engage the child's attention, which can be further maintained by softly whistling or humming a nursery rhyme.

Depending upon the visual system maturation, the pediatric population can be classified into three broad categories:

1. Infants and toddlers (up to 3 years)
2. Preschool children (3 years to 5 years)
3. School going children (above 6 years)

Vision Assessment in Infants and Toddlers

Infant—3 Months

Behavioral responses play a key role in vision assessment in preverbal children. An infant since birth exhibits a blink reflex in response to stimuli such as bright light, sound, and corneal stimulation.

The light reflex can be elicited even in premature babies over 29 weeks of gestational age. It is best performed in a dim-lit room with a well-focused bright light. Its presence is suggestive of an intact visual pathway up to the level of the superior colliculus and efferent pathway till the iris sphincter. It is a reliable indicator of the presence of visual function. Another behavior seen in the infants that can aid in the estimation of the visual potential is a change in the palpebral opening stimulated by the changes in the illumination of the room. When the lights are dimmed, the infant opens its eyes wide and closes them when they are brought up back.

The vestibulo-ocular reflex (VOR) is elicited by suddenly turning the head sideways as the infant fixes an object of interest. A normal doll's eye response is indicated by the movement of the eyes in the direction opposite to that of head rotation.

Objective tests that can help to assess the status of visual function in infants are:

- *Optokinetic nystagmus (OKN):* Assessment of the presence or absence of OKN in response to a patterned rotating drum or a drifting stimulus presented on a computer screen can be used to objectively assess visual functions. A grating pattern of black and white stripes is shown either on a computer screen or by using a drum rotating at 8–10 rpm. The normal response consists of a slow following movement followed by compensatory fast movement, i.e., saccades in the opposite direction. The visual angle subtended by the smallest strip width that elicits this response gives the measure of the resolution acuity. The infant is required to be attentive and hold both eyes open for the entire duration of the test. Various studies have reported that the OKN acuity is at least 6/120 in a neonate and improves quite rapidly over the initial few months of life reaching a level of 6/6 by 20 months of age. The test must be cautiously interpreted as cases with cortical blindness can show this phenomenon.
- *Visually evoked response (VER):* It is an electrophysiological test that records the cortical response to a given visual stimulus. This aids in assessing the state of the visual system beyond the retinal ganglion cells. Depending on the stimulus used, it can be a flash VER that is best for young infants with an inability to fixate any object. This gives a good estimate of the macular functions and integrity of the visual pathway. In the pattern reversal VER a patterned stimulus that evokes a steady-state VER is used. The spatial frequency is then changed at a fixed intensity of illumination. The amplitude and latency of the response generated are measured for each spatial frequency which provides a rough estimate of the visual acuity. As the size of the pattern target decreases, there is a corresponding decrease in the VER amplitude and the visual acuity threshold is the smallest check size that results in a measurable response. It is reported that infants aged 1 month, elicit a visual acuity of 6/120 which matures to provide detection of 6/6–6/12 targets by 6 months to 1 year of age. The advantages of using this for measuring visual acuity in infants are the speed of the test, absence of any response by the child, and can be a good indicator of the macular function **(Table 2)**.

However, due to the vast discrepancy in the values of visual acuity obtained by OKN, VER, and the lack of standardization, these tests are primarily a research technique and are not often employed in clinical or screening settings.

TABLE 2: Expected visual acuity at different ages.

Age (months)	*Optokinetic nystagmus*	*Preferential looking test*	*Visually evoked response*
1	6/120	6/120	6/120
6	6/30	6/30	6/6–6/12
12	6/12	6/36	6/6
36	6/6	6/6	6/6

3–6 Months

- *Fixation behavior* assesses the ability of an infant to fixate on an object of interest. The fixation reflex starts developing at 33 weeks of intrauterine life and matures by 2 months after birth. The test can be done by observing as the infant fixes and follows a light stimulus, bright objects like toys or examiners face. The test is performed binocularly at first followed by monocular testing by covering one eye with an occluder or hand. A resistance to occlusion of either eye may depict a preferential fixation with that eye and poor vision in the other eye. A central, steady, and maintained fixation with corneal light reflex falling at the center of the pupil with no oscillatory movements and ability to keep the eyes fixed when either is covered indicates good central visual acuity (6/9–6/6). A centered steady nonmaintained fixation indicates subnormal vision (6/60–6/36) whereas an unsteady central fixation implies poor vision (<6/60). An infant showing eccentric fixation is expected to have very poor visual acuity (counting fingers at 1 m). Though this test can be used to recognize amblyopia especially when compared to the other eye, it is not a very good predictor of visual acuity.

In a patient with suspected malalignment, a cover test can be performed to observe the movement of the other eye.

- *Bruckner's test*: In infants who do not cooperate for the cover test, the Bruckner's reflex can be elicited to assess the presence of small angle strabismus or anisometropia. This involves the illumination of the pupil with a direct ophthalmoscope at a distance sufficient to illuminate both the eyes simultaneously. If strabismus is present, the deviated eye will have lighter (brighter) reflex than the better eye. Assessment of the reflex is done with both undilated and dilated pupils. This test detects but does not measure the magnitude of deviation. It can also be used to comment on the media opacities and the presence of anisometropic amblyopia.
- *Menace response* is a type of blink reflex wherein the subject closes the eyes and turns away his trunk as a protective response from a rapidly approaching object. A menace reflex is elicited by a threatening hand gesture heading toward the eye in infants with normal visual apparatus by 5 months of age. The neural pathway of this reflex is composed of the optic nerve (II) and the facial nerve (VII). It is mediated by the tectobulbar fibers of the midbrain passing from the optic tract to accessory nuclei and from there to the spinal cord and lower motor neurons that innervate the head and neck.

6–12 Months

- *Preferential looking test* is based on the principle that a child will always preferably look at a pattern stimuli compared to a plain field. This occurs as long as the pattern is resolvable.

Teller's acuity card test is a behavioral test for measuring the grating acuity and is a modification of the PLT. The test consists of a visual assessment using a set of 17 cards by the name of Teller's acuity cards. Each rectangular card measuring 55 cm by 25 cm consists of a gray background with a 12.5 cm^2 with a striped black and white pattern printed to one side of it with a centrally placed peephole. The stripe width which is the spatial frequency of the test grating varies from card to card. The average luminance of the stripes are exactly matched to the luminance of the surrounding gray color so that when the patient is unable to resolve the test grating, the card will appear as homogeneous gray (same space-average luminance). The procedure requires the patient to be comfortably seated in the parent's lap as the cards are projected. The observer watches through the hole at the center and records the behavioral response of the child like head-turning, pointing, and any verbal response in older children. An independent examiner records whether the response of the child is right or wrong to assess the visual acuity. The finest grating pattern that a child can make out denotes the visual acuity. The advantages of the test are that it is a rapid test, is easy to administer, and is a reliable method for quantification of the visual acuity in unco-operative, preverbal children. The cost of the equipment is also low and the tester can interact with the child between the cards thus maintaining the interest. The disadvantage of the test is that it only tests the near visual acuity, there is a large variability of acuity scores in normal infants and the cards must be kept clean and free of dirt and smudges that could attract the infant's attention away from the grating target. Also, as it overestimates the grating visual acuity when compared to Snellen's recognition acuity, it may fail to detect amblyopia.

- *Catford drum test* that measures the detection acuity was introduced by Catford and Oliver in 1971 to assess the vision of children below 3 years of age when a subjective response cannot be elicited. Catford drum is a motor-driven drum consisting of oscillating black dots of varying sizes on a white background projected through a rectangular aperture measuring 4 cm by 6 cm. The patient is seated 60 cm from the drum and is instructed to observe the dots with the other eye occluded. The smallest dot that elicits a pendular eye movement gives the estimate of visual acuity. As the target is moving, this method also overestimates the visual acuity when compared to Snellen's recognition acuity and, hence, is not reliable as a screening measure for amblyopia.

1–3 Years

- *Cardiff acuity test:* This test developed at Cardiff, UK is designed to measure visual acuity in toddlers and older children with visual impairment. It is based on the principle of preferential looking and uses vanishing optotypes to measure recognition, resolution, and detection thresholds altogether. The Cardiff acuity cards are rectangular with the target drawn on one side leaving the other edge plain. The targets are drawn with white outline bordered by two black bands each having a width half of the white band on a gray background. The average luminance of the target is the same as the gray background so that the pattern is visible only till a certain distance depending on the subject's visual acuity, after which it disappears (vanishes) to blend with the gray background. The test can be done at 50 cm and 1 m. The result is read as Snellen's denotations but this test overestimates the visual acuity in comparison to letter recognition acuity.

- *Sheridan's ball test:* 10 styrofoam balls of progressively decreasing sizes are rolled up to 3 m on a well-illuminated contrasting floor. The pursuit eye movements are observed. The smallest ball that the child can fixate gives a rough measure of visual acuity.
- *Worth's ivory ball test:* Ivory balls measuring 0.5–2.5 inches rolled on the floor till a distance of 3 m and the child is asked to retrieve them. The visual acuity is measured from the smallest ball that can be recognized by the child.
- *Coin test:* The child is shown coins of decreasing sizes and is expected to pick only those he can visualize.
- *Miniature toy test:* Two sets of miniature toys are used, one with the child and other with the examiner. The examiner shows a toy from his set to the child from a distance of 10 ft and the child is instructed to pick the matching toy from his set.
- *Dot visual acuity test:* An illuminated box with black dots of different sizes is shown to the child in a dark room. The smallest size of the dot identified by the child is taken as the visual acuity.
- *Boek candy bead test:* Beads of different colors and sizes are shown to the patient at a distance of 40 cm and the smallest bead matched by the child is used to denote the visual acuity.

Preschool Age Group 3–5 Years

While, it is difficult for children <5 years of age to be tested with adult letter visual acuity charts, tests have been developed that are more "child friendly" yet provide accurate visual acuity.

- *Allen's picture card test:* This comprises of seven optotypes for recognition at a distance of 15 ft for a 3-year-old child and 20 ft for 4-year-old child.
- *Sheridan's letter test:* It uses five letters H, O, T, V, X, and A, U are added in seven letter set and C, L in the nine letter set. The test is performed at 3 m. The examiner shows cards having letters of varying sizes. Child points at one of the cards identical to the examiner's card (lap card). Snellen's equivalent of 6/6–6/60 can be estimated using this method. Lipman's letter test is a similar test that uses only four letters H, O, T, and V.
- *Tumbling E test:* This test uses E optotype of different sizes oriented in all four directions. The test is performed mono-ocularly at a distance of 6 m. The child is asked to indicates the orientation of the E.
- *Sjogren's hand and arrow tests:* These are the direction identification tests used in a similar way as the Landolt's ring test and Tumbling E test.
- *Lea symbols chart* uses four symbols—house, heart, square, and circle instead of letters in 15 lines and is performed at 3 m. The test also has the four picture/symbol Lea recognition cards which are given to the child to point to and identify the symbol shown on the chart. The Lea symbols chart consist of lines of four different symbols, arranged in combinations of five symbols per line. The symbols on each line are smaller than those on the line above. The Lea symbols chart distance visual acuity test are very useful for children 3–4 years and older.

5 Years and Above

- *Snellen's test types:* The charts were introduced in 1862 by Herman Snellen, a Dutch physician and is still the most commonly used test for distance visual acuity assessment. It is based on the principle that two points are visualized as separate when they subtend an angle of 1 minute at the nodal point of the eye. It consists of a series of black letters on a white illuminated background. The standard distance for measuring the visual acuity is 6 m (20 ft) and normal acuity is designated as 6/6. The size of each letter (optotype) on the 6/6 line is designed in such a way that each letter fits into a square subtending an angle of 5 minutes of arc at the nodal point of the eye and every individual limb of the letter subtends an angle of 1 minute each. If the subject is unable to recognize the letters of the 6/6 line from a distance of 6 m, he is tested with larger optotype in the lines above, that have this critical dimension of 1 minute of arc at a distance >6 m.
- *Landolt's test types:* This based on the same principle as Snellen's test with the only difference that instead of letters broken circles are used as the optotypes. Unlike Snellen's test where the letters have to be recognized, Landolt's rings use the detection of the correct orientation of the break in the circle as the endpoint and measures the minimal separable acuity.
- *LogMAR charts:* LogMAR stands for logarithm of the minimum angle of resolution. It is a specially designed chart to enable a more precise measure of visual acuity as compared to Snellen's chart and other tests as they have a regular progression of size and spacing of lines. Each line comprises five letters in sloan font which are equally legible one from another which are read at the distance of 4 m. As the chart's name suggests the visual acuity is scored with reference to the logarithm of the minimum angle of resolution. An observer who can resolve details as small as 1 minute of visual angle scores LogMAR 0 since, the base-10 logarithm of 1 is 0.

POINTS TO REMEMBER

- A tailored approach is needed to assess the visual system in infants and children as the standard tests used for adults are not appropriate for the pediatric subjects.
- The visual acuity in a normal neonate is inferior to an adult and a rapid improvement occurs in the first postnatal year. Hence, the visual status is not static. This calls for serial follow-up visits.
- The visual development in an infant is highly plastic and responsive to environmental changes. As these longitudinal changes are not linear, a single vision assessment cannot reliably predict the future vision outcome.
- Behavioral reflexes and fixation behavior test are the most commonly used methods for estimating the vision in infants below 6 months of age.
- Objective tests such as VER and OKN may be useful in preverbal infants and older children with severe visual impairment but an ambiguity exists in the interpretation and age-matched norms for these tests.
- Most of the tests done in infants and toddlers such as PLTs use mobile grating targets and measure only the resolution acuity. These may overestimate the visual acuity and fail to detect amblyopia and macular pathologies.

SUGGESTED READING

1. Boothe RG, Dobson V, Teller DY. Postnatal development of vision in human and nonhuman primates. Annu Rev Neurosci. 1985;8:495-545.
2. Dobson V, Teller DY. Visual acuity in human infants: A review and comparison of behavioral and electro-physiological studies. Vision Res. 1978;18(11):1469-83.
3. Dobson V. Visual acuity testing in human infants: From laboratory to clinic. In: Simons K (Ed). Early visual development, normal and abnormal. New York: Oxford University Press; 1993. p. 318.
4. Jacobson SG, Mohindra I, Held R. Visual acuity of infants with ocular diseases. Am J Ophthalmol. 1982;93(2):198-209.
5. Kushner BJ, Lucchese NJ, Morton GV. Grating visual acuity with Teller cards compared with Snellen visual acuity in literate patients. Arch Ophthalmol. 1995;113(4):485-93..
6. McDonald MA, Dobson V, Sebris SL, Baitch L, Varner D, Teller DY. The acuity card procedure: A rapid test of infant acuity. Invest Ophthalmol Vis Sci. 1985;26(8):1158-62.
7. von Noorden GK, Campos EC. Binocular vision and ocular motility: theory and management of strabismus, 6th edition. Missouri, United States: Mosby, A Harcourt Health Sciences Company; 2002.

CHAPTER 3

Management of Refractive Errors in Children

Yogesh Shukla

INTRODUCTION

Early in life, the two eyes of infants normally grow in a highly co-ordinated manner toward an ideal refractive state, a process called "emmetropization". Evidence from many different species indicates that emmetropization is an "active" process that is regulated by visual feedback by the eye's effective refractive state. For example, making the eyes of young animals artificially myopic with positive lenses or hyperopic with negative lenses, produces compensating ocular growth, that within certain operational limits, eliminates the imposed refractive error.

The refractive state of the eye is dependent on the relationship between the axial length and the combined refractive power of the cornea and the lens. Axial length changes from 17 mm at birth to 23.8 mm in adult. To compensate for this increase in axial length, the cornea and lens flatten, so that the mean refractive power of cornea and lens decreases from 51.0 (D) and 35.0 (D) in the newborn to adult values of 44.0 (D) and 18.0 (D) respectively. With such remarkable changes occurring in these parameters, it is gratifying that the refractive state of the eyes remains fairly stable.

Premature infants are recognized to be more myopic than full term infants; the reason described is due to the more convexity of lens. The mechanism responsible for this lenticular myopia is unclear.

At birth, a full term infant, on the other hand, is hyperopic. In one study, 75% normal infants were hyperopic (ranging from +1.0 to +10.0 D) and 25% were myopic (from -1.0 to -12 D). These large variations are not clearly understood. Another group of studies indicate gradual decrease in hyperopia up to 4 years of age; thereafter, a myopic shift occurs toward emmetropization.

Changes in refractive errors vary widely from individual to individual making it impossible to predict the ultimate refractive error. It is generally believed that if myopia presents before 6 years of age, then the child is at a greater risk of progression to high myopia (>5.0 D).

Astigmatism is more common in infancy than in general adult population. "Against-the-rule (ATR)" astigmatism predominates and is present in >70% of infants. Corneal curvature is the major component of infantile astigmatism. Longitudinal studies have shown a dramatic decrease in astigmatism with age, with most pronounced changes occurring by 2 years of life. Most of this astigmatism disappears by 4–6 years of life. There is alteration in type of astigmatism also; with predominance of "with-the-rule (WTR)" axis. Infants with higher degrees of astigmatism, may not revert to normalcy, specifically if the axis is oblique.

World Health Organization (WHO) report published in 2011, estimated 153 million global cases of visual impairment resulted from uncorrected or under corrected refractive errors with 19 million of these falling in age group of 6–16 years. Recent, WHO reports indicate that refractive errors are the first cause of visual impairment and second cause of visual loss worldwide as 43% visual loss is due to refractive errors. Visual impairment due to uncorrected or improperly corrected refractive errors have a major impact on children's scholastic, psychologic, and cognitive development. It is therefore, imperative that we understand correctly and clearly the management of these errors.

Before we discuss each refractive error, we must know the natural history of these errors, as there are significant changes when eye is developing and emmetropization is in progress, when some errors come and go.

NATURAL HISTORY OF REFRACTIVE ERRORS

There is now a general agreement that the range of refractive errors is wider at birth and in the first year of life than in later childhood. Most infants are hyperopic at birth and the average cycloplegic refraction is around +2.0 D with a standard deviation of +2.0 D. There is not much change in refractive state in first 3 months being static or slight decrease. From 3 months to 12 months, there is rapid emmetropization with a decrease of 1.0 D hyperopia by 1 year of age. This is followed by a slower change until 2 years for hyperopes and 4–5 years for myopes.

A few infants are myopic at birth and most of these will eventually emmetropize. The rate of emmetropization is proportional to the initial error. Those who begin close to emmetropia or close to standard error show gradual change, while those who have higher ametropia show greater and faster change.

There is also higher prevalence of astigmatism at birth with as many as 70% of full-term newborns having astigmatism of 1.0 D or more. In most cases, there is decrease in the degree of astigmatism by 4 years of life. Of the large scale studies, 30% have 1.0 D or more of astigmatism by 2 years, 24% by 4 years, and only 17% at 6–7 years. With regard to the type of astigmatism, WTR, ATR, and oblique astigmatism are all more common in children than adults. Of these types, oblique astigmatism is least common. There is a general agreement that all types of astigmatism decrease with infants losing most of their astigmatism by 2 years.

Anisometropia is more common in infants than adults. Studies suggest that 15–30% infants have anisometropia of >1.0 D, and of these 7–11% have spherical anisometropia of 1.0 D or more by 4 years of life. Some children lose anisometropia while some gain it during this period. The anisometropia is due to different rates of emmetropization between the two eyes, it is transient and disappears by 4 years of age. These "transient" anisometropias are of low level, around 2.0 D or less and may not lead to amblyopia. Higher levels of anisometropia of 3.0 D or more are likely to remain and is amblyogenic.

After the rapid period of emmetropization which happens by 3–4 years of age, there is less change occurring between 4 and 6 years. It is to be remembered that the axial growth of the eye is rapid by 3 years when it almost nearly assumes the normal configuration of an adult eye. Rarely, hyperopia may continue regress up to 10–12 years of age.

CLINICAL IMPLICATIONS OF EMMETROPIZATION

The above stated "naturally occurring" refractive errors and their transformations have a consequent clinical implications. A big question to be asked is "Will this particular child's refractive error emmetropize?" Although the majority of children will emmetropize, this is not true for all. We would like to be able to predict those who will fully emmetropize, as there is less likely a need to prescribe spectacles, at least in early childhood. But those who are less likely to emmetropize and have a residual high refractive error, would need glasses. There is evidence that children with high refractive error, above the normal range discussed above, are less likely to emmetropize. The above natural history and emmetropization have a big impact on the future course and management of these errors.

Certain guidelines are presented by the American Academy of Ophthalmology (AAO) and is the preferred pattern of practice in children who present before 3 years of age (**Table 1**). But, there is discrepancy between the AAO

TABLE 1: Guidelines for refractive correction in infants and young children [American Academy of Ophthalmology (AAO) Guidelines-2012].

Condition	***Refractive error in Diopter***		
	Age 1 year	***Age 2 years***	***Age 3 years***
Isoametropia: (Equal refractive error in both eyes)			
Myopia	–5.0 or more	–4.0 or more	–3.0 or more
Hyperopia (no deviation)	+6.0 or more	+5.0 or more	+4.0 or more
Astigmatism	3.0 or more	2.5 or more	2.0 or more
Anisometropia:			
Myopia	–4.0 or more	–3.0 or more	–2.0 or more
Hyperopia	+3.0 or more	+2.5 or more	+1.5 or more
Astigmatism	2.5 or more	2.0 or more	2.0 or more

guidelines and some other studies mentioned earlier. Hyperopic anisometropia of even 1.0 D, myopic anisometropia of 2.0 D, and astigmatic anisometropia (of any variety) of 1.5 D, after the age of 3 years, is amblyogenic. Moreover, these figures are more research oriented and statistically important but in clinical practice, usually children after 3 years are brought for consultation for any refractive problem, except when tropias are manifested. Furthermore, the above guidelines are a starting point of refractive problems and their treatment schedule, but far larger number of children belong to preschool age and above.

Choice of cycloplegic agent for refraction - see **Table 1** in Chapter 1.'

HYPEROPIA

Physiologic or simple hyperopia is the most common type of hyperopia. Overall prevalence of hyperopia is about 10% in children. Most full-term infants are mildly hyperopic, around +2.0 D.

Rapid emmetropization is taking place in infants and by 6 months about 10% remain hyperopic and by 1 year of age only 3.6% are hyperopic. Hyperopia of >4.5 D at 1 year of age and >3.5 D at 3 years of age is likely to remain. Infants with >3.0 or 3.5 D of hyperopia are 13 times more likely to develop strabismus by 4 years, if left untreated. There is no gender difference. Family history increases the risk of hyperopia. Hyperopia has been found to be associated with smoking during pregnancy, prematurity, low-birth weight, and juvenile diabetes. It is also reported that intelligence scores are less in hyperopic than myopic children.

Classifications

- Etiological
  - Axial—short eyeball
  - Curvature—flat cornea
  - Index—change in refractive index of lens
  - Positional: (1) posture (2) dislocation of lens

- Absence of crystalline lens—aphakia
- Accommodation loss (functional) old age; third N palsy, use of cycloplegic drugs, and medications
- *Consecutive*: Due to overcorrection of myopia

▪ Clinical
- Total
- Manifest
- Absolute
- Facultative
- Latent

▪ Types of hyperopia
- *Simple*: Biological alterations in eye ball.
- *Pathological*: Associated with comorbidities like mal development of eyes (microphthalmos and nano-ophthalmos), corneal or lenticular changes, chorioretinal or orbital inflammations, neoplasms, or neurological diseases. These will be discussed in their respective chapters.

From practical point of view, the understanding of clinical classification is necessary as it has bearing on the treatment. Let us understand by an example. Suppose, unaided visual acuity (VA) is 6/9 Oculus Uterque (OU) on Snellen chart. Manifest refraction yields OU +4.0 D. A cycloplegic refraction reveals +6.0 D. "Postcycloplegic test" shows placing +1.0 in front of each eye, improves vision to 6/6 Snellen. The explanation is as follows: the plain refraction showed +4.0 D which is "manifest hyperopia". The hyperopia revealed after cycloplegia is +6.0 D and this is "total hyperopia". The difference between these two is the "latent hyperopia" of +2.0 D, which is revealed only after cycloplegia. Of the manifest hyperopia, +3.0 D, is inherently corrected by accommodation and is termed as "facultative hyperopia". The remaining, +1.0 D, which cannot be corrected by accommodation and needed correction of +1.0 D, is the "absolute hyperopia". Normally, the latent hyperopia is of +1.0 D only but in cases of high hyperopia, there is excessive ciliary tone and latent hyperopia is more. Therefore, in moderate to high hyperopias, full cycloplegia is important as these children have excessive ciliary tone and can go into ciliary spasm on continued near work.

Clinical Features

- *Ocular asthenopia*: Redness, watering, irritation, lack of interest in reading, and tiredness of eyes
- Headaches
- Blurring of vision after long hours of work
- Diminished VA—in selected cases.

Management: Simple Hyperopia

By far, most of hyperopia is of simple variety and thus our focus will be directed toward this type of hyperopia. Mild hyperopia, i.e., <2.0 D does not need any treatment in children well into teen age. It is only the moderate (3–6 D) and high hyperopia (>6.0 D) which needs attention.

Moderate hyperopia: In a landmark study entitled "vision in preschool—hyperopia in preschool (VIP-HIP)" hypothesized that children with moderate uncorrected hyperopia, would have greater difficulty in near activities like reading and writing that would deter their performance in school. For this, they administered the "test of preschool early literacy" (TOPEL) to a group of children with 1.0 D or less of hyperopia compared with a group of age-matched children with 3–6 D of uncorrected hyperopia.

The TOPEL is a standardized, widely used test. It tests the reading, learning of words, and writing abilities. The average TOPEL score of 3–5 years children is 90–110. A score of <90 predicts difficulty in learning to read and write. The current AAO preferred practice patterns recommends that children aged 3 years with bilateral hyperopia of +4.0 D or more, should receive corrections.

There are several factors to consider when deciding whether to prescribe glasses for a child with moderate hyperopia without esotropia or reduced VA. First, the acceptance of children to wear glasses with no symptoms. Secondly, the cost of spectacles when the parents think that they are not needed. Thirdly, the sociopsychological impact on children wearing glasses. Lastly and more importantly, early correction of moderate hyperopia, interfere with emmetropization, possibly consigning them to a lifetime of hyperopia are mandatory in these children (For the age-related cycloplegic choice of drug - see **Table 1** in Chapter 1). At this time, there is insufficient evidence to recommend that all children with moderate hyperopia be prescribed spectacles. Spectacles should be prescribed for children with moderate hyperopia associated with esophoria/tropia or reduced VA. These children usually have insufficiency of accommodation or accommodative lag and need correction. The best way is to give the "best subjective correction" after a postcycloplegic test. If associated with excessive "accommodative convergence (AC)" (abnormal AC/A ratio), then a bifocal with +3.0 near addition is given.

Children with anisometropic hyperopia have uniocular amblyopia in the higher hyperopic eye and are then treated as per the amblyopia treatment schedule. If by any chance, a child of around 3 years is referred by a pediatrician for delayed milestones, particularly motor deficiency, and a cycloplegic refraction reveals moderate hyperopia, a corroboration with delayed motor activity can be attributed to hyperopia and in such cases a "partial correction" of one-third of hyperopia can be initiated as emmetropization is still in progress.

As the child grows, the hyperopia weans and in some cases even up to 12 years age and cycloplegic refraction is continued every year to monitor the power of glasses. Yearly cycloplegic refraction is also recommended in every child with moderate hyperopia, as the power of glasses may need increment depending upon the load on eyes and the waning amplitude of accommodation. Some may not require correction who have good amplitude of accommodation and follow the near work rules. But as age advances into teens, the need for glasses may arise for near work, and these patients should be advised to come for consultation whenever they feel any symptoms.

In author's clinical opinion, since the hyperopia will never increase, moderate hyperopic children, with asthenopic symptoms, are advised to change the reading habits, minimize computer work, and stop use of mobile phones. If symptom persists, usually in accommodative insufficiency, "best subjective correction" for near is prescribed.

High hyperopia: Children who have persistent high hyperopia (>6.0 D) have diminished vision (bilateral ametropic amblyopia) and visuomotor and visuocognitive deficiencies. These are difficult to treat. Such children have poor accommodation and many times severe amblyopia which is refractory to treatment. Nonetheless, maximum tolerated hyperopic correction should be given to start with and then gradually increased. High hyperopias, in contrast to moderate hyperopia, usually do not reduce with age and any such notion can be misleading for treatment.

■ MYOPIA

Myopia has emerged from ancient Greek word "muopia" from myein meaning "to shut" and "opos" meaning "eye".

Myopia is the most common refractive error and so prevalent that it has attracted the maximum number of studies worldwide. Looking at the worldwide figures, a whopping 70–90%prevalence exists in some Asian countries, 30–40% in Europe and USA, and only 10–20% in Africa. The increase in the incidence of myopia and the futile measures to prevent its progression have generated a deep interest into its factors of pathogenesis, prevention, and management. Hence, this subject will be dealt in detail.

Etiopathogenesis

We have seen earlier in the chapter, that only 20–25% infants are born with myopia and most of it emmetropize by 5–6 years of age. It is generally agreed that if myopia persists by age 6 years, it is most likely to progress. There are numerous reasons speculated for causation and progression of myopia. It would be prudent to discuss them in brief, as they have bearing on the management.

- *Role of peripheral vision and retinal image degradation:* Research on the effect of "peripheral" or "off-vision" showed that peripheral form deprivation can produce axial myopia at the central fovea, even in the presence of potentially clear images in the central retina and that an intact fovea is not essential for the recovery from experimentally-induced refractive errors. There are several explanations for how the peripheral image quality affect foveal refractive state. One is that the expansion of globe occurs all over, influenced by peripheral form degradation and the foveal region becomes part of it. Another theory is that the vision dependent growth signals are pooled across a large area of retina. The major part of signals originate from the larger peripheral area and have a dominant effect on overall eye growth. It has been reported that individuals who are more hyperopic in the periphery, presumably because of the geometry of the eye or the shape of posterior globe, are more prone to development of myopia at the fovea than individuals who manifest relative myopic state at the periphery.
- *Genetics and heredity:* Heredity is an unarguably the most significant factor in the causation and progression of myopia. Though all types of refractive errors have some genetic base, but maximum genetic loci have been identified with myopia. The knowledge on genetic background of myopia has expanded dramatically in last few years. The Genome-Wide Association Studies (GWAS) have successfully identified many common genetic variants (mutations) associated with myopia. Like many other traits, myopia has a complex etiology that is influenced by an interplay of genetic and environmental factors. Evident by GWAS, myopia is likely to be caused by many genes, each contributing to a small effect to the overall myopia risk. But still, the exact mechanisms by which these genes function in a retina-to-sclera signaling cascade and potential pathways are yet to be elucidated. Also, the interplay between the genetic factors and environmental factors like near work and outdoor exposure is now well established.

  Early linkage studies, candidate gene studies, and GWAS enabled studies have identified >200 genes and 25 chromosomal loci responsible for myopia progression; out of this 22 are on autosomal chromosome and 3 on X-linked chromosome. Polygenic (multiple gene involvement) risk factors with these genetic understanding indicate that persons with high genetic risk have 40 times increased risk of myopia than persons with low genetic risk.

  Another study called Genome-Environment-wide Interaction Studies (GEWIS) assessing the genetic plus education interaction, identified nine other variant loci. As evidence, it meant that persons with profound genetic risk with higher education (more near work), appeared more susceptible to developing myopia. As technology improves, we can probably identify more genetic variants and pinpoint the causative genes.

  Myopia can also accompany many systemic or ocular syndromes (syndromic myopia). The secondary syndromic myopias are generally monogenic (involvement of single gene) and have a wide spectrum of presentations. A number of inherited retinal dystrophies also present with myopia, most strikingly X-linked retinitis pigmentosa caused by mutation in the *RPGR* gene. Other ocular disorders strongly associated with myopia are ocular albinism, congenital stationary night blindness, and

Wagner vitreoretinopathy. Most genes causing syndromic myopia have not yet been implicated in common forms of myopia but some genes like collagen type 2 alpha (COL2 A1) and fibrillin-1 (FBN 1) have clear contribution in myopia causation.

- *Nutrition:* Like so many dietary deficiencies linked with diseases, myopia has been also linked with low protein diet. Other factors like hyperinsulinemia, insulin resistance, insulin-like growth factors, carbohydrate metabolism disturbances, etc., all have hypothetical attributions to myopia.
  Vitamin-D has been found to be deficient in large number of studies in patients with high myopia but the association is not statistically significant.
- *Myopia and near-work:* Myopia has been strongly linked with close work. Studies evaluating association between myopia and near work have produced inconsistent results. Firstly, amount of near work to have significant impact on myopia progression has not been quantified. Secondly, the type of near work is not defined. Does only reading and writing have an impact or any kind of near work is a contributory factor. One important factor which emerged from "COMET" study (Correction of Myopia Evaluation Trial) that accommodative insufficiency was noted in large number of cases with myopia progression. Another interesting inference deduced from some studies is 9–10 hours of near work can be compensated with 2–3 hours of outdoor activity. The risk of any "go" signal may not be relevant, if there is sufficient "stop" signal to counter it. Thus, the amount of outdoor activity may provide the stop signal.
  On similar basis, the use of "over convergence", in causation and progression of myopia, is under debate. The pressure on the globe of contracting muscles for long durations may increase myopia. It is now clear that environmental factors are driving the myopia epidemic in recent years. To date, the most influential and consistent environmental factor are near work. Studies have shown individuals going for higher education have double the myopia prevalence compared to those who leave school early.
  Genome studies in individuals doing extensive near work and progressive myopia, found that persons with certain genes like *APLP-2, DNAH9, GJD2,* and *ZMAT4* variations, have strong association of developing myopia involved in higher education (see suggested reading).
- *Intelligence and myopia:* Certain confounding factors may be considered such as high IQ and type A personality. Children involved in outdoor activities are more cheerful and extrovert; a personality trait not found in children confined to room. Correlation between long hours of study and intelligence has not been defined. Children studying for longer hours may not necessarily be intelligent!
- *Outdoor activity:* The evolution of eyes has been going on for millions of years. The human eye, as many experts suggest, was not "programmed" for so much of near work. The environment to which human eye was adapted does not match our present environment. Its function was to view landscapes, mountains, and meadows; as our ancestors lead a nomadic life. The stress of constant near work has increased the load on our eyes and the prevalence of myopia. The hypothesis of outdoor life is in corroboration with lowest prevalence of myopia in African and Arctic regions, where people mostly lead life of hunting and wandering outdoors.
- *Gender variability:* Controversy exists in the gender variance in the epidemiology of myopia. One study showed that girls were more affected than boys, probably because of less hours of outdoor activity than boys, but this has not proved convincing but in models produced for evaluating myopia, the number of hours of outdoor/sports activity was inversely proportional to the progression of myopia.
- *Illumination:* Does studying or working in dim light causes myopia? People working with candle of lantern light over centuries has not shown increase in incidence of myopia. How much light is optimum for near work to avoid "eye-strain" has not been carefully investigated. In olden days, most of the work was done in daylight and whatever close work was done in dim illumination was compensated by an ample outdoor life. Good illumination increases the "depth of focus", and improves near vision, and less strain on accommodation, but does it contributes as a deterrent for myopia, is not known.
- *Biochemical changes:* With increased production and activation of matrix metalloproteinases (MMP) and decreased activity of their regulators, the biological mechanisms of eye growth and refractive development are well characterized, a result of many careful studies that have been carried out over the years. As the outermost coat of the eye, the sclera has the ultimate impact on the restraint or facilitation of eye growth, thus, any changes in its biochemistry, ultra structure, gross morphology, and biomechanical properties are critical in refractive error development, particularly myopia.

The sclera consists of extracellular matrix of interwoven lamellae of collagen and elastic fibrils, interspersed with proteoglycans and glycoproteins. Sandwiched between the lamellae are the cell bodies, scleral fibroblasts, which are responsible for the synthesis and degradation of the scleral extracellular matrix. The scleral collagen fibrils are primarily composed of type 1 collagen, interspersed with smaller amounts of at least 11 other collagen types. The interfibrillar spaces contains many enzymes and regulators that are of great importance for the structure and function of the scleral extracellular matrix. These include collagen regulator and degrading enzymes, regulators from MMP, range of cytokines, and members of transforming growth-factor-beta family (TGF-β). The fibroblast is the resident cell of the scleral matrix, and therefore, responsible for the production, organization, and regulation of the scleral structure matrix. A large proportion of scleral fibroblasts, comprises of fully-differentiated "myofibroblasts", which have the potential to contribute to biomechanical regulation within the sclera. Highly myopic eyes have shown that apart from thinning of collagen fibers, there is active scleral collagen loss and mucopolysaccharide depletion. The process and causes of this matrix degradation are well documented, the tissue inhibitors of MMP's [tissue inhibitors of metalloproteinase (TIPM)].

The defining feature of the sclera in a highly myopic eye is its significant thinning with the thickness approaching half that of the sclera in an emmetropic eye. The structural changes in the sclera make them more susceptible to distending, when exposed to the normal intraocular pressure overtime. The tendency of sclera tissue to buckle under physiological load suggests that the biochemical factors underlying scleral remodeling and ultrastructural changes in myopia lead to a consequent biomechanical weakness in sclera, which overtime, results in ocular elongation and myopia development.

Classification

The classification is simple and based on cause or the clinical appearance.

- *Axial:* The increase in the overall axial length of the eyeball.
- *Curvature:* The increase in the corneal curvature results in myopia.
- *Index:* Increase in the refractive index of the refracting elements of the eye, mainly crystalline lens.

Clinically, myopia can be classified as:

- Simple
- Degenerative
- Nocturnal
- Induced
- Quasi-myopia
- Pseudomyopia.

Simple or Progressive Myopia

This is perhaps the most prevalent of all type of myopia. Simple or progressive myopia, usually emerges at young age and continues to grow till the end of teen age. We have seen above that infantile of myopia of more than 3.0 D will usually not emmetropize and may become progressive. Also myopia which has appeared at 5 or 6 years of age, will generally progress. There may be a spurt of myopia progression usually at puberty and late teens. Rarely, myopia once set, may not progress.

Management

The high prevalence of myopia as a significant public health problem, emphasize the importance of finding solutions that's slow or control myopia progression. The mainstay of treatment options of spectacles, contact lenses or for that matter refractive surgery, do not control the accompanying eye growth or retard the physiological changes associated with the abnormal eye growth. Newer therapies by pharmacological agents are now being explored for control of myopia. Attempts to reverse the biochemical changes in sclera are also being explored. Newer surgical techniques to strengthen the sclera and prevent its elongation are also under experimentation.

Treatments that are currently available for myopia control will be discussed.

Pharmaceutical Agents

Atropine: Atropine molecule, a plant derivative, is a nonselective muscarinic receptor blocking agent. The role of atropine in control of myopia progression has been well documented. Use of 1.0% and 0.5% atropine drops has shown promise but ocular side-effects have discouraged its use. Consequently, interest shifted to use of much lower concentrations of atropine which also showed to reduce myopia progression. The original justification for using 0.01% atropine for myopia control was based on findings from atropine treatment of myopia 2 (ATOM 2) studies. This study conducted by Chia et al. in 2016, showing a 5 years study of treatment of myopia with 0.01% atropine is the most authentic study so far. Another recent study with equal value was the low-concentration atropine for myopia progression (LAMP) study by Yam et al. in 2019, which used 0.05%, 0.025%, and 0.01% atropine.

The results showed that even with 0.01% atropine proved to be equally effective.

The treatment is initially given for 2 years and then an observation period of 1 year is interposed. If the myopia shows signs of progression, then the treatment is resumed and continued for 12–15 years of age. The therapeutic regime consists of one drop daily in both eyes. Very minimal side effect on pupils and accommodation is noted. In the authors view who have been treating children on 0.01% atropine for last 4 years, none of children have complained of any discomfort. The author advices to continue drops till teenage which is usually the cut-off age for myopia progression. An increase of myopia of 1 D or more in 1 year is an indication to initiate therapy, which is now a standard treatment protocol for progressive myopia. As of results, all studies have shown a 50% reduction in axial growth of eyes. The only drawback is the rebound increase of myopia on stopping the drug.

The exact mechanism of action of low-dose atropine is not very clear, although the up and down regulation of retinal and scleral muscarinic receptors with influence on the scleral matrix has been postulated. One theory is that atropine creates generalized depression in retinal functions, indicated electroretinography (ERG) studies, initiating release of dopamine from cellular stores, which counters the factors associated with axial growth. Similar mechanism has also been reported of its action on scleral fibroblasts, which we know has significant effect on extracellular matrix.

Pirenzepine: Pirenzepine is a selective M-1 muscarinic receptor blocking agent. Its use in management of myopia progression has been under investigation for almost a decade. It holds promise that it could supplant atropine as an antimyopia treatment, but with fewer side effects. Pirenzepine is reported to have reduced mydriatic and cycloplegic effects in humans. Thus, it has merit over atropine which raises long-term safety concerns. Studies have shown that 2% pirenzepine gel, given twice daily, reduced the progression of myopia by almost 30–50% as compared to the controls. The drug is Food and Drug Administration (FDA) approved. With 2% concentration, the gel has been found to have clinically acceptable safety profile. Its mechanism of action has been shown to inhibit experimental myopia progression through modulation of MMP's and TIMP expression.

Other antimuscarinic drugs: Two other known antimuscarinic drugs used extensively in ophthalmic practice, tropicamide and scopolamine, have also been reported to slow down myopia progression. In a recent study nightly administration of 1% tropicamide, reduced myopia by approximately 50%. But the study was not randomized and long-term follow-up is awaited. This drug, though, holds promise as with only night time instillation, the pupillary dilation wears off by morning and the cycloplegic action is of short duration.

Scopolamine is similar to atropine in side effects and the long-term studies are lacking.

Other miscellaneous drugs: Intraocular pressure (IOP) lowering drugs have also been clinically tested for control of myopia, motivated by the data, though equivocal, linking myopia with increased IOP. Beta-blockers have been studied most extensively. In one of best designed study using timolol maleate, no evidence in regression of myopia was found in a 2 years period.

Epinephrine also lowers IOP and has been tried as an antimyopic agent. Though the results are inconsistent, but no serious long-term studies have been conducted so far.

Collagen and Proteoglycans

A different approach to strengthen sclera and prevent myopia progression is to target prevention of "degradation of sclera tissue" which occurs during myopia development. Collagen content in sclera is significantly reduced with thinning of fibers, loss of tissue, and overall reduction in sclera thickness.

The caffeine metabolite, 7-methylxanthine, a nonselective adenosine antagonist, has been shown to increase collagen fibril diameter and prevent loss of collagen fibril gradient. In long-term human trials, it has been shown to reduce significantly axial elongation. It is available commercially and can be given in 400 mg daily divided doses.

Other potential targets to increase collagen content and quality of collagen include cyclic-adenosine-monophosphate, guanosine-monophosphate, and bone-morphogenetic proteins.

Spectacles

The magic of treatment still lies with the spectacles. A child who does not see anything on the school board is exuberantly delighted when his/her vision becomes clear and crisp on wearing simple glasses. Spectacle correction is the mainstay of management of myopia, not only for vision clarity but it helps to control the progression also. But, it is easier said than done! There are lot of queries which surround the prescription of spectacles.

To prescribe or not to prescribe spectacles in small amounts of myopia has entered into lots of debate. As previously mentioned, even small of myopia (0.5 to 1.0 D) have the propensity of myopia progression in many children, especially detected by age 5 years. The author has a protocol of following such children every 6 month for 1 year; if no progression, then child is called for yearly consultation and any increase in numbers is given. If the progression is 1.0 or more, then atropine 0.01% is started.

Secondly, the family history is very important. If either of the parent is grossly myopic, then rapid progression of myopia is imminent; and review of myopia progression is monitored every 6 months. Consensus is now gathering to give correction on detection of myopia, not to wait for myopia to progress and cause symptoms.

What to prescribe: Full correction is the rule, in any type of myopia, whenever it is detected.

In phorias: If the patient has a phoria, the refractive status and type of phoria should be determined. In case of exophoria, full correction should be given to facilitate accommodative convergence. In case of esophoria, which may be due to use of excessive fusional convergence which is common in uncorrected high myopes, care should be taken not to over prescribe minus lenses, which can increase the eso deviation. A common practice in children is to remove glasses for near which should be discouraged.

Contact Lens

There has been a historical change in the quality and material used in contact lenses, since, they first came into existence in 1950s. There is a big inventory from which a doctor can pick and choose the right type of lens needed. All contact lenses of routine use are meant to replace spectacles, but we will discuss lenses which also serve to retard the progression of myopia.

The possibility that myopia progression can be controlled "optically" has seen a recent upsurge in interest in this field.

- *Defocus contact lenses:* Also known as "defocus incorporated soft contact (DISC) lens". Also known as "dual focus" soft lenses, these have significantly less power at the periphery compared to the center, and it is thought that this "peripheral defocus" may reduce the tendency for excessive lengthening of the eyeball.

A recent study showed myopia progressed more slowly in 25% of DISC lenses group, accompanied by less axial elongation. More recently, Cooper Vision (USA) has released the MiSight lens, a soft multifocal contact lens which has concentric rings in periphery for myopia correction for distance and a plus addition in center to decrease accommodation.

- *High oxygen content lenses:* Studies have shown that children using soft lenses of low oxygen content especially in very young patient are at risk of myopia progression probably due to corneal changes, diminution in vision and defocused image.

Some studies comparing myopic progression among low Dk/t hydrogel lenses and silicone hydrogel lens wearers have shown that contact "material" also affects myopic progression, although the relative contribution of physical properties versus physiological properties (corneal oxygen level) has not been yet clearly defined.

If a child has to wear a contact lens for myopia correction, a high water content with high Dk value comprising of a material with the above qualities should be used.

Orthokeratology

Orthokeratology or "Ortho-k" is a technique of fitting of specially designed gas-permeable contact lenses that reshapes cornea. The cornea is gently reshaped while the lenses are worn overnight and the vision remains clear during the day after the lenses are removed in the morning. This is a temporary effect and effective only till the lenses are worn. Furthermore, the development of new base material for "rigid" gas—permeable lenses, with higher levels of oxygen permeability, opened up possibility of orthokeratology becoming an effective, dependable, and comfortable.

It is postulated that 6 μm flattening of corneal curvature results in 1 D of changed vision. Therefore, a specially shaped lens can be used to lightly press on the cornea causing it to gradually flatten and configure it to a correct shape for a clear-focused vision. This therapy is also known as "corneal refractive therapy" (CRT).

Orthokeratology and CRT are theoretically different terms. CRT uses a specific brand of corneal reshaping lens and has a proprietary lens design and fitting procedure. Though technically different from orthokeratology, the ultimate purpose is similar and produces comparable results.

Another technique employed in orthokeratology is to use gas permeable rigid lenses with increasing base curves over a period of time. The principle is to gradually flatten the cornea with different lens designs which would gently press the cornea, over a period of time. On removing the lens, the result wanes off in 72 hours.

Surgical Options

- *Refractive surgery:* Refractive surgery in children is controversial and very few studies are in literature to comment upon. Fortunately, the population of children requiring surgery is very small. Refractive surgery can be an option with anisometropic amblyopia that is refractory to standard treatment or for those children who have high bilateral refractive error who cannot wear spectacles or contact lenses presumably because of behavioral or developmental problems. Since, we do not know reaction of a child's eye to laser surgery and since progressive myopia is basically an axial growth anomaly, correcting corneal curvature will not have permanent effect.
- *Scleral strengthening procedures:*
    - *Posterior scleral reinforcement (PCR):* The surgery consists of "buckling" the posterior sclera to control the bulge of posterior sclera. Both donor sclera tissue and synthetic material have been used. Owing to the invasive nature of the procedure, it is only reserved for severe cases and posterior staphylomas.
    - *Collagen cross-linking:* Similar to the corneal procedure, collagen cross-linking (C3R) has been tried on sclera also. But the difficulty by which riboflavin and UVA or blue light needs to be delivered for extended periods of time, makes this invasive procedure unsuitable in general public. Some of the difficulty has been solved by using fibro-optic flexible delivery system which is still experimental.
    - *Sub-Tenon's injections of hydrogel material* or implants are under study. Sub-Tenon's injection of hydrogel comprising "acrylated hyaluronic acid" has successfully prevented posterior axial growth in guinea pigs.

Special Types of Myopia

Unilateral Myopia

A child may not complain in small to moderate amounts of myopia, but cases rapidly loose binocular fusion and become exotropic or present with asthenopic symptoms. Since, we do not know the trend of myopia progression, it is always prudent to give spectacles early and strongly advise parents to consult at regular intervals.

Quasi Myopia

Progressive blurring of vision does not always mean that myopia is progressing. When a child who is wearing high minus lenses are brought to the clinic with complaints of diminished vision or headaches, two important aspect should be looked for.

Firstly, the position of the spectacles and secondly the "pantoscopic tilt" of the pecks (pantoscopic tilt is the angle of the spectacle frame from the vertical). It is common for heavy spectacles to slide down the nose; this will change the effective power of the lenses, as the vertex distance increases, and will have reduced distance vision or stress on accommodation. Similarly, too much tilting of frame or wrongly mounted frame on the nose will change the effective power and produce symptoms.

Pseudomyopia

Pseudomyopia is a condition when the patient complains of blurred vision at distance and the manifest refraction reveals minus lenses, but the factual position is different! A cycloplegic refraction shows "hyperopia". One of the most prevalent notion is that cycloplegic refraction is not needed in cases of myopia. This is unfortunately misleading. Cycloplegic refraction is as important in myopia as in hyperopia. It should be taken a mental note that cycloplegic refraction should be done routinely in all cases of suspected refractive error, at least for the first time.

Over-corrected Myopia

Complaints of ocular asthenopia by a myope are unusual but not rare. If a myopic child complains of eye strain, an overcorrection should be suspected. A minus overcorrection can provoke symptoms due to over accommodative effort. The symptoms would increase on near work, as the accommodative need is more.

If the current glasses show more minus lenses than manifest refraction, then overcorrection is present. If the manifest shows more minus than cycloplegic refraction, then ciliary spasm is present.

A symptomatic myope, who has been wearing overcorrection, may have so much of ciliary spasm that it is not always possible to rectify easily. The overcorrection has to be weaned gradually in steps.

A very pertinent question will still haunt the reader that is why an overcorrection of just 1.0 or 1.5 D minus, triggers asthenopic symptoms; whereas a hyperopic child of similar refraction of same age remains asymptomatic. This is because a hyperope had this condition since birth and has well adapted to it (remember all hyperopes of this degree do not have tropia or amblyopia). He has learned unconsciously, a comfortable balance between the accommodation required to see clearly and the convergence needed to maintain fusion. Actually, he uses fusional divergence to counter the excessive accommodative-convergence.

As the child grows older, the hyperopia gradually decreases and so his accommodative demand and the accompanying convergence. But for a myope who has been abruptly overcorrected produces an accommodative convergence, to which, being a myope, was not accustomed! To counter the overconvergence, the patient tries to counteract by fusional divergence. The tug-a-war, subsequently, creates the asthenopic symptoms.

Night Myopia

During nightfall or in dim light, our refractive state shifts toward near sightedness. This night myopia has been known for almost two centuries, but only recently it has gained importance. Though its cause has not been fully explained, but being a distinct clinical entity it should be understood.

Three separate factors operate at night when the pupils dilate, viz. accommodation, spherical aberration, and chromatic aberration. But for all practical purposes, it is the accommodative element which matters most. At night or in extremely dim illumination, there is loss of retinal image contrast. A low contrast of image is incapable of stimulating the accommodation to focus; so it simply drifts into a resting state. This resting state is not "zero" accommodation, but an "attempt to focus". This results in myopic state. The typical symptoms are blurred image with surrounding "halos". The halos represent defocused retinal image.

Management deals with estimating the night myopia and then giving the appropriate lenses.

The easiest and simplest way of estimating the night myopia is to do a retinoscopy in a fully "darkened" room at 1 meter distance with the person's minus correction in place. The extra minus lenses needed to neutralize the error present, gives the final correction. Children rarely need this correction and is narrated here for academic interest. Another reason when children should be encouraged to read in good illumination.

ASTIGMATISM

The visual system is not very sensitive to uncorrected astigmatism in the first year of life but from 1 year onward, there is evidence that uncorrected astigmatism, particularly oblique astigmatism, is associated with meridional amblyopia. Literature suggests that almost 45% of children between 6 months and 2 years of age will have 1.0 D or more of astigmatism, but this is bilateral, transient, and drops to 8–10% by 3–4 years of age. Persistent astigmatism of 1.5 D or more after 4 years of age is associated with poor VA, such that for every diopter increase in cylinder there is half-line decrease in VA. In older children, where astigmatism is first corrected between 5 and 12 years of age, a range of visual functions (recognition acuity, grating acuity, vernier acuity, contrast sensitivity, and stereo acuity) is impaired, indicates that correction of astigmatism of 1.5 D or more after 5 years of age may be too late for development of optimal visual functions. Similarly, Atkinson and colleagues state that we should correct astigmatism of 1.0 or more as early as 2 years to optimize visual functions. If we were to correct astigmatism of 1.0–1.5 D according to Atkinson and colleagues by 2 years of age, then we might find ourselves prescribing to almost 45% of children who normally have 1.0–1.5 D astigmatism by 2 years of age. This would not be clinically reasonable.

Management

We know that a large number of children are born with astigmatic eyes which decreases rapidly by 1 year of age and most of it is gone by 4–5 years of age. But in some cases, it remains or even increases with the increase in ametropia with age. A study done by a group of ophthalmologists "Risk factors for astigmatism in preschool children: A multi-ethnic Pediatric Eye Disease and Baltimore Pediatric Eye Disease Stud" showed that preschool children, aged 6 years with myopia >1.0 D are five times more prone to develop astigmatism and hyperopia of >2.0 D are two times more prone to develop astigmatism. This goes well with previously mentioned study that as myopia increases with age, so does the astigmatism.

Cylindrical anisometropia (aniso astigmatism) is a potent risk factor for amblyopia. And high bilateral isoastigmatism is also a cause of "ametropic amblyopia", where both eyes become amblyopic. Therefore, early detection of refractive error is a key for successful management of such problems. In a study, early corrected children before 4 years, 45% gained a VA of 20/20 (6/6) or better and only 22% gained VA of 6/6 or better whose error was corrected after 8 years of age.

We have learned that any symmetrical astigmatism of >1.5 D and oblique astigmatism of even 1.0 D should be corrected before 4–6 years of age as they are amblyogenic. Astigmatism appearing after 7 years onward, astigmatism should be fully corrected to allow development of higher visual functions and avoidance of asthenopic symptoms.

ANISOMETROPIA

Management: We have already seen that 1.0 D hyperopic or 2.0 D of myopic and 1.5 D of cylindrical anisometropia is enough to cause amblyopia in younger age group. Due to shift toward myopia after 6 years of age or so, anisometropia becomes more prevalent in myopes. This anisometropia reflects a difference in rate of eye growth between the two eyes. But interestingly, hyperopes were also likely to develop anisometropia. The mechanism for hyperopic anisometropia is not clear.

Different parts of world have different prevalence of refractive errors and therefore, treatment cannot be standardized. We do not have a broad based study on this issue in Indian population but a study done in United States on Indian population shows a high prevalence of 15%. Children at 12 years age with anisometropia may not necessarily have been anisometropic at age 6 years, and as this may tend to increase with increase in ametropia, therefore, treatment should be initiated.

Also, there is a strong association of anisometropia with increased interocular differences in axial length, but not corneal curvature. Thus, in author's clinical experience, that even anisometropic myopia of even 0.5 D be corrected, as this may be enough to trigger progressive myopia and subsequent increased anisometropia.

Anisometropia is the only identifiable amblyogenic factor in 37% of cases and present concomitantly with strabismus in additional 24% of clinical populations (PEDIG study). Since, such a large pediatric population is affected from amblyopia due to anisometropia, treatment schedule of anisometropia is directed toward management of amblyopia.

Anisometropia developing after age 6 or 7 years, may not be amblyogenic but may affect higher visual functions like stereoacuity and contrast sensitivity. In the author's clinical experience, most of these children with even smaller levels of anisometropia complain of ocular asthenopia and headaches, and a thorough cycloplegic refraction is mandatory.

ANTIMETROPIA

The term antimetropia is a rare subset of anisometropia, in which one eye is hyperopic and other myopic. The prevalence of naturally occurring antimetropia is extremely low, about 0.1% in large pediatric population, and typically associated with amblyopia in the hyperopic eye. This is because of unequal anatomical development of the two eyes. The condition is well recognized and management is typically on the lines of amblyopia.

WILL EARLY PRESCRIPTION OF SPECTACLES IMPROVE VISUAL FUNCTION OR FUNCTIONAL VISION?

By "visual function" we mean the physical measures of the sensory capability of the visual system such as VA or contrast sensitivity; while "functional vision" refers how the child performs his vision related tasks with whatever vision he/she has.

With regard to visual function, there are studies in which they used spectacle correction from age 6 months to 4 years. The incidence of strabismus and amblyopia was reduced, and VA was found 6/12 or better than the control group at age 4 years. But, this again is a research study, but practically children do not come for consultation before 3–4 years of age, and it is practically difficult also for children under 3 years to wear spectacles constantly. Except strabismus, consultation is not sought early.

There is clinical evidence that amblyopia due to high isometropic hyperopia responds to treatment with refractive correction, although the time course varies from one to several years and the VA achieved was 6/9 or better. Clinical studies conclude that moderate improvements can be obtained for children who already have bilateral refractive amblyopia due to hyperopia, but do not indicate whether we can completely prevent amblyopia by even earlier spectacle prescription. In author's view, general concept developing all over the world is that "photo screening" procedure is very effective in diagnosing refractive errors at an early age and early intervention will help in managing amblyopia. The only problem is of compliance of spectacle wearing in very young children.

In cases, where uniocular amblyopia is detected early due to hyperopia and spectacle correction is not feasible, occlusion of the good eye, as per the guidelines, can be adopted till the child accepts spectacles. Vision impairment due to other types of refractive errors, when detected early, the above-mentioned schedule should be followed.

With regard to functional vision, studies have shown that young children with uncorrected hyperopia or astigmatism perform poorly on some tests. The results of studies show that 4–5 years old with high uncorrected hyperopia of 4.0 D or more and astigmatism of 2.0 or 1.5 D or more had poor visuomotor and visuocognitive skills than normal children. Importantly, after the children with these high ametropias were prescribed glasses, their visuomotor skills improved considerably.

We have learned that any symmetrical astigmatism of >1.5 D and oblique astigmatism of even 1.0 D should be corrected before 4–6 years of age as they are amblyogenic. Astigmatism appearing after 7 years onward should be fully corrected to allow development of higher visual functions.

SUMMARY

- Management of refractive errors is different in children than in adults.
- The process of "emmetropization" should be well understood, as modulation of eyes is taking place and refractive errors come and go up to 12 years of age.
- In case of early detection of any error, the amount and type of error is important, as it may be amblyogenic.
- Cycloplegic refraction is key to detection of any error and should be continued up to 21 years of age.
- Hyperopias should not be misunderstood; as they are a source of multiple complaints in children.
- Any child with complaints of ocular asthenopia or headaches, needs full cycloplegic evaluation and if any hyperopia of >3.0 D is detected in preschool or school going child, "accommodative lag" should be looked for and subjective near correction should be given.
- As mentioned, anisometropias and astigmatism are strong amblyogenic factors and should be fully corrected.
- Myopia, whenever detected, should be fully corrected.
- Myopia continuing from infancy or appearing by age 6 years is usually progressive and should be closely monitored.
- Low-dose atropine has proved to be a strong deterrent to progressive myopia, and should be started and continued up to teen age.
- Correction of even small degrees of hyperopia, anisometropias, or astigmatism should be done as they have impact on other visual functions apart from VA.

SUGGESTED READING

1. Abrahamsson M, Sjostrand J. Natural history of infantile anisometropia. Br J Ophthalmol. 1996;80(10):860-3.
2. Adler D, Millodot M. The possible effect of undercorrection on myopic progression in children. Clin Exp Optom. 2006;89(5): 315-21.
3. American Academy of Ophthalmology. Pediatric ophthalmology/ strabismus panel. Amblyopia. San Francisco: American Academy of Ophthalmology; 2007.p. 28.
4. American Optometric Association. (2010). Care of the patient with Hyperopia. [online] Available from https://fdocuments.in/document/care-of-the-patient-with-hyperopia.html; www.aoa.org; [Last accessed August, 2021].
5. Atkinson J, Braddick O, French J. Infant astigmatism-Its disappearance with age. Vision. Res. 1980;20(11):891-3.
6. Chai XB, Shin SR, Chen DF, Zhang Q, Jin ZB. An overview of myopia genetics. Exp Eye Res. 2019;188:107778.
7. Chia A, Lu QS, Tan D. Five year clinical trial on atropine for the treatment of myopia 2: Myopia control with atropine 0.01% eyedrops. Ophthalmology. 2016;123(2):391-9.
8. Ciner EB, Kulp MT, Maguire MG, Pistilli M, Candy TR, Moore B. Visual function of moderately hyperopic 4- and 5-year old children in the vision in preschoolers-Hyperopia in preschoolers study. Am J Ophth. 2016;170:143-52.
9. Ciner EB. Management of refractive errors in infants, toddlers and preschool children. Probl Optom. 1990;2:394-419.
10. Congdon NG, Patel N, Esteso P, Chikwembani F, Webber F, Msithini RB, et al. The association between refractive cutoff for spectacle provision and visual improvement among school-aged children in South Africa. Br J Ophthamol. 2008;92(1):13-8.
11. Deng L, Gwiazda JE. Anisometropia in children from infancy to 15 years. Invest Ophthalmol Vis Sci. 2012;53(7):3782-7.
12. Dobson V, Harvey EM, Miller JM, Clifford-Donaldson CE. Anisometropia prevalence in highly astigmatic school-aged population. Optom Vis Sci. 2008;85(7):512-9.
13. Fan Q, Wojciechowski R, Kamran M, Cheng CY, Chen P, Zhou X, et al. Education influences the association between genetic variants and refractive error: A meta-analysis of five Singapore studies. Hum Mol Genet. 2014;23(2):546-54.
14. Gwiazda J, Bauer J, Thorn F, Held R. Meridional amblyopia does result from astigmatism in early childhood. Clin Vis Sci. 1986;1:145-51.
15. Gwiazda J, Hyman L, Hussein M, Everett D, Norton TT, Kurtz D, et al. A randomized clinical trial of progressive addition lenses versus single vision lenses on the progression of myopia in children. Invest Ophthalmol Vis Sci. 2003;44(4):1492-500.
16. Gwiazda J, Thorn F, Bauer J, Held R. Emmetropization and progression of manifest refraction followed from infancy to puberty. Clin Vis Sci. 1993;8:337-44.
17. Harvey EM, Dobson V, Clifford-Donaldson CE, Green TK, Messer DH, Miller JM. Prevalence of astigmatism in native American infants and children. Optom Vis Sci. 2010;87(6):400-5.
18. Harvey EM, Dobson V, Miller JM, Clifford-Donaldson CE. Changes in visual function following optical treatment of astigmatism-related amblyopia. Vision Res. 2008;48(6):773-8.
19. Hutchinson AK, Rychwalski PJ, Stahl E. Refractive surgery in children: Narrow indications and improved quality of life. Am Acad Ophthalmol. 2013.
20. Ingram RM, Traynar MJ, Walker C, Wilson JM. Screening for refractive errors at age 1 year: a pilot study. Br J Ophthalmol. 1979;63(4):243-50.
21. Jones LA, Mitchell GL, Mutti DO, Hayes JR, Moeschberger ML, Zadnik K. Comparison of ocular component growth curves among refractive error groups in children. Invest Ophthalmol Vis Sci. 2005,46(7):2317-27.

22. Klimek DL, Cruz OA, Scott WE, Davitt BV. Isoametropic amblyopia due to high hyperopia in children. J AAPOS. 2004;8(4):310-3.
23. Kulp MT, Ciner E, Maguire M, Moore B, Pentimonti J, Pistilli M, et al. Uncorrected hyperopia and preschool early literacy: Results of vision in preschoolers-Hyperopia in Preschoolers (VIP-HIP) Study. Ophthalmology. 2016;123(4):681-9.
24. Mayer DL, Hansen RM, Moore BD, Kim S, Fulton AB. Cycloplegic refractions in healthy children aged 1 through 48 months. Arch Ophthalmol. 2001;119(11):1625-30.
25. McKean-Cowdin R, Varma R, Cotter SA, Tarczy-Hornoch K, Borchert MS, Lin JH. Risk factors for astigmatism in preschool children: A multi-ethnic Pediatric Eye Disease and Baltimore pediatric eye disease studies. Ophthalmology. 2011;118(10): 1974-81.
26. Miao Z, Li L, Meng X, Guo L, Cao D, Jia Y, et al. Modified posterior scleral reinforcement as a treatment for high myopia in children and its therapeutic effect. Biomed Res Int. 2019;2019: 5185780.
27. Mirshahi A, Ponto KA, Hoehn R, Zwiener I, Zeller T, Lackner K, et al. Myopia and level of education: results from the Gutenberg health study. Ophthalmology. 2014;121(10):2047-52.
28. Monga S, Dave P. Spectacle prescription in children: Understanding Practical approach of Indian ophthalmologists. Indian J Ophthalmol. 2018;66(5):647-50.
29. Nishimura M, Wong A, Cohen A, Thorpe K, Maurer D. Choosing appropriate tools and referral criteria for vision screening of children aged 4-5 years in Canada: a quantitative analysis. BMJ Open. 2019;9(9):e032138.
30. O'Donoghue L, Julie F McClelland, Logan NS, Rudnicka AR, Owen CG, Saunders KJ. Profile of anisometropia and aniso astigmatism in children: Prevalence and association with age, ocular biometric measures, and refractive status. Invest Ophthalmol Vis Sci. 2013;54(1):602-8.
31. O'Keefe M, Nolan L. Lasik surgery in children. Br J Ophthalmol. 2004;88(1):19-21.
32. Pediatric Eye Disease Investigator Group. The Clinical profile of moderate amblyopia in children younger than 7 years. Arch Ophthalmol. 2002;120(3):281-7.
33. Ramessur R, Williams KM, Hammond CJ. Risk factors for myopia in a discordant monozygotic twin study. Ophthalmic Physiol Opt. 2015;35(7):643-51.
34. Shukla Y. Management of Refractive Errors and Prescription of Spectacles. New Delhi: Jaypee Brothers Medical Publishers (P) Ltd. 2015.
35. Tkatchenko AV, Tkatchenko TV, Guggenheim JA, Verhoeven VJ, Hysi PG, Wojciechowski R, et al. APLP2 regulates refractive error and myopia development in Mice and Humans. PloS Genet. 2015;11(8):e1005432.
36. Yam JC, Jiang Y, Tang SM, Law AKP, Chan JJ, Wong E, et al. Low- concentration atropine for Myopia Progression (LAMP) study: a randomized, double-blinded, placebo-controlled trial of 0.05%, 0.025%, and 0.01% atropine eye drops in myopia control. Ophthalmology. 2019;126(1):113-24.

4 CHAPTER

Accommodative Anomalies in Children

Yogesh Shukla

INTRODUCTION

Accommodation is one of the greatest virtues we use to see clearly and comfortably. There are quite a number of visual problems which arise while using the eyes for near work, where accommodation comes into effect; but unfortunately, this aspect has been least studied and even disregarded. Ocular asthenopia and host of related problems arising on near work, have never been addressed scientifically and attributed to anomalies in accommodation. More so, such problems have never been even thought to arise in children as their accommodation is assumed to be great and flawless. This is a big misbelief which we have nurtured for all along. Though this concept has been studied for many years and we have now a clear understanding of the accommodative mechanism, but it is rarely clinically applied in practice. Symptoms on near work such as headaches, asthenopia, watering, blurring, redness, lack of concentration, etc., occur frequently in children, and every test is done from refraction to ocular motility to find the cause, except accommodative tests.

The knowledge of how the neuronal accommodative system functions is still limited. The general consensus that young children or teenagers, with strong accommodative amplitudes are immune to accommodative anomalies, is misleading. Way back in 1912, Duane stated that the amplitude of accommodative is quite high in young children. Since then, for almost a century, it has been universally approved that accommodation in young children is extremely flexible and resistant to fatigue. Though this old data is still what we normally believe, the ocular accommodation in children is not as sufficient or efficient as we expect. There is no simple standard procedure which includes all accommodative facets for examination. The accommodative system is therefore, not routinely examined because of lack of such method and more so because of the concept that there cannot be any fallacy of accommodation in children. Young school children may have an insufficient accommodative ability that causes subjective symptoms when reading. Excluding all pathological or pharmaceutical entities, a "general weakness" in a child is enough to cause near work dysfunctions. Therefore, it is prudent and mandatory to look carefully and seriously into any complaints arising out of near work in children.

A proper cycloplegic refraction is primary to all complaints, whether or not the visual acuity is normal. After a correct lens prescription, if the complaints persist, then a thorough accommodative tests should be performed. Accommodative spasm is not infrequent in an uncorrected hyperope, especially if the person is involved in excessive, long near work as in computer work. The ordeal of "computer vision syndrome" is now well documented. But, we rarely go into the tests for accommodative anomalies arising in this syndrome.

But, it may come as a surprise that accommodation is not as efficient in children as expected. Number of studies have now clearly stated that in case of above symptoms, a thorough accommodative tests should also be carried out. Subjective symptoms usually emerge around 6–7 years of age, when children start getting extensively involved in near work, and there is a clear relation between accommodative parameters and these symptoms. Because accommodative dysfunctions may result in varied visual and asthenopic symptoms, it is of utmost importance to identify this dysfunction to prevent unnecessary visual problems. Therefore, clear standards for diagnosing an accommodative dysfunction need to be further refined. Studies have shown that accommodative training, in cases of dysfunction, is an effective method in alleviating the symptoms.

BASICS OF ACCOMMODATION

- Anatomically, three parts in the eye are involved in the accommodative process, i.e., (1) ciliary muscles-circular and meridional, (2) the zonules, and (3) the crystalline lens.

  By far, most of attention has been through a single window—the lens in the accommodative mechanism; very little focus has been given to the muscles which are the primary partner in this process. It is now becoming evidently clear that accommodative anomalies, especially in children, are primarily situated in the muscles.
- The characteristics of effective "accommodative stimuli" is the first step in our understanding of accommodative system. There are a number of "different" accommodative

stimuli which stimulate accommodation to varying degrees. These are:

- Blur of the object
- Proximity of the target
- Changing target size
- Chromatic aberration
- Convergence of eyes
- Spatial frequency.

These are all different stimuli to accommodation with "Blur" of object having the greatest impact as stimuli, though independent of visual acuity.

An important implication is the completely different character of these stimuli which can act together as well as independently.

AMPLITUDE OF ACCOMMODATION

The ability to focus a visual target at varying distances is known as accommodation and is present to some extent from birth, but improves rapidly by first 6 months of life. It is believed that a small child is able to focus from infinity down to very close to the eyes because of high level of accommodation. However, it is to be noted that accommodation and convergence are not automatically linked from the start. The amount of accommodation in diopters, needed to clearly focus an object from infinity to the nearest point possible, is the "amplitude of accommodation".

The accommodative function is normally expressed by describing the accommodative amplitude and its dioptric value. However, the accommodative function is more complicated than that. The accommodative system is complex and comprises of not only the amplitude but number of other functions; any of them can be underdeveloped and can give rise to ocular symptoms. Therefore, the object of this article is to apprise the reader of various facets of accommodative system and the implications it has on the subjective symptoms in a child.

DIFFERENT FACETS OF ACCOMMODATION

- Amplitude of accommodation
- Tonic accommodation (TA)
- Lag of accommodation
- Convergence accommodation
- Accommodative facility
- Relative accommodation.

These facets differ greatly from each other with regard to function. They require different methods of measurement and are not explained by the same dioptric value. There is no method in use that describes the complete accommodative function nor we use the same measuring system for different dioptric results. Furthermore, dysfunction of each envisages different set of symptoms.

Let us review each of these facets.

- *Amplitude of accommodation:* As already stated, it is the total accommodative power of the eye and is expressed in dioptric equivalent and is reciprocal to the distance of the object from the eye. As age advances, the power of accommodation deteriorates, and the ability to see clearly at near diminishes. As a matter of fact, this ability or facet of accommodation, is most relevant to the clinician and thus is the only one tested clinically in routine practice.
  Amplitude tests:
  - *Donders push-up method:* This uses the Royal Air Force (RAF) ruler (also known as prince ruler). In this, a ruler about 50 cm in length has markings on one side in cms and other side in diopters. A sliding box is mounted on the ruler in which letter lines conforming to Snellens optotype size to be read from near. The subject holds the ruler with one end mounted on nose and holds the other end with the hand. A +3.0 D lens is placed in front of eyes to pull up the range of accommodation to 35 cm. The reading card or box is moved away till the print blurs and pulled up near till the print blurs again. The difference between the two readings gives the amplitude of accommodation.
  - *Sheard's method:* Here, minus lenses are added at far distance target, monocularly or binocularly, until blur at distance occurs. The power of lenses used, gives the amplitude.
- *Tonic accommodation:* Tonic accommodation or dark accommodation (DA) is a passive state of accommodation in the absence of any stimulus. This occurs when the eye is in complete darkness or when it is looking at a bright empty field. Basically, it is the inherent tone of the ciliary muscles when the eye at rest. Ironically, the resting "tone" varies in different situations or differs in refractive errors. This tonic state of accommodation or the "resting state tone" of the ciliary muscles can be unearthed only after total cycloplegia. Another way of measuring is by using an objective "infrared optometer".
- *Lag of accommodation:* The amount by which the accommodative response of the eye is less than the dioptric stimulus to accommodation is defined as the "accommodative lag". Clinical measurement of accommodative lag at near is typically done by dynamic retinoscopy. This is an objective method in which the patient views a near point target, while the examiner uses lenses to neutralize the fundal glow.
- *Convergence accommodation:* Convergence accommodation is normally described by the ratio between convergence-accommodation and convergence, or the CA/C ratio. The ratio is the measure of the effect of change in convergence on accommodation. It is expressed as the change in accommodation (Diop.) for each change in convergence in prism D.
- *Accommodative facility:* "Accommodative facility" is the ability to rapidly change the power of the crystalline lens to various focus distances while maintaining a requisite angle of convergence (binocularly) or eliminating the

influence of convergence (monocularly). This ability is important while changing the fixation from near to distance and back again.

Clinically, accommodative facility can be measured using lenses that stimulate accommodation (minus lenses) or inhibit accommodation (plus lenses). Any combination can be used for evaluation, but experience has shown that ±2 D is a reasonable choice. The procedure uses ±2 D lens pair mounted on a "flipper frame". A flipper is a frame on which two plus and two minus lenses are mounted **(Fig. 1)**. The subject focuses through one pair of lenses at an object at fixed distance (say 40 cm). When the object is clearly focused, a "flip" of the frame is quickly performed to bring the other pair in front of eyes, and the person focuses through them. This is then again repeated; and the number of cycles completed in 1 minute is noted as the "accommodative facility" in "cycles/min" (cpm).

Normative data on children have been collected by number of researchers. The results of the flipper test in children aged 6–12 years were 5.0 ± 2.5 cpm, in one study and 4.0 ± 2.5 cpm in another study.

The cutoff parameter for reduced facility to show symptoms is <3 cpm.

The facility testing is important and has bearing on the symptoms where children complain in difficulty in focusing on the board and then reading/writing at near.

- *Relative accommodation:* The total amount of accommodation which can be exerted while the convergence remaining fixed is called the "relative accommodation". This can be either "positive relative accommodation (PRA) or negative relative accommodation (NRA)." PRA is the amount of accommodation in excess of the accommodation needed for convergence and NRA is the amount of accommodation less than needed for convergence. In other words, the least amount of accommodation or maximum relaxation of accommodation with which one can see clearly at a fixed distance is the NRA and the maximum accommodation used over and above the need at a fixed distance is called PRA. To assess this flexibility, a simple test is used. With a vergence stimulus fixed at 40 cm, positive lenses with 0.25 D increment are put in front of both eyes and the first sign of blur is noted. The amount of plus lenses used will give the value of NRA. Similarly, now minus lenses are used with increasing power in 0.25 D steps, binocularly, till the first sign of blur is noted. The increased amount of stimulus at this point is the PRA.

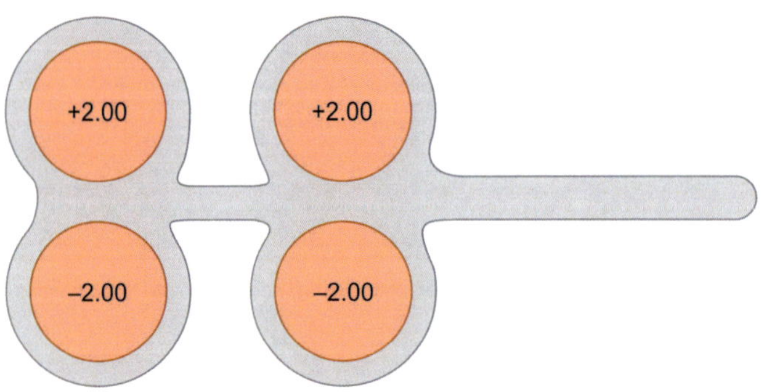

Fig. 1: Flipper frame.

Tests for PRA and NRA are very helpful in determining accommodative dysfunctions in children. A low NRA reveals accommodative spasticity; while a low PRA suggests that the focusing mechanism may be prone to tiring after concentrated near work.

It would be not out of place to discuss about the accommodative convergence/accommodation ratio (AC/A) ratio; as it is linked with accommodation. Due to the near vision reflex complex, a certain amount of convergence is expected when accommodation is in force. The relation between the dioptric change in accommodation and the prismatic change in convergence is called the AC/A ratio. In simple terms, the AC/A ratio describes how much convergence is activated by an accommodative change of 1 D. Normally a convergence of 3–5 PD occurs when 1 D of accommodation is exerted. An AC/A of 10 or more is termed as high ratio while an AC/A ratio of <3 is termed as low.

Tests for PRA and NRA are very helpful in determining accommodative dysfunction. A low NRA reveals accommodative spasticity; a low PRA, on the other hand, suggests that the focusing system is prone to tiring after concentrated near work.

PRACTICAL DYSFUNCTIONS

The accommodative system at young age is quite flexible and resistant to fatigue. However, in clinical practice, accommodative dysfunction can occur in children and young people. Often children and teenagers complain of certain symptoms which appear when doing near work. The refractive system is usually emmetrope or slightly ametropic, but that is not always in relation to the complaints. Unfortunately, there does not exist, as mentioned earlier, no simple, single standard procedure which might include all facets of accommodative dysfunction. Because of this reason and because we do not have any clear cut method of treating accommodative problems, the accommodative system is not routinely examined. But, it is of great importance to identify any accommodative dysfunction, if any complaints exist, so that unnecessary near vision problems may be prevented. It is also important to identify any accommodative dysfunction or deficiency in school going children, because this has a bearing on the performance of children in school. Because the focusing system of eyes has contribution in the learning process, any accommodative deficiency can make it unnecessarily difficult for the child to read and write and develop in studies. If the child's accommodative deficiencies are not resolved, he/she may develop dislike any near work and develop lack of interest in studies. Therefore, we need to find a simple and easy-to-use method that identifies an accommodative dysfunction.

It is difficult to group together accommodative dysfunctions, as the boundaries are often unclear. However, clinically it is useful to separate anomalies of accommodation into five distinct syndrome categories:

1. Insufficiency of accommodation
2. Infacility of accommodation
3. Fatigue of accommodation
4. Spasm of accommodation
5. Paresis of accommodation

These five syndromes constitute different accommodative disorders, having slightly different symptoms, having different impact on accommodative function.

A brief description of each would be helpful in identifying and treating the disorders.

An important aspect is that of symptoms related to accommodative dysfunction must be clearly recognized and understood. Most of times, the clinician concentrates only on the refractive anomalies and attributes all symptoms to the refractive problem. It should be remembered that all symptoms need not be due to refractive error; time should be devoted to enquire about all symptoms specially arising from near work and tests should be employed to determine the type of accommodative anomaly.

Understanding the symptoms is of paramount importance in recognizing any accommodative anomaly.

Asthenopia is a cardinal symptom which stands out prominently in accommodative deficiencies. Asthenopia is a term used to describe eye-strain or symptoms arising from use of eyes for near work.

Though asthenopia is used loosely to describe all types of symptoms but scientifically explaining, it means purely eye strain and comprises of red eyes, frequent rubbing and irritation of eyes, and disinterest in doing near work after a certain time. Other symptoms arising of accommodative strain are headaches, diplopia, blurring, vertigo, and drowsiness.

As asthenopia is the flagbearer of any ocular morbidity, it would be not out of place to illustrate the reasons of asthenopia. Asthenopia, per se, can occur in the following conditions:

- Accommodative insufficiency
- Accommodative infacility
- Accommodative fatigue
- Accommodative spasm
- Dyslexia
- Hysteria
- Ocular inflammations
- Phorias-ocular motility disorders
- Latent nystagmus
- Aniseikonia
- *Refractive errors*: Astigmatism; hyperopia; and anisometropia
- Accommodative paresis.

It thus becomes mandatory to recognize these conditions by exclusion and look for the accommodative reasons carefully.

Since, this article is dedicated to accommodative problems, let us briefly discuss the five syndromes which occur clinically:

1. *Insufficiency of accommodation:* It is a condition in which the amplitude of accommodation is chronically below the lower limits of expected amplitude of accommodation for the person's age. Classically, insufficiency of accommodation is a physiological phenomena of advancing age and very rare in children. But studies have shown that this problem is not too uncommon in children. In one study, children aged 10–15 years, with low accommodative amplitude, had severe complaints of asthenopia, headaches, diplopia, and difficulty in reading. Therefore, the clinical recognition of accommodative insufficiency is important in preventing unwanted frustration in school going children. The clinician should keep his mind open where such accommodative insufficiency is suspected, especially in circumstances of certain syndromes or the child is on drugs for psychological disorders.
2. *Infacility of accommodation:* As previously discussed, this is a condition in which a rapid change of accommodation from far to near and vice-versa is failing and raises symptoms of asthenopia. It differs from insufficiency in that clear vision is eventually achieved, albeit after some time. If changing fixation from distance to near takes >1 second, an abnormal condition is likely to be present. Children who need to change fixation rapidly from distance to near, as is commonly done in school in viewing blackboard and then writing at near, start complaining of ocular pain or headaches after long hours in school.
3. *Fatigue of accommodation:* Fatigue of accommodation is described as the inability of ciliary muscle to maintain contraction while viewing a near target with a resulting blurring of the object and shift of accommodation toward far point. Normally, in young children, the amplitude is so much in reserve that this condition is rare. If in a child, there is doubt of such a situation, then a thorough cycloplegic refraction is warranted to weed out hyperopia or astigmatism. Still, the reading habits and light source should also be enquired into.
4. *Spasm of accommodation:* Spasm of accommodation is a constant or intermittent involuntary and

inappropriate ciliary contraction. It may be unilateral or bilateral. Symptoms include distance and/or near blur, visual distortion, constant brow ache, or headaches, and sometimes diplopia. Also, a dynamic retinoscopy shows no change.

5. *Paresis of accommodation:* Paresis of accommodation could be partial or complete.

The most common cause of paresis is use of cycloplegic drops whether deliberate or inadvertent. It is to be understood that the use of cycloplegic drops used for refraction have a duration of effect; but it may not be surprising if the effect continues well beyond the stipulated time frame. In every case of suspected cycloplegic used, whether at your clinic or elsewhere, the type and date of refraction must be enquired.

Accommodative paresis can also be functional, owing to weakness, or fatigue of ciliary muscles.

Near work performance can also be hampered due to certain accommodative syndromes, neurological disorders, use of certain sedatives, anticholinergic drugs, antipsychotic drugs, hysteria, etc. The "accommodative facility" can be inherently deficient despite the amplitude being normal; thus, a thorough tests of various facets of accommodation should be done to arrive at a correct diagnosis of accommodative problem.

ACCOMMODATIVE THERAPY

Accommodative dysfunctions are not an uncommon visual anomaly in children and the symptoms typically occur during near work. Out of the dysfunctions mentioned above, accommodative "insufficiency" and accommodative "infacility" are the most common dysfunctions encountered in children. After ruling out neurological, pharmaceutical, and general health issues, the standard treatment of accommodative dysfunction is generally orthoptic exercises or addition of plus lens for near.

In cases of accommodative insufficiency, what is needed is a proper distance correction with an addition of appropriate plus lenses for near. Orthoptic exercises to strengthen vergence or accommodation by "push-up" technique should also be employed.

A plus lens add are recommended in cases of excessive "lag of accommodation", "very low PRA", or "fatigue of accommodation". The prescription can be either in form of normal reading glasses or bifocals.

Orthoptic exercise is a sequence of activities individually prescribed and monitored by the clinician to develop efficient visual skills and processing. "Flipper" method is one of the extremely efficient methods aimed at developing accommodative efficiency and "push-up" exercise to strengthen vergence and accommodation. Use of synoptophore is a time tested machine for orthoptic exercises, but the patients regular attendance are doubtful; even home-based exercises have proved to be equally effective and should be relied upon.

There is a scientific and clinical evidence to support the efficiency of using facility therapy techniques to strengthen or improve accommodative functions.

CONCLUSION

With all said and done, near work complaints and problems are on the increase in children, because of computers and mobile game gadgets, and as a vigilant clinician it is imperative that we take the near vision complaints of children seriously and make a conscience effort to look for accommodative anomalies. Asthenopic and related symptoms are a major problem in school-going children. With the inception of computers and other gadgets for near work, the unseen problems arising out of constant and continuous near work are on the rise. Parents wander from pillar to post, seeking respite from their child's constant complaints from near work; but inspite of best spectacle correction and avoidance of excessive near work, the complaints continue. Studies have shown that majority of these problems arise from defects in accommodation, even in a young child. Therefore, various aspects of accommodation deficiencies have to be studied clinically, detected, and treated to ameliorate the symptoms.

SUGGESTED READING

1. Atchison DA. Accommodation and presbyopia. Ophthalmic Physiol Opt. 1995;15(4):255-72.
2. Banks MS. The development of visual accommodation during early infancy. Child Dev. 1980;51(3):646-66.
3. Beers AP, van der Heijde GL. Age-related changes in the accommodation mechanism. Optom Vis Sci. 1996;73(4):235-42.
4. Bobier WR, Guinta A, Kurtz S, Howland HC. Prism induced accommodation in infants 3 to 6 months of age. Vision Res. 2000;40(5):529-37.
5. Bobier WR, Sivak JG. Orthoptic training of subjects showing slow accommodative responses. Am J Optom Physiol Opt. 1983;60(8):678-87.
6. Cacho P, Garcia A, Lara F, Seguí MM. Diagnostic signs of accommodative insufficiency. Optom Vis Sci. 2002;79(9):614-20.
7. Chiu NN, Rosenfield M. Tonic accommodation, tonic vergence, and surround propinquity. Ophthalmic Physiol Opt. 1994;14(3):290-2.
8. Chrousos GA, O'Neill JF, Lueth BD, Parks MM. Accommodation deficiency in healthy young individuals. J Pediatr Ophthalmol Strabismus. 1988;25(4):176-9.
9. Fisher RF. The mechanics of accommodation in relation to presbyopia. Eye. 1988;2:646-9.
10. Garcia A, Cacho P, Lara F, Megías R. The relation between accommodative facility and general binocular dysfunction. Ophthalmic Physiol Opt. 2000;20(2):98-104.
11. Goldstein JH, Schneekloth BB. Spasm of the near reflex: A spectrum of anomalies. Surv Ophthalmol. 1996;40(4):269-78.
12. Goss DA. Clinical accommodation testing. Curr Opin Ophthalmol. 1992;3(1):78-82.
13. Hung GK, Ciuffreda KJ. Sensitivity analysis of relative accommodative and vergence. IEEE Trans Biomed Eng. 1994;41(3):241-8.

14. Kedzia B, Pieczyrak D, Tondel G, Maples WC. Factors affecting the clinical testing of accommodative facility. Ophthalmic Physiol Opt. 1999;19(1):12-21.
15. Kruger PB, Aggarwala KR, Bean S, Mathews S. Accommodation to stationary and moving targets. Optom Vis Sci. 1997;74(7):505-10.
16. Leat SJ, Gargon JL. Accommodative response in children and young adults using dynamic retinoscopy. Ophthalmic Physiol Opt. 1996;16(5):375-84.
17. Marran LF, De Land PN, Nguyen AL. Accommodative insufficiency is the primary source of symptoms in children diagnosed with convergence insufficiency. Optom Vis Sci. 2006;83(5):281-9.
18. Matsuo T, Ohtsuki H. Follow-up results of a combination of accommodation and convergence insufficiency in school-age children and adolescents. Graefes Arch Clin Exp Ophthalmol. 1992;230(2):166-70.
19. McLin LN Jr, Schor CM, Kruger PB. Changing size (looming) as a stimulus to accommodation and vergence. Vision Res. 1988;28(8):883-98.
20. Miwa T, Tokoro T. Dark focus of accommodation in children with accommodative esotropia and hyperopic anisometropia. Acta Ophthalmol (Copenh). 1993;71(6):819-24.
21. O'Leary CI, Evans BJW. Criteria for prescribing optometric interventions: literature review and practitioner survey. Ophthalmic Physiol Opt. 2003;23(5):429-39.
22. Owens DA, Wolf-Kelly K. Near work, visual fatigue, and variations of oculomotor tonus. Invest Ophthalmol Vis Sci. 1987;28(4):743-9.
23. Pigion RG, Miller RJ. Fatigue of accommodation: changes in accommodation after visual work. Am J Optom Physiol Opt. 1985;62(12):853-63.
24. Rosenfield M, Cohen AS. Push-up amplitude of accommodation and target size. Ophthalmic Physiol Opt. 1995;15(3):231-2.
25. Russell GE, Wick B. A prospective study of treatment of accommodative insufficiency. Optom Vis Sci. 1993;70(2):131-5.
26. Scheiman M, Herzberg H, Frantz K, Margolies M. Normative study of accommodative facility in elementary school children. Am J Optom Physiol Opt. 1988;65(2):127-34.

CHAPTER 5

Amblyopia

Edward Kuwera, Courtney L Kraus, Oded Lagstein, Adrianna Jensen

BRIEF HISTORY

The first mention of "*amblyopia*" dates back to the fifth century BC to the old Greek civilization where hippocrates used the word to indicate conditions which resulted in decreased visual acuity (VA) in seemingly healthy eyes. The old Greeks also defined "*strabismus*" as a disorder of eye movements and position. By today's standards, their treatment options would be seen as bizarre, but it was a start in the treatment of amblyopia. More than a thousand years later, in the Byzantine empire, around the year 900 AD, there was the first mention of occlusion for the treatment of strabismus in history. In the 13th century, the first eye hospital was established in France, and in the 16th century a German physician designed special hoods to put them over one's head to treat strabismus. In 1722, a French ophthalmologist by the name Charles de Saint-Yves wrote that covering a nonstrabismic eye will cause the deviated eye to immediately look straight ahead—something now known as the cover test. He also proposed that the nonstrabismic eye should be covered in order to restore the correct eye position of the deviated eye. Later in 1743, George Comte de Buffon described that the weaker eye regains its strength with occlusion of the good eye, which is why he is considered a founder of occlusion therapy for amblyopia. The first idea to treat strabismus (and amblyopia) surgically came in the 18th century by John Taylor, although his surgical techniques on eye muscles were later recognized as fraud. About 100 years later, Germans Stromeyer and Dieffenbach, and Belgian Cunier were the first to have performed proper surgery for correcting strabismus. It was also then noted by Ludwig Boehm that the surgery to correct strabismus also improved amblyopia.

At the beginning of the 20th century, occlusion therapy was repopularized. Sattler started to use a patch as we know today, although he suggested occlusion for at least several days without a break—contrary to what we do now. What Sattler happened to infer correctly was that occlusion is most effective in children up to the age of 6–8 years. Weckert suggested using a spectacle occluder instead of an eyepatch, and this was generally more tolerated by children than an eyepatch. In the coming decades, the benefits, duration, and side effects of occlusion therapy became more and more recognized. By the 20th century, more sophisticated forms of occlusion were introduced, though ophthalmologists had already come to agree that refractive correction was as important as occlusion itself. Improvements in surgical techniques made the correction of strabismus much safer. Alternatives to occlusion via "penalization" was introduced to clinical practice, and this represents an appealing alternative for those who have difficulty tolerating conventional occlusion.

INTRODUCTION

Amblyopia is a disorder of visual development and early diagnosis of visual dysfunction associated with amblyopia is crucial to allow for treatment to begin at a stage where the neurological pathways are still amenable to stimulation, recovery, and reversal of cortical damage. All children should have periodic visual screenings, as the potential for successful treatment of amblyopia is greatest in young children. If not promptly recognized or treated, a plethora of functional deficits may result and persist into adulthood with far reaching impacts on productivity and quality of life. The resulting morbidities from strabismic amblyopia include:

- *Psychosocial repercussions:* Interference with social contact and cosmetic distress. Children begin to develop a negative attitude toward classmates with strabismus as early as the age of 6 years. This attitude adversely affects interpersonal relationships, self-image, schoolwork, participation in sports, and only intensify in the teenage and adult years.
- *Increased risk of impairment of the sound eye:* The lifetime risk of impairment to the sound eye is estimated to be 1:100–1:1,000 from accidental trauma or other etiologies such as macular degeneration and retinal vein occlusion.
- *Impaired binocular function:* There is reduced, or absent, stereopsis which can affect visual-motor skills, and even restrict careers such as aviation.

Anisometropic amblyopia was defined as amblyopia in setting of anisometropia of 0.50 D or more spherical equivalent or difference in astigmatism between eyes of at least 1.50 D in any axis that persists after 4 weeks of spectacle use. Strabismic amblyopia was defined as amblyopia in the presence of either a heterotropia at distance and/or near fixation, or a history of strabismus surgery (or botulinum toxin injection) in the absence of refractive error meeting the criteria for combined-mechanism amblyopia.

Current standards of care in the treatment of amblyopia are based on the work of two study groups that conducted randomized clinical trials to define optical treatment protocols. There is the UK-based Monitored Occlusion Treatment of Amblyopia Study (MOTAS), and the US-based Pediatric Eye Disease Investigator Group (PEDIG). The strengths of these studies include a large cohort, broad age groups, different types of amblyopia in a wide range of acuities, certified examiners, and standardized acuity testing protocols. The primary limitation in both studies is the lack of control subjects.

OPTICAL TREATMENT

Refractive correction is the first step in treating amblyopia of any variety and has been part of the standard inclusion criteria in studies by PEDIG for additional treatments for amblyopia (i.e., patching and atropine). Amblyopia, regardless of etiology, is treated in order to improve VA and binocularity in an ultimate attempt to equalize and maximize VA between the eyes. This goal can be achieved by various means including patching and atropine penalization, but in the treatment of anisometropic amblyopia, the use of glasses or contacts to correct for the difference in refractive error between eyes, is the foundation of treatment.

For the treatment of anisometropic amblyopia, refractive correction has been shown to improve the vision in majority of children, regardless of age of detection. In children 3 to <7-year-old treated with refractive correction alone, VA improved an average of 2.9 lines, improving at least two lines in 77% of subjects. Refractive correction by itself is also effective at significantly improving VA in patients with bilateral refractive amblyopia with improvement at 1 year averaging 3.9 lines and greater improvement seen in patients with worse initial binocular acuity.

In the treatment of strabismic amblyopia, the first step is also to identify any significant refractive error through a full cycloplegic refraction and begin spectacle correction. Fielder et al. discovered that the acuity in many children improved significantly with correction of refractive error alone, and this is true even in the absence of anisometropia. After 18 weeks, the acuity of the amblyopic eye in children 3–7 years of age improved on average 3.2 lines with 88% of children improving two or more lines. Improvements in acuity after 18 weeks seem to occur regardless of the angle of deviation at distance or near at presentation, regardless of whether eye alignment improved following treatment. This effect was greater in pure strabismic amblyopia than combined forms of strabismus with anisometropia (3.2 vs. 2.3 lines)—implying that residual optical blur was probably not a critical factor. However, this difference is not observed with Bangerter foils, atropine, or patching therapies. Refractive correction alone was also beneficial in treatment-naive older children (7–17 years old) with anisometropic, strabismic, or combined amblyopia. After 24 months, VA improved two lines or more in 36% and 20% of children 7–12 years old and 13–17 years old, respectively. How VA can improve with refractive correction alone in the context of pure strabismic amblyopia, regardless of whether eye alignment improved or not following treatment, is largely unknown. Classic teaching is that early-onset strabismus leads to suppression or the development of anomalous retinal correspondence. Additionally, there are measurable central and peripheral scotomas, up to 20° in size. The larger the angle, typically, the greater the suppression scotoma, and the depth and extent of suppression was similar in strabismic and nonstrabismic patients. Interocular suppression appears to be the key factor in all types of amblyopia, as enhancing binocular interaction is the basis for reducing suppression and improving acuity. As optical correction mostly results in mild improvement in ocular alignment in combined or pure strabismic amblyopia, one possible explanation for best corrected visual acuity (BCVA) improvement with this treatment is that the amblyopic eye fixates during some activities and takes advantage of the better focus. The treatment effect of optical correction was similar to the use of atropine or Bangerter filters. Nonetheless, spectacle correction is the reasonable first step in treating combined or strabismic amblyopia before initiating other therapies.

Recommendations for initiating spectacles when they have never been used before and with no prior amblyopia treatment is based on PEDIG eligibility criteria:

Refractive error ≥1.00 D of astigmatism in the amblyopic eye
≥1.00 D spherical equivalent anisometropia
or ≥+2.00 D spherical equivalent hyperopia in either eye

Full-time spectacle wear is suggested for a minimum of 14 weeks. We recommend follow-up every 6–9 weeks for a minimum of 18 weeks, or until acuity plateaus before initiating occlusion therapy. Once improvement is <1 line compared to the prior visit and if there is still residual amblyopia, begin occlusion.

Studies of refractive correction generally utilized best *spectacle* correction, however, contact lenses are another option in children and have been shown to improve VA in both myopes and hyperopes. Contact lenses may also provide the benefit of reduced aniseikonia in large refractive errors, as the effect of magnification/minification is decreased when the corrective lens is placed at the corneal plane as opposed to the usual plane of spectacle wear. They play a unique role in the correction of anisometropic amblyopia due to extremely high refractive error.

OCCLUSION THERAPY

Direct occlusion, or patching of the dominant eye, is a standard treatment for all types of amblyopia. Occlusion has been found to be more effective than refractive correction alone. The deficient accommodative response of the amblyopic eye is also better treated by occlusion, since, it is mediated by foveal stimulation. A meta-analysis of part-time versus full-time occlusion therapy revealed no statistically significant differences, and is why full-time patching is no longer recommended in the treatment of amblyopia.

The general rule-of-thumb is 2 hours of patching for mild amblyopia (BCVA 20/40 or better in the amblyopic eye), 4 hours for moderate amblyopia (BCVA 20/50–20/100 in the amblyopic eye), and 6 hours for severe amblyopia (BCVA worse than 20/100 in the amblyopic eye).

There seems to be no difference in BCVA improvement with or without near activities in children aged 3–7 years with 2 hours of patching per day.

The recommended amount of occlusion time may be divided throughout the day to ease the burden on the patient and caregiver. The child may also be rewarded, or encouraged to patch, by allowing for enjoyable, but normally restricted, activities to be done during this time.

We recommend adhesive pediatric eye patches applied directly to the skin, followed by spectacle wear to minimize the chances of "peeking", or cheating, by the child. For children who have sensitive skin, there are sensitive skin patches, or nonadhesive forms of occlusion such as concave patches, or cloth-type patches that fit over spectacles. However, these require a cooperative patient who will not cheat by looking out of the dominant eye while patching. Be sure to maintain safety precautions in a child who has moderate to severe amblyopia during the early stages of treatment, at least until vision has improved to a degree that the child can safely navigate their environment.

OPTICAL PENALIZATION

For children who cannot tolerate direct patching or atropine for various reasons, we have dubbed optical penalization "patch glasses". The concept behind this is fogging of the dominant eye by refractive overcorrection (over-plusing). This type of therapy is most useful for patients with ocular conditions such as latent nystagmus (in which the nystagmus worsens under complete occlusion). The amount of refractive overcorrection is suggested to be anywhere between +1.25 D and +3.00 D, of which we recommend anywhere from +2.00 D to +3.00 D, using the clinician's own judgment depending on the density of amblyopia and other comorbidities that may be present in the child's medical history. We suggest more overcorrection for healthy children with moderate to severe amblyopia, and less for children with significant medical conditions, or less severe amblyopia. As with nonadhesive patches, this treatment requires a cooperative child who will not peek with their dominant eye.

PHARMACOLOGICAL PENALIZATION

Atropine is a very potent and long-acting anticholinergic drug that is both a mydriatic and cycloplegic. It is administered to the dominant eye on a regular interval to change the refractive status of the eye and blur images sufficiently enough to promote use of the amblyopic eye. Much work has been done over the years through clinical trials to determine the optimal strength and frequency of this medication. This method of treatment provides another option for parents and children who may not be able to adhere to other therapies. A shift in fixation preference to the amblyopic eye is not a necessary requirement for improvement with atropine treatment. The benefit of atropine is improved reliability since, it is directly administered by the care giver, and its effects are long-lasting, requiring little to no monitoring. It is important to note the common side effects of atropine includes light sensitivity, tachycardia, dry mouth, and rarely fever, and facial flushing. Initially, atropine may result in an increase in the angle of esotropia.

We recommend the use of atropine 1% in patients who are unable to tolerate occlusion therapy, or those who are not adherent to spectacle wear. It is most efficacious in patients who have hypermetropia, and less useful for myopia or emmetropia. This is because a hyperopic eye will have decrease in acuity across all distances when it is unable to accommodate, whereas myopes will still have some degree of useable vision at near, and emmetropes at distance. For children who have refractive error and refuse glasses, a 1–2 week course of daily atropine in both eyes can ease acceptance and promote their use. Once glasses are worn consistently, the atropine can be stopped in the amblyopic eye, and tapered to 2–3 times a week in the dominant eye. As with occlusion therapy, be sure to maintain safety precautions in a child who has moderate to severe amblyopia during the early stages of treatment, at least until vision has improved to a degree that the child can navigate their environment safely. In a strongly dominant eye, the patient will not reap as much of a benefit with this treatment modality.

Atropine 1% on weekends has been shown to be as effective as daily patching for 2 hours, as well as daily atropine in moderate amblyopia with acuity in the range of 20/40–20/80. Weekend atropine with full refractive correction is also shown to be effective for severe amblyopia in children ages 3–7 years. Much like with refractive correction alone, there is improvement in acuity of the deviated eye, even when there is no change to ocular alignment. The reason for this is not completely understood.

NONMEDICAL PATCHING ALTERNATIVES

Bangerter Foil

These are plastic neutral density filters of varying opacities that can be applied to spectacles in order to reduce image quality, contrast sensitivity, and luminance entering the dominant eye. This promotes binocular balance and reduces suppression of the amblyopic eye. When worn for 3–4 hours daily, Abrams et al. reported improvements in motor fusion and acuity, along with a decrease in the angle of strabismus using a 0.1 foil. In patients who developed motor fusion, this was maintained beyond 13 months after cessation of amblyopia treatment. We recommend this treatment for patients with mild to moderate strabismic amblyopia, when treatment with patching or atropine penalization is unsuccessful or impossible.

Liquid Crystal Glasses

An alternative to traditional patching is liquid crystal glasses (LCG) which provide intermittent occlusion built into spectacles the child is already wearing. The child's refractive correction is inserted into a carrier frame that has a tinted set of liquid crystal lenses for each eye. When activated and in the "ON" position, the lens of one eye becomes darkened and opaque, serving to occlude that eye. As opposed to traditional patching, which is prescribed for a defined period of uninterrupted occlusion (i.e., 2 hours daily), LCG utilize intermittent occlusion, generally a cycle of 30–40 seconds "ON"/occluded out of each minute. The daily wearing period is designated to provide a given amount of occlusion, for instance a 4-hours wearing period for 2 hours of occlusion if the glasses have a 30 second "ON"/30 second "OFF" cycle.

SYSTEMIC MEDICAL ALTERNATIVES AND ADJUNCTS

In addition to therapies restricted to the eyes, systemic medical therapies have been explored as a means of treating amblyopia either alone or combined with traditional occlusion therapies. One of the most extensively studied therapies is levodopa/levodopa-carbidopa. This agent appears to *decrease* the threshold for plasticity of the visual cortex, lessening the active suppression interfering with binocularity of neurons when deprivation is initiated.

Levodopa/carbidopa has been investigated in clinical scenarios as an adjunct to occlusion therapy, with benefits in some studies showing greater visual improvement as compared to occlusion alone, improved fusion (suggesting a smaller central suppression scotoma), greater maintenance of the effects of occlusion when therapy was discontinued, as well as increased contrast sensitivity. VA also improved slightly in the dominant eye in some patients while on levodopa. No significant effect has been seen in more recent studies in patients with residual amblyopia when levodopa is used with continued patching, in contrast to earlier studies that appeared more promising in patients who had already maxed out their amblyopia therapy.

Cytidine-5'-diphosphocholine, which crosses the blood-brain barrier and becomes part of cell membrane phospholipids, has been investigated as another centrally-acting therapy for amblyopia. Use of this agent in older individuals outside the critical period of visual development has led to improvement in VA, visual evoked potentials (VEPs), and contrast sensitivity in both amblyopic and fellow eyes. Many of the subjects were anisometropic or mixed amblyopes, so this therapy may hold some promise for anisometropic amblyopia in the future.

Other agents of interest include gamma-aminobutyric acid (GABA) inhibitors and the selective serotonin reuptake inhibitors (SSRIs). Fluoxetine appears to restore some visual functioning to amblyopic animals and recover plasticity in the adult rat visual cortex.

Transcranial magnetic stimulation (TMS) is another experimental form of treatment for amblyopia. It has been reported that repetitive stimulation of the visual cortex may temporarily have some effect on contrast sensitivity and acuity of the amblyopia eye. However, the long-term effects of TMS are still largely unknown.

Furthermore, a study done by Shuai et al. investigating adults with amblyopia found that anisometropic amblyopia and strabismic amblyopia are likely injured in different pathways, adding to the complexity of its management. The author's experience is to offer adults the current standards of care who are motivated and willing to try. They can be monitored every 6–12 months and are better able to keep track of their own goals than children.

DICHOPTIC TRAINING

This type of training involves presenting a different visual stimulus to each eye independently, followed by a task that requires integrating the two stimuli together to promote binocular function and balance. This is done by reducing contrast in the sound eye to a point that reduces suppression of the amblyopic eye. Birch and colleagues studied the effects of binocular versus sham games in children ages 3–<7 years with improvement in the binocular but not the sham group's VA, but with no significant effect on stereoacuity. Some members of each study group also patched but in the patients who were compliant (i.e., completed at least 50% of intended treatment time), a similar improvement was demonstrated regardless of whether the patient patched or not. Subsequent studies have compared iPad-based falling blocks game to more traditional amblyopia treatment methods—namely patching and refractive correction. In both younger (ages 5–12 years) and older (ages 13–18 years) children, there was greater improvement in VA with part-time patching than with iPad therapy. However, compliance with iPad therapy was a major issue, especially maintaining the child's interest and there was concern that effectiveness may be masked by poor compliance.

DIG RUSH

Pediatric Eye Disease Investigator Group then developed a more engaging game, Dig Rush, which was investigated specifically in anisometropic amblyopia, comparing game play with glasses to glasses alone. Slightly more than half of iPad participants had >75% adherence, improved from the falling blocks game, yet there was no difference between spectacles only and spectacles plus iPad groups in VA or stereoacuity. As compliance was better here than in the falling blocks studies, it is likely that the dichoptic stimulus game method as it currently exists lacks strong support for effectiveness. However, participants in this study were 7–12, and it is hoped that perhaps this therapy would be effective in a younger group aged 4–6 years. A study of this age group is currently still in process.

SURGICAL INTERVENTION

The decision to proceed with strabismus surgery before, or after the completion of amblyopia therapy has been debated, especially in children under the age of 7 years where they are most susceptible. Early surgery may also have little benefit for children who have intermittent or variable strabismus, and in these cases, conservative methods should be tried first. Traditionally, it is taught that amblyopia therapy should be completed to its maximal benefit before considering strabismus surgery. This is thought to improve physiological mechanisms that fine-tune and stabilize alignment after surgery. Binocular vision and stereopsis require appropriate eye alignment early in infancy, ideally corrected before 1 year of age. Any delays will result in deficiencies of stereopsis but fusion may continue to develop normally up to 21 months of age. There was a multicenter study done that reported children who underwent surgery before 20 months of age had better outcomes in stereopsis as compared to children who had surgery at 49 months of age. The group that underwent early intervention required a higher number of surgeries overall. There are other studies that also suggest aligning the eyes earlier lead to improvements in amblyopia. To the author's knowledge, there are no prospective randomized controlled trials on early versus late surgery in strabismic amblyopia.

The use of adjustable sutures is another debatable topic. A study done by Leffler et al. did not find lower reoperation rates in children who underwent adjustable strabismus surgery. His group did find that younger age, esotropia, hypermetropia, and botulinum toxin injections were associated with higher rates of postoperative abnormal binocularity. Surgery on the superior oblique and use of botulinum toxin were associated with higher rates of reoperation. However, a recent meta-analysis by Choi et al. found improved success rates in primary and secondary surgery using adjustable techniques in pediatric esotropia and exotropia. The author's experience is that families seem to appreciate the option of adjustable surgery, since, it allows them to directly observe the efforts involved in achieving a good result as possible after surgery.

We recommend continuing with amblyopia therapy, if the reader decides to do surgery prior to its completion, typically giving the patient a 1–2 week holiday to recover from the initial discomfort of surgery. Ultimately, the choice to perform early versus late surgery, or the use of adjustable sutures, will depend on the surgeon's level of comfort with the above procedures, along with considerations of the child's health and comorbidities.

SURGICAL ALTERNATIVES: REFRACTIVE SURGERY

Despite parent's and practitioner's best attempts, compliance with refractive correction and patching or penalization therapies can be poor, and in some patients not effective enough to adequately address amblyopia. In large refractive differences between eyes, diplopia, and aniseikonia from refractive correction can make compliance even more difficult. In cases, where more conservative options have been exhausted and/or are not appropriate, refractive surgery can provide an alternative means to treat anisometropia and anisometropic amblyopia, and in some cases, surgery can provide superior results in terms of BCVA and binocular function compared to contact lens use.

Though refractive surgery in an adult population is generally aimed at achieving uncorrected visual perfection, the purpose of refractive surgery in an anisometropic amblyope is to resolve or lessen the difference in refractive error between the two eyes, expecting that refractive correction may still be necessary, though more tolerable. Most studies have used either ketamine sedation or general anesthesia in order to obtain the best and safest results.

LASIK

Laser in-situ keratomileusis (LASIK) is effective in treating anisometropic amblyopia in both adult and pediatric populations, leading to improvement in BCVA and in some instances, uncorrected VA (UCVA) to a level greater than preoperative BCVA. Adverse effects of LASIK include induced astigmatism, in addition to development of haze at the flap-stroma interface, diffuse lamellar keratitis, flap striae, interface deposits, epithelial ingrowth, and Bowman wrinkles.

ADVANCED SURFACE ABLATION TECHNIQUES: PHOTOREFRACTIVE KERATECTOMY AND LASER-ASSISTED SUBEPITHELIAL KERATECTOMY

Photorefractive keratectomy (PRK) and laser-assisted subepithelial keratectomy (LASEK), both advanced surface ablation (ASA) techniques represent another attractive option in treating anisometropic amblyopia in spectacle and contact lens noncompliant or intolerant patients. PRK and LASEK have been shown to safely address refractive errors and enhance BCVA in both hyperopic and myopic children and to enhance stereopsis in myopic patients. Improved VA and stereopsis have also been found in children treated with PRK compared to traditional treatment with glasses or contacts, which may indicate not only the effect of PRK compared to glasses/contacts but also the implied and guaranteed 100% compliance with refractive correction once, surgery has been performed.

PHAKIC INTRAOCULAR LENSES

If the patient has a large refractive error, e.g., high myopia up to 20 D, phakic intraocular lenses (pIOLs) are a consideration. These lenses can be either anterior chamber lenses or posterior chamber lenses. pIOLs tend to provide a more stable and predictable BCVA compared to PRK and LASIK and may be superior when patients have myopia of -8 D or more.

The use of pIOLs has also been specifically studied in special needs children including those with neurobehavioral disorders in whom spectacle wear can be particularly challenging. Tychsen and colleagues described how in cases of profound visual impairment from large magnitude ametropia, neurobehavioral disorders are exacerbated, making social interaction more difficult, and causing issues with visual attention and motor skills-deemed "visual autism". Children with the implantation of pIOL for anisometropia or high isoametropia universally demonstrated improvement in uncorrected distance VA, an important measure in these children as spectacle or other corrective lens wear is untenable. Additionally, a majority of those patients with neurobehavioral disorders were noted to have improved interaction and/or attentiveness/visual awareness, and were overall less fearful in interactions with their environment.

CLEAR LENS EXCHANGE AND LENS EXTRACTION WITHOUT IMPLANTATION

Clear lens exchange/extraction (CLE) with or without IOL implantation is a possibility for patients with anterior chambers too shallow for pIOLs or with very high refractive errors (more than 15.0 D of myopia). Regression is less with this technique and likely related to increased axial length in younger patients. CLE may not achieve as good final VA as excimer laser, but Aloi and colleagues noted that these results may be the result of poor initial VA and visual comorbidities in studied patients.

TREATMENT FAILURE

There are many factors that affect the prognosis for visual recovery in an amblyopic eye, along with a high variability of treatment response, regardless of age. Although up to 90% of children achieve some improvement in VA with different treatment modalities, either alone or in combination, 15–50% fail to achieve normal acuity. Several modifiable factors include:

- Early detection—the duration of amblyopia can be reduced with proper screening programs.
- Proper optical correction—repeating a cycloplegic refraction to determine if there is any residual uncorrected hyperopia. Eyes with highly pigmented irides may require a stronger cycloplegic agent (e.g., atropine 1%).
- Adherence to treatment—ensuring proper communication with caregivers and their understanding of amblyopia and the urgency of its treatment. Consider providing written instructions. Another study showed that 4-year-old children presented with an educational cartoon prior to beginning occlusion therapy demonstrated improvement to adherence.
- Social deprivation and perceived restriction of the child's activities—explain that children can continue to play and socialize as tolerated, limited only by the degree of amblyopia.

Risk of recurrence for successfully treated amblyopia is estimated in about 25% of patients within the first year off treatment in children under the age of 8 years. Recurrence of amblyopia is defined as two consecutive measurements of acuity in the amblyopic eye that is 2 logMAR levels worse than post-treatment. There was a greater risk when 6 or more hours of daily patching was abruptly stopped, instead of tapering to 2 hours. In these patients, we have had good results tapering to 2 hours for at least a month, followed by 1 hour a day for 1 month, then 1 hour every other day for 1 month before stopping.

Atropine 1% penalization used 2 times per week was also shown to improve VA over 4 months of use for children who failed patching therapy, especially in younger children with worse amblyopia.

When therapy has been discontinued, patching may still be restarted at any point in time after a decrease in best corrected acuity is identified, provided there has been no significant change in refractive error. A short course of patching for 2 hours a day with a taper should improve vision to its best corrected acuity at baseline. For these reasons, it is recommended to follow patients every 3–4 months for the first year after cessation of therapy to allow for detection and retreatment of any recurrence of amblyopia.

CONCLUSION

Refractive correction is the most important initial step to take. Part-time occlusion and weekend atropine have similar efficacy even for severe amblyopia. We recommend occlusion therapy of 2 hours for mild amblyopia, 4 hours for moderate amblyopia, and 6 hours for severe amblyopia. When compliance or socioeconomic concerns exist, it is possible to initially utilize shorter treatments and progressively increase treatment duration. Pharmacologic penalization is a possible substitute when occlusion is unsuccessful. Optical penalization and Bangerter foils may be good alternatives as well, but cheating may hinder their effect. Pharmacologic penalization is a possible substitute when occlusion is unsuccessful. Optical penalization, LCG, and Bangerter foils may be good alternatives as well, but cheating may hinder their effect. Pharmacotherapy, TMS, and dichoptic therapy are all still under investigation, and more studies need to be done to determine the role of these interventions in strabismic amblyopia. Until more information is obtained to recommend consistent and generalizable guidelines for their use, refractive correction, occlusion therapy, and optical penalization are the mainstays of treatment.

SUGGESTED READING

1. Abrams MS, Duncan CL, McMurtrey R. Development of motor fusion in patients with a history of strabismic amblyopia who are treated part-time with Bangerter foils. J AAPOS. 2011;15(2):127-130.
2. Alió JL, Grzybowski A, Romaniuk D. Refractive lens exchange in modern practice: when and when not to do it? Eye Vis (Lond). 2014;1:10.
3. Babu RJ, Clavagnier SR, Bobier W, Thompson B, Hess RF. The regional extent of suppression: strabismics versus nonstrabismics. Invest Ophthalmol Vis Sci. 2013;54(10):6585-93.
4. Birch EE, Li SL, Jost RM, Morale SE, De La Cruz A, Stager D Jr, et al. Binocular iPad treatment for amblyopia in preschool children. J AAPOS. 2015;19(1):6-11.
5. Chen AM, Cotter SA. The Amblyopia Treatment Studies: Implications for Clinical Practice. Adv Ophthalmol Optom. 2016;1(1):287-305.
6. Choi B, Nayeni M, Malvankar M, Sharan S. The Use of Adjustable Sutures in Pediatric Strabismus Surgery: Systematic Review and Meta-Analysis. Invest Ophthalmol Vis Sci. 2020;61(7):4593.
7. Cotter SA, Foster NC, Holmes JM, Melia BM, Wallace DK, Repka MX, et al. Optical treatment of strabismic and combined strabismic-anisometropic amblyopia. Ophthalmology. 2012;119(1):150-8.
8. Hess RF, Mansouri B, Thompson B. Restoration of binocular vision in amblyopia. Strabismus. 2011;19(3):110-8.
9. Holmes JM, Beck RW, Kraker RT, Astle WF, Birch EE, Cole SR, et al. Risk of amblyopia recurrence after cessation of treatment. J AAPOS. 2004;8(5):420-8.
10. Holmes JM, Manny RE, Lazar EL, Birch EE, Kelly KR, Summers AI, et al. A Randomized Trial of Binocular Dig Rush Game Treatment for Amblyopia in Children Aged 7 to 12 Years. Ophthalmology. 2019;126(3):456-66.
11. Ing MR, Okino LM. Outcome study of stereopsis in relation to duration of misalignment in congenital esotropia. J AAPOS. 2002;6(1):3-8.
12. Korah S, Philip S, Jasper S, Antonio-Santos A, Braganza A. Strabismus surgery before versus after completion of amblyopia therapy in children. Cochrane Database Syst Rev. 2014;10(10):CD009272.
13. Kraus CL, Culican SM. New advances in amblyopia therapy I: binocular therapies and pharmacologic augmentation. Br J Ophthalmol. 2018;102(11):1492-6.
14. Leffler CT, Vaziri K, Schwartz SG, Cavuoto KM, McKeown CA, Kishor KS, et al. Rates of Reoperation and Abnormal Binocularity Following Strabismus Surgery in Children. Am J Ophthalmol. 2016;162:159-66.
15. Leguire LE, Komaromy KL, Nairus TM, Rogers GL. Long-term follow-up of L-dopa treatment in children with amblyopia. J Pediatr Ophthalmol Strabismus. 2002;39(6):326-46.
16. Manh VM, Holmes JM, Lazar EL, Kraker RT, Wallace DK, Kulp MT, et al. A Randomized Trial of a Binocular iPad Game Versus Part-Time Patching in Children Aged 13 to 16 Years with Amblyopia. Am J Ophthalmol. 2018;186:104-15.
17. McGraw PV, Barrett BT, Ledgeway T. Optical treatment of strabismic amblyopia. Ophthalmic Physiol Opt. 2019;39(5):309-12.
18. Milla M, Piñero DP. Characterization, passive and active treatment in strabismic amblyopia: a narrative review. Int J Ophthalmol. 2020;13(7):1132-47.
19. Noorden GK. The History of Strabismology. Am Orthopt J. 2002;52:123.
20. Osborne DC, Greenhalgh KM, Evans MJE, Self JE. Atropine Penalization Versus Occlusion Therapies for Unilateral Amblyopia after the Critical Period of Visual Development: A Systematic Review. Ophthalmol Ther. 2018;7(2):323-32.
21. Paysse EA, Tychsen L, Stahl E. Pediatric refractive surgery: corneal and intraocular techniques and beyond. J AAPOS. 2012;16(3):291-7.
22. Pediatric Eye Disease Investigator Group. A randomized trial of near versus distance activities while patching for amblyopia in children aged 3 to less than 7 years. Ophthalmology. 2008;115(11):2071-8.
23. Pediatric Eye Disease Investigator Group. The clinical profile of moderate amblyopia in children younger than 7 years. Arch Ophthalmol. 2002;120(3):281-7.
24. Pediatric Eye Disease Investigator Group. The course of moderate amblyopia treated with atropine in children: experience of the amblyopia treatment study. Am J Ophthalmol. 2003;136(4):630-9.
25. Repka MX, Cotter SA, Beck RW, Kraker RT, Birch EE, Everett DF, et al. A randomized trial of atropine regimens for treatment of moderate amblyopia in children. Ophthalmology. 2004;111(11):2076-85.
26. Repka MX, Kraker RT, Beck RW, Birch E, Cotter SA, Holmes JM, et al. Treatment of severe amblyopia with weekend atropine: results from 2 randomized clinical trials. J AAPOS. 2009;13(3):258-63.
27. Repka MX, Kraker RT, Dean TW, Beck RW, Siatkowski RM, Holmes JM, et al. A randomized trial of levodopa as treatment for residual amblyopia in older children. Ophthalmology. 2015;122(5):874-81.
28. Rutstein RP, Quinn GE, Lazar EL, Beck RW, Bonsall DJ, Cotter SA, et al. A randomized trial comparing Bangerter filters and patching for the treatment of moderate amblyopia in children. Ophthalmology. 2010;117(5):998-1004.
29. Scheiman MM, Hertle RW, Beck RW, Edwards AR, Birch E, Cotter SA, et al. Randomized trial of treatment of amblyopia in children aged 7 to 17 years. Arch Ophthalmol. 2005;123(4):437-47.
30. Seol BR, Yu YS, Kim SJ. Effect of 4-Month Intermittent Atropine Penalization in Amblyopic Children for Whom Patch Therapy Had Failed. J Pediatr Ophthalmol Strabismus. 2017;54(6):375-80.
31. Shuai L, Leilei Z, Wen W, Shu W, Gangsheng L, Yinglong L, et al. Binocular treatment in adult amblyopia is based on parvocellular or magnocellular pathway. Eur J Ophthalmol. 2020;30(4):658-67.
32. Simonsz HJ, Kolling GH, Unnebrink K. Final report of the early vs. late infantile strabismus surgery study (ELISSS), a controlled, prospective, multicenter study. Strabismus. 2005;13(4):169-99.
33. Simonsz-Tóth B, Joosse MV, Besch D. Refractive adaptation and efficacy of occlusion therapy in untreated amblyopic patients aged 12 to 40 years. Graefes Arch Clin Exp Ophthalmol. 2019;257(2):379-89.
34. Spierer A, Raz J, Benezra O, Herzog R, Cohen E, Karshai I, et al. Treating amblyopia with liquid crystal glasses: a pilot study. Invest Ophthalmol Vis Sci. 2010;51(7):3395-8.
35. Stewart CE, Fielder AR, Stephens DA, Moseley MJ. Design of the Monitored Occlusion Treatment of Amblyopia Study (MOTAS). Br J Ophthalmol. 2002;86(8):915-9.
36. Stewart CE, Moseley MJ, Fielder AR, Stephens DA; MOTAS Cooperative. Refractive adaptation in amblyopia: quantification of effect and implications for practice. Br J Ophthalmol. 2004;88(12):1552-6.
37. Stewart CE, Moseley MJ, Stephens DA, Fielder AR. Treatment dose-response in amblyopia therapy: the Monitored Occlusion Treatment of Amblyopia Study (MOTAS). Invest Ophthalmol Vis Sci. 2004;45(9):3048-54.
38. Taylor K, Elliott S. Interventions for strabismic amblyopia. Cochrane Database Syst Rev. 2014;(7):CD006461.
39. Tychsen L, Hoekel J, Ghasia F, Yoon-Huang G. Phakic intraocular lens correction of high ametropia in children with neurobehavioral disorders. J AAPOS. 2008;12(3):282-9.
40. von Noorden GK. Binocular Vision and Ocular Motility: Theory and Management of Strabismus. Missouri: Mosby Incorporated; 1996.
41. Wang J, Neely DE, Galli J, Schliesser J, Graves A, Damarjian TG, et al. A pilot randomized clinical trial of intermittent occlusion therapy liquid crystal glasses versus traditional patching for treatment of moderate unilateral amblyopia. J AAPOS. 2016;20(4):326-31.
42. Yazdani N, Sadeghi R, Momeni-Moghaddam H, Zarifmahmoudi L, Ehsaei A, Barrett BT. Part-time versus full-time occlusion therapy for treatment of amblyopia: A meta-analysis. J Curr Ophthalmol. 2017;29(2):76-84.

CHAPTER 6

Conjunctival Inflammatory and Allergic Disorders in Children

Ahmad Kheirkhah, Vadrevu K Raju

INTRODUCTION

The conjunctiva is a delicate, translucent mucous membrane covering anterior surface of the sclera, and posterior surface of the eyelids. It consists of the palpebral conjunctiva, fornices, and bulbar conjunctiva. This tissue's primary function is to provide a mucous layer to the tear film and provide immune cells and bactericidal and virucidal agents to protect the ocular surface. The conjunctiva consists of a nonkeratinizing squamous epithelial layer, which has mucin secreting goblet cells intercalated within it, and substantia propria, which provides connective tissue support and lymphoid tissue. The substantia propria has two layers; the outer lymphoid layer, which is absent at birth and develops several months later, and an inner fibrous layer. The conjunctiva is highly vascularized and is supplied by the marginal tarsal arcades, peripheral tarsal arcades, and the anterior ciliary arteries. The conjunctival veins drain into the superior and inferior ophthalmic veins and the anterior ciliary veins. The conjunctival innervation is supplied by the first and second divisions of the trigeminal nerve. These nerves comprise the infratrochlear branch of the nasociliary nerve, the lacrimal nerve, the supratrochlear and supraorbital branches of the frontal nerve, and the infraorbital nerve from the maxillary division of the trigeminal nerve.

Conjunctivitis is inflammation of the conjunctiva. Conjunctivitis in children can have infectious and noninfectious etiologies, and an eye examination can help to determine the possible cause. Typical symptoms of conjunctivitis are redness in the eye, foreign body sensation, tearing, pain, and sometimes matting of eyelashes. Signs of conjunctivitis include dilation of conjunctival vessels causing conjunctival hyperemia, edema of the conjunctiva called chemosis, and conjunctival discharge. Conjunctival inflammation typically produces a follicular or a papillary reaction. Follicles represent focal lymphoid hyperplasia without a central vessel and appear pale at the surface and red at the base. Papillae represent focal dilated conjunctival vessels with edema and inflammation. They appear red at the surface and pale at the base. Follicles are more prominent in the inferior fornix and papillae are more commonly seen in the upper tarsal conjunctiva. We will discuss various causes of infectious, allergic, and immune conjunctivitis in children in this chapter.

INFECTIOUS CONJUNCTIVITIS

Bacterial Conjunctivitis

The common bacteria responsible for bacterial conjunctivitis in children are *Streptococcus pneumoniae*, *Haemophilus influenzae*, *Staphylococcus aureus*, and *Moraxella catarrhalis*. The hyperacute form of bacterial conjunctivitis is caused by *Neisseria gonorrhoeae* or *Neisseria meningitidis*.

Risk factors for bacterial conjunctivitis include contact with contaminated fingers, fomites, or oculogenital contact with someone who is infected. Ocular diseases, including dry eye, dacryocystitis, blepharitis, and anatomic abnormalities of the ocular surface and lids can predispose to bacterial infection. Additionally, disruption of the natural conjunctival epithelial barrier due to ocular trauma, contact lens wear, recent ocular surgery, exposed sutures, ocular foreign bodies, chronic use of topical medications, or immune suppressed state may also lead to bacterial conjunctival infections. Newborns are often infected during passage through the birth canal via vaginal delivery by infected mothers or from caregivers.

- *Pathophysiology*: Bacterial conjunctivitis can result from direct infection through the compromised epithelial surface except for certain organisms such as *N. meningitidis*, *Haemophilus aegyptius*, and *Corynebacterium diphtheria* which can penetrate the intact epithelium. Abnormal proliferation of the native conjunctival flora or the spread of infection from the organisms colonizing the nasal and sinus mucosa can lead to conjunctival infection. These bacteria can infiltrate the conjunctival epithelial layer and substantia propria. Proteases, collagenases, coagulases, and fibrinolysis combined with toxins produced by bacteria such as *Staphylococcus* and *Pseudomonas* species further lead to disruption of the conjunctival tissue and bacterial entry.

- *Symptoms and signs:* Patients present with symptoms of red and watery eyes, purulent or mucopurulent discharge, sticking of eyelids, matting of the eyelashes, and foreign body sensation. The signs include eyelid edema, conjunctival injection, purulent or mucopurulent discharge, ocular pain, and a papillary reaction in the conjunctiva, which gives a velvety red appearance to the conjunctiva. Bacterial conjunctivitis can be clinically subcategorized based on presentation as acute, hyperacute, and chronic conjunctivitis.

Hyperacute Bacterial Conjunctivitis

Neisseria gonorrhoeae and *N. meningitidis* cause hyperacute bacterial conjunctivitis. This type of conjunctivitis is most common in neonates and occasionally in sexually active adolescents. The most striking feature is a copious amount of thick yellowish/greenish purulent discharge, marked chemosis, severe hyperemia, eyelid edema, and occasional conjunctival membrane formations. These bacteria, which are highly virulent, can penetrate the intact corneal epithelium, and cause keratitis and resultant corneal melting and perforation. Immediate Gram staining and cultures are critical in cases of hyperacute conjunctivitis. Systemic therapy with single dose intramuscular or intravenous ceftriaxone is indicated. Intensive topical antibiotics are used, and frequent saline lavages to remove the purulent discharge need to be performed on a frequent basis. Corneal involvement is not infrequent as these bacteria are highly virulent and infect an intact corneal epithelium. Concurrent infections with other sexually transmitted diseases such *as Chlamydia trachomatis* need to be investigated and treated simultaneously.

Acute Bacterial Conjunctivitis

Acute bacterial conjunctivitis in children is usually caused by *S. aureus*, *S. pneumoniae*, and *H. influenzae*. Other pathogens responsible for the acute disease are *Pseudomonas aeruginosa*, *M. catarrhalis*, *Streptococcus viridans*, and *Proteus mirabilis*. The disease course of acute bacterial conjunctivitis usually lasts for 7–10 days. Diagnosis is predominantly clinical and does not need bacterial cultures or Gram stains unless in atypical cases such as hyperacute conjunctivitis, chronic nonresponding cases, and neonatal conjunctivitis. It is a contagious condition, and hence proper handwashing and isolation should be followed. Excuse for school or daycare for at least 4–5 days or until the discharge is stopped, should be provided. Mild bacterial infections resolve on their own within a time frame of 7–10 days; however, topical antibiotic treatment has been shown to speed resolution and improve the clinical and microbiological remission time. Commonly used antibiotics are broad-spectrum antibiotics such as ophthalmic erythromycin ointment, bacitracin ointment, neomycin/polymyxin B/bacitracin ointment, fluoroquinolone eye drops, and tobramycin eye drops, in day time and ointments at night time. The dose schedule depends upon the severity of infection. Supportive treatment with cold compresses and artificial tears and oral anti-inflammatory tablets is helpful.

Severe acute conjunctivitis may require oral broad spectrum antibiotics in addition to local drops.

Chronic Bacterial Conjunctivitis

The common causes of chronic bacterial conjunctivitis are *C. trachomatis*, *Staphylococcus* species, and *Moraxella* species. *C. trachomatis* is an obligate intracellular bacterium responsible for three different conjunctivitis syndromes—(1) inclusion conjunctivitis (neonatal and adult), (2) trachoma, and (3) lymphogranuloma venereum.

Neonatal inclusion conjunctivitis occurs around 1 week of age in neonates born to mothers infected with *C. trachomatis*. In older children and adolescents, it can cause trachoma and adult inclusion conjunctivitis. We will discuss the neonatal chlamydial infection in a separate section below. The adult inclusion conjunctivitis is caused by *C. trachomatis* serotypes D-K. Adult inclusion conjunctivitis usually occurs in sexually active adolescents and adults. It can be found in association with chlamydial urethritis, vaginitis, or cervicitis. The disease is transmitted through the hand-to-eye spread of infected genital secretions. The incubation period is 1–2 weeks. Patients present with mild redness of eyes, scant mucoid discharge, sticking of eyelashes, and foreign body sensation. The signs include conjunctival follicular reaction, scant mucopurulent discharge, and preauricular lymphadenopathy. Corneal involvement can follow conjunctivitis and can present as corneal infiltrates and superior limbal pannus. Severe cases may have a chronic relapsing course, which may lead to corneal scarring.

Trachoma is caused by *C. trachomatis* serotypes A-C; it is a severe blinding condition in endemic areas in developing countries. It is the result of chronic multiple-repeated infections. The recurrent infections lead to tarsal follicular conjunctivitis, limbal follicles, papillary hypertrophy, tarsal scarring, corneal microerosions, neovascularization, and in late stages cicatrization of the conjunctiva, cornea, and eyelids **(Fig. 1B)**.

Lymphogranuloma venereum is caused by *C. trachomatis* serotypes L1, L2, and L3. It presents as mild conjunctivitis with scant discharge but has preauricular, parotid, and submandibular lymphadenopathy. Diagnosis of chlamydial conjunctivitis is made by isolating the organism via culture from conjunctival scrapping and swab. Giemsa stain will demonstrate basophilic intracellular inclusions. Polymerase chain reaction (PCR), direct fluorescence antibody test, and enzyme immune assays from conjunctival swab have also been used for diagnosis. Treatment of chlamydial conjunctivitis includes systemic treatment with antibiotics such as oral azithromycin 1-g single dose or a course of oral erythromycin 50 mg/kg/day in four divided doses for 2 weeks or oral doxycycline 100 mg twice a daily for 7 days in children above 8 years of age. Investigation for coinfection with gonorrhea must be performed and treated accordingly. Treatment of sexual partners is recommended.

Staphylococcal species are other causes of chronic bacterial conjunctivitis. The eyelid margin and surrounding skin harbor staphylococcal bacteria and thus staphylococcal infection can be challenging to eradicate. The staphylococcal toxins lead to a hypersensitivity reaction, which causes immune-mediated chronic blepharokeratoconjunctivitis (BKC), which is discussed in detail below. *Moraxella lacunata* is a gram-negative diplobacillus which causes chronic angular conjunctivitis with maceration of the outer and inner canthal areas. It presents as chronic follicular conjunctivitis and keratitis. It responds well to topical erythromycin.

Management: Bacterial conjunctivitis is usually self-limiting and lasts 1–2 weeks but may evolve into chronic conjunctivitis, if the course lasts longer than 4 weeks. Topical antibiotics have shown to speed recovery, reduce the risk of further ocular complications, and prevent chronicity. There has not been any significant difference in outcomes reported when comparing the various available broad-spectrum antibiotic eye drops or ointments to manage bacterial conjunctivitis. Typically, the prescription depends on local availability, patient allergies, resistance patterns, and costs. In chronic or refractory cases, conjunctival swabs to guide the exact etiology to target the specific organism are indicated. *Chlamydia* and *Neisseria* infections need systemic treatments, as described above. Chronic staphylococcal conjunctivitis needs adequate lid hygiene and often systemic treatment for associated eyelid disease.

Viral Conjunctivitis

Viral conjunctivitis is another important cause of ocular morbidity. Adenoviruses account for most cases of viral conjunctivitis. Other common viruses causing conjunctivitis are herpes simplex, herpes zoster, and molluscum contagiosum.

Adenovirus Conjunctivitis

Adenovirus is a DNA virus with different serotypes that can cause conjunctivitis such as epidemic keratoconjunctivitis (serotypes 8, 19, and 37), pharyngoconjunctival fever (serotypes 3 and 7), acute hemorrhagic conjunctivitis (serotypes 11 and 21), and acute follicular conjunctivitis (serotypes 1, 2, 3, 4, 7, and 10).

The patient presents with eyelid swelling, conjunctival redness, tearing, mucoid discharge, and severe foreign body sensation. Signs include conjunctival hyperemia, mixed follicular and papillary reaction in the conjunctiva, conjunctival membranes, petechial conjunctival hemorrhages, and preauricular lymphadenopathy. In some patients, after 3–5 days, focal superficial epithelial keratitis develops, followed by immune-mediated focal subepithelial corneal infiltrates. Severe acute foreign body sensations are highlighted in some cases. After 3–4 weeks, the subepithelial infiltrates subside and form scarring, which may persist for an extended period and may cause irregular astigmatism. Acute conjunctivitis could be associated with systemic symptoms of fever and sore throat.

Diagnosis: Diagnosis is usually clinical; history of contact with someone suffering from a similar condition could often be elicited. Diagnosis can be confirmed by PCR or enzyme-linked immunosorbent assay (ELISA) on conjunctival swabs.

Management: All patients should be instructed to avoid sharing personal items such as towels, sheets, and pillows and avoid close personal contact for approximately 2 weeks. They need to practice frequent handwashing to avoid spread. Children should be excused from school or daycare for 2 weeks to avoid the spread of the disease. Treatment is mostly symptomatic comprising of anti-inflammatory eye drops, artificial tears, and cold compresses. Oral analgesics and anti-inflammatory can be given. Conjunctival membranes sometimes need to be removed for comfort and to avoid symblepharon. Topical corticosteroids are used for severe keratitis and severe symptoms like lid edema and chemosis, and to prevent scarring from keratitis. However, topical corticosteroids should be used with caution as they may lengthen the period of virus shedding and cause recurrences. After the acute stage has subsided, steroids can be used for subepithelial immune keratopathy.

Herpes Simplex Conjunctivitis

Herpes simplex virus (HSV) conjunctivitis can be caused by either HSV1 or HSV2. Most commonly, HSV1 causes infection above the waist, and HSV2 causes infection below the waist. However, either virus can cause disease at either location. The infection source is children with primary disease, adults with recurrent disease, and children and adults as asymptomatic carriers. Primary HSV illness is manifested in only approximately 1–6% of the patients infected with the virus. Primary HSV infection involves mostly skin and mucosal surfaces. It may manifest as a nonspecific upper respiratory tract infection. HSV spreads from the infected skin and mucosal epithelium via sensory nerve axons to establish latent infection in the associated sensory nerve ganglia, including the trigeminal ganglion. Reactivation of the virus may follow in any of the three branches of the trigeminal nerve [ophthalmic nerve (V1), maxillary nerve (V2), and mandibular nerve (V3)]. Neonates can get infected with HSV via infection through the birth canal or postpartum from caregivers and cause neonatal ocular herpes. This is discussed in a separate section below.

Primary ocular herpes may present as vesicular eyelid lesions, preauricular lymphadenopathy, acute follicular conjunctivitis, occasional conjunctival pseudomembrane formation, and dendritic ulcers of the cornea, which are the hallmark of HSV keratitis (***see*** **Fig. 6A**). Conjunctival dendrite has also been reported, but it is extremely rare (***see*** **Fig. 7**).

Corneal involvement with dendritic epithelial keratitis may occur; however, stromal disease or uveitis is rare in primary ocular HSV infection. HSV infections are most commonly unilateral; however, bilateral disease can occur, especially in association with atopic disease or immune suppression. Recurrent HSV infection occurs via reactivation of the latent virus in the sensory ganglion, which travels down the nerve axons to the sensory nerve endings and affects the ocular surface epithelium. Trigger for reactivation may include stress, other acute viral or febrile illnesses, ultraviolet exposure, surgery, or trauma. Recurrent HSV infection can present as vesicular blepharoconjunctivitis, superficial punctuate keratitis (SPK), dendritic ulcers, and geographical ulcers (***see* Fig. 6B**). Clinically, it could be indistinguishable from the primary infection; however, corneal stromal disease and uveitis are not uncommon.

Diagnosis: Diagnosis is usually clinical; however, in complex cases, laboratory diagnosis can be made by scrapings from the conjunctival, corneal, or skin lesions for Giemsa staining, which shows multinucleated giant cells and intranuclear inclusions. Antigen detection by PCR, ELISA, and/or viral cultures can be performed on conjunctival swabs, corneal scraping, and skin lesions.

Management: HSV blepharoconjunctivitis is treated with oral acyclovir TID. The dose depends on the weight and age. Acyclovir has a wide safety margin, and a dose of 40–80 mg/kg/day is tolerated. In children up to 18 months of age, 100 mg TID; in children 18 months–3 years of age, 200 mg TID; in children 3–5 years of age 300 mg TID; and in older than 6 years, 400 mg TID is recommended. The oral treatment must be continued for at least 2 weeks. Topical treatment with acyclovir ointment 3%, trifluridine 1% eye drops, and ganciclovir 0.15% ophthalmic gel should be used in combination. It usually takes 2 weeks for dendritic ulcer to heal and topical should be continued for 1 week more, though in tapering doses. Recurrent disease with corneal involvement may need long-term prophylactic treatment with oral acyclovir. Once stromal involvement or uveitis occurs, steroids have to be combined with specific antiviral treatment. The course of treatment, in such cases, depends upon the severity and the slit-lamp findings. In any case, topical antivirals and steroids have to be continued for 4–6 weeks, in reduced doses.

Recurrences are a major concern in herpes simplex keratitis. Statistics show that, once infected, there 25% chance of recurrence; twice recurrence, chances are 50%; and multiple recurrences can occur with more recurrences. In cases where multiple recurrences have occurred, the cornea is usually severely scarred and keratoplasty is the only remedy.

Herpes Zoster Virus Conjunctivitis

Varicella-zoster virus (VZV) is a herpes virus that can cause varicella (chickenpox) and herpes zoster. After the primary infection, the virus can remain latent in the sensory ganglion. Its reactivation causes signs and symptoms of herpes zoster. Herpes zoster ophthalmicus is rare in children as it is associated with reducing antibodies to VZV unless they are immune compromised. However, it still has been reported in otherwise healthy children. Children who have had varicella infection before 1 year of age have an increased incidence of developing zoster as compared to those who have varicella after the first year of life. Ocular involvement of herpes zoster presents as vesicular rash or ulceration of eyelids with lid edema, confined to a single dermatome, bulbar conjunctival injection, watery discharge, and a follicular reaction of the conjunctiva. Corneal involvement and anterior uveitis are most likely to occur if the nasociliary branch of cranial nerve V (tip of the nose) is involved. Excruciating pain in and around eyes and frontal headache, is the hallmark of early onset, even before vesicular eruptions appear. The vesicular eruptions last for 1 week, get converted into papules, and finally crusting occurs in 2 weeks. The person is in infective phase until the crusting occurs.

Treatment with oral acyclovir in healthy children is recommended to reduce the severity and duration of ocular inflammation. Intravenous antiviral agents (famciclovir, valacyclovir, or acyclovir) are indicated in immunocompromised patients or individuals with severe disseminated disease. Antiviral medications should be started within 72 hours of the onset of symptoms.

Epstein-Barr Virus Conjunctivitis

Epstein-Barr virus is a herpes virus that causes infectious mononucleosis. Findings include fever, lymphadenopathy, sore throat, and hepatic involvement. Conjunctivitis is the most common ocular finding. Corneal involvement with nummular keratitis may also occur. Diagnosis is performed by detecting immunoglobulin M antibodies to viral capsid antigens or positive results on the heterophile antibody test. Ocular treatment is with cold compresses and lubricant eye drops, and anti-inflammatory drops.

Molluscum Contagiosum Conjunctivitis

A DNA poxvirus causes molluscum contagiosum. It presents with single or multiple umbilicated skin lesions. Lesions close to the eyelid margin can release viral particles onto the conjunctival surface, resulting in follicular conjunctivitis. Chronic lesions can cause keratopathy and vascularization. Multiple facial lesions can be present in immunocompromised children. The diagnosis is clinical. Most of the time, these lesions undergo self-resolution; however, persistent lesions can be treated with incising each lesion and debriding the central core and curettage. Cautery and cryotherapy can also be used but should be performed with caution, as this can lead to depigmentation of the skin and loss of eyelashes **(Fig. 2)**.

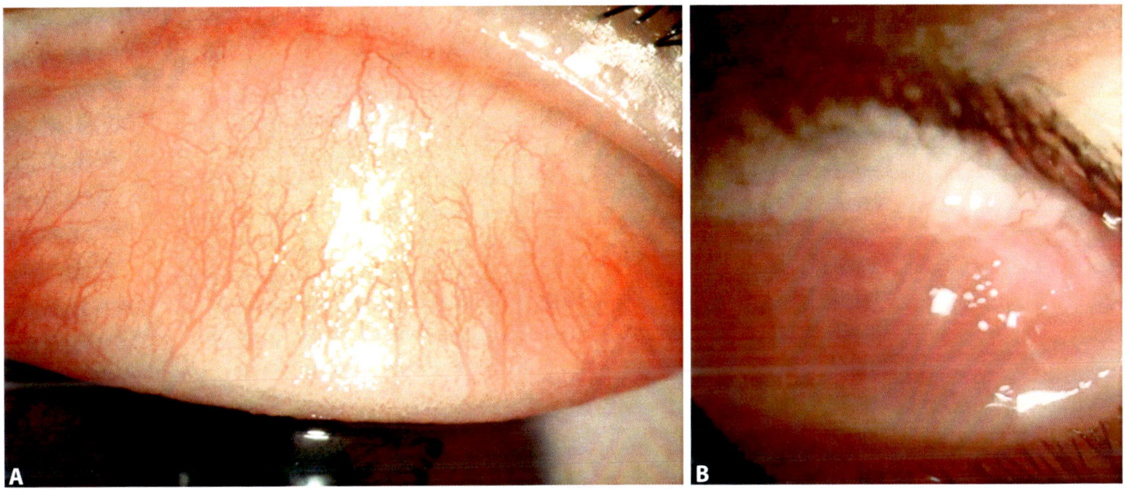

Figs. 1A and B: (A) Micropapillae in the upper palpebral conjunctiva in a patient with seasonal allergic conjunctivitis; (B) Numerous large follicles in the inferior palpebral conjunctiva in a 16-year-old female with chlamydial conjunctivitis.

ALLERGIC CONJUNCTIVITIS

Allergic conjunctivitis is subdivided into different types that include seasonal allergic conjunctivitis (SAC), perennial allergic conjunctivitis (PAC), vernal keratoconjunctivitis (VKC), and atopic keratoconjunctivitis (AKC).

Seasonal Allergic Conjunctivitis

Seasonal allergic conjunctivitis is the most common form of allergic conjunctivitis. Symptoms primarily occur in spring and fall and are triggered by contact with specific airborne allergens such as pollens, flowers, weeds, and trees. SAC occurs due to a type I hypersensitivity response with conjunctival activated mast cells due to allergen cross-linking of the surface immunoglobulin E (IgE) receptors resulting in degranulation of the mast cells and release of histamine, leukotrienes, proteases, prostaglandins, cytokines, and chemokines. All these substances cause vascular leakage, resulting in further cellular infiltration of eosinophils and neutrophils, leading to conjunctival and periorbital edema. Patients present with ocular itching, red and watery eyes, and boggy-appearing conjunctiva. Symptoms are typically bilateral, although one eye may be more affected than the other. Patients often have concomitant clinical history of atopy and other seasonal allergies. On examination, there is mild-to-moderate conjunctival injection, the papillary reaction on the tarsal conjunctiva, and moderate chemosis. Corneal involvement is rare. There may also be allergic shiners present, a blue to purple discoloration of lower eyelids secondary to venous stasis from nasal congestion. Acute allergic response is noted in some individuals with severe chemosis, itching, and lid swelling **(Fig. 1A)**.

Management

Allergen avoidance is a crucial measure in managing allergic conjunctivitis. Essential management of SAC also involves informing patients to avoid eye rubbing, which can cause mechanical mast cell degranulation. Cold compresses can help to reduce edema and alleviate symptoms. Refrigerated artificial tears can help to dilute and wash out the offending allergens. If the patient wears contact lenses, they should be informed to reduce or halt usage until symptoms resolve as allergens may adhere to the lenses. Allergen avoidance through filtering systems, barriers, special cleaning products, and vacuum sweepers can be of immense help to allergic patients.

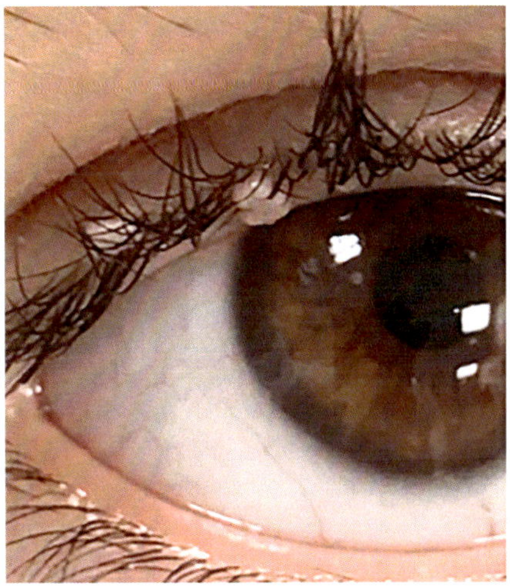

Fig. 2: Molluscum contagiosum of the eyelid margin in a 6-year-old child.

The topical treatment of SAC should begin at least 2–4 weeks before the patient's local pollen season to optimize symptomatic relief. The agent of choice for treating SAC is an antihistamine eye drop with mast cell-stabilizing properties (dual-acting agents) such as olopatadine, azelastine, ketotifen, alcaftadine, or bepotastine. Itching relief should be evident within 24–72 hours of application, and the most common side effects are dry eyes and a burning sensation. Other classes of eye drops include vasoconstrictor/antihistamine combinations and direct mast cell stabilizers. In severe cases, topical steroids can be considered.

Perennial Allergic Conjunctivitis

Perennial allergic conjunctivitis is less common than SAC and presents with a relatively mild ocular condition that persists year-round rather than in SAC's seasonal nature. This difference in timing is attributable to the fact that the allergens implicated in PAC are indoor (i.e., house-dust, mites, animal dander, or mold) rather than outdoor (i.e., pollens) and thus are chronically present. Like SAC, patients with a history of atopy and known allergies should be of suspicion for having PAC. New environmental changes such as moving to a new home or work environment may also trigger PAC's onset. As with SAC, PAC also involves an immediate-type hypersensitivity response, but the resultant inflammation is more chronic because it is continuously present. The year-round symptoms associated with PAC are the result of chronic mast cell activation and Th2 lymphocyte infiltration. Increased mast cells are detected in both the tarsal conjunctival epithelium and substantia propria, with both mucosal and connective-tissue-type mast cell phenotypes. Besides, mast cells, eosinophils, neutrophils, and T cells are present, suggesting that several cell-mediated processes contribute to PAC's chronic inflammation.

Diagnosis

Perennial allergic conjunctivitis is differentiated from SAC by its time course and chronicity. PAC is a milder form of allergic conjunctivitis with similar ocular itching symptoms, redness, and edema, but while SAC has an acute or subacute onset that corresponds to a pollen season, PAC is year-round and often secondary to indoor allergens.

Management

Allergen avoidance or removal is key to managing all types of allergic conjunctivitis. PAC treatment is identical to that of SAC (see above), except topical treatment may need to be prescribed for more extended periods until the environmental exposure can be reduced.

Vernal Keratoconjunctivitis

Vernal keratoconjunctivitis is a chronic bilateral, seasonal allergic inflammatory disease of the eye, primarily involving the tarsal and bulbar conjunctiva. It is a chronic disease with episodes of acute exacerbations. It is more common in males and is more prevalent in subtropical zones of Mediterranean areas, Central and West Africa, the Middle East, Japan, the Indian subcontinent, and South America. Children with VKC are more likely to have other atopy forms, such as asthma and allergic rhinitis. The age of onset of VKC is typically before 10 years. Most children outgrow VKC during puberty. An IgE-mediated type I hypersensitivity reaction with concomitant Th2-associated lymphocyte alteration is believed to underlie the pathogenesis of VKC. Th2 lymphocytes are responsible for both hyperproduction of IgE and interleukin 4, and differentiation and activation of mast cells and eosinophils. Mast cells and basophils cause the immediate reaction by releasing histamine and by recruitment of inflammatory cells such as lymphocytes and eosinophils upon exposure to an allergen. The predominant cell types involved in VKC include mast cells, T cells, eosinophils, basophils, and macrophages. Eosinophils are the dominant cell type responsible for several long-term complications in cases of VKC.

Diagnosis

Vernal keratoconjunctivitis presents with bilateral conjunctival redness, severe itching, ropy mucoid discharge, and foreign body sensation. The symptoms decrease during colder months and usually disappear in adulthood. It is classified into three forms—(1) tarsal or papillary form, (2) limbal form, and (3) mixed form. The tarsal form is characterized by predominantly tarsal conjunctival papillae, which are variable in size from 0.1 to 5 mm and are discrete and flat-topped. Histopathologically, the papillae consist of the hyperplastic conjunctival epithelium with capillary hypertrophy and core presence of eosinophils, mast cells, and neutrophils. Multiple confluent papillae in the tarsal conjunctiva give it a "cobblestone" appearance. The limbal form represents gelatinous limbal papillary hyperplasia, which gives the limbus a thickened appearance. These may also be associated with Horner-Trantas dots which are whitish discrete excrescence on the limbus, made of eosinophils and epithelial cells. The limbal form may also have superficial corneal neovascularization. Grayish-white lipid deposition at the peripheral superficial corneal stroma is seen in patients with limbal VKC which resembles an arcus and is called a pseudogerontoxon.

The mixed form has characteristics of both the palpebral form and limbal form. Increased pigmentation in the interpalpebral conjunctiva has also been noted in patients with VKC. Patients with VKC can have waxing and waning course and acute exacerbations **(Figs. 3A to D)**.

Severe VKC can cause corneal complications causing decreased visual acuity. Corneal involvement in VKC can present as superficial keratopathy with punctuate epithelial erosions in the initial stages, which progress to coarse epitheliopathy and macroerosions or shallow corneal ulcers called "shield ulcers". A large demographic study by Bonini et al., has shown that 90% of patients with VKC have superficial keratopathy, and 10% can have a shield ulcer. Cameron grading system has been used to grade shield ulcers as grade 1, ulcer with a transparent base; grade 2, translucent base with or without opaque white or yellow deposits; and grade 3, ulcer with elevated plaque. Another corneal complication noted in VKC is keratoconus. Management of the first two grades consists of local steroid and immune suppressive therapy; but grade 3 may require debridement with amniotic membrane treatment.

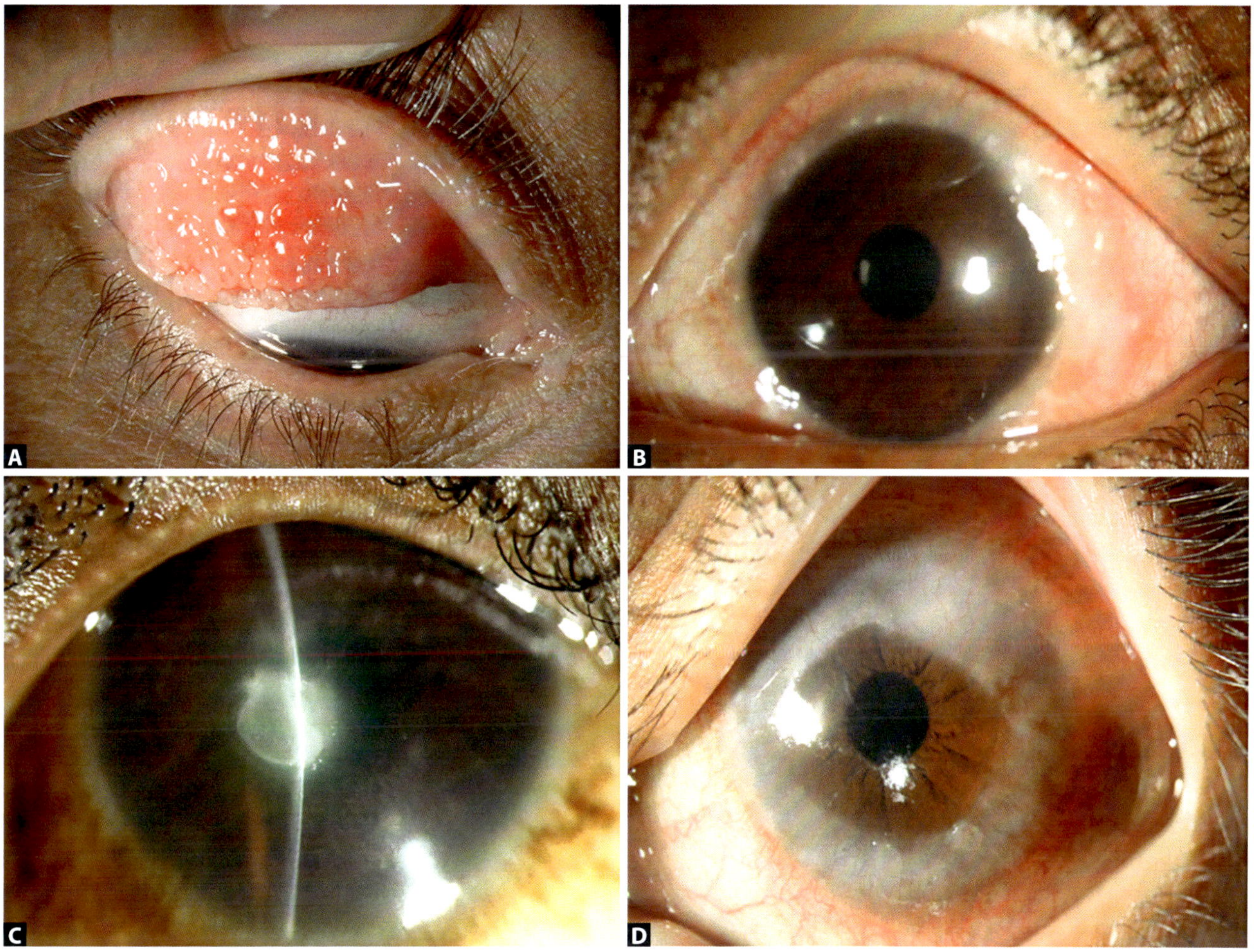

Figs. 3A to D: Vernal keratoconjunctivitis. (A) Large cobblestone papillae on the superior palpebral conjunctiva; (B) Limbal thickening with gelatinous appearance of the limbus along with white colored tiny spots representing Horner-Trantas dots on the superior limbus; (C) Shield ulcer; (D) Limbal stem cell deficiency.

The prevalence of keratoconus in VKC varies in different studies ranging from 0.7 to 6%. The possible theory behind the mechanism of keratoconus in VKC has been postulated to be frequent eye rubbing. Excessive eye rubbing possibly releases inflammatory mediators, which cause stromal keratocyte apoptosis and lead to thinning of the cornea.

Another vision-threatening corneal complication in severe recurrent and long-standing VKC is limbal stem cell deficiency (LSCD). It has been shown to have a prevalence of 1.2%. Recurrent chronic limbal inflammation results in a poor stromal support to the stem cells by affecting the microenvironment of the limbal stem cell niche and causes LSCD. VKC can also cause eyelid complications such as ptosis, which could either be mechanical due to large cobblestone papillae or due to disinsertion of the levator palpebrae superioris muscle due to frequent rubbing.

Management

Management of VKC involves long-term treatment and proper counseling of parents about this disease's chronic nature and recurrent acute exacerbations. Nonpharmacologic therapies include avoiding known allergens or triggers, avoiding eye rubbing, cold compresses, and artificial tears. First-line pharmacological approaches include topical dual-acting agents (mast cell stabilizers with antihistamine properties) such as olopatadine, ketotifen, azelastine, epinastine, bepotastine, and alcaftadine used daily throughout the affected season. For patients with VKC refractory to initial treatment, short-term topical corticosteroids such as loteprednol 0.5%, fluorometholone 0.1%, prednisolone 0.12% or 1%, and dexamethasone 0.1% may be prescribed. Follow-up is paramount as side effects of corticosteroid use can cause other complications such as glaucoma, cataracts, and secondary infections. Supratarsal injection of steroids such as triamcinolone acetate has been used for severe refractory cases of VKC. Studies have shown that topical cyclosporine A in different concentrations and topical tacrolimus ointment have beneficial effects in alleviating signs and symptoms of refractory VKC. Occasionally, complications of VKC may need surgical management. Giant papillae which cause recurrent corneal erosions can be removed with surgical shave excision or cryotherapy. Grade 3 shield ulcers which are refractory to medical treatment may be treated with superficial debridement and amniotic membrane transplantation. Systemic immunomodulatory therapy with cyclosporine A, azathioprine, and molecular antagonist of IgE omalizumab has also been shown to have a role in recalcitrant disease. Practically, in cases of moderate-to-severe VKC, an initial course of steroids for 2 weeks, in combination with specific dual-acting antiallergic drops, is usually the standard mode of management. Topical steroids are then stopped and rest treatment is continued for the whole season. Topical tacrolimus ointment (0.03%) three to four times-a-day, in combination with antiallergic drops, as first line, has also proved effective in many cases.

Atopic Keratoconjunctivitis

Atopic keratoconjunctivitis is a bilateral chronic inflammation of the conjunctiva and lids commonly associated with atopic dermatitis. This condition is more commonly seen in young adults in their 20s and may progress into the 5th decade; however, it can affect children as well.

Atopic conjunctivitis is usually associated with a history of other allergic disorders such as atopic dermatitis, asthma, or allergic rhinitis. Often, there is a family history of atopic diseases. Pathophysiology of AKC involves both a chronic degranulation of the mast cell-mediated by IgE, and immune mechanisms mediated by Th1- and Th2-lymphocyte-derived cytokines. Moreover, eosinophils and other inflammatory cells play a role.

Diagnosis

It presents with symptoms of severe itching of eyes, watering, redness, blurry vision, and photophobia. The lids and periocular skin may show eczematous changes, thickening of the lid margin, cracking of the lateral canthal area, madarosis, and even cicatricial ectropion in severe cases. The conjunctiva shows injection, papillary reaction especially in the inferior conjunctival fornix, fornix shortening, and symblepharon in severe cases. Corneal changes in AKC consist of punctate epitheliopathy, persistent epithelial erosions, corneal scarring, and neovascularization and are the primary causes of decreased vision in AKC. The diagnosis of AKC is based on typical clinical features. AKC can be differentiated from VKC by its age of onset, which is later in AKC than in VKC, and the pattern of symptoms, which are perennial in AKC but more in summer and spring in patients with VKC. Eyelid involvement with cicatricial changes in the eyelid is more common in AKC than in VKC. The conjunctival papillae are more commonly seen in the inferior conjunctiva in AKC and upper tarsal conjunctiva in VKC. Corneal involvement mainly presents as corneal neovascularization in AKC and as shield ulcer in VKC. Anterior and posterior subcapsular cataracts have also been described in AKC. Atopic conjunctivitis is almost always associated with lid eczema **(Fig. 4)** and usually with eczematous lesions on other parts of face.

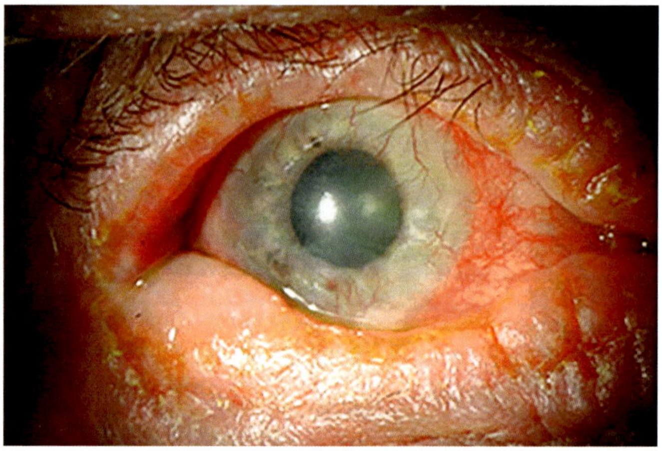

Fig. 4: Atopic keratoconjunctivitis.

Management

Treatment of AKC is multifaceted with preventive measures such as avoiding allergens and environmental triggers as well as topical and systemic medications. The involvement of other specialists, such as dermatologists and allergists, is essential for successful management. As described in the VKC section, topical treatment with antihistaminic and mast cell stabilizers is used for mild disease. Topical steroids are used for severe disease. Topical tacrolimus dermatologic ointment 0.03% can be used for periocular skin disease and has been used off label for the eye disease. Topical cyclosporine 0.05% eye drops have also been shown to be beneficial in alleviating symptoms. Patients with severe refractory AKC unresponsive to topical and systemic corticosteroids may require treatment with systemic cyclosporine, tacrolimus, or omalizumab.

NEONATAL CONJUNCTIVITIS

Any conjunctivitis occurring within 4 weeks of birth is termed as neonatal conjunctivitis or ophthalmia neonatorum. Neonatal conjunctivitis can be caused by a chemical agent, bacterial infection, or viral infection. The incidence of the disease ranges between 1.6 and 12% in different studies and geographical locations. The incidence of ophthalmia neonatorum is high in areas where sexually transmitted diseases are common, and the healthcare is inadequate. The neonates are usually infected via direct contact with the causative organism during passage through the birth canal. Infection can also ascend to the uterus in cases of prolonged rupture of membranes; thus, neonates delivered via cesarean section can also get infected.

Chemical Conjunctivitis

Chemical conjunctivitis develops within 1–2 days of birth. It is commonly caused by the administration of topical agents used for prophylaxis of infectious conjunctivitis. Silver nitrate 1% had been used as prophylaxis for infectious conjunctivitis in developing countries and was the most common cause of chemical conjunctivitis. It is rarely seen now as erythromycin is commonly used for prophylaxis. Conservative management typically results in gradual resolution of symptoms within a few days.

Neisseria Gonococcal Conjunctivitis

Newborns of mothers with gonococcal infection of perigenital area, who do not receive, prophylaxis have a high likelihood of developing gonococcal conjunctivitis. The prevalence of gonococcal conjunctivitis in neonates depends on the prevalence of gonococcal infection, prenatal screening, and infection treatment among pregnant women. Prophylaxis with a topical antibiotic to prevent gonococcal conjunctivitis in newborns is commonly indicated in most countries. Erythromycin 0.5% ophthalmic ointment in each eye in a single application at birth has been found to be the most used prophylactic agent. The neonates with gonococcal conjunctivitis typically exhibit symptoms within 2–5 days of birth. This type of conjunctivitis has an aggressive course with copious purulent discharge, conjunctival hyperemia, chemosis, and matting of lashes. Gonococci can penetrate intact corneal epithelium and cause rapid corneal infiltrates, melting, and even endophthalmitis. Systemic infection can also cause sepsis, arthritis, and meningitis. Diagnosis of gonococcal infection is made by Gram stain, culture, and PCR from conjunctival swabs. Neonates with gonococcal conjunctivitis are treated with a single dose of intramuscular or intravenous ceftriaxone 25–50 mg/kg. Ceftriaxone should be used cautiously in neonates with hyperbilirubinemia. Gonococcal infection in neonates is an ophthalmic emergency and treatment with intensive topical antibiotics, hourly saline lavages to clean the copious discharge, and parenteral antibiotics indicated in case of corneal involvement. Concurrent infection with other sexually transmitted diseases is common, and hence investigations for concurrent infections such as chlamydia should be performed. The mother and her sexual partner should also be treated.

Neonatal Chlamydial Conjunctivitis

Chlamydia trachomatis is an intracellular bacterium that causes neonatal conjunctivitis by infecting the newborn via contamination through the birth canal. Symptoms are usually seen around 5–14 days after birth. Conjunctivitis can be unilateral or bilateral. The clinical presentation of neonatal chlamydial infection differs from that in older children and adults. Neonatal chlamydial infection presents with a greater amount of mucopurulent discharge, pseudomembrane formation on the palpebral conjunctiva, and the lack of typical follicular reaction due to the absence of lymphoid tissue in the conjunctiva at this age. Although typical conjunctivitis is mild and responds to topical treatment, severe conjunctivitis can lead to conjunctival scarring and corneal neovascularization and scarring. Diagnosis is made by isolating chlamydia by culture from conjunctival cells obtained by conjunctival swabs. Giemsa staining demonstrates intracellular inclusion bodies. PCR and direct fluorescence antibody test can also be used. Chlamydial conjunctivitis can be associated with systemic infections like otitis media or pneumonitis.

Chlamydial conjunctivitis is treated with oral erythromycin 50 mg/kg/day in four divided doses for 2 weeks or oral azithromycin 20 mg/kg/day one dose daily for 3 days. Infantile hypertrophic pyloric stenosis (IHPS) has been reported in infants treated with oral erythromycin and azithromycin, especially under 6 weeks of age and hence infants treated with either of these medications should be followed for signs and symptoms of IHPS. To avoid this potential complication, azithromycin 1% eye ointment is used three to four times a day for 1 week. The mother and her sexual partner should be treated with a single dose of azithromycin 1 g and investigated for other sexually transmitted diseases.

Other Neonatal Bacterial Conjunctivitis

Other causes of bacterial conjunctivitis in neonates include *S. aureus, Strep. pneumoniae, Strep. viridans, Enterococcus* species, and *Haemophilus* species. Such bacterial conjunctivitis typically presents at 5–14 days of life and can be unilateral or bilateral. Broad-spectrum topical antibiotics are used for treatment.

Neonatal Herpetic Conjunctivitis

Neonatal herpes infection can be caused by HSV1 and HSV2. Neonates can become infected while passing through the birth canal or via ascending intrauterine infection. HSV1 can also be transmitted through the oral secretions of caregivers. Symptoms are usually seen within the first 2 weeks of life. Manifestations include eyelid vesicles and erythema, conjunctivitis, keratitis, and anterior uveitis. The keratitis can involve all layers of the cornea and does not follow the typical adult pattern of keratitis. Ocular infection can be associated with a systemic disease, including pneumonitis, dermatitis, hepatitis, and meningoencephalitis. Diagnosis can be established by PCR testing of conjunctival swabs, corneal scraping, or skin vesicles fluid. The recommended regimen for newborns treated for known or suspected neonatal herpes is acyclovir 20 mg/kg intravenously every 8 hours for 14 days if the disease is limited to the skin and mucous membranes. Simultaneously, local acyclovir eye ointment, four times a day, for 2 weeks is used.

Kawasaki Conjunctivitis

Kawasaki disease is also called mucocutaneous lymph node syndrome. It is primarily a vasculitis mediated by IgA and affects children younger than 5 years of age. Kawasaki disease is a generalized vasculitis that affects medium-sized arteries. It is characterized by systemic inflammation that manifests as persistent fever, erythema of mucous membranes, bilateral nonexudative conjunctivitis, rash, swelling and redness of the hands and feet, and cervical lymphadenopathy. Conjunctivitis is bilateral and nonexudative, and typically begins within days of fever onset. It is present in >90% of patients with Kawasaki disease. Photophobia is common. The conjunctivitis of Kawasaki disease tends to spare the limbus. The second most common ocular finding is the presence of anterior uveitis.

Management

Treatment with high-dose aspirin and intravenous immunoglobulin (IVIg) is the primary treatment for Kawasaki disease and helps in reducing the risk of coronary artery aneurysms, the most significant complication of this disease.

LIGNEOUS CONJUNCTIVITIS

Ligneous "woody" conjunctivitis is a rare disorder due to the autosomal recessive inheritance of mutations in the plasminogen gene. The disease itself is triggered upon exposure to irritants, infection, and ocular surgery. The nature of the mutation causes a deficiency in plasminogen. The conjunctiva in these patients is particularly sensitive and susceptible to external irritants and trauma, especially in young children. Any conjunctival damage triggers wound healing involving fibrin deposition in the first step to act as a scaffold for further tissue repair. In normal conditions, the plasma protein plasmin eventually degrades this fibrin scaffolding. However, because plasmin is derived from plasminogen, the latter's deficiency in ligneous conjunctivitis causes accumulation of fibrin, causing the formation of hard, "woody" pseudomembrane. Attempts to surgically excise these ligneous membranes may further exacerbate this process and worsen the condition.

Diagnosis

Diagnosis is confirmed by decreased serum plasminogen type I and histopathology of the membranes demonstrating fibrin-rich pseudomembrane. The tissue should also be assessed for amyloid, which can present similarly. A familial genetic history or involvement of another mucosal site would further support the diagnosis.

Management

No consensus exists on a single treatment for ligneous conjunctivitis. The most evidential support paradigm is topical plasminogen or plasminogen activator (tPA) followed by the excision of membranes. Then, an intensive topical heparin regimen is used until wound healing is complete. Secondary therapies include topical fresh frozen plasma, corticosteroids, or cyclosporine-A with amniotic membrane. Patients should be frequently assessed for recurrence as trauma, and subsequent pseudomembrane formation may occur postoperatively. Providing protective eyewear like polycarbonate glasses may act as prophylaxis for further conjunctival injury.

GIANT PAPILLARY CONJUNCTIVITIS

Giant papillary conjunctivitis (GPC) is a form of the ocular inflammatory disease characterized by "giant" papillae (1 mm or larger in diameter) on the superior tarsal conjunctiva. GPC is most often associated with contact lens wear; however, it may occur with ocular prosthetics, exposed sutures, exposed scleral buckles, glaucoma filtering blebs, and keratinized corneal scars. GPC most likely develops from the combination of mechanical trauma to the superior tarsal conjunctiva and an immunologic response by the conjunctiva to deposit on the contact lens surface.

Diagnosis

The most common symptoms of GPC include itchiness, blurry vision, excessive mucus production, foreign body sensation, irritation, and excessive lacrimation, and often blood tinged. Signs include giant papillae on the tarsal plate, conjunctival hyperemia, and thick mucus deposits in both the tear film and the medial canthal region. It appears that there is a shorter time to onset of GPC in soft contact lens wearers compared to rigid contact lens wearers.

Management

Contact lens wear is responsible for the initial trauma and inflammatory reaction in most cases of GPC and thus temporary contact lens wear discontinuation is the first step of management. Contact lens holiday should be for at least 2–4 weeks or until symptoms and signs resolve. Reinitiation of contact lenses should preferably include daily disposable or short-time disposable soft contact lenses. Removal of the inciting agent, such as a broken suture or exposed scleral buckle, will lead to resolution of the related GPC. Antiallergic therapies may be used to treat GPC during the temporary contact lens discontinuation period. These include topical antihistaminic agents, mast cell stabilizers, or dual-acting agents. Persistent symptoms may benefit from mild topical steroids such as loteprednol 0.5% or fluorometholone 0.1%. Topical nonsteroidal anti-inflammatory drugs could also be used. In rare instances, patients with recalcitrant disease may require immunomodulatory treatment with topical tacrolimus. Occasionally, the giant papillae need surgical excision or cryotherapy for a persistent disease.

BLEPHAROKERATOCONJUNCTIVITIS

Blepharitis is a lid margin disease that can involve the anterior lid margin which includes the lash follicles or the posterior lid margin which includes meibomian glands. The manifestations of blepharitis can extend to the ocular surface, causing conjunctivitis and corneal disease, which encompasses BKC. The proposed pathogenesis of BKC is a delayed hypersensitivity type IV reaction to foreign microbial pathogens such as *S. aureus* and *Propionibacterium acne*. Demodex mites may also have a role in causing severe

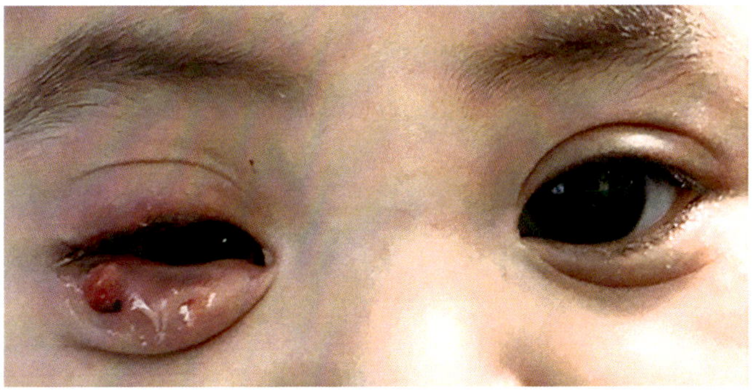

Fig. 5: Multiple chalazia with blepharitis.

blepharitis. BKC is more commonly seen in female children, the age of onset is 4–5 years. It may be associated with recurrent chalazia and styes **(Fig. 5)**. It is associated with ocular rosacea in 12% of the cases.

Diagnosis

Symptoms include conjunctival redness, extreme photophobia, eye rubbing, watering, and blurry vision. Signs include lid margin disease with blepharitis, chalazia, inspissated meibomian ducts, crusting and collarettes, and telangiectasia of the lid margin. Severe disease can cause notching the lid margins and loss of lashes. Conjunctiva presents with injection, tarsal papillary reaction, tarsal follicles, and phlyctenules. Corneal signs include punctate epitheliopathy, marginal keratitis with infiltrates usually seen at 4, 8, 10, and 2 o'clock positions where the lid margin meets the cornea. Severe recurrent disease can cause diffuse involvement of the cornea with superficial scarring and neovascularization. Patients may also have facial skin changes such as a papular rash on the cheeks and nose, as well as acne, which raise suspicion of rosacea. Recurrent chronic disease in children with corneal scarring can cause induced astigmatism and amblyopia.

Management

It is essential to explain to the families of children with BKC that this is a chronic inflammatory condition with exacerbations and remissions. Long-term treatment is necessary. The initial treatment of acute exacerbations is with lid scrubs with diluted baby shampoo twice daily. Warm compresses for 10 minutes two to three times a day should be used. After the warm compress, lid massages to open the clogged meibomian glands should be performed. This treatment targets opening the plugged up meibomian glands and clearing them of bacteria and oily debris. Bacitracin and erythromycin ophthalmic ointment applied to lid margins at bedtime may help to limit colonization with *Staphylococcus* and other microflora. Corneal involvement will need treatment with soft topical corticosteroids such as loteprednol 0.5%, fluorometholone 0.1%, or prednisolone 0.12% to control the inflammatory corneal infiltrates and neovascularization. If the disease is not controlled with soft

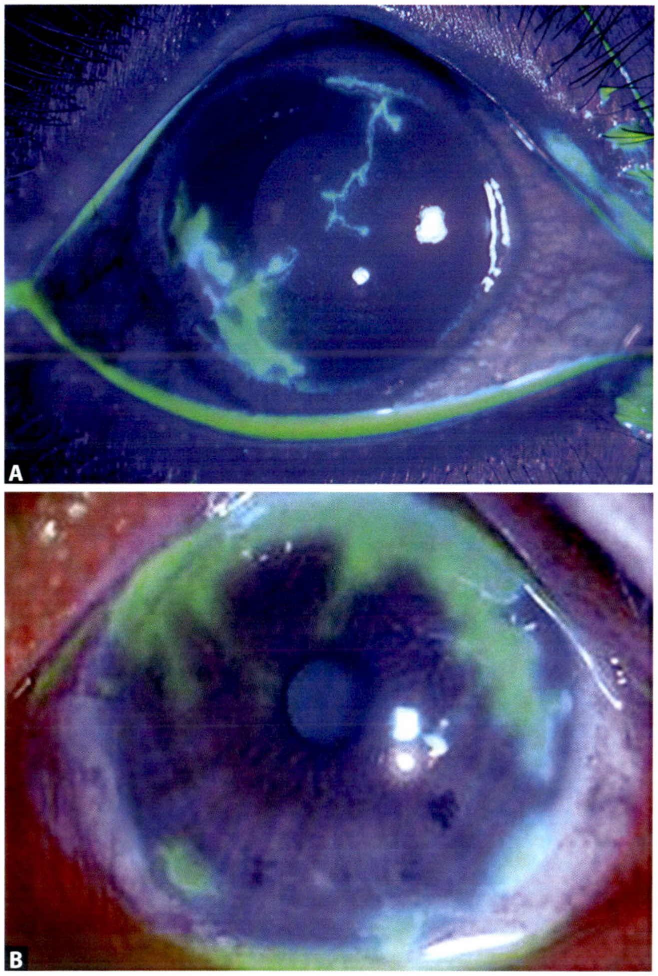

Figs. 6A and B: (A) Dendritic corneal ulcer; (B) Geographical corneal ulcer.

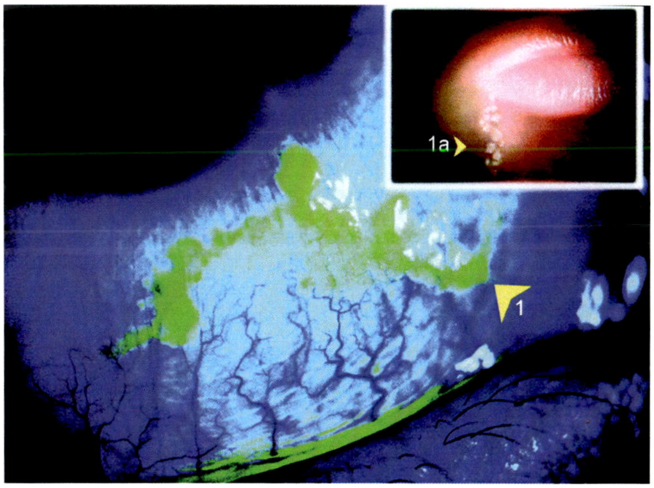

Fig. 7: Conjunctival dendrite in primary HSV.
(Adapted from Br J Ophthalmol. 2004;88(4):590-1)

steroids, more potent steroids such as prednisolone 1% or dexamethasone 0.1% are needed. Steroids should be slowly tapered to avoid recurrences. Topical azithromycin eye drops have been shown to be effective in BKC in some studies. Systemic antibiotic treatment is needed in severe disease. Erythromycin 20 mg/kg/day for 3 months, azithromycin

5 mg/kg/day for 5 days, or doxycycline 100 mg daily for 3 months in children above 12 years of age may be needed in severe disease with recurrences. Longer duration of treatment with azithromycin, and repeated cycles of treatment have also been described. Treatment with dietary supplements with oral omega-3 fatty acids such as flaxseed oil has also been shown to improve meibomian gland disease in children with BKC. Long-term treatment with continued lid hygiene and warm compresses is needed in these patients to prevent a recurrence. Appropriate refraction to look for induced astigmatism from corneal scarring and amblyopia treatment is essential.

SUGGESTED READING

1. Al-Amri AM. Long-term follow-up of tacrolimus ointment for treatment of atopic keratoconjunctivitis. Am J Ophthalmol. 2014;157(2):280-6.
2. Ang MJ, Papageorgiou KI, Chang SH, Kohn J, Garneau HC, Goldberg RA. Topical plasminogen as adjunctive treatment in recurrent ligneous conjunctivitis. Ophthalmic Plast Reconstr Surg. 2017;33(2):e37-9.
3. Azari AA, Barney NP. Conjunctivitis: a systematic review of diagnosis and treatment. JAMA. 2013;310(16):1721-9.
4. Bonini S, Coassin M, Aronni S, Lambiase A. Vernal keratoconjunctivitis. Eye (Lond). 2004;18(4):345-51.
5. Brémond-Gignac D, Nischal KK, Mortemousque B, Gajdosova E, Granet DB, Chiambaretta F. Atopic keratoconjunctivitis in children: clinical features and diagnosis. Ophthalmology. 2016;123(2):435-7.
6. Cameron JA. Shield ulcers and plaques of the cornea in vernal keratoconjunctivitis. Ophthalmology. 1995;102(6):985-93.
7. Choi DS, Djalilian A. Oral azithromycin combined with topical anti-inflammatory agents in the treatment of blepharokeratoconjunctivitis in children. JAAPOS. 2013;17(1):112-3.
8. De Freitas D, Martins EN, Adan C, Alvarenga LS, Pavan-Langston D. Herpes zoster ophthalmicus in otherwise healthy children. Am J Ophthalmol. 2006;142(3):393-9.
9. Gokhale NS, Samant R, Sharma V. Oral cyclosporine therapy for refractory severe vernal keratoconjunctivitis. Indian J Ophthalmol. 2012;60(3):220-3.
10. Heffler E, Picardi G, Liuzzo MT, Pistorio MP, Crimi N. Omalizumab treatment of vernal keratoconjunctivitis. JAMA Ophthalmol. 2016;134(4):461-3.
11. Jones SM, Weinstein JM, Cumberland P, Klein N, Nischal KK. Visual outcome and corneal changes in children with chronic blepharokeratoconjunctivitis. Ophthalmology. 2007; 114(12): 2271-80.
12. Kenny SE, Tye CB, Johnson DA, Kheirkhah A. Giant papillary conjunctivitis: A review. Ocul Surf. 2020;18(3):396-402.
13. Kheirkhah A, Zavareh MK, Farzbod F, Mahbod M, Behrouz MJ. Topical 0.005% tacrolimus eye drop for refractory vernal keratoconjunctivitis. Eye (Lond). 2011;25(7):872-80.
14. La Rosa M, Lionetti E, Reibaldi M, Russo A, Longo A, Leonardi S, et al. Allergic conjunctivitis: a comprehensive review of the literature. Ital J Pediatr. 2013;39:18.
15. Leonardi A, Castegnaro A, Valerio AL, Lazzarini D. Epidemiology of allergic conjunctivitis: clinical appearance and treatment patterns in a population-based study. Curr Opin Allergy Clin Immunol. 2015;15(5):482-8.
16. Liu S, Pavan-Langston D, Colby KA. Pediatric herpes simplex of the anterior segment: characteristics, treatment, and outcomes. Ophthalmology. 2012;119(10):2003-8.
17. Ramphul K, Mejias SG. Kawasaki disease: a comprehensive review. Arch Med Sci Atheroscler Dis. 2018;3:e41-5.
18. Reddy JC, Basu S, Saboo US, Murthy SI, Vaddavalli PK, Sangwan VS. Management, clinical outcomes, and complications of shield ulcers in vernal keratoconjunctivitis. Am J Ophthalmol. 2013; 155(3):550-9.
19. Rousta ST. Pediatric blepharokeratoconjunctivitis: is there a 'right' treatment? Curr Opin Ophthalmol. 2017;28(5):449-53.
20. Schuster V, Seregard S. Ligneous conjunctivitis. Surv Ophthalmol. 2003;48(4):369-88.
21. Sheikh A, Hurwitz B. Topical antibiotics for acute bacterial conjunctivitis: a systematic review. Br J Gen Pract. 2001;51(467): 473-7.
22. Singhal D, Sahay P, Maharana PK, Raj N, Sharma N, Titiyal JS. Vernal Keratoconjunctivitis. Surv Ophthalmol. 2019;64(3):289-311.
23. Varu DM, Rhee MK, Akpek EK, Amescua G, Farid M, Garcia-Ferrer FJ, et al. Conjunctivitis preferred practice pattern. Ophthalmology. 2019;126(1):P94-P169.
24. Viswalingam M, Rauz S, Morlet N, Dart JK. Blepharokeratoconjunctivitis in children: diagnosis and treatment. Br J Ophthalmol. 2005;89(4):400-3.
25. Workowski KA, Bolan GA. Centers for Disease Control and Prevention. Sexually transmitted diseases treatment guidelines, 2015. MMWR Recomm Rep. 2015;64(RR-03):1-137.
26. Zloto O, Gharaibeh A, Mezer E, Stankovic B, Isenberg S, Wygnanski-Jaffe T. Ophthalmia neonatorum treatment and prophylaxis: IPOSC global study. Graefes Arch Clin Exp Ophthalmol. 2016;254(3): 577-82.

CHAPTER 7

Disorders of Pediatric Cornea and Management

Namrata Sharma, Rasik Vajpayee, Rinky Agarwal, Mohamad Ibrahime Asif, Priyadarshini KM

INTRODUCTION

Cornea is an avascular, aspheric, and transparent tissue that classically consists of five layers—(1) epithelium, (2) bowman layer, (3) stroma, (4) Descemet membrane (DM), and (5) endothelium **(Table 1)**. Recently, a sixth layer or the pre-Descemet layer (Dua's layer) has been described by Harminder Singh Dua. The adult cornea measures 9-11 mm vertically and 11-12 mm horizontally with an approximate thickness of 500-600 microns at the center and gradually increasing toward the periphery. The normal human cornea at birth has a horizontal diameter of 9.5-10.5 mm which grows to adult size of 12 mm by 2 years. The refractive index of the cornea is 1.376 and the refractive power of the cornea is 40 D-44 D which constitute two-thirds of the total refractive power of the eye. The neonatal cornea has a mean keratometry of 48 D, which progressively decreases and stabilizes over the next 4.5 years. The nutrition for the cornea depends on glucose diffusion from aqueous humor and oxygen through the tear film. The peripheral cornea also receives nutrient supply from the limbal circulation.

EMBRYOLOGY

Understanding the development of cornea and anterior segment structures is important for better comprehension of congenital corneal anomalies. Various cell lineages are involved in the development of cornea and anterior segment

TABLE 1: Different layers of the cornea and their features.

Layer	***Features***
Epithelium	It is 40–50 μm thick and consists of 4–6 layers (superficial squamous cells—1–2 layers; wing cells—2–3 layers; a single layer of columnar basal cells). Along with tear film, it forms a clear optical surface. Tight junctions provide a barrier to stromal hydration. Limbal stem cells proliferate and differentiate to form superficial cells in approximately 7–14 days. The 50 nm thick basement membrane composed of type IV collagen is secreted by the basal cells. Basal cells express keratin 5/14, however, keratin 3/12 is specifically expressed in the epithelium. Various markers of limbal stem cells are p63, ABCG2, keratin 19, and vimentin but no keratin 3/12
Bowman layer	This is rather an acellular condensation of the anterior-most stroma. It is 12–15 μm thick and does not regenerate when disrupted. It is primarily made of collagen I and III
Stroma	Constitutes 90% of the thickness, regularly arranged collagen lamellae, proteoglycans (decorin—dermatan sulfate and lumican—keratan sulfate) along with fibroblasts. Type I (major) and V collagen are intertwined with type VI collagen. Corneal transparency is maintained by keeping the water content at 78% by epithelial, endothelial barriers, and endothelial pumps (Na-K ATPase)
Pre-Descemet layer	It is an acellular layer of 15 μm thick consisting of 5–8 lamellae of type I collagen. Despite being thin, it has high resistance (could resist 200 KPa of pressure)
Descemet membrane (DM)	It is the basement membrane for endothelium consisting of anterior banded and posterior nonbanded zone. 3 μm at birth, increases to 10–12 μm in adults (posterior nonbanded zone is continuously laid by the endothelium). It is primarily composed of collagen type IV and VIII and laminin. DM ends as Schwalbe line where trabecular meshwork starts
Endothelium	It consists of a monolayer of interdigitated, hexagonal cells. If a cell gets damaged, the defect is covered by the enlargement of the surrounding cells. Corneal endothelial cell density is 6,000 cells/mm^2 at birth which falls by 26% in the first year and 26% in the next 11 years, following it decreases at an average of 0.6%/year. These cells are attached by hemidesmosome to Descemet and between them by tight junctional complex which acts as a barrier. There are also metabolic pumps to draw water osmotically from the cornea and maintain transparency

TABLE 2: Embryological origin of different structures of the cornea and anterior segment.

Origin	*Structures*	*Time of development*
Epidermal ectoderm	Corneal epithelium	6th week
Neural crest (neuroectoderm)	Keratocytes, scleral fibroblasts, and endothelial cells	6th week
Neural crest-derived mesenchymal cells	Corneal stroma, endothelium, trabecular meshwork, and iris	7th to 8th week
Surface ectoderm	Lens	Starts at 25 days of gestation

(Table 2). Neural crest-derived mesenchyme migrates in three waves between the primitive corneal epithelium and lens vesicle during the 7th week of gestation. The first wave of migration forms the corneal endothelium, the second wave differentiates into keratocytes to form corneal stroma, and the third wave gives rise to iris. During the 8th week, the keratocytes form five to eight layers of collagen lamellae and the endothelium forms the DM. Impaired differentiation of neural crest-derived tissues could result in various anomalies such as Peters anomaly. Till the 7th month, there will be an accumulation of proteoglycans leading to the well-developed cornea. During the early stage of development, hyaluronan is the major glycosaminoglycan (GAG) which is slowly replaced by keratan sulfate, chondroitin sulfate, and dermatan sulfate as the cornea develops.

CLASSIFICATION OF PEDIATRIC CORNEAL OPACITIES

The differential diagnosis of congenital and neonatal corneal opacities has been traditionally described using the acronym STUMPED (Sclerocornea, Tears in Descemet membrane, Ulcers, Metabolic diseases, Peters' anomaly, Endothelial dystrophies, Dermoids). As it had certain inaccuracies due to its broad nature, recently a new classification system has been proposed **(Table 3)**.

TABLE 3: Traditional and novel classification of congenital and neonatal corneal opacities.

Traditional (STUMPED)	*Novel classification*
Sclerocornea Tears in Descemet membrane • Congenital (infantile) glaucoma • Forceps injury and other trauma Ulcers • Viral • Bacterial • Fungal • Neurotrophic Metabolic diseases • Mucopolysaccharidoses • Mucolipidoses Peters' anomaly Endothelial dystrophies • Congenital hereditary endothelial dystrophy • Posterior polymorphous dystrophy Dermoids	*Primary corneal disease*: • Corneal dystrophies – Congenital hereditary endothelial dystrophy – Posterior polymorphous corneal dystrophy – Congenital hereditary stromal dystrophy – X-linked endothelial corneal dystrophy • Corneal dermoid • Peripheral sclerocornea • CYP1B1 cytopathy *Secondary corneal disease:* • *Congenital* – Kerato-irido-lenticular dysgenesis - Iridocorneal adhesions - Lens fails to separate from cornea - Lens separates but fails to form - Thereafter - Lens separates and forms, but there is - Late corneal apposition - Lens fails to form – Irido-trabecular dysgenesis - Primary congenital glaucoma. - Intracorneal cyst - Axenfeld-Rieger syndrome - Congenital aniridia • *Acquired* – Infection - Viral - Bacterial – Trauma - Forceps injury - Amniocentesis injury – Metabolic - Mucolipidosis IV

CONGENITAL PEDIATRIC CORNEAL DISORDER

Sclerocornea

Sclerocornea refers to peripheral whitening or scleralization of the cornea that may extend toward the visual axis **(Fig. 1)**. It is a nonprogressive, sporadic (can be familial/autosomal dominant/autosomal recessive form—mutation in KERA gene), usually bilateral (90% cases) condition. Opacification is smooth, white and vascular similar to the sclera, involving full-thickness of the cornea, predominantly in the peripheral circumferential area than the central. The cornea is relatively flatter (<43D) in 80% cases. Contrary to the uniform, parallel, and organized lamellar structure of corneal collagen, histologically, the cornea in sclerocornea is like a sclera with an irregular arrangement of thickened collagen fibers, and decreased diameter of collagen fibrils in posterior stroma. The DM and the underlying endothelium may be attenuated or absent.

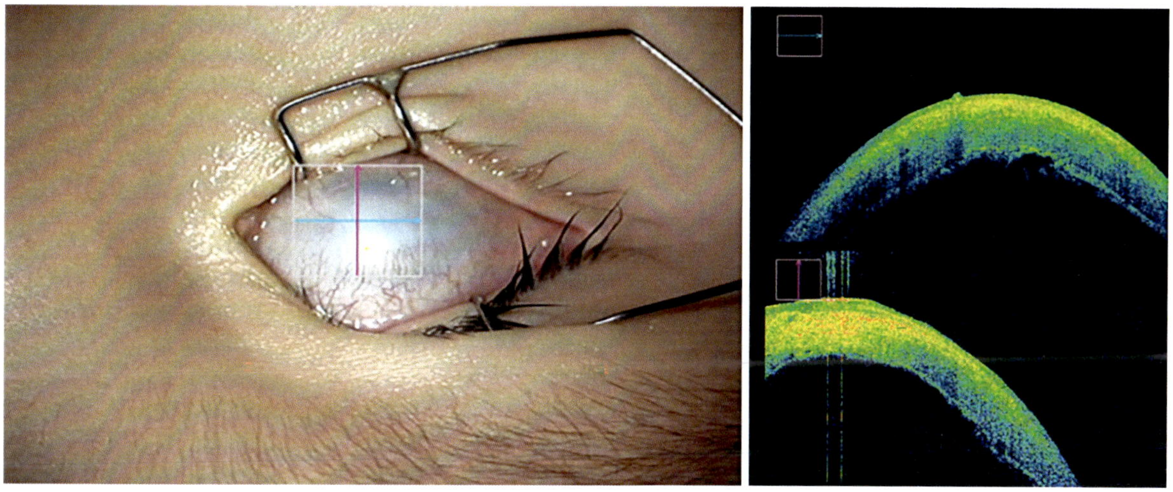

Fig. 1: Total sclerocornea, seen under iOCT-equipped microscope. (iOCT: intraoperative optical coherence tomography)

Waring and Rodrigues classified sclerocornea into four groups:

1. Isolated peripheral sclerocornea
2. Sclerocornea plana
3. Sclerocornea associated with anterior chamber cleavage anomalies
4. Total sclerocornea (most common form)

Ocular associations include microcornea, microphthalmos, blue sclera, coloboma, aniridia, ectopia lentis, cataract, glaucoma, and systemic associations such as cerebellar anomalies, Dandy-Walker cyst, polydactyly, cryptorchidism, ear deformities, osteogenesis imperfecta, and various other syndromes. Ultrasound biomicroscopy (UBM) and anterior segment optical coherence tomography (ASOCT) could be a help in diagnosis of any associated structural abnormalities, identification of pupil and thereby facilitating surgical planning. Penetrating keratoplasty (PKP) should be planned if vision acuity is affected significantly and other ocular structures are relatively normal as surgical outcomes are very poor.

Trauma to Descemet's Membrane

Iatrogenic DM rupture can occur due to forceps or vacuum-assisted childbirth. These ruptured areas heal spontaneously but usually leave a hypertrophic ridge that can cause high astigmatism leading to dense amblyopia. Congenital glaucoma can present with similar clinical findings **(Table 4)**. Intrauterine ocular trauma during diagnostic amniocentesis in second trimester may also result in congenitally opacified cornea.

TABLE 4: Differentiating features between birth trauma and congenital glaucoma.

Birth trauma	*Congenital glaucoma*
Forceps or vacuum extraction-induced globe compression	Due to raised intraocular pressure
DM rupture are usually vertical/ oblique—due to instrumental (forceps) delivery	DM rupture are usually horizontal/concentric to the limbus known as Haab striae
Left eye more commonly affected due to left occipitoanterior head crowning position	Either/ both eyes could be affected
Corneal edema appears in the immediate postpartum period	Corneal edema appears few weeks after birth
Corneal diameter, intraocular pressure, and optic nerve head are normal	Enlarged corneal diameter, elevated IOP, and optic nerve head cupping are present singly or in combination
Lesser incidence of photophobia	Photophobia commonly present
Other signs of periocular trauma such as eyelid coloboma, iris abnormalities, cataract, or retinal detachment may be present	These are absent

Long-standing corneal decompensation due to raised intraocular pressure (IOP) and/or presence of DM tears **(Fig. 2)** can result in corneal opacification that may require corneal transplant **(Fig. 3)**, either PKP or Descemet stripping automated endothelial keratoplasty (DSAEK).

Primary Congenital Glaucoma

It is evident at birth or within first few years of life. Various genes such as CYP1B1 and MYOC are associated with primary congenital glaucoma (PCG). The newborns present with a triad of epiphora, photophobia, and blepharospasm.

Corneal Ulcers and Inflammation

Herpes simplex virus (HSV) keratitis is usually contracted during delivery through infected birth canal. Mostly, it is caused by HSV-2 (80%). They represent as primary infection that can recur later in life. Systemic dissemination and central

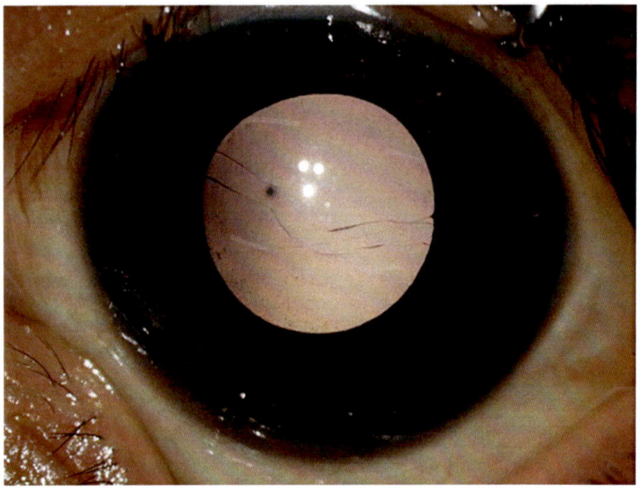

Fig. 2: Haab striae.

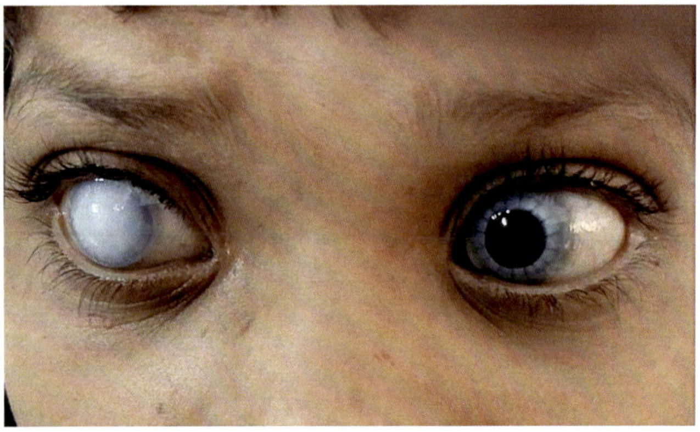

Fig. 3: Child with bilateral PCG showing failed PKP graft in right eye and a clear PKP graft in left eye.

nervous system involvement are common. Bacterial keratitis is rare to appear at birth. Infection with *Neisseria gonorrhoeae* can produce serious ocular and systemic complications in neonates and systemic treatment is mandatory to avoid these. Neurotrophic keratitis can occur in cases of Riley-Day syndrome (familial dysautonomia) due to generalized dysfunction of autonomic nervous system. Decreased corneal sensation and sterile ulceration are common and may be present at birth.

Metabolic Diseases

- *Mucopolysaccharidosis*: They are inherited lysosomal storage disorders, leading to accumulation of GAGs in various corneal cells leading to corneal clouding **(Table 5)**. PKP or deep anterior lamellar keratoplasty (DALK) may be considered after assessing the visual potential as optic nerve and retinal pathologies can coexist **(Fig. 4)**. Besides, the deposits might accumulate in the graft also. Some regression in corneal clouding occurs following successful bone marrow transplantation. Enzyme replacement therapy and gene therapy are upcoming modalities.
- *Mucolipidosis*: They are autosomal recessive disorders with inherited abnormalities of carbohydrate and lipid metabolism. They are due to defect in lysosomal acid hydrolase enzymes leading to intracytoplasmic accumulation in the epithelium and can present with varying degrees of corneal clouding **(Table 6)**.
- *Tyrosinemia*: Autosomal recessive disorder due to defect in soluble hepatic cytosol tyrosine aminotransferase (chromosome 16). Only type II (Richner-Hanhart syndrome)

TABLE 5: Differentiating features between various mucopolysaccharidosis.

	Hurler/Gargoylism syndrome	***Maroteaux-Lamy syndrome***	***Scheie syndrome***	***Morquio syndrome***	***Hunter syndrome***
Inheritance	AR	AR	AR	AR	XLR
Deficiency	Alpha-1-iduronidase	Arylsulfatase B	Alpha-1-iduronidase	Galactosamine-6-sulfate sulfatase/ beta-galactosidase	Iduronate sulfatase
Onset	Within the first few years	Within the first few years	From birth but vision decreases by 2nd decade	Usually after 10 years old	Doesn't present as corneal opacity
Ocular	Diffuse punctate stromal opacities, Significant corneal clouding	Punctate corneal opacities almost always present at birth, narrow-angle glaucoma	Thickened or edematous cornea, prominent in the periphery. Associated glaucoma	Corneal opacities are seen in 10% cases	Corneal opacity might occur later in life in the mild form
Systemic	Mental retardation, large head, abnormal facies, dwarfism, joint contractures, hepatosplenomegaly, deafness, hirsutism, cardiac and CNS defects	Mild facial abnormalities, skeletal changes like kyphosis, genu valgum, protuberant sternum, hydrocephalus	Claw hand deformities, valvular (aortic valve) heart diseases	Dwarfism, joint laxity, valvular (aortic valve) heart diseases	Clinically appears like Hurler but deafness and cardiac defects are common

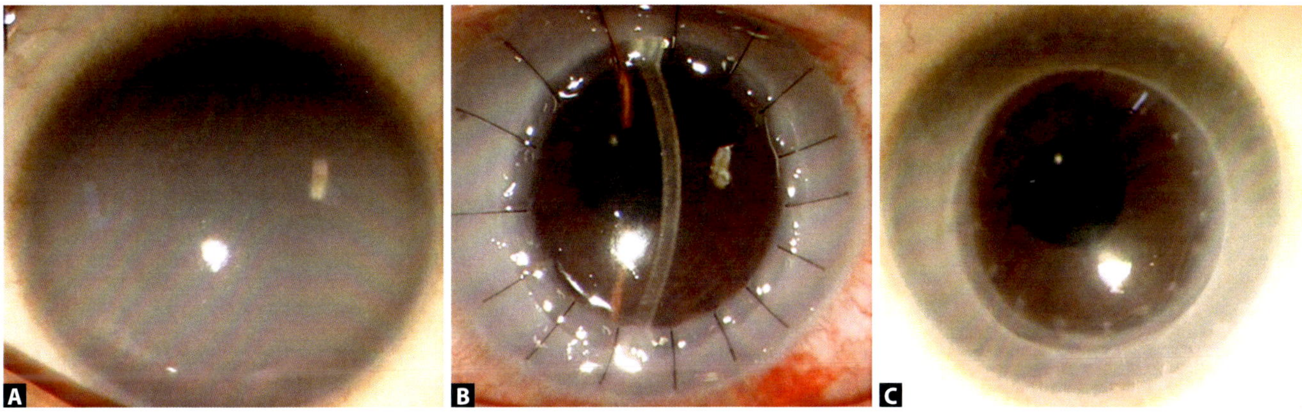

Figs. 4A to C: A child with Hurler's syndrome showing corneal opacification (mucopolysaccharidosis) in right eye (A), improvement in corneal clarity after DALK at 3 months (B) and 3 years (C) postoperatively.

TABLE 6: Ocular features of various mucolipidosis (MLS).

MLS-I, MLS-II (I cell disease) and MLS-III (Pseudo-Hurler polydystrophy)	These do not cause any severe corneal diseases and usually do not require any ocular treatment
MLS-IV	This type is present with significant corneal opacity present from birth. Episodic eye pain is seen due to epithelial irregularities caused by accumulation of abnormal material. Other associated findings include retinal degeneration, cherry red spot, optic atrophy, cataract, and attenuated vessels. They have profound psychomotor retardation without skeletal/facial deformity *Management*: Any keratoplasty procedure carries poor prognosis due to resurfacing by the abnormal epithelium. Allograft limbal stem cell transplantation may be an option

is associated with corneal opacity. It is characterized by a triad of mental retardation, dendriform lesions of the cornea, and hyperkeratotic lesions of palms and soles. It usually appears in first few months of age and it is important to distinguish this from herpes keratitis. Bilateral involvement, morphology (lack of terminal bulbs and poor staining of the lesion, consistent inferocentral location), normal corneal sensitivity, lack of response to antiviral treatment (persisting >6 weeks), and exacerbation with increased protein intake and systemic associations should raise the suspicion of tyrosinemia. Child should be advised tyrosine and phenylalanine restricted diet which would resolve corneal lesions.

- *Cystinosis*: Autosomal recessive disorder is caused by a mutation in CTNS gene in chromosome 17, leading to defect in the cystine transport with intracellular accumulation of free cystine, thereby resulting in crystalline deposition in various tissues (eyes, kidneys, bone marrow, and lymph nodes). These needle-shaped crystals appear around 2 years of age in cornea (epithelium, stroma, and endothelium) and conjunctiva. They start anteriorly and in periphery and later involve the entire cornea, leading to irritation, pain, and photophobia. Lubricating eye drops and therapeutic bandage contact lenses (BCL) could be useful in providing symptomatic relief. Topical cysteamine solution 0.5% administered every 1–2 hourly could be useful in dissolving the cystine accumulated. It is also useful post-PKP to prevent redeposition.
- *Fabry disease*: X-linked recessive disorder due to lack of the enzyme alpha-galactosidase A leading to deposition of sphingolipids within lysosomes. It is characterized by angiokeratomas of skin along with multisystem involvement. Ocular manifestations include corneal opacities (90%, earliest and most consistent changes), conjunctival vessel tortuosity (60%), retinal vessel tortuosity, and cataract (Fabry cataract—spoke-like posterior capsular cataract). In advanced cases, fine, curvy, or whorl-like superficial corneal opacity (cornea verticillata) can be seen. They are not present at birth but can occur as early as 6 months of age. Enzyme replacement therapy is available for Fabry disease.

Peters' Anomaly

It is a congenital corneal disorder, usually bilateral (80%), asymmetrical, and sporadic with a central leukomatous corneal opacity **(Figs. 5 and 6)** and an associated defect in posterior stroma, DM, and endothelium. Bowman layer might also be absent centrally. Iris adhesions can extend to the margins of this defect. There is increased incidence of glaucoma (50–80%) due to defects in angle development. There are two types of Peter syndrome—type I and II **(Table 7)**. Peter anomaly when associated with intellectual disability, short stature, heart defects, nervous system defects, external ear abnormalities, cleft lip, and palate refers to Peter-plus syndrome. Systemic malformations could be associated with genetically transmitted syndromes such as

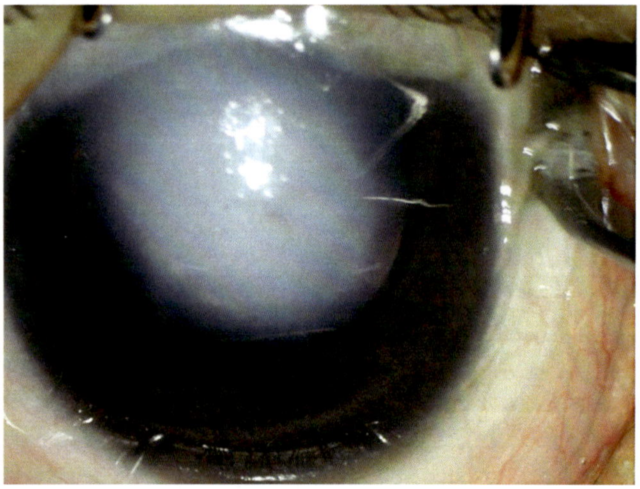

Fig. 5: Type 1 Peters' anomaly.

Kivlin syndrome and Pfeiffer syndrome. Hence, children with this anomaly should be screened for systemic malformations especially midline body structures like the heart and pituitary gland. **Table 8** depicts features differentiating Peters' anomaly from sclerocornea. Definite ocular management of Peters' anomaly includes PKP though in few cases with small, localized opacity attempt of optical iridectomy could be done. Outcomes of PKP are better in type 1 Peter than in type 2.

Axenfeld-Rieger Syndrome

It is a bilateral, developmental disorder with autosomal dominant mode of inheritance. It can be caused by mutations in genes FOXC1, PITX2, or PAX6. Traditionally, three eponyms are used pertaining to this—Axenfeld anomaly (peripheral anterior segment defects), Rieger anomaly

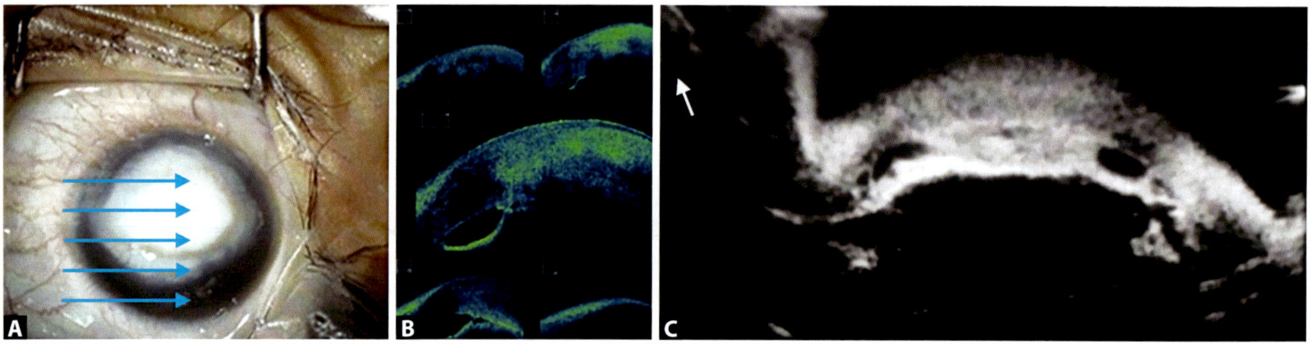

Figs. 6A to C: Type 2 Peters' anomaly showing central corneal opacity, membranous cataract, and keratolenticular adhesions as seen on iOCT and UBM.
(iOCT: intraoperative optical coherence tomography; UBM: ultrasound biomicroscopy)

TABLE 7: Types of Peters' anomaly.

Type 1	*Type 2*
Corneal opacity along with iridocorneal adhesions. No keratolenticular contact or cataract	Type 1+ lens abnormalities (keratolenticular adherence, cataractous lens)
Associated ocular anomalies—microcornea, sclerocornea, infantile glaucoma, and vitreoretinal abnormalities rare. However, systemic associations are rare	• Associated ocular anomalies—microphthalmia with PHPV, microcornea, sclerocornea, cornea plana, coloboma, aniridia, and optic atrophy • Systemic associations—poly/syndactyly, Wilms tumor, craniofacial dysplasia, cardiac defects, CNS anomalies, pulmonary hypoplasia, and ear abnormalities
Predominantly unilateral involvement with less dense opacity	Predominantly bilateral with denser opacity
Good visual potential	Poor visual potential when compared to type 1

TABLE 8: Differentiating features between Peters' anomaly and sclerocornea.

Peters' anomaly	*Sclerocornea*
Opacity predominantly involves the central cornea with clear periphery	Opacity more pronounced peripherally. A variant can involve the total cornea
Iris strands attach to the posterior corneal defect/leukoma	Usually not seen
Mostly sporadic. Autosomal dominant/recessive, PITX2, FOXC1, CYP1B1, and PAX6 are genes involved	Sporadic (can be familial/AD/AR form) KERA gene is involved
Better prognosis with PKP compared to sclerocornea	Worse prognosis than Peter

(peripheral anterior segment defects + iris changes), and Rieger syndrome (ocular + systemic developmental defects). Rarely, Peter syndrome may also be associated with this. Ocular structures involved are the peripheral cornea, anterior chamber angle, and iris. Ocular features include posterior embryotoxon, thread-like to broad iridocorneal adhesions obscuring the scleral spur and inserting at the posterior part of the trabecular meshwork, iris defects ranging from mild thinning to large defects, corectopia, and ectropion uveae. The angles are usually open beyond the iridocorneal adhesions. >50% patients develop glaucoma usually in late childhood. Most associated systemic features are dental abnormalities (microdontia, hypodontia/anodontia) and facial anomalies (maxillary hypoplasia with midface flattening, hypertelorism, telecanthus, micrognathia, mandibular prognathism, receding upper lip, and prominent lower lip). Other less common are pituitary defects, cardiac defects, umbilical, middle ear deafness, and mental deficiency. The primary concern should be the detection and management of glaucoma. Medical management should be initiated, however, in infantile cases and refractory to medical management, trabeculectomy or drainage devices should be planned. In children with opacities involving the central cornea, PKP can be planned.

CYP1B1 Cytopathy

Mutations in the CYP1B1 gene are usually known to cause PCG. However, these have also been reported in rare cases of congenital corneal opacification. CYP1B1 cytopathy can be associated with iridocorneal and/or keratolenticular adhesion, posterior embryotoxon (prominent anteriorly displaced Schwalbe line) and iris hypoplasia. Histopathologic findings include loss of central Bowman layer, DM, and endothelium as well as cellular stromal infiltration. Corneal transplantation has a good survival rate, but the visual prognosis is guarded due to progressive glaucoma.

Congenital Aniridia

It is defined by the classic clinical triad of iris hypoplasia, foveal hypoplasia, and nystagmus. Although the disease manifests throughout the eye, it is often classified among the anterior segment dysgeneses. The iris abnormalities can range from the near complete absence of iris, with the development of only a short iris stump, to mild iris transillumination defects, or pupillary anomalies. Additional features include cataract (50–85%), glaucoma (30–50%), and keratopathy (20%). Aniridic keratopathy is caused by progressive limbal stem cell deficiency (LSCD), usually starting in the first decade of life.

Intracorneal Cyst

Rarely, intracorneal cyst can be found inside the corneal stroma. The mechanism remains unknown; however, glaucoma may be associated. Central anterior stromal thinning may be misinterpreted as clearing of corneal opacity. PKP may be undertaken but the prognosis depends on associated ocular signs and features.

Corneal Dystrophies

Corneal dystrophies that could present as congenital corneal opacities are congenital hereditary endothelial dystrophy (CHED), posterior polymorphous corneal dystrophy (PPCD), congenital stromal corneal dystrophy, and X-linked endothelial dystrophy **(Table 9)**. Management involves DSAEK in cases of CHED/PPCD if there is no significant

TABLE 9: Differentiating features between types of dystrophies at birth.

Congenital hereditary endothelial dystrophy	***Posterior polymorphous corneal dystrophy***	***Congenital stromal corneal dystrophy***	***X-linked endothelial dystrophy***
Autosomal recessive	Autosomal dominant	Autosomal dominant	X-linked
Mutations in the *SLC4A11* gene	Mutations in COL8A2, ZEB1	Mutations in decorin (DCN) gene	—
Diffuse, nonbullous severe corneal edema (thickness increased by two to three times) leading to bluish-gray ground glass appearance	Varying degree of corneal edema seen. Endothelial vesicles, geographic shaped lesions, and broad endothelial bands could be seen on the posterior corneal surface	Diffuse clouding with flake-like opacities throughout stroma. Corneal thickness is normal/ slightly thickened	Mild cases and asymptomatic carriers present with endothelial lesions resembling moon craters and subepithelial band keratopathy
Corneal clouding presents at birth usually	Onset in first or second decade with slow progression of corneal clouding over a decade	Corneal changes are present at birth and are stationary	Severe lesions present at birth with significant bilateral corneal clouding with a ground glass/milky appearance
Corneal thickness increased	Stromal edema can be seen	Corneal thickness normal or increased	—
No associated symptoms like epiphora/photophobia	Epiphora and photophobia with subsequent clouding of cornea, glaucoma, irregular astigmatism, and steep cornea	Asymptomatic	—

stromal scarring in the visual axis. Performing surgery at early age could improve visual development and potentially avoid amblyopia. If significant stromal scarring is present in visual axis, PKP is preferred. Rarely, PPCD can recur in graft.

Congenital Dermoids

They are congenital overgrowth of normal tissues in an abnormal location (choristoma). Three grades have been described based on the extent of involvement (Mann grading):

1. *Grade 1*: Most frequent type; single, small (usually <5 mm diameter) in the inferotemporal limbus generally involving superficial structures, present at birth and may enlarge during puberty. One-third cases could have associated syndrome complex such as Goldenhar syndrome (triad of epibulbar dermoid, preauricular appendages, and pretragal fistulas).
2. *Grade 2*: Larger, cover a part or entire cornea but does not involve DM or endothelium **(Figs. 7 and 8)**.
3. *Grade 3*: Most severe type; rarest; anterior segment is involved in this type.

Management depends of the grading. Grade 1 dermoid can be managed conservatively (except when inducing irregular astigmatism, amblyopia unresponsive to conservative management, progressive dellen, inadequate lid closure, and aesthesis). Surgical intervention ranging from simple excision to lamellar/penetrating grafts might be required for larger dermoids **(Figs. 8A and B)**.

Corneal Keloids

They are rare and usually occur following ocular trauma and perforations. Congenital corneal keloids are bilateral and have been described in Lowe syndrome, Rubinstein-Taybi syndrome, and ACL (acromegaly, cutis verticis gyrate, and corneal leukoma) syndrome. They may represent failure of normal differentiation of the corneal tissue. This must be distinguished from congenital dermoids **(Table 10)**.

Abnormalities of Corneal Size and Shape

- *Microcornea*: It refers to corneal diameter <10 mm (< 9 mm in newborns). It is commonly inherited as autosomal

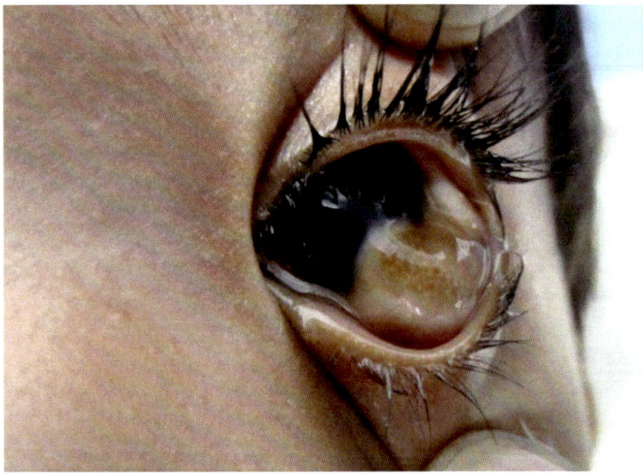

Fig. 7: Congenital dermoid.

TABLE 10: Differential diagnosis of dermoids.

Dermoid	*Keloid*	*Salzmann nodules*
They are yellowish-white elevated nodule containing hair follicles, sebaceous glands, sweat glands, bones, cartilages, or teeth, situated in the inferotemporal limbus usually. It can be central with often associated satellite lesions	They are chalky white solid masses with glistening appearance and the texture is usually gelatinous. Definitive diagnosis made with a corneal biopsy	They are multiple, bluish-white superficial corneal nodules usually seen in mid peripheral cornea. They are not present at birth and are usually associated with chronic ocular inflammation

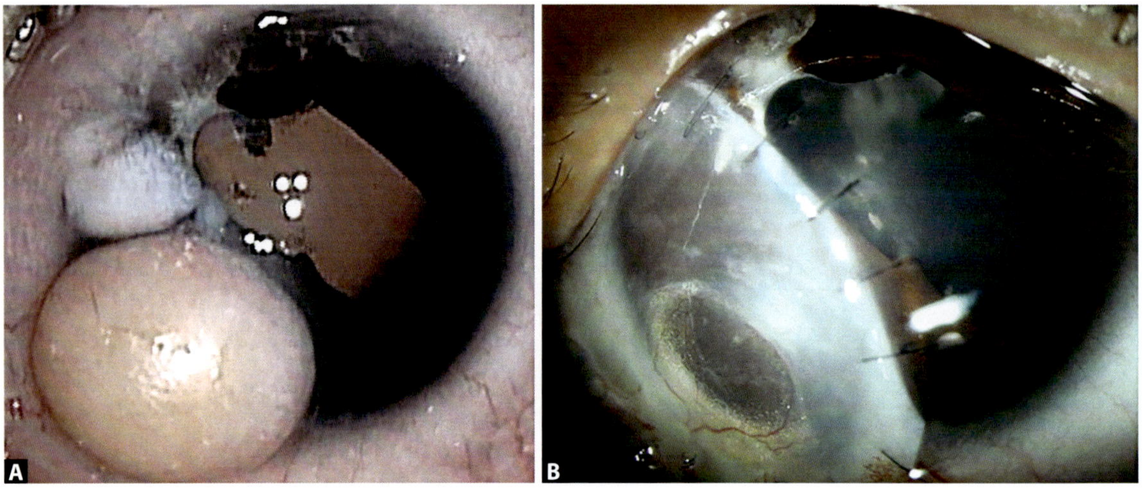

Figs. 8A and B: Lamellar keratoplasty for congenital dermoid.

dominant trait with mutation in the *PAX6* gene. This could be due to arrest of corneal growth during the 5th month of gestation. These corneas are relatively flat resulting in hyperopia and closed angles. Although microcornea occurs as isolated anomaly, it could be associated with congenital cataracts, anterior segment dysgenesis (PAX6 mutations), persistent fetal vasculature, and optic nerve hypoplasia. Ehlers-Danlos syndrome, myotonic dystrophy, and achondroplasia could be significant systemic associations. Associated refractive error, cataract, and glaucoma should be appropriately managed to prevent dense amblyopia.

- *Megalocornea*: It refers to bilateral, nonprogressive enlargement of the cornea usually >13 mm diameter (>12 mm in neonates). It is inherited as X-linked recessive trait with mutation in the CHRDL1 gene (chordin-like 1). This could be due to failure of growth of the anterior tips of optic cup to close leaving relatively large space for the cornea. This condition should be differentiated from PCG **(see Table 4)**. Arcus juvenilis, glaucoma, iris translucency, ectopia lentis, and cataract could be associated. Down syndrome, Alport syndrome, osteogenesis imperfecta, Marfan syndrome, tuberous sclerosis, dwarfism, ichthyosis, craniofacial anomalies, hypotonia, and intellectual disability are few nonocular associations. Similar to microcornea, associated refractive error, glaucoma and lens abnormalities should be addressed appropriately to prevent amblyopia. There can be zonular weakness and large capsular bag which would affect the centration of intraocular lens (IOL). Glued IOL or ACIOL placement could be difficult. Iris claw lens/suture fixation of IOL could be a viable option.
- *Cornea plana*: It refers to a congenitally flat cornea in which the radius of curvature is <43D (usually in the range of 30–35D). It is inherited as autosomal dominant/recessive trait with mutation in the KERA gene (12q22). It is often associated with high hyperopia (+10 D), sclerocornea, or microcornea. Other ocular associations include cornea clouding, angle-closure/open-angle glaucomas, and colobomas. Ehlers-Danlos syndrome is a known association. Refractive error management should be appropriately done in all cases and lamellar or full-thickness keratoplasty may be indicated if corneal clarity is compromised. Corneal transplantation holds high risk of rejection and postsurgical glaucoma.
- *Posterior keratoconus*: It is a rare developmental condition classified as an anterior cleavage syndrome. It can also be considered as the mildest variant of Peters' anomaly. It is unilateral, sporadic, nonprogressive, and noninflammatory condition of cornea characterized by local conical, internal protrusion of the posterior corneal curvature without protrusion of the anterior surface. It can be either generalized (keratoconus posticus generalis) or localized (keratoconus posticus circumscriptus) and may be associated with subtle anterior curvature irregularities which could result in irregular astigmatism and amblyopia that must be addressed at an early age.
- *Keratoglobus*: It is a congenital corneal ectatic disorder characterized by bilateral symmetric thinning and anterior protrusion of the cornea, the site of maximal thinning being mid-periphery. Keratometry values measure well into the 50–60 D range. Iron lines, Vogt striae, and apical scarring are typically absent. However, spontaneous breaks in DM and acute corneal hydrops occur in approximately 10% of eyes. It can be associated with brittle cornea syndrome and Ehlers-Danlos syndrome. These children are prone to phthisis bulbi secondary to spontaneous or post-traumatic globe/corneal rupture. Management involves effective refractive correction and wearing of protective eyewear. Corneal transplantation may be necessary for tectonic and optical purposes and is complicated by a mismatch between host and donor thickness.
- *Congenital anterior staphyloma and keratectasia*: In this condition, there is anterior protrusion of the cornea lined posteriorly by uveal tissue. Keratectasia refers to a similar protrusion san the uveal tissue. These may be a result of abnormal migration of neural crest cells into the developing cornea or any intrauterine corneal inflammations and infections. Associated corneal thinning and scarring can lead to poor fixation and dense amblyopia.
- *Congenital absence of cornea*: This represents an extreme deviation of normal corneal structure and may be associated with agenesis of anterior segment structures and anophthalmos. In ablepharon or complete cryptophthalmos, the cornea remains exposed since birth due to absence of eyelids on the globe.

ACQUIRED PEDIATRIC CORNEAL DISORDERS

While many corneal disorders acquired in early and late childhood are specific to pediatric population, others present similar to adults.

Dystrophies

It includes a group of corneal inherited disorders that are usually bilateral, symmetric, and slowly progressive, not related to systemic or environmental factors **(Figs. 9 to 11)**. Details are mentioned in **Table 11**.

Allergic Disorders

Seasonal Allergic Conjunctivitis and Perennial Allergic Conjunctivitis

Allergic conjunctivitis commonly occurs due to ocular irritation (type I hypersensitivity reaction) caused by circulating aeroallergens. It affects children and younger adults more

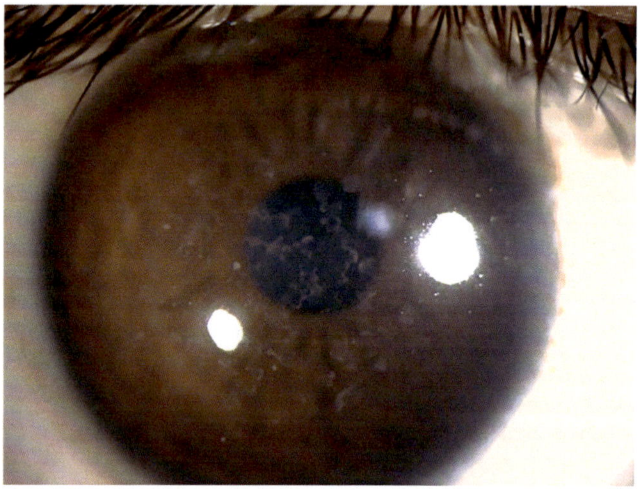

Fig. 9: Granular dystrophy.

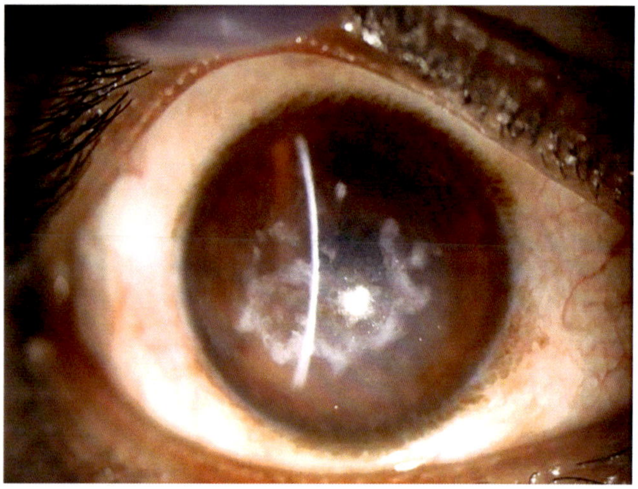

Fig. 10: Macular dystrophy.

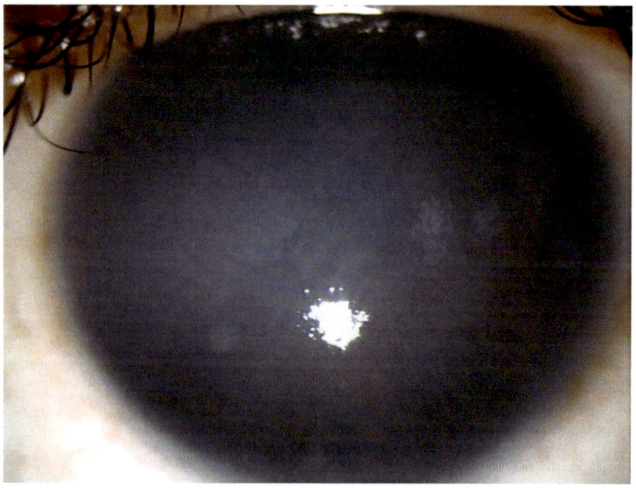

Fig. 11: Congenital hereditary endothelial dystrophy.

commonly. Seasonal allergic conjunctivitis (SAC) usually peaks at certain time of the year (spring and summer), inciting factor being an outdoor allergen (pollen), and perennial allergic conjunctivitis (PAC) is present throughout the year and is usually triggered by an indoor allergen (animal dander, dust mites, mold, air pollutants, and feathers). Watering, redness, and itching and puffy eyelids are the major presenting complaints, ocular pruritus being the cardinal symptom. Discharge is typically clear and watery, with symptoms being bilateral. Examination shows eyelid edema with mild congestion/hyperemia, chemosis, and papillary reaction on eyelid eversion. Avoidance and decreasing exposure to the allergen, cold compresses, preservative free lubricants, topical antihistaminics, and mast cell stabilizers are the mainstay of management. Low potency steroids (loteprednol 0.5% and fluorometholone) can also be used over a short course to reduce symptoms.

Vernal Keratoconjunctivitis

Vernal keratoconjunctivitis (VKC) is a chronic bilateral conjunctival inflammatory condition found in individuals predisposed to atopy. It presents before 10 years of age lasting 2–20 years until puberty. It shows a male predominance in younger population and is prevalent in residents of dry, hot climates with a significant history of other atopic manifestations. Tarsal conjunctiva shows neutral proteases tryptase- and chymase-positive MCs (MCTC), basophils, eosinophils, neutrophils, and mononuclear cells in hyperplastic epithelium, which are responsible for the allergic response and corneal erosions and ulcers occurring in VKC. Symptoms include severe itching and photophobia, with associated foreign body sensation, thick mucus discharge, and mechanical ptosis. Clinically, it is of three types—(1) papillary VKC (classic "cobblestone" flattened, discrete tarsal papillae >1 mm in size associated with ropy discharge), (2) limbal VKC (more gelatinous or confluent limbal papillae associated with Horner-Trantas spots, collections of epithelial cells and eosinophils, found around the limbus) **(Fig. 12)**, and (3) mixed VKC that shows features of both limbal and papillary VKC. Pseudogerontoxon (so named due to its resemblance to arcus senilis) can also be seen in the peripheral cornea as a superficial stromal gray-white deposition of lipids. Mediators from the inflamed tarsal conjunctiva can cause punctate epithelial keratitis that coalesces to give rise to frank epithelial erosions. These result in a plaque containing fibrin and mucous deposits over the defect, which impairs epithelial healing and causes neovascularization. This is called shield ulcer and has its lower border in the upper half of visual axis. Cameron has classified it into three grades and managed accordingly as given in **Table 12**. Due to long-standing corneal inflammation, VKC can lead to corneal opacity, irregular astigmatism, and keratoconus all of which can ultimately result in amblyopia in children.

Treatment is as follows:
- Avoidance of allergens and use of cold compresses
- Preservative-free artificial tears for symptomatic relief and wash-off of toxins

TABLE 11: Corneal dystrophies in children.

Dystrophy	*Inheritance*	*Clinical features*	*Light microscopy*	*Electron microscopy*	*Management*
Meesmann juvenile epithelial dystrophy	Autosomal dominant, mutation in corneal keratin (K3 or K12)	Intraepithelial microcysts or vesicles primarily in the visual axis and in the midperiphery, children are usually asymptomatic	Epithelial microcysts consisting of degenerated epithelial cells, thickened basement membrane, increased glycogen in basal epithelial cells	Collections of granular and filamentary material ("peculiar substance") within the cytoplasm of epithelial cells	Lubricating ointments and BCL for minute erosions, rarely surgical intervention
CDB-I or Reis-Bücklers corneal dystrophy (RBCD)	Autosomal dominant, variant of GCD	Recurrent corneal erosions beginning in childhood followed by early and fairly marked visual loss from corneal scarring	Region of Bowman's membrane and basement membrane is replaced with a fibrocellular scar tissue that has an undulating "sawtooth" configuration	Ultrastructural deposits of rod-like bodies	Lubricants and BCL, superficial keratectomy or PTK for painful erosions, DALK and PKP for deeper scarring and opacities
CDB-II or Thiel–Behnke corneal dystrophy	Autosomal dominant	Similar to CDB-I, however, vision loss occurs at later age in life	Similar to CDB-I	"Curly" fibers appear in the region of Bowman's membrane	Similar to RBCD
Granular corneal dystrophy (GCD)	Autosomal dominant; conservative mutation in transforming growth factor beta (TGFB1) on chromosome 5q31	Small discrete well-demarcated greyish white opacities in the central anterior stroma with intervening clear areas, later coalesce and extend into the periphery. Three morphological types namely, (1) drop-shaped, (2) bread crumb-shaped and (3) ring-shaped. Mild photophobia in early stages with loss of vision in 5th decade	Eosinophilic hyaline deposits which stain bright red with Masson trichrome and weakly with periodic acid Schiff and keratoepithelin	Homogeneous moth-eaten pattern in the inner structures. Hyperreflective round or trapezoidal deposits in the corneal stroma on confocal microscopy	Superficial keratectomy or PTK for lesions involving the superficial 100 μm, anterior lamellar keratoplasty or PKP for lesions beyond 100 μm
Lattice corneal dystrophy	Autosomal dominant disorder associated with (Arg124Cys) mutation in TGFB1 gene	Discrete, ovoid/round subepithelial opacities, anterior stromal white dots and refractile filamentary lines, panstromal haze as disease advances. Recurrent corneal erosions in 1st to 2nd decade of life	Irregular, eosinophilic amyloid deposits distorting configuration of stromal lamellae Green birefringence and red-green dichroism on polarizing filter	Electron dense fibrils of 80–100 Å diameter	Similar to GCD
Macular corneal dystrophy	Autosomal recessive, mutations in the N-acetylglucosamine 6-O-sulfotransferase gene (CHST6) on chromosome 16 (16q22.1)	Stromal opacities with indistinct margins and hazy intervening stroma, the lesions extend till limbus with central lesions being more anterior than peripheral ones, associated stromal thinning and abnormal endothelium	Degeneration of the basal epithelial cells, and focal epithelial thinning over the accumulated material, Bowman's layer may be irregular, thinned, or absent in some areas	Accumulation of glycosaminoglycans in keratocytes, extracellular matrix and endothelial cells, guttae and infiltration of posterior nonbanded layer of DM with vesicular and granular material	Similar to CDB

Contd...

Contd...

Dystrophy	Inheritance	Clinical features	Light microscopy	Electron microscopy	Management
Congenital stromal corneal dystrophy	Autosomal dominant, mutations involving Decorin gene on chromosome 12q21.33	Focal white stromal opacities in addition to diffuse stromal haze in the central anterior stroma, diminution of vision along with searching nystagmus and dense amblyopia	Normally aligned collagen fibrils alternate with randomly arranged fibrils (radially arranged with 1/2 the normal diameter)	Increased reflectivity of the stroma on confocal microscopy	PKP should be planned as early as possible to avoid amblyopia
Posterior polymorphous corneal dystrophy	Autosomal dominant; three locus of genes (COL8A2, ZEB1)	• Incidentally diagnosed, vesicle-like lesions involving DM and endothelium, band lesions or diffuse opacities • Endothelial guttae corneal edema, PAS, iris atrophy with or without corectopia and elevated IOP	Severe cases show signs of chronic edema, subepithelial fibrosis and band keratopathy	Focal areas of endothelium containing large squamous epithelial cells with large numbers of tonofilaments attached to prominent desmosomal intercellular junctions. Abnormal posterior nonbanded zone appears like a second DM	Most patients are asymptomatic and do not require active management
Congenital hereditary endothelial dystrophy	Autosomal recessive; mutations in SLC4A11 gene (locus 20p13-12)	Severe corneal edema and scarring in childhood. Gray-blue, ground-glass haziness of cornea within the first week to 6 months of age with limited progression over the next few decades	Thickened epithelium, subepithelial fibrosis, calcification and varying loss of Bowman's membrane, thickened stroma with severe lamellar disorganization and visible pockets of interstitial fluid	Abnormal posterior nonbanded zone of DM, endothelium is either absent or demonstrates a reduced number of cells that are predominantly vacuolated and dystrophic	Most children require corneal transplantation in early life. While PKP is commonly performed, DSAEK is recently rising as an effective alternative
X-Linked endothelial corneal dystrophy (XECD)	X-linked, mapped to the genetic locus Xq25, affects males much more severely than females	Moon crater-like changes in the endothelium to diffuse haze or milky, ground-glass appearance. Depending on visual acuity, nystagmus may be present	Irregular thinning of the epithelium and Bowman's layer, thickened and irregular DM with loss of endothelial cells or atypical multilayering	Subepithelial amorphous deposits of granular material consistent with BSK and abnormal anterior banded zone	PKP is the preferred surgical treatment for children with significant corneal clouding and BSK

(BCL: bandage contact lens; BSK: band-shaped keratopathy; corneal dystrophy of Bowman's membrane; DALK: deep anterior lamellar keratoplasty; DM: Descemet membrane; GCD: granular corneal dystrophy; IOP: intraocular pressure; PAS: peripheral anterior synechiae; PAS: periodic acid-Schiff; PKP: penetrating keratoplasty; RBCD: Reis–Bücklers' corneal dystrophy)

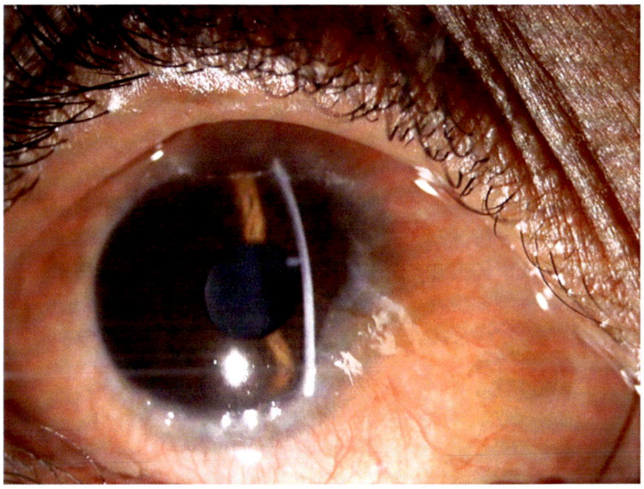

Fig. 12: Horner-Trantas dots in VKC.

TABLE 12: Cameron classification of shield ulcers.

Grades	*Characteristics*	*Management*
Grade 1	Ulcer with transparent base	Medical management including supratarsal steroid injection
Grade 2	Translucent base/ opaque white/yellow deposits	Debridement of ulcer with medical management ± amniotic membrane transplantation (AMT)
Grade 3	Elevated plaque above the level of adjacent normal epithelium	Debridement + AMT ± PTK

(PTK: penetrating keratoplasty)

- Topical antihistamines (olopatadine, ketotifen, epinastine, or azelastine) can be used for symptomatic relief. Topical mast cell stabilizers (cromolyn sodium) can be used to prevent further degranulation of mast cells and release of histamine and other chemotactic factors.
- Topical nonsteroidal anti-inflammatory drugs (NSAIDs) block prostaglandin biosynthesis and can be used as additive drugs to reduce hyperemia and pruritus.
- Topical decongestants cause vasoconstriction and can be employed to relieve ocular erythema. However, these have no effect on allergic inflammatory response.
- For seasonal exacerbation, short-term pulse dose of topical steroids (dexamethasone 0.1%, prednisolone phosphate 1%, or difluprednate 0.05%) eight times a day up to 1 week and then tapered.
- Topical calcineurin inhibitors (cyclosporin A 0.05% up to four times/day and tacrolimus 0.3%) in chronic, unresponsive cases can be utilized as steroid sparing drugs.
- Immunotherapy, whether via the subcutaneous route or the intranasal or sublingual route, should be considered in the treatment of persistent severe cases refractory to conventional treatment.
- Systemic immune suppression, in conjunction with a pediatric rheumatologist, is indicated for severe cases of ocular allergy unresponsive to topical treatment where progressive cicatrization is vision-threatening.

Atopic Keratoconjunctivitis (AKC)

It is a bilateral chronic inflammation of the conjunctiva and lids in association with atopic dermatitis. This can secondarily affect the cornea in the form of corneal ulceration, superficial punctuate keratitis, and corneal neovascularization. It consists of both type I and IV hypersensitivity reaction. The disease typically begins in late teens but may present until fourth or fifth decade of life. Around 95% of atopic keratoconjunctivitis (AKC) patients also have eczema and 87% have history of asthma. Majority are diagnosed by 5 years of age with male predominance. As in VKC, mast cells and eosinophils are present in conjunctival epithelium with an increase in CD4:CD8 ratio with elevated serum IgE. Symptoms are itching, watering, mucous discharge, redness, decreased vision, photophobia, and pain. Clinical signs include:

- Skin—periocular scaling, flaking dermatitis with a reddened base (eczema), Dennie-Morgan lines, and allergic shiners (darkness and swelling underneath the eyes).
- Lid margins—cicatricial ectropion, lagophthalmos, lateral canthal ulceration, madarosis, meibomitis, keratinization, punctal ectropion, entropion, and trichiasis.
- Conjunctiva—pale white edema with papillary reaction more prominent in inferior fornix, subepithelial fibrosis, fornix shortening and symblepharon, erythema and chemosis in bulbar conjunctiva, and lower tarsal conjunctiva.
- Cornea—superficial punctate keratitis, neovascularization, persistent epithelial defect, and filamentary keratitis.

Other associations of AKC include herpetic keratitis, keratoconus, and atopic cataracts. The treatment involves use of topical steroids, antihistamines, mast cell stabilizers, and immunomodulators. Avoidance of allergens and a multifaceted treatment approach are required with involvement of a physician/an allergist. Associated uncontrolled vision threatening corneal complications indicate the need for oral steroids.

Giant Papillary Conjunctivitis (GPC)

It is a noninfectious inflammatory disorder involving the superior tarsal conjunctiva, characterized by presence of papillae >0.3 mm in diameter. The risk factors inciting giant papillary conjunctivitis (GPC) are hydrophilic/rigid-gas permeable contact lens (CL) wear, glaucoma filtering blebs, exposed sutures, ocular prosthetics, and extruded scleral buckles. Clinical features include mild hyperemia of the upper tarsal conjunctiva, conjunctival translucency and opacification, and ropy whitish mucoid discharge concentrated in the medial and inferior fornix. Papillae, with cobblestone appearance, ranging from 0.3 to 1.75 mm occur with continued exposure to inciting agents in the upper fornix. Conjunctiva shows increase in the number of goblet cells with interpapillary clefts having nongoblets cells secreting mucin. Substantia propria is infiltrated with eosinophils and basophils, increased number of lymphocytes, mast cells, and plasma cells. The pathogenesis of GPC involves the combined effect of mechanical trauma and subsequent immune response to antigens or environmental factors. Primary treatment involves immediate removal of the inciting factor. In children with keratoconus or anisometropia, CL wear cannot be totally discontinued owing to resulting handicap and risk of amblyopia. In such cases, daily disposable lenses, modifying the patient's routine use, and care of CLs can be done. Lens should be assessed for deposits and preservatives used in CL solutions need to be modified. Medical management advocates use of topical corticosteroids for the initial inflammatory phase, NSAIDs, mast cell stabilizers, and histamine receptor blockers.

Phlyctenular Keratoconjunctivitis

It is a type IV hypersensitivity reaction, which occurs commonly in response tuberculoprotein and staphylococcal antigen, commonly presenting in the teenage years. Sensitization of the cornea or conjunctiva to a microbial antigen and a repeat exposure to the same antigen results in phlyctenule formation. Corneal phlyctenules typically occur at the limbus with an intense conjunctival injection and undergo necrosis forming marginal ulcer typically triangular in shape with its base toward the limbus, resolving with scarring. Management involves treating the inciting cause (tuberculosis/staphylococcal blepharitis). Short-term course of topical steroids can be used to reduce inflammation. Later topical steroid sparing agents such as cyclosporine A are advocated. Long-term treatment involves preventing recurrences through exogenous sources.

Traumatic

Children are particularly prone to ocular injuries due to their physically active nature and unsupervised child play.

Traumatic Corneal Perforation

It is full thickness defect of the cornea, mostly occurring due to injury with sharp objects **(Fig. 13)** but can also occur after globe rupture secondary to blunt trauma. Although difficult to obtain in preverbal and preschool going children, all attempts should be made to obtain a good history about the nature and the mode of the injury. The extent of the injury should be assessed; posterior segment examination by ultrasound and radiological imaging to rule out intraocular foreign body should be done. Corneal perforation repair is an emergency and is usually done under general anesthesia. The goal of surgery is restoration of globe integrity and salvaging vision. Corneal wounds are usually closed using 10–0 nylon interrupted sutures. If there is rupture in the anterior lens capsule, lens aspiration can be done along with primary closure. In injuries associated with iris tissue prolapse, the tissue should be reposited and preserved unless necrosed. A water-tight closure of wound with burial of suture knots in the stroma is done. Longer and widely spaced sutures are placed in the periphery to ensure corneal flattening with shorter and closely placed sutures centrally. In case of difficulty in apposition due to loss of tissue, cyanoacrylate glue can be used along with BCL. Postoperatively topical antibiotics, steroids, and cycloplegics are given to reduce inflammation. Early suture removal can be planned depending on the age and healing response for faster refractive stability and optical correction. Sometimes, rigid CL and PKP may be required to battle corneal astigmatism in these cases.

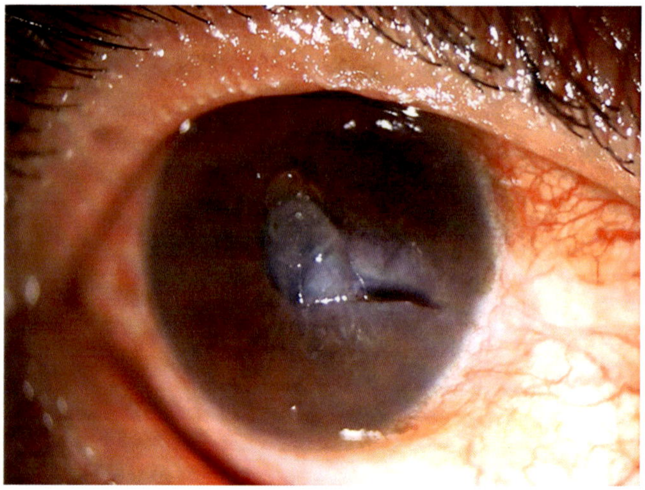

Fig. 13: Traumatic corneal perforation.

TABLE 13: List of common acids and alkalis causing injury.

Alkalis	*Acids*
• Ammonium hydroxide	• Sulfuric acid
• Sodium hydroxide	• Sulfurous acid
• Potassium hydroxide	• Hydrofluoric acid
• Magnesium hydroxide	• Acetic acid
• Calcium hydroxide	• Hydrochloric acid

Chemical Injury

Chemical injuries remain a frequent cause of ocular morbidity in children particularly from developing countries. Common alkalis and acids causing injury are listed in **Table 13**. In thermochemical injuries resulting from accidental firecracker bursts and battery blasts, the child is usually a bystander and not an active participant. Alkali injury causes formation of calcium soaps which precipitate and limit ocular penetration. Acid injuries cause damage to ocular tissues by dissociated

TABLE 14: Dua's grading of chemical injury.

Grade	*Clock hours of limbal involvement*	*Conjunctival involvement*	*Analog scale*	*Prognosis*
I	0	0%	0/0%	Very good
II	<3	<30%	0.1–3/1–29.9%	Good
III	>3–6	>30–50%	3.1–6/30–50%	Good
IV	>6–9	>50–75%	6.1–9/ 51–75%	Good to guarded
V	>9<12	>75<100%	9.1–11.9/75.1–99.9%	Guarded to poor
VI	12	100%	12/100%	Very poor

protons and deeper penetration of ocular tissues. The prognosis of chemical injuries depends on its grading (Dua's grading) as given in **Table 14**. Analog scale in the same table shows limbal involvement in clock hours/% conjunctival involvement. Children are usually uncooperative or irritable after chemical injuries; hence, a complete examination of both eyes should be done under general anesthesia.

Following is the immediate treatment line for acute presentation of chemical injury.

- Thorough irrigation with double eversion of fornices till the pH normalizes and sweeping the fornices with glass rod to prevent symblepharon formation
- Preservative free topical antibiotics, corticosteroids, and preservative free lubricants
- Topical ascorbate to reduce the incidence of corneal thinning and ulceration
- Topical sodium citrate 10% to prevent and retard the progression of ulcers
- Cycloplegic agents to reduce pain and posterior synechiae formation
- Umbilical cord serum and blood serum in grade III, IV, and V chemical injuries
- Amniotic membrane transplantation (AMT) to enhance epithelialization and reduce inflammation in severe chemical injury. While postoperative complications are rarely encountered, graft dislodgement can occur due to habitual rubbing of eyes in children. Use of a symblepharon ring or Cartella shield may help in preventing this
- Tenonplasty flaps, conjunctival flaps, and oral mucosal epithelial cell transplantation can also be used to promote epithelialization.

Inflammatory

Peripheral Ulcerative Keratitis

It is an autoimmune condition which occurs in association with immune-mediated and rheumatic diseases. History of underlying connective tissue disorder should be elicited and correlated with systemic exacerbation. The most common associated disease is rheumatoid arthritis/juvenile idiopathic arthritis in children. The initial lesion occurs in a zone 1–2 mm within the limbus as a crescent-shaped epithelial defect with stromal thinning with vaso-occlusion of associated limbal vessels. The leading edges are undermined and the ulcer progresses circumferentially. It may be unilateral or bilateral and may be associated with scleritis. Symptoms include pain, watering, redness and photophobia, and decrease in visual acuity due to associated iritis and irregular astigmatism. Complete systemic work-up including complete blood count, erythrocyte sedimentation rate, rheumatoid factor, antinuclear antibodies, antineutrophil cytoplasmic antibodies, X-ray chest and sacroiliac joint, liver enzymes, serum angiotensin convertase enzyme and calcium, hepatitis C, urine, and stool examination is to be done to diagnose the underlying disease. Definitive management involves identifying the underlying disorder and advocating systemic management as advised by rheumatologist. Local therapy includes topical steroids, preservative free lubricants, and topical cyclosporine. Surgically excision or recession of the adjacent conjunctiva can promote healing of ulcer. Impending perforation or perforated peripheral ulcerative keratitis (PUK) can be treated with tectonic patch grafts.

Mooren's Ulcer

A PUK, in the absence of an underlying etiology is termed as Mooren's ulcer and hence, a diagnosis of exclusion. A bilateral aggressive presentation which progresses rapidly from the periphery to center is commonly seen in younger population. It represents the final common pathway of immune response to various insults occurring in the cornea in susceptible patients. The immune components diffuse from the limbal vessels into the inflamed corneal stroma, with ulcer occurring in the periphery. The clinical presentation is same as PUK, except scleritis is hardly ever seen. Local management is also similar to PUK. Systemic immunosuppression can be given in bilateral severe Mooren's ulcer not responding to conventional topical therapy and surgical management.

Marginal Staphylococcal Keratitis

It is a type III hypersensitivity reaction that occurs due to immune response triggered by chronic staphylococcal colonization in eyelids. The lesions occur 1–2 mm from the limbus permitting a clear lucid interval between the lesion and the limbus. Children present with pain, photophobia, irritation, and congestion. The catarrhal lesions occur typically in the 2, 4, 8, and 10 o' clock positions where the lid margin crosses the limbus. Spontaneous resolution occurs in 2–3 weeks. Topical corticosteroids are the mainstay of management. Lid hygiene along with antibiotic ointment for eyelid margin should be advocated to treat staphylococcal blepharitis and prevent recurrences.

Scleritis

It is a chronic, painful condition which presents with edema and cellular infiltration of the sclera. In children, posterior scleritis is more commonly prevalent than anterior scleritis. Among anterior scleritis, nodular scleritis is the most common presentation. Most common cause is idiopathic, but scleritis associated with granulomatosis polyangiitis and tuberculosis has also been described. Children with posterior scleritis present with severe inflammation, orbital involvement, lid signs, and restriction of extraocular movements, and may be associated with anterior scleritis. Necrotizing scleritis, however, is extremely rare in children. Peripheral cornea can rarely be affected due to extension of inflammatory process from the sclera. The mainstay of treatment is with topical and systemic steroids and treatment of the underlying condition.

Immune-mediated Diseases

Immune-mediated diseases prevalent in children are Steven-Johnson syndrome (SJS), toxic epidermal necrolysis (TEN), and erythema multiforme (EM) **(Table 15)**. These are type 4 hypersensitivity reactions which occur following immune mechanism to certain drugs (NSAID, sulfonamide drugs, and anticonvulsants) or following a viral infection. The ocular and dermatologic manifestations occur after a prodrome of fever and myalgia headache. Acute phase is characterized by nonspecific mononuclear inflammation of the cornea and conjunctiva followed by a cicatricial chronic phase. It can range from mild hyperemia to sloughing of the mucosal surfaces. The inciting agent should be identified and avoided in the future to prevent life-threatening complications. Topical steroids, preservative free lubricants, and regular sweeping of fornices to prevent symblepharon formation constitute acute phase management. AMT extending into the fornices can be considered in patients with extensive mucosal erosion. Prognosis remains grim in severe cases due to poor ocular surface hindering successful corneal transplantation.

TABLE 15: Classification of SJS, TEN and EM.

Classification	*Involvement*
Bullous EM	<10% BSA
SJS	<10% BSA
SJS-TEN	10-30% BSA
TEN with spots	>30% BSA
TEN without spots	10% BSA

(BSA: body surface area; EM: erythema multiforme; TEN: toxic epidermal necrolysis (TEN); SJS: Stevens-Johnson syndrome)

Infective

Ophthalmia Neonatorum

It refers to inflammation of conjunctiva in the first month of life. The various etiology, symptoms, and management have been tabulated below **(Table 16)**. Cornea should always be examined after fluorescein staining in children presenting with this condition as gonococcal and herpetic conjunctivitis can cause keratitis in neonates. Also, the former has a rapid progression and can also be systemically dangerous. The condition should also be differentiated from congenital nasolacrimal duct obstruction and dacryocystitis. These children need urgent pediatric referral and hospital admission depending on the severity. Besides, the mother should also be evaluated for any genital tract infections.

Trachoma

Trachoma, once a leading cause of preventable blindness, has been eliminated from India since 2017 (elimination criteria—prevalence of active infection below 10 years of age <5%). The causative organism is *Chlamydia trachomatis* serovars A, B, Ba, and C. As the organism is transmitted by vectors such as flies, children remain at high risk of acquiring the infection. Acute trachoma conjunctivitis manifests as follicular conjunctivitis in the superior palpebral conjunctiva with papillary hypertrophy. Chronic inflammation results in cicatricial findings such as Arlt's line (linear white scar parallel to eyelid margin in the superior tarsal conjunctiva), entropion, trichiasis, diffuse punctal epithelial keratopathy with superficial pannus, and Herbert's pits (pigmented lesions in the superior limbus representing resolved follicles). The World Health Organization (WHO) grading of trachoma is detailed in **Table 17**. Treatment includes SAFE strategy (surgery for trichiatic lashes, antibiotics—single dose azithromycin for active disease, facial cleanliness, and environmental improvement to prevent spread).

Microbial Keratitis

Pediatric microbial keratitis is more dangerous in children due to a greater inflammatory response in them. Viral **(Fig. 14)** and bacterial etiologies are more common in children comparison to fungal. Various risk factors for acquiring microbial keratitis in children include trauma, CL wear, and ocular disease such as VKC, chronic blepharitis, ocular rosacea, eyelid abnormalities, corneal anesthesia, and systemic diseases such as systemic immunodeficiencies, hypoxic encephalopathy, measles, severe prematurity, SJS/TEN, vitamin, or protein energy deficiencies. Iatrogenic causes such as sutures, and topical steroids should also be ruled out. HSV recurrences are reported to occur more frequently in the pediatric population, with up to 80% of pediatric patients experiencing recurrences within as little as 15 months of the first episode. Examination under general anesthesia for corneal scraping for Gram and potassium

TABLE 16: Ophthalmia neonatorum: Etiology, symptoms, and management.

Etiology	*Symptoms*	*Management*
Chemical conjunctivitis	• Due to use of 2% silver nitrate used to prevent gonococcal conjunctivitis • Transient redness, resolves in 24–48 hours	Self-resolving; 0.5% erythromycin has replaced silver nitrate
N. Gonorrhoeae	Occurs 2–5 days after birth; serosanguinous discharge progressing to thick purulent discharge, conjunctival membranes, lid edema, and chemosis; can penetrate intact corneal epithelium and cause ulceration if untreated	• Single dose ceftriaxone 125 mg IM (or) • Injection cefotaxime 25 mg/kg IV/IM every 8–12 hours for 7 days (or) • Oral fluoroquinolones • Hourly irrigation of eyes with saline along with topical fluoroquinolones
Other bacterial (*H. influenzae, S. aureus, Strep. pneumoniae*, and *P. aeruginosa*)	Occurs 5–8 days after birth; lid edema chemosis, purulent discharge	• Gram-positive cocci—eye ointment tetracycline 1%/erythromycin 0.5% • Gram-negative bacilli—eye ointment tobramycin 0.3%/ciprofloxacin 0.5%
Chlamydia	Occurs 5–14 days after birth; can also be hyperacute; presents with mild mucopurulent palpebral conjunctivitis, moderate lid edema, and chemosis.	Oral erythromycin ethylsuccinate suspension 50 mg/kg/day in three to four divided doses for 14 days
Viral—herpes simplex	Occurs 6–14 days after birth; eyelid edema and serous discharge ± vesicular lesions on skin/lid margins	• Eye ointment acyclovir 5% five times/day for no >14 days to avoid epithelial toxicity • Systemic acyclovir 30 mg/kg/day for 10 days

TABLE 17: WHO grading system for trachoma.

Grade	*Definition*
Trachomatous inflammation—follicular (TF)	≥5 follicles ≥0.5 mm in the upper tarsal conjunctiva
Trachomatous inflammation—intense (TI)	Pronounced inflammatory thickening of the upper tarsal conjunctiva obscuring >1/2 of normal deep tarsal vessels
Trachomatous scarring (TS)	Scarring in tarsal conjunctiva
Trachomatous trichiasis (TT)	At least one eyelash rubbing the cornea
Corneal opacity (CO)	Visible opacity over the pupil

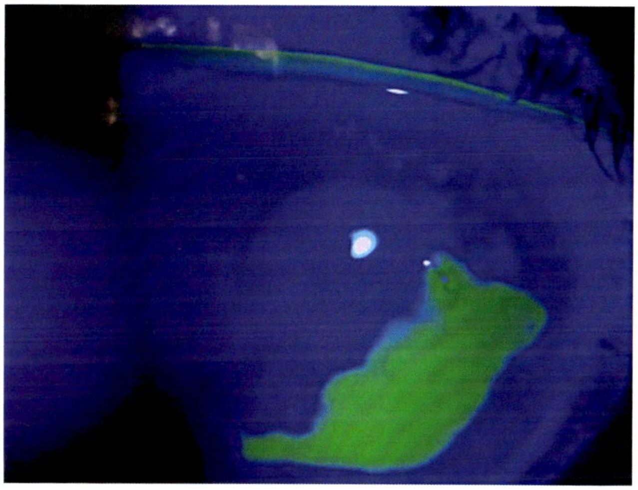

Fig. 14: Geographic ulcer in HSV keratitis.

hydroxide staining and bacterial and fungal culture may be required in young children and neonates. The various etiological presentations and their management are tabulated in **Table 18**.

Ectatic Disorder

Keratoconus is the most common ectatic disorder of the cornea that presents in early childhood **(Fig. 15)**. It refers to bilateral (90%, asymmetric) noninflammatory conical-shaped protrusion of the cornea commonly associated with its progressive steepening and irregular thinning. Keratectasia secondary to corneal trauma and keratitis has also been reported in literature. Although the mechanism remains unknown, keratoconus is characterized by changes in corneal collagen structure and organization that cause biomechanical instability with subsequent development of irregular astigmatism, progressive myopia, corneal thinning, and central corneal scarring, all of which can lead to mild to marked impairment in visual acuity. The onset is most common during adolescence and puberty, although it can occasionally be present in children as young as 4 years, especially in the setting of chronic eye rubbing. It is typically progressive until the third or fourth decade of life, when it usually arrests. Corneal hydrops associated with keratoconus has been described in children as young as 6 years of age. Although there remains a greater incidence of keratoconus in relatives of patients with the disorder, epigenetic and environmental factors certainly play a role in expression and progression of keratoconus. Clinical presentation, diagnosis, and management are similar to adult patients **(Table 19)**. However, it has to be remembered that keratoconus tends to be more severe and rapidly progressive in children, especially those with central cones, which are more common in this population and more visually significant than peripheral

TABLE 18: Etiology, clinical features, and management of microbial keratitis.

Feature	***Bacterial***	***Viral***	***Fungal***
Organisms	*P. aeruginosa*, *S. aureus*, α-hemolytic streptococci, gonococcal	Herpes simplex	*Fusarium* and *Alternaria*
Onset	Acute	Acute	Long-standing
Symptoms	Excessive mucopurulent discharge, pain redness with excessive photophobia, diminution of vision	Pain, redness, and diminution of vision	Redness, watering, pain, and diminution of vision, wherein symptoms are relatively lesser than signs
Signs	Large central or paracentral epithelial defect with dense suppurative stromal infiltrate ± necrosis with intense stromal edema	• *Primary:* – *Epithelial keratitis*: Small vesicles, dendritic ulcer, and geographic ulcer • *Recurrences:* – *Stromal involvement*: Immune mediated, necrotizing, and neurotrophic – *Endotheliitis*: Disciform, diffuse, and linear	Epithelial defect with fluffy cotton-wool like infiltrate with fuzzy margins ± satellite lesions ± hypopyon
Management	• Combined therapy with fortified aminoglycoside and cephalosporin or monotherapy with fluoroquinolone eye drops every 5 minutes—1st day, then every 30minutes—2nd day and then tapered. A loading dose of a drop every 5 minutes for the first 30 minutes for severe ulcers. • Systemic antibiotics for perforation, extensive infection, scleritis, or endophthalmitis	• *Epithelial keratitis*: Topical acyclovir, prophylactic antibacterial agents • *Stromal and endothelial keratitis*: Topical and oral acyclovir + topical corticosteroid • *Neurotrophic keratitis*: Cautious use of topical acyclovir, steroids and other anti-inflammatory medications • Preservative-free lubricants, BCL, AMT, tarsorrhaphy, or conjunctival flaps	• Topical natamycin 5% ± topical azoles • Systemic antifungals for perforation, extensive infection, scleritis, or endophthalmitis

(AMT: amniotic membrane transplantation; BCL: bandage contact lenses)

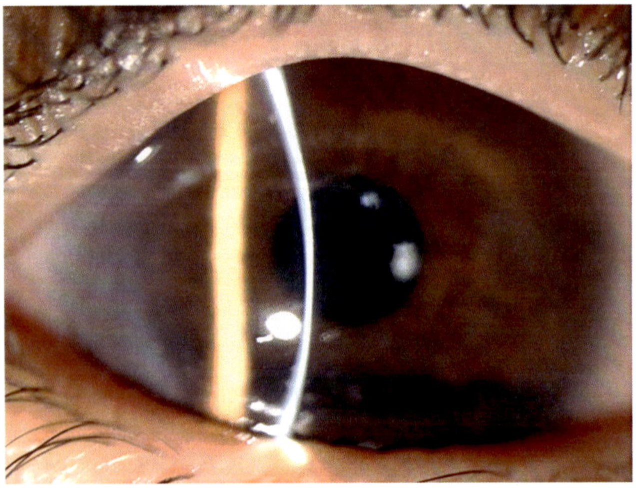

Fig. 15: Keratoconus.

cones. Low threshold should be maintained for collagen cross-linking in view of rapid progression. Standard procedure (epithelium-off Dresden protocol) is preferred in children as it has been shown to be successful in most studies. A close follow-up (every 1–3 months rather than 6–12 months as is done in adults) is required to monitor progression and repeat procedures may be necessary.

Iatrogenic

Contact Lens-induced Corneal Changes

Children are usually prescribed CLs for large refractive errors, symptomatic anisometropia, irregular astigmatism, or ocular surface disease, particularly during the critical period for amblyopia. The choice of CL depends on the indication, intended wearing schedule, and lens material and its design features necessary to achieve the therapeutic or refractive goals. Similar to adults, children remain at risk of acquiring CL-related complications such as microbial keratitis (*P. aeruginosa*, *Acanthamoeba*, and fungi), discomfort, dry eye, GPC, punctate keratopathy, corneal hypoxia, edema, deep stromal opacities and neovascularization, and reactivation of herpes. Risks for adverse events are higher in teenagers, especially in late adolescence due to poor CL hygiene and wearing schedule. Overnight wear, failing to wash hands before lens handling, choice of cleaning, disinfection and storage solutions, adherence to recommended replacement schedule, and practices with regard to use of solutions and storage cases are risk factors for CL-associated microbial keratitis. Complication rates can be decreased by appropriate education of children regarding CL use and replacement and by actively involving the guardians in CL schedule.

TABLE 19: Keratoconus in children.

Ocular associations	*Systemic associations*
• Atopic dermatitis • Ocular allergic tendencies • Retinitis pigmentosa • Blue sclera • Leber congenital amaurosis	• Magnesium deficiency • Down's syndrome • Turner syndrome • Marfan syndrome • Ehlers–Danlos syndrome • Mental retardation • Osteogenesis imperfecta • Pseudoxanthoma elasticum

Histopathology:
- Epithelium shows central thinning, with irregular or thickened basement membrane, reduced basal epithelial density and defects in the Bowman layer
- Decreased subbasal nerve density
- Stromal scarring and apoptosis in proximity to breaks in the Bowman layer, loss of stromal collagen lamellae and altered collagen fibril orientation, decreased keratocyte density, particularly in the central anterior stroma
- Descemet membrane and endothelium are generally unaffected, except in cases with corneal hydrops, although elongation of endothelial cells with pleomorphism can occur

Clinical signs:
- Conical protrusion of the cornea with stromal thinning
- *Fleischer ring*: Iron line partially or completely surrounding the cone
- *Vogt's striae*: Fine vertical lines in the posterior stroma
- *Munson's sign*: V-shaped conformation of the lower lid produced by the ectatic cornea in downgaze
- *Rizzuti's sign*: A sharply focused beam of light near the nasal limbus seen on illumination of temporal limbus

Tools for diagnosis and monitoring progression:
- Computer-assisted videophotokeratoscopy (VKG)
  - Placido disk-based computer videokeratoscopes
  - VK indices (Central K, I-S and KISA) are significantly increased in keratoconus patients and unaffected relatives of keratoconus patients
- Orbscan
  - Slit scanning with Placido-based topography analysis
  - Increase in maximum posterior elevation compared with the best fit sphere (BFS)
  - Irregularity in the central 3 mm and 5 mm zones
  - Displacement of the corneal apex
  - Decrease in thinnest-point pachymetry
  - Increase in the mean simulated keratometry minimum value
- Pentacam
  - Scheimpflug principle
  - Similar to Orbscan
- Ocular response analyzer
  - Excessive higher order aberrations
  - Lower values of corneal hysteresis and corneal resistance factor

Amsler-Krumeich classification:
- *Stage I*:
  - Eccentric corneal steepening
  - Induced myopia and/or astigmatism <5 D
  - Mean keratometry ≤48 D
  - Vogt's striae, no scars
- *Stage II*:
  - Induced myopia and/or astigmatism >5 D, <8 D
  - Keratometry ≤53 D

Contd...

Contd...

  - Absence of scarring
  - Minimal apical corneal thickness >400 μm
- *Stage III*:
  - Induced myopia and/or astigmatism >8D, <10D
  - Keratometry >53D
  - Absence of scarrring
  - Minimal apical corneal thickness 300–400 μm
- *Stage IV*:
  - Refraction not measurable
  - Keratometry >55D
  - Central scars, perforation
  - Minimal apical corneal thickness <300 μm

Treatment:
- *Preventing progression*: Collagen cross linking
- *Optical correction*:
  - *Early stages*: Spectacle correction and soft contact lens
  - *Moderate stages*: Rigid CL, rarely intracorneal ring segments
  - *Severe stages*: Deep anterior lamellar keratoplasty and penetrating keratoplasty

Radiation Keratopathy

Children may be administered radiation therapy in the form of external beam radiotherapy or brachytherapy for various ocular (retinoblastoma) and extraocular (rhabdomyosarcomas) tumors as well as other head and neck tumors (non-Hodgkin's lymphomas, nasopharyngeal carcinomas, osteosarcomas, and juvenile nasopharyngeal angiofibromas). This can cause both acute and late toxicity to ocular structures.

- *Acute toxicity*: Conjunctival inflammation, chemosis and tear film instability, and dry eye sensation. Acute radiation keratopathy can be transient and negligible and present with superficial punctate keratitis, stromal keratitis, stromal scarring, and corneal edema, and treatable with anti-inflammatory and lubricant drops.
- *Late toxicity*: Eyelid abnormalities, LSCD, dry eye (lacrimal gland and meibomian gland obliteration and decreased conjunctival mucous production), decreased corneal sensation, neurotrophic corneal ulcers, melting, perforation, neovascularization, and scarring. The management is symptomatic and prevention difficult in most of the cases.

Drug-induced Corneal Changes

They are mentioned in **Table 20**.

Degenerations

Arcus Juvenilis/Anterior Embryotoxon

Usually, arcus is an age-related degenerative change occurring in the peripheral cornea due to lipid deposition in the DM and subsequently at Bowman's layer. It starts as a gray to yellow arc, first in the inferior cornea followed by the superior cornea later forming a complete ring. The arcus

TABLE 20: Drug-induced corneal changes.

Amiodarone, aminoquinoline, tamoxifen, nonsteroidal anti-inflammatory drugs, and antineoplastic drugs	Vortex pattern corneal epithelial deposits
Chlorpromazine	Corneal opacification (diffuse, interpalpebral, and radiating from optic axis), corneal stromal pigment dusting, and corneal edema
Clofazimine	Brown to reddish brown fine granular lines in the inferior cornea, conjunctival pigmentation
Topical gentamicin and tobramycin	Superficial punctate lesions, delayed reepithelialization, corneal ulceration, conjunctival pseudomembranes, and papillary conjunctivitis
Topical fluoroquinolones (particularly ciprofloxacin)	White crystalline corneal epithelial deposits of drug precipitates

has a diffuse central border and a sharp peripheral border separated from limbus by a lucent zone. Histochemically, the opacity is made up of cholesterol, cholesterol esters, phospholipids, and neutral glycerides. Commonly, it has no visual significance, and thus requires no treatment. However, patients under the age of 40 years with corneal arcus (arcus juvenilis or anterior embryotoxon) have an increased risk of coronary artery disease and should be evaluated for hyperlipoproteinemia (nephrotic syndrome, hypothyroidism, increased cholesterol intake, obstructive jaundice, diabetic ketoacidosis, and lecithin cholesterol acyltransferase deficiency).

Band-shaped Keratopathy

Band-shaped keratopathy is a type of corneal degeneration characterized by the deposition of calcium at the level of Bowman's layer. These deposits are gray or white and are located within the palpebral fissure, separated from the limbus by an area of clear cornea. The band appears like a "Swiss cheese" pattern, with holes within the band representing corneal nerves penetrating through Bowman's layer. The calcification is generally denser peripherally and often fades more centrally. In children, BSK may be associated with chronic uveitis such as in juvenile rheumatoid arthritis or in hypercalcemic states such as chronic renal failure. While early stages are asymptomatic, later stages can present with decreasing vision, foreign body sensation, tearing, or photophobia and require disodium ethylene diamine tetra-acetic acid chelation with or without an excimer laser to produce a smoother more regular ocular surface. Phototherapeutic keratectomy is especially helpful if Bowman's layer has been damaged or destroyed.

Ocular Surface Disorder

Any ocular surface disease can result in punctate keratopathy, recurrent corneal erosions, corneal ulcers, and perforations. Aqueous tear deficiency can be seen in congenital alacrima (aplasia or hypoplasia of lacrimal gland with or without salivary gland involvement), ectodermal dysplasia, cystic fibrosis, Sjogren's syndrome, juvenile rheumatoid arthritis, and after exposure to radiation for orbital or nasopharyngeal tumors. Meibomian gland dysfunction can be witnessed in pediatric blepharoconjunctivitis, pediatric rosacea, and CL use. Multifactorial tear film dysfunction can be seen in ocular graft versus host disease after bone marrow transplant, SJS/TEN, after chemical injury, nutritional deficiencies, and allergic eye disease. These can also lead to LSCD. LSCD can also be associated with congenital aniridia, CL wear, antiglaucoma medications, and use of mitomycin-C during surgery. Neurotrophic corneal disease can result from damage to trigeminal nucleus, root, ganglion, or any segment of its ophthalmic branch. Infectious diseases such as HSV and varicella zoster virus keratitis and other conditions such as congenital corneal anesthesia, familial dysautonomia (Riley-Day syndrome), Moebius syndrome, iatrogenic injuries (surgeries for tumors or fractures), topical medications (beta-blockers, NSAIDs, and trifluridine) and chemical injuries can also lead to neurotrophic disease in children. Exposure keratitis secondary to eyelid abnormalities can occur in Moebius syndrome, Graves' disease, ichthyosis, xeroderma pigmentosum, trachoma, after surgical repair of congenital ptosis, and due to abnormal tonic activity of orbicularis oculi in intensive care unit admissions.

Nutritional Disorders (Vitamin A Deficiency)

Vitamin A deficiency affects mucosal surfaces throughout the body thereby resulting in keratinizing metaplasia in the epithelial lining of lungs, and intestines in severe cases. Ophthalmic manifestations are mentioned in **Box 1**. Causes of vitamin A deficiency in children include protein-energy malnutrition, chronic liver disorders, malabsorption syndromes (cystic fibrosis), and diarrhea (measles infection). It is unlikely in >6 months of age group unless the lactating mother is deficient in vitamin A. Bitot's spots are dry scaly

BOX 1: Classification of xerophthalmia.

- XN night blindness
- X1A conjunctival xerosis
- X1B Bitot's spots
- X2 corneal xerosis
- X3A corneal ulceration/keratomalacia <one-third of corneal surface
- X3B corneal ulceration/keratomalacia >one-third of corneal surface
- XS corneal scar
- XF xerophthalmic fundus

TABLE 21: Management of xerophthalmia.

Nutritional supplementation:	
• <6 months of age	• Oral 50,000 IU vitamin A
• 6–12 months of age	• Oral 100,000 IU vitamin A
• >12 months of age with severe xerophthalmia	• Oral 200,000 IU vitamin A (110 mg retinol palmitate or 66 mg retinol acetate)
• Women of childbearing age with severe xerophthalmia	• Oral 200,000 IU vitamin A
• Women of reproductive age with night blindness or Bitot's spots	• 5,000–10,000 IU daily for four weeks, not exceeding 10,000 IU daily or weekly dose of 25,000 IU

*Additional dose 2 weeks later to boost liver reserves
*Children at highest risk should receive repeated dosing at 4–6-month intervals
*Parenteral administration of 100,000 IU or 55 mg water-miscible retinol palmitate for children with severe anorexia, edematous malnutrition, septic shock, or inability to take oral supplementation.

Ophthalmic management (as and when required):
- Topical lubricants and antibiotics
- Keratoplasty (poor visual outcome)
- Bandage contact lens ± cyanoacrylate/fibrin glue
- Amniotic membrane transplantation

patches in the interpalpebral area of the bulbar conjunctiva occurring due to metaplasia of conjunctival epithelium. Corneal ulcers in vitamin A deficiency have sharp margins, majorly occur in the lower half of the cornea and are frequently bilaterally symmetrical. Keratomalacia refers to sloughing or softening of cornea due to its necrosis. This can be aggravated by vitamin A deficiency as well as concomitant infection *(P. aeruginosa)* and trauma. The age group most at risk of blinding corneal disease (X2 and X3) is between 6 months and 3 years of age, while conjunctival disease (X1A and X1B) is more common in older children (between 3 and 6 years). The diagnosis of xerophthalmia constitutes a medical emergency, and prompt treatment with massive supplementation of vitamin A is required **(Table 21)**.

Systemic Disorders

Corneal findings reported in pediatric age group in numerous systemic disorders are mentioned in **Table 22**. Management depends on the underlying cause and clinical presentation.

CHALLENGES IN EXAMINATION AND MANAGEMENT OF PEDIATRIC CORNEAL DISORDERS

There are specific issues and approaches when a child has a corneal problem. Obtaining accurate history from children is difficult and most history will come from the parents or other caregivers; however, all verbal children must be encouraged to add their perspectives to parents' narrative. Clinical examination is always challenging due to the playful and easily distractable, thereby uncooperative, nature of children. Examination of an infant can be facilitated by feeding immediately before or during the examination, use of pacifiers, and swaddling in parents' arms. Toddlers (age 18–36 months) and preschoolers (≥3 years) can be engaged with colorful toys with sounds or motion to enable examination. They are best seated on parents' lap for safety and cooperation. It is always preferable to start with the affected eye in a unilateral process lest the child resists further assessment. Also important is to know what we are looking for prior to starting the examination. A low intensity light should be used initially and if required, the illumination can be gradually increased. Constantly encouraging the child during the examination and coaching him/her about the progress and duration of the examination may be helpful. As many corneal conditions (corneal dystrophies and keratoconus) have a hereditary component, a quick slit lamp examination of parents and cooperative siblings can guide further details. Routine clinical photography as well as high-resolution photographs, which are useful to document findings and monitor progression, are not always possible in pediatric patients. Slit lamp cameras can be used for cooperative children and video capture techniques and smart phone flash light photographs can be employed for children unable to maintain focus. Children usually cooperate for B-scan ultrasound and gross posterior segment pathologies can thus be assessed reasonably in children. However, low threshold should be maintained for performing examination under anesthesia (EUA), especially for peripheral fundus examination and corneal scraping. Noncontact procedures (ASOCT, specular microscopy, and noncontact tonometry) should be preferred over contact procedures (UBM, confocal microscopy, and applanation tonometry) in children. Younger children can be cajoled for serial corneal topography and optical biometry assessment. If uncooperative, mobile hand-held autokeratometers/refractometers, and A-scan can be undertaken during EUAs. If available, intraoperative OCT can also be utilized. Compliance with medical therapy and follow-up is a major issue in children. Parents may lose interest due to need for repeated EUAs and child may not always be fit for general anesthesia. Surgical interventions require extensive parental counseling. Refractive surgeries are generally considered unsafe in children and therefore rarely performed unless indicated for high anisometropic amblyopia. The growing nature of the pediatric eye makes prediction of postoperative refractive error unpredictable and myopic progression can be anticipated in a large number of children. PKP is an extremely challenging procedure in children because of various intraoperative morphologic and functional aspects such as less surgical space due to small globe size, anteriorly displaced iris lens diaphragm, positive vitreous pressure, and decreased rigidity of cornea and sclera. Postoperative complications such as severe inflammatory

TABLE 22: Pediatric corneal changes in systemic disorders.

Disorder	***Pathogenesis***	***Corneal and ocular surface manifestation***
Syndromic associations		
Down's syndrome	Trisomy 21	Keratitis, VKC, keratoconus, conjunctivitis, and blepharitis
Stüve-Wiedemann syndrome	Ocular dysautonomia	Alacrima or hypolacrimation, corneal hypoesthesia, decreased blink reflexes, neurotrophic keratopathy, and corneal opacities
Alport syndrome	Abnormal type 4 collagen	PPCD, arcus juvenilis, fine punctate corneal opacities, megalocornea, microcornea, keratoconus, ring abscesses, and endothelial pigmentation
Lowe syndrome	Error in inositol phosphate metabolism	Corneal keloids (excess fibrovascular proliferation to leaked amino acids after trauma)
Wilms tumor	Nephroblastoma	Aniridic keratopathy (poor corneal epithelial cell adhesion and migration, and LSCD)
Dermatological disorders		
Psoriasis	Autoimmune hyperproliferative disorder	• Punctate keratitis, corneal erosions, melt, neovascularization, and opacities • Dry eyes, blepharitis, and conjunctivitis
Epidermolysis bullosa	Defective basement membrane protein	Bullous keratopathy, corneal erosions, corneal scarring, pannus, LSCD, lacrimal duct obstruction, pseudopterygia, and microphthalmos
Kindler syndrome	Abnormal cell adhesion	Recurrent corneal erosions, corneal scarring, thickened corneal nerves, blepharitis, and keratoconjunctivitis
Ichthyoses	Abnormal keratinocyte differentiation	Exposure keratopathy (2° to eyelid defects), posterior corneal stromal opacities, corneal ulceration, neovascularization, and scarring, defective tear film, and recurrent AKC
Conradi-Hünermann-Happle syndrome	Abnormal emopamil binding protein	Anterior segment dysgenesis and posterior embryotoxon
Keratitis-ichthyosis-deafness (KID) syndrome	Abnormal connexin 26 protein	Vascularizing keratitis, recurrent corneal erosions, ulceration, neovascularization, pannus and scarring, MGD, LSCD, and KCS
Sjögren-Larsson syndrome	Defective fatty aldehyde dehydrogenase	Inferiorly located vascularized grayish corneal stromal opacities
Richner-Hanhart syndrome	Tyrosine accumulation	Bilateral circular opacities, corneal pseudodendrites, recurrent redness, tearing, pain, and photophobia
Xeroderma pigmentosum	Abnormal nucleotide excision repair	Corneal neovascularization, and scarring, conjunctivitis, dry eye, ectropion, blepharitis, OSSN, and LSCD
Pachyonychia congenita	Abnormal keratin 6a	Corneal epithelial defects and opacities
Proteus syndrome	Mutation in AKT1	BSK
Ectodermal dysplasia	Defects in ectodermal derivatives	Lacrimal gland hypoplasia, dry eyes, KCS, corneal pannus, blepharitis, and LSCD
Hematological disorders		
Leukemia	Neoplasm of leukocytes	• Limbal infiltration, corneal infiltration and ring ulceration, and keratic precipitates • Keratitis due to immunosuppression, epithelial changes from chemotherapy, or dry eye
Multiple myeloma	Hypergammaglobulinemia	Needle like stromal deposits, BSK, and prominent corneal nerves
Postbone marrow transplantation	Ocular graft versus host disease	Severe dry eye, keratopathy, and corneal scarring
Metabolic disorders		
Wilson's disease	Copper accumulation	KF rings (golden-brown or green rings in deep corneal periphery)
Gout	Uric acid accumulation	Tophi in corneal epithelium and stroma (fine, refractile yellow crystals of monosodium urate)
Cystinosis	Cystine accumulation	Cystine deposits in cornea leading to erosions, peripheral neovascularization, and punctate/filamentary/band keratopathy

Contd...

Contd...

Disorder	***Pathogenesis***	***Corneal and ocular surface manifestation***
Fabry disease	Ceramide trihexoside deposition	Vortex keratopathy/cornea verticillata (inferiorly located bilateral whitish to golden brown whorl-like opacities in epithelial and subepithelial layers of cornea)
Hyperlipoproteinemia	Cholesterol deposition	Arcus juvenilis (gray/white/yellowish circumferential peripheral corneal band due to lipid infiltration of corneal stroma)
Homocystinuria	Homocysteine accumulation	Anterior staphylomas
Porphyrias	Porphyrin accumulation	Keratitis (due to eyelid abnormalities
Endocrine disorders		
Graves' disease	Hyperthyroidism	Exposure keratopathy (2° to eyelid retraction), dry eye, and superior limbic keratoconjunctivitis
Kearns-Sayre syndrome	Hypercalcemia (hyperparathyroidism)	Exposure keratopathy (due to lagophthalmos), dry eye, and BSK
Addison's disease	Adrenal insufficiency	Corneal ulcers and keratoconjunctivitis
MEN 2A and 2B	Catecholamine excess	Enlarged cornea nerves
Diabetes mellitus	Hyperglycemia	Diabetic keratopathy (punctate keratopathy, recurrent erosions, persistent epithelial defects, and neurotrophic keratopathy) due to aqueous tear deficiency, reduced corneal sensation, and delayed wound healing
Musculoskeletal disorders		
Crouzon syndrome and Apert syndrome	Proptosis	Exposure keratopathy
Goldenhar syndrome and Treacher Collins syndrome	Errors in morphogenesis	Epibulbar dermoids, irregular corneal astigmatism, and amblyopia
Ehlers–Danlos syndrome (EDS)	Defect in collagen synthesis	Keratoglobus, keratoconus, acute hydrops, and xerophthalmia
Osteogenesis imperfecta	Defect in collagen synthesis	Corneal thinning, keratoconus, megalocornea, and posterior embryotoxon
Marfan's syndrome	Defective fibrillin-1	Corneal flattening, thinning, and astigmatism
End organ damage		
Pancreatic disorders	Hyperglycemia, malabsorption	Diabetic keratopathy and vitamin A deficiency (cystic fibrosis)
Liver disorders	Multiple metabolic abnormalities	Xanthelasma, xerophthalmia, KF ring, pseudo KF ring, posterior embryotoxon, and corneal clouding
End-stage renal disease	Calcium and apatite deposition	BSK
Autoimmune disorders		
Rheumatoid arthritis and systemic lupus erythematosus	Chronic inflammation	KCS (2° Sjögren syndrome), chronic keratitis, and corneal melt
Wegener granulomatosis	Necrotizing vasculitis	Bilateral peripheral ulcerative keratitis
Antiphospholipid antibody syndrome	Vascular thrombosis	Limbal keratitis and filamentary keratitis
Systemic infections		
Tuberculosis	*Mycobacterium tuberculosis* infection	Interstitial keratitis, corneal phlyctenules, and phlyctenular keratoconjunctivitis
Congenital syphilis	*Treponema pallidum* infection	Interstitial keratitis
COVID-19	SARS CoV-2 infection	Keratoconjunctivitis, subepithelial infiltrates, and overlying epithelial defects

(AKC: atopic keratoconjunctivitis; BSK: band-shaped keratopathy; KF ring: Kayser-Fleischer ring; KCS; keratoconjunctivitis sicca; LSCD: limbal stem cell disease; MGD: Meibomian gland dysfunction; OSSN: ocular surface squamous neoplasia; PPCD: posterior polymorphous corneal dystrophy; VKC: vernal keratoconjunctivitis) reaction, secondary glaucoma, graft rejection, and suture-related complications though more common, are frequently missed in children due to their inability to report them timely. Besides, despite a clear graft, suboptimal visual gain is common due to amblyopia. It is, therefore, advisable to perform lamellar procedures in children due to their inherent advantages. For example, anterior lamellar procedures reduce the risk of graft rejection, retain structural integrity, and require less stringent donor criteria, while DSAEK is associated with improved safety profile, accelerated wound healing, structurally stronger globe, and minimal astigmatism when compared to PKP. Identification and scoring of DM are difficult and chances of lens touch remain high in pediatric DSAEK. Keratoprosthesis is a last resort option in children due to poor lifetime prognosis and known complications such as retroprosthetic membrane formation, and infections (keratitis and endophthlamitis). Postoperative follow-up is tedious and vigorous attempts should be made to combat amblyopia in children.

CONCLUSION

Diagnosis and management of pediatric corneal disorders are challenging and require a great level of expertise. Poor compliance, surgical complexities, and extensive parental counseling and cooperation are required for handling them successfully.

SUGGESTED READING

1. Agarwal R, Nagpal R, Todi V, Sharma N. Descemetocele. Surv Ophthalmol. 2021;66(1):2-19.
2. Agarwal R, Sen S, Kashyap S, Dada T, Nag T, Gupta V, et al. Correlation of histopathology of trabecular meshwork with clinical features in primary congenital glaucoma. Br J Ophthalmol. 2020:bjophthalmol-2020-316346.
3. Alkemade PP. Dysgenesis Mesodermalis of the Iris and the Cornea: A Study of Rieger's Syndrome and Peters' Anomaly. Assen, Netherlands: Van Gorcum; 1969.
4. American Academy of Ophthalmology. External diseases and cornea. Basic and Clinical Sciences Course 2007-2008. San Francisco: American Academy of Ophthalmology; 2007
5. Ashworth JL, Biswas S, Wraith E, Lloyd IC. Mucopolysaccharidoses and the eye. Surv Ophthalmol. 2006;51(1):1-7.
6. Bastuji-Garin S, Rzany B, Stern RS, Shear NH, Naldi L, Roujeau JC. Clinical classification of cases of toxic epidermal necrolysis, Stevens-Johnson syndrome, and erythema multiforme. Arch Dermatol. 1993;129:92-.
7. Biswas S, Munier FL, Yardley J, Hart-Holden N, Perveen R, Cousin P, et al. Missense mutations in COL8A2, the gene encoding the alpha 2 chain of type VIII collagen, cause two forms of corneal endothelial dystrophy. Hum Mol Genet. 2001;10:2415-23.
8. Busin M, Beltz J, Scorcia V. Descemet-stripping automated endothelial keratoplasty for congenital hereditary endothelial dystrophy. Arch Ophthalmol. 2011;129(9):1140-6.
9. Cameron JA. Shield ulcers and plaques of the cornea in vernal keratoconjunctivitis. Ophthalmology. 1995;102(6):985-93.
10. Charlton KH, Binder PS, Wozniak L, Digby DJ. Pseudodendritic keratitis and systemic tyrosinemia. Ophthalmology. 1981;88(4): 355-60.
11. Colby K. Corneal Diseases in Children, 1st edition. Philadelphia: Springer International Publishing; 2017.
12. Cotran PR, Bajart AM. Congenital corneal opacities. International ophthalmology clinics. 1992;32(1):93-105.
13. Dua HS, Faraj LA, Said DG, Gray T, Lowe J. Human corneal anatomy redefined: a novel pre-Descemet's layer (Dua's layer). Ophthalmology. 2013;120(9):1778-85.
14. Dua HS, King AJ, Joseph A. A new classification of ocular surface burns. Br J Ophthalmol. 2001;85:1379-83.
15. Fledelius HC, Sandfeld L, Rasmussen ÅK, Madsen CV, Feldt-Rasmussen U. Ophthalmic experience over 10 years in an observational nationwide Danish cohort of Fabry patients with access to enzyme replacement. Acta ophthalmologica. 2015;93(3):258-64.
16. François J, Feher J. Light microscopical and polarisation optical study of the lattice dystrophy of the cornea. Ophthalmologica. 1972;164(1):1-18.
17. Hahn TW, Sah WJ, Kim JH. Phototherapeutic keratectomy in nine eyes with superficial corneal diseases. Refract Corneal Surg. 1993;9(2 Suppl.):S115-8.
18. Henriquez AS, Kenyon KR, Dohlman CH, Boruchoff SA, Forstot SL, Meyer RF, et al. Morphologic characteristics of posterior polymorphous dystrophy. A study of nine corneas and review of the literature. Surv Ophthalmol. 1984;29:139-47.
19. Héon E, Mathers WD, Alward WL, Weisenthal RW, Sunden SL, Fishbaugh JA, et al. Linkage of posterior polymorphous corneal dystrophy to 20q11. Hum Mol Genet. 1995;4:485-8.
20. Holland EJ, Daya SM, Stone EM, Folberg R, Dobler AA, Cameron JD, et al. Avellino corneal dystrophy. Clinical manifestations and natural history. Ophthalmology. 1992;99(10):1564-8.
21. Injarie AM, Narang A, Idrees Z, Saggar AK, Nischal KK. Ocular treatment of children with Stuve-Wiedemann syndrome. Cornea. 2012;31(3):269-72.
22. Irani AM, Schwartz LB. Neutral proteases as indicators of human mast cell heterogeneity. Monogr Allergy. 1990;27:146-62.
23. Iwamoto T, Stuart JC, Srinivasan BD, Mund ML, Farris RL, Donn A, et al. Ultrastructural variation in granular dystrophy of the cornea. Albrecht Von Graefes Arch Klin Exp Ophthalmol. 1975;194(1):1-9.
24. Jen M, Nallasamy S. Ocular manifestations of genetic skin disorders. Clin Dermatol. 2016;34(2):242-75.
25. Jing Y, Kumar PR, Zhu L, Edward DP, Tao S, Wang L, et al. Novel decorin mutation in a Chinese family with congenital stromal corneal dystrophy. Cornea. 2014;33(3):288-93.
26. Jones ST, Zimmerman LE. Histopathologic differentiation of granular, macular and lattice dystrophies of the cornea. Am J Ophthalmol. 1961;51:394-410.
27. Kim YW, Choi HJ, Kim MK, Wee WR, Yu YS, Oh JY. Clinical outcome of penetrating keratoplasty in patients 5 years or younger: peters anomaly versus sclerocornea. Cornea. 2013;32(11):1432-6.
28. Krachmer JH. Posterior polymorphous corneal dystrophy: a disease characterized by epithelial-like endothelial cells which influence management and prognosis. Trans Am Ophthalmol Soc. 1985;83:413-75.
29. Laganowski HC, Sherrard ES, Kerr Muir MG. The posterior corneal surface in posterior polymorphous dystrophy: a specular microscopical study. Cornea. 1991;10:224-32.
30. Laganowski HC, Sherrard ES, Muir MG, Buckley RJ. Distinguishing features of iridocorneal endothelial syndrome and posterior polymorphous dystrophy: value of endothelial specular microscopy. Br J Ophthalmol. 1991;75:212-6.
31. Leonardi A, Abatangelo G, Cortivo R, Secchi AG. Collagen types I and III in giant papillae of vernal keratoconjunctivitis. Br J Ophthalmol. 1995;79(5):482-5.
32. Liskova P, Tuft SJ, Gwilliam R, Ebenezer ND, Jirsova K, Prescott Q, et al. Novel mutations in the ZEB1 gene identified in Czech and

British patients with posterior polymorphous dystrophy corneal dystrophy. Hum Mutat. 2007;28:638.
33. Majumder PD, Ali S, George A, Ganesh S, Biswas J. Clinical profile of scleritis in children. Ocul Immunol Inflamm. 2019;27(4):535-9.
34. Mann I. Developmental abnormalities of the eye. CUP Archive. United Kingdom: British Medical Association; 1957.
35. Mannis M, Holland E. Cornea. 4th edition. Philadelphia: Elsevier; 2016.
36. Nischal KK. A new approach to the classification of neonatal corneal opacities. Curr Opin Ophthalmol. 2012;23(5):344-54.
37. Pietruszyńska M, Zawadzka-Krajewska A, Duda P, Rogowska M, Grabska-Liberek I, Kulus M. Ophthalmic manifestations of atopic dermatitis. Postepy Dermatol Alergol. 2020;37(2):174-9.
38. Polack FM, Bourne WM, Forstot SL, Yamaguchi T. Scanning electron microscopy of posterior polymorphous corneal dystrophy. Am J Ophthalmol. 1980;89:575-84.
39. Rathi VM, Murthy SI, Bagga B, Taneja M, Chaurasia S, Sangwan VS. Keratoglobus: An experience at a tertiary eye care center in India. Indian J Ophthalmol. 2015;63(3):233-8.
40. Reddy JC, Basu S, Saboo US, Murthy SI, Vaddavalli PK, Sangwan VS. Management, clinical outcomes, and complications of shield ulcers in vernal keratoconjunctivitis. Am J Ophthalmol. 2013;155(3):550-9.
41. Sharma N, Agarwal R, Jhanji V, Bhaskar S, Kamalakkannan P, Nischal KK. Lamellar Keratoplasty in Children. Survey of Ophthalmology. 2020;65(6):675-90.
42. Sharma N, Priyadarshini K, Agarwal R, Bafna R, Nagpal R, Sinha R, et al. Role of microscope-intraoperative optical coherence tomography in paediatric keratoplasty: A comparative study. Am J Ophthalmol. 2021;221:190-8.
43. Stark WJ, Chamon W, Kamp MT, Enger CL, Rencs EV, Gottsh JD. Clinical follow-up of 193 nm ArF excimer laser photokeratectomy. Ophthalmology. 1992;99(5):805-12.
44. Streeten BW, Qi Y, Klintworth GK, Strauss JA, Bennett K. Immunolocalization of beta ig-h3 protein in 5q31-linked corneal dystrophies and normal corneas. Arch Ophthalmol. 1999;117(1):67-75.
45. Stretton S, Gopinathan U, Willcox MD. Corneal ulceration in pediatric patients. Pediatric Drugs. 2002;4(2):95-110.
46. Thylefors B, Dawson CR, Jones BR, West SK, Taylor HR. A simple system for the assessment of trachoma and its complications. Bull World Health Organ. 1987;65(4):477-83.
47. Traboulsi EI, Maumenee IH. Peters' anomaly and associated congenital malformations. Archives of Ophthalmology. 1992; 110(12):1739-42.
48. Waring 3rd GO, Rodrigues MM. Ultrastructure and successful keratoplasty of sclerocornea in Mietens' syndrome. Am J Ophthalmol. 1980;90(4):469.
49. Weisenthal RW, Krachmer JH. Posterior polymorphous corneal dystrophy: ten years of progress. In: Cavanagh HD (Ed). The cornea: transactions of the World Congress on the Cornea III. New York: Raven; 1988.
50. Witschel H, Fine BS, Grutzner P, McTigue JW. Congenital hereditary stromal dystrophy of the cornea. Arch Ophthalmol. 1978;96(6):1043-51.

8

CHAPTER

Pediatric Uveitis

Vishali Gupta, Nitin Kumar Menia, Aniruddha Agarwal

INTRODUCTION

Managing children with uveitis is a challenge for the ophthalmologists. Pediatric uveitis is a potentially blinding eye disease and the ophthalmologist must make use of all his experience, time, and resources to treat the disease. The parents can be very apprehensive and need special care and counseling to allay the fears of child going blind due to the disease. Uveitis in children is less prevalent than in adults and accounts for <10% of all the uveitis cases. The prevalence of pediatric uveitis can be up to 27.9 per lakh population, as seen in a population-based study from Finland. Pediatric uveitis can have varied presentations and protean manifestations. The variations are influenced by geographic locations and ethnicity. While Behçet's disease (BD) is common in Middle Eastern countries, uveitis associated with juvenile arthritis is more common in European countries. Some entities like pediatric tubercular uveitis are mostly seen in Asian countries like India.

The management of uveitis in children is difficult because of its various presentations, chronicity, recurrences, and risk of amblyopia. It requires multiple therapies, a multispecialty approach, and an impeccable coordination between the uveitis specialist, pediatric ophthalmologist, and pediatric rheumatologist. Children may be asymptomatic, present with a white eye, despite severe ocular inflammation, and may be uncooperative for a comprehensive eye examination thus posing challenges in management. Smaller children may require multiple examinations under anesthesia and examination of anterior segment can be difficult under an operating microscope. The uveitis in pediatric population can be very severe, difficult to manage and refractory to treatment leading to blinding complications. Also, in spite of successful treatment, children with uveitis can develop amblyopia and severe visual loss. Pediatric uveitis can occur either sporadically or in association with systemic diseases. An effective strategy can help to detect an underlying medical disorder and its appropriate management. Pediatric uveitis can be broadly divided into two broad categories, (1) infectious and (2) noninfectious uveitis. We, here in, describe the uveitic entities commonly seen in children, their diagnosis, and management with a brief overview of treatment of these entities.

The type of uveitis according to their anatomical position is listed in **Table 1**.

NONINFECTIOUS UVEITIS

Juvenile Idiopathic Arthritis-associated Anterior Uveitis

Juvenile idiopathic arthritis (JIA) is defined as an idiopathic arthritis of at least 6 weeks duration in a child with age <16 years. Uveitis is one of the cardinal manifestations in JIA. The JIA-associated anterior uveitis is one of the most common forms of uveitis in children. The incidence of the

TABLE 1: Anatomical classification of the specific uveitic entities showing the primary site of inflammation.

Type of uveitis	*Anterior*	*Intermediate*	*Posterior*	*Panuveitis*
	Juvenile Idiopathic arthritis	Pars planitis	Tuberculosis	Tuberculosis
	Tubulointerstitial nephritis and uveitis		Sarcoidosis	Vogt-Koyanagi-Harada disease
			Toxoplasma retinochoroiditis	Sympathetic ophthalmia
			Toxocariasis	Behcet's disease
			Acute retinal necrosis	
			Masquerades	

disease shows a slight predominance in females with a 3:2 female to male ratio. The disease can have a longer course in females while the affected males, have a more severe involvement. Certain risk factors such as female gender, antinuclear antibody (ANA) test positivity, occurrence of articular disease before 6 years of age, and oligoarticular arthritis predispose to development of uveitis in JIA. The JIA-associated uveitis can precede the joint disease (3–7% of cases). The intraocular inflammation in JIA is a smoldering, nongranulomatous, and chronic anterior uveitis. The children with JIA-associated uveitis may be asymptomatic and uveitis may get incidentally detected on a routine screening examination. However, few of the patients can present with severe visual loss and complications secondary to a chronic undetected disease. The clinical signs include band-shaped keratopathy (BSK), cellular reaction, flare, posterior synechiae, complicated cataract, and hypotony with cyclitic membrane formation **(Figs. 1A and B)**. Chronic inflammation can lead to secondary glaucoma due to damage to trabecular meshwork and formation of anterior and posterior synechiae. Posterior segment complications include epiretinal membrane formation and hypotony-related maculopathy and neuropathy.

A differential diagnosis of JIA-related uveitis should be considered in a young child with joint involvement and ocular inflammation. Investigations include ANA testing, erythrocyte sedimentation rate estimation, rheumatoid factor, and a complete hemogram.

Treatment includes topical corticosteroids, cycloplegic drugs, oral corticosteroids, and immunosuppressive drugs in cases with mild disease. While severe disease requires oral corticosteroids and recurrent disease warrants systemic immunosuppression. Control of intraocular inflammation and achieving quiescence is central to the management of JIA-associated disease. As a smoldering inflammation accompanied by systemic and ocular recurrences is common, these patients require to be on systemic immunosuppression to prevent chronic side effects of topical (cataract and glaucoma) and systemic corticosteroids (osteoporosis, retarded growth, and Cushingoid syndrome). Methotrexate is the most used drug in the long-term control of intraocular inflammation; however, its therapeutic concentration in plasma builds up after 5–6 weeks of administration. Acute flare up of inflammation needs to be managed with topical and oral corticosteroids. The standard pediatric dosage of methotrexate is 10 mg/m^2/week, administered either orally or parenterally (intramuscular/subcutaneous).

The patients need to be monitored with liver function tests and complete blood counts for hepatotoxicity and bone marrow suppression, respectively. Other drugs which are used in JIA-associated uveitis are azathioprine (AZA), cyclosporine (CYC), tumor necrosis factor-alpha (TNF-α) inhibitors (adalimumab) and monoclonal antibody against CD20 (rituximab). However, these drugs can have serious adverse effects and need to be administered under close supervision of a pediatric rheumatologist and the patients need to be monitored frequently for any adverse events.

Pars Planitis

Pars planitis is defined as intermediate uveitis of unknown etiology. This entity is not associated with any systemic disorder and is a diagnosis of exclusion. Clinical findings in pars planitis include vitritis, vitreous membranes, snowballs, and snow banking. Chronic inflammation can lead to fibrosis, and membrane formation in the pars plana region leading to secondary tractional retinal detachment. Chronic inflammation can cause peripheral neovascularization and lead to vitreous hemorrhage. Chronic low-grade inflammation can also lead to secondary cataract, glaucoma, and cystoid macular edema.

The approach to a patient with pars planitis requires a step ladder approach, which includes topical and periocular steroids, oral corticosteroids, immunosuppressive drugs, cryotherapy, and vitrectomy. Mild anterior segment

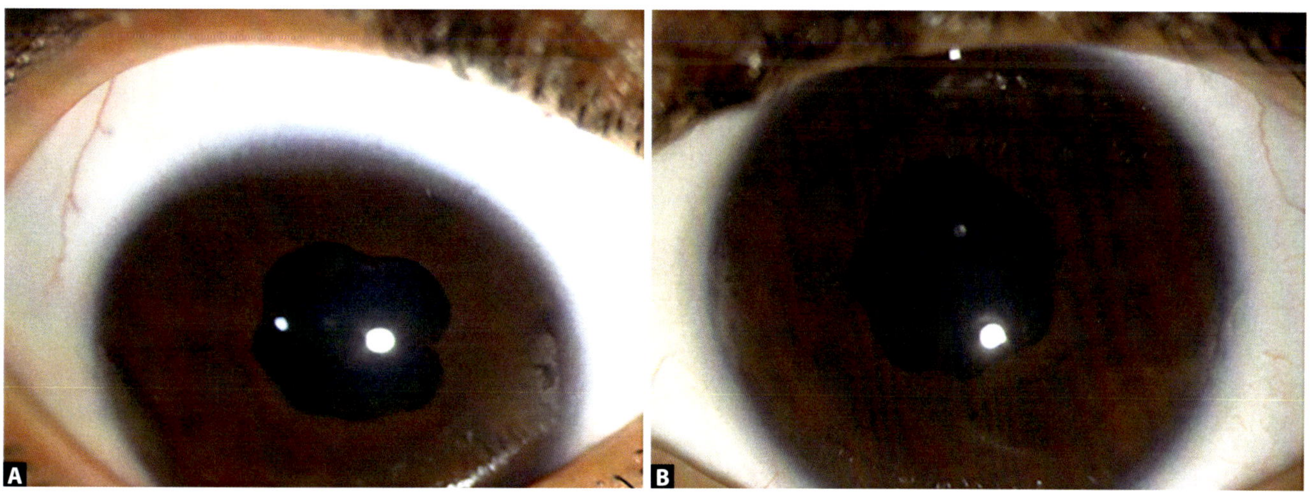

Figs. 1A and B: Slit lamp photograph of both eyes of a 10-year-old female showing band-shaped keratopathy, posterior synechiae, and complicated cataract.

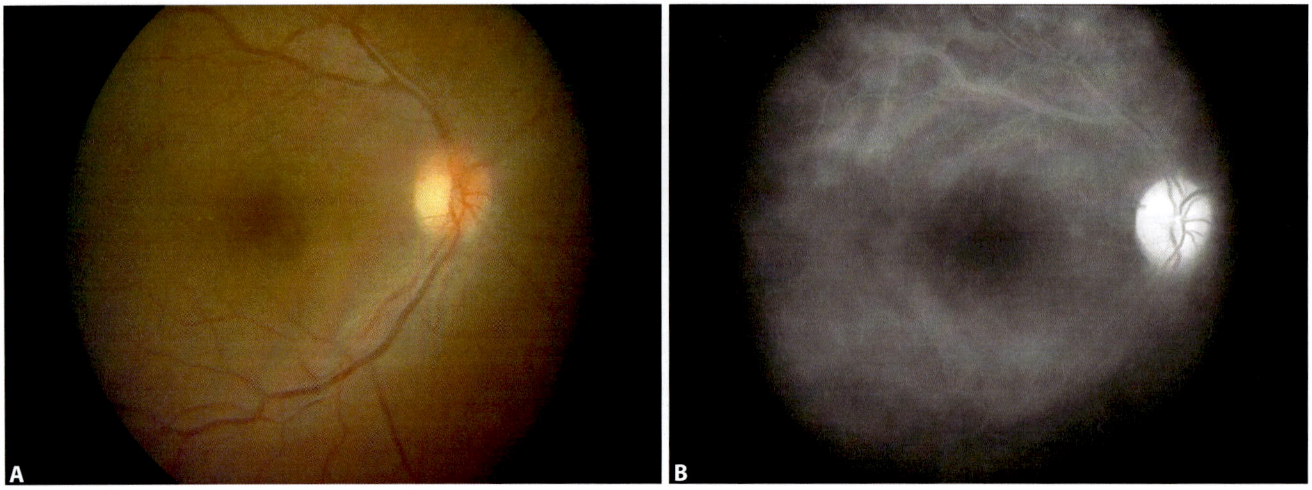

Figs. 2A and B: (A) A 9-year-old male with bilateral vitritis and disk swelling; (B) Fundus fluorescein angiography showing diffuse vascular leakage suggestive of Behcet's disease (right eye shown here).

inflammation requires topical corticosteroids, cystoid macular edema can be managed with periocular steroids, while vitreous hemorrhage and tractional retinal detachment may require pars plana vitrectomy, however, recurrences are managed with oral corticosteroids and immunosuppressive drugs.

Behçet's Disease

Behçet's disease is seen commonly in adults in the third decade of life. However, children can also be affected. Kitiachi et al., reported that almost 50% of the patients in an international retrospective study belonged to Middle Eastern countries highlighting that the ethnic background played an important role in the disease. The onset of uveitis in BD develops at a mean age of 10–15 years. The disease is a multisystemic inflammatory disease, which involves the retinal veins (vasculitis), and patients have oral and genital ulcers. BD may involve other systems like gastrointestinal, neurological, and vascular systems. Unlike adult BD, there are no accepted diagnostic criteria for diagnosis of pediatric uveitis. Majority of the children develop uveitis between 3 months of onset of the systemic disease, however, uveitis can be the only presenting manifestation of BD. Patients from endemic region are reported to have family history suggestive of a genetic predisposition.

Behçet's disease presents as a bilateral, recurrent, nongranulomatous panuveitis, and vasculitis. The anterior segment manifestations in BD include hypopyon uveitis, iridocyclitis, complicated cataract and secondary glaucoma. While posterior segment involvement occurs in form of vitritis, periphlebitis, retinitis, retinal hemorrhages, and optic disk pallor **(Figs. 2A and B)**. Vasculitis is one of the most devastating manifestations of BD and can lead to macular ischemia and optic disk hypoperfusion. Cystoid macular edema can develop in most cases and cause severe visual loss. The diagnosis of BD is based on typical clinical features (oral ulcers, genital ulcers, and uveitis). Fundus fluorescein angiography in BD can show a characteristic "fern-like" pattern with diffuse vascular leakage. Human leukocyte antigen B51 (HLA B51) testing has been employed to aid in the diagnosis.

Treatment includes management of anterior segment inflammation with topical steroid drops and cycloplegic drugs. The posterior segment inflammation can be very severe in BD and lead to severe visual loss. Control of severe inflammation requires oral corticosteroids and intravenous methylprednisolone pulse therapy. Immunosuppression is the cornerstone in the management of BD-related uveitis as recurrences are common and subclinical inflammation may threaten vision. The commonly used immunosuppressive drugs are AZA, CYC, methotrexate, and cyclophosphamide. The introduction of biological agents (anti-TNF α) in the treatment of BD has led to lesser recurrences, better control of inflammation, and limitation of daily dose of oral corticosteroids. Infliximab is the drug of choice (first line drug) for BD-related uveitis (acute episodes and recurrences).

Sarcoidosis

Sarcoidosis is a chronic inflammatory multisystem disease. Uveitis secondary to sarcoidosis is relatively rare in children. Older children (8–15 years) are more commonly affected, pulmonary involvement and posterior uveitis are more common in this age group. Younger children (under 5 years) mostly present with a triad of anterior uveitis, arthritis, and skin lesions. Sarcoid-related uveitis presents as granulomatous uveitis with mutton-fat keratic precipitates (KPs), iris nodules, cellular reaction, flare, posterior synechiae, vitritis, snowballs, and snowbanking. Retinal vasculitis (periphlebitis with a "candle wax dripping" like picture), sarcoid granulomas, and tubercles are also seen in ocular sarcoidosis.

Laboratory testing in suspected ocular sarcoidosis includes serum lysozyme, liver function tests, and serum calcium levels. Serum angiotensin-converting enzyme levels are less reliable in children as its levels can be physiologically elevated and the results can be misleading. Liver function tests can be deranged in sarcoidosis, due to subclinical involvement of liver (occult sarcoid granulomas). A contrast-enhanced computed tomography of chest should be obtained and biopsy of any abnormally enlarged lymph nodes should be carried out in consultation with a pediatric pulmonologist to establish a tissue diagnosis. The anterior segment inflammation is managed with topical and periocular steroids, while posterior segment disease requires oral corticosteroids and immunosuppressive drugs to avoid recurrent inflammation.

Tubulointerstitial Nephritis and Uveitis Syndrome

Tubulointerstitial nephritis and uveitis syndrome (TINU) is a rare disease, and uveitis in TINU constitutes approximately 1.7% of all adult uveitis cases. Children are more susceptible to develop TINU as compared to adults. A slight female preponderance is common. Older children are more predisposed to develop TINU. The disease is characterized by a concurrent acute tubulointerstitial nephritis and bilateral acute anterior uveitis. The uveitis can either precede, occur spontaneously, or follow renal involvement. The systemic symptoms for diagnosis include weight loss, fever, abdominal pain, and arthralgias. Renal dysfunction as evidenced by deranged renal functions is the most important diagnostic criteria for TINU. The various parameters, which are increased include raised serum urea and creatinine levels, increased proteinuria, microhematuria, glycosuria, and increased urinary beta-2 microglobulin levels. The definitive diagnosis is confirmed by a renal biopsy.

While the typical presentation is an acute bilateral anterior uveitis, in atypical cases, bilateral posterior and panuveitis can occur. Anterior segment involvement is a nongranulomatous form of uveitis. Vitritis, papillitis, macular edema, chorioretinitis, and multifocal choroiditis can be the varied posterior segment presentations of TINU. Anterior segment inflammation can be managed with topical steroids while posterior uveitis and panuveitis require oral corticosteroids and immunosuppressive drugs. In majority of the cases, immunosuppression is needed for management of the renal disease. Chronic renal dysfunction despite adequate systemic therapy (oral corticosteroids and immunosuppression) is common.

Vogt-Koyanagi-Harada Disease

Vogt-Koyanagi-Harada (VKH) disease occurs rarely in children. Females are predominantly affected, as in seen in adults. The disease is a bilateral granulomatous panuveitis with systemic manifestations. Neurological (headache and neck rigidity), integumentary (skin depigmentation), and auditory (tinnitus and sensorineural deafness) manifestations are seen commonly. Pediatric VKH disease consists of the four phases as seen in adults. The phases are the prodromal phase, acute uveitic phase, convalescent, and chronic recurrent phase. Acute uveitic phase presents with bilateral granulomatous anterior uveitis, vitritis, exudative retinal detachment, and optic disk edema **(Figs. 3A and B)**. The findings in convalescent stage include depigmentation of choroid, loss of retinal epithelial cells leading to a typical "sunset-sign", perilimbal vitiligo (Sugiura's sign), and skin depigmentation.

Complications such as cataract, secondary glaucoma, subretinal fibrosis, and choroidal neovascular membrane develop in the chronic recurrent phase of VKH disease leading to severe visual loss. Severe acute inflammation and recurrences require high dose oral corticosteroids and

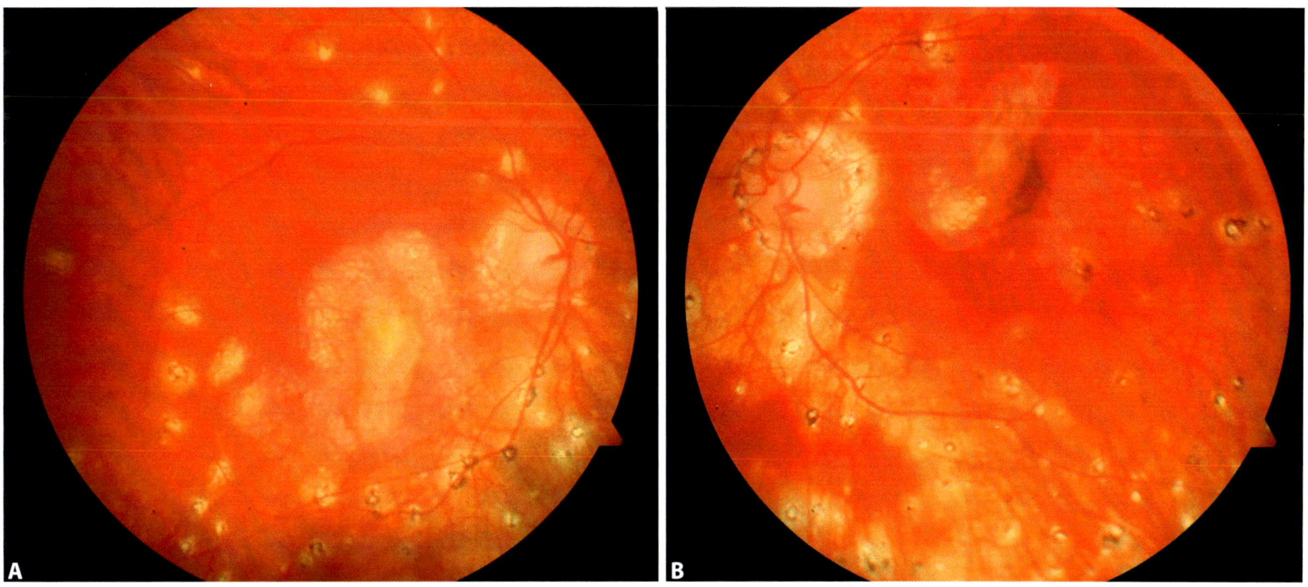

Figs. 3A and B: Fundus photographs of both eyes of a 12-year-old female in chronic convalescent stage of Vogt-Koyanagi-Harada disease showing nummular scars and "sunset-glow" sign.

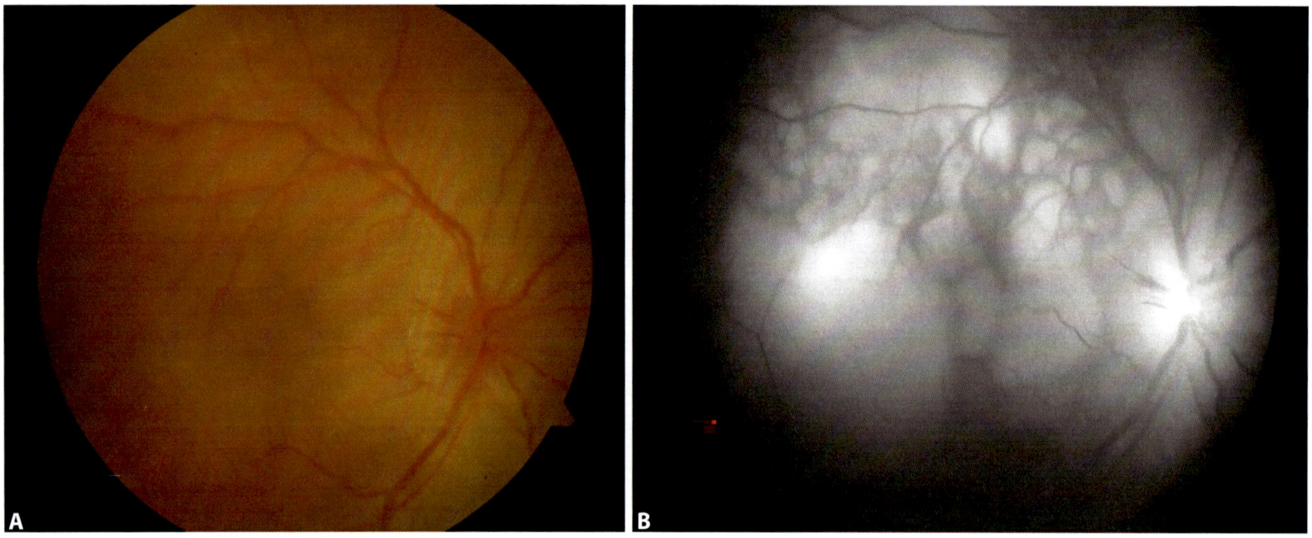

Figs. 4A and B: (A) Following penetrating trauma to left eye, a 7-year-old male presented with right eye decreased vision, fundus photograph disk showed disk edema and pockets of subretinal fluid; (B) Fundus fluorescein angiography showed massive disk hyperfluorescence and pooling of dye suggestive of sympathetic ophthalmia.

intravenous methylprednisolone pulse therapy, while to control the chronic inflammation, the patients need to be started on immunomodulatory therapy.

Sympathetic Ophthalmia

Sympathetic ophthalmia (SO) is a rare form of bilateral granulomatous panuveitis incited by ocular penetrating and ocular surgery. It is a dreaded disease, which can severe bilateral visual loss. Although majority of cases occur within the first year of ocular trauma or surgery, the disease can occur within a range of days to years. The incidence of pediatric SO ranges from 0.2 to 0.5% following trauma and approximately 0.01% following intraocular surgery. The findings include mutton-fat KPs, cellular reaction, flare, posterior synechiae, complicated cataract, vitritis, subretinal fluid pockets, and papillitis **(Figs. 4A and B)**. In one-third patients, subretinal yellowish white nodules, known as Dalen-Fuchs nodules, are seen.

Treatment includes frequent topical steroids to control anterior segment inflammation, posterior segment inflammation is managed with oral corticosteroids and intravenous methylprednisolone therapy. Control of chronic inflammation and prevention of recurrences require immunosuppression. The drug most used is AZA, however, methotrexate can also be used in a once weekly dosage.

INFECTIOUS UVEITIS

Toxoplasma Retinochoroiditis

Toxoplasma retinochoroiditis (TRC) is the most common cause of posterior uveitis worldwide. Similar to adults, pediatric TRC is a major cause of infectious posterior uveitis. The causative agent is *Toxoplasma gondii,* which infects almost one-third of the world population. *T. gondii* is an obligate intracellular parasite. Felines (cats) are the definite host and humans are the intermediate host. Human beings are infected by the ingestion of fruits, vegetables, and uncooked foods contaminated by oocysts (the cyst form of the organism), which are excreted in the cat feces.

The TRC presents as a focal necrotizing retinochoroiditis. The choroid is involved secondarily to the retinal involvement. The typical lesion seen in TRC is a "headlight in fog appearance" characterized by a retinochoroiditis lesion with overlying vitritis. An active lesion is a yellowish-white lesion, oval or round lesion, and close to the edge of a pigmented old scar **(Figs. 5A and B)**. Multiple satellite lesions can be seen in some cases. Atypical, large widespread, multifocal lesions are seen in immunocompromised children. Anterior segment findings in TRC include a granulomatous reaction (mutton-fat KPs), cellular reaction, flare, and posterior synechiae. Some cases present with a raised intraocular pressure (IOP) due to associated inflammation of trabecular meshwork. The posterior segment manifestations include active vasculitis known as "Kyrieleis arteritis" associated with active lesions and optic nerve involvement (neuroretinitis) in rare cases. Complications secondary to chronic inflammation include complicated cataract, secondary glaucoma, epiretinal membrane, choroidal neovascular membrane formation, and tractional retinal detachment.

The diagnosis of TRC is a clinical one. However, laboratory investigations can aid in the diagnosis of TRC. Serological tests previously used in diagnosis were Sabin-Feldman test, complement fixation test, agglutination test, indirect immunofluorescence test, and enzyme-linked immunofluorescence test. Polymerase chain reaction (PCR) is an important tool for the detection of TRC, and has been recently used in the analysis of ocular samples.

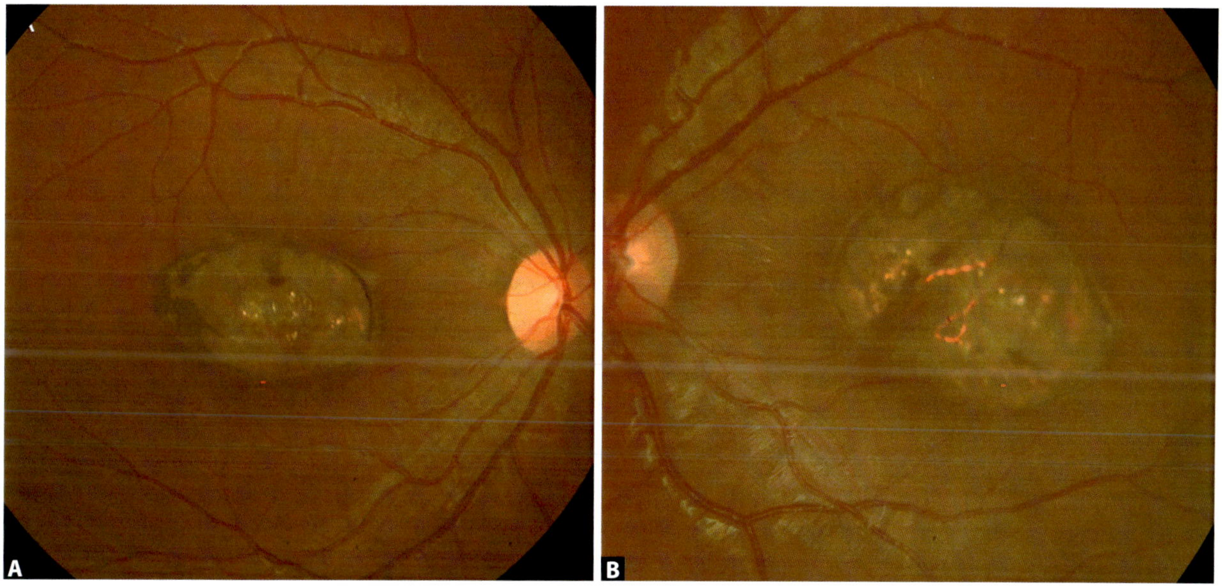

Figs. 5A and B: Fundus photographs of a 5-year-old male child showing congenital, bilateral toxoplasma scars.

The treatment of ocular TRC includes administration of antibiotics such as pyrimethamine, sulfadiazine, trimethoprim, and sulfamethoxazole. These drugs act by inhibition of DNA synthesis. The combination of trimethoprim and sulfamethoxazole is most commonly used drug for treatment of acute active disease and to prevent recurrences. Combination of intravitreal clindamycin and dexamethasone can also be used as monotherapy. Other less commonly used systemic antibiotics include azithromycin and atovaquone. Oral clindamycin is rarely used nowadays due to serious systemic side effects such as pseudomembranous enterocolitis.

Toxocariasis

Ocular toxocariasis is a rare cause of primarily unilateral infectious uveitis. The causative agents implicated are parasitic nematodes, *Toxocara canis* and *Toxocara cati*. The parasites live in the small intestines of dogs and cats, respectively. Systemic form of toxocariasis is known as visceral larva migrans and produces a self-limiting disease with fever, cough, malaise, hepatomegaly, irritability, and anorexia. While systemic toxocariasis occurs in younger children (<5 years of age) and ocular toxocariasis occurs in relatively older children.

Humans contract the disease by ingesting foods contaminated with eggs and larvae of the parasites. The three presentations characteristic of toxocariasis are a peripheral inflammatory granuloma, posterior pole granuloma, and an endophthalmitis-like picture. The peripheral toxocara granuloma presents as a whitish elevated lesion with size almost the size of the optic disk. Inflammatory process in a peripheral lesion can involve the pars plana region (pars planitis). Granulomas at the posterior pole can have varied presentations such as visual loss, exotropia, esotropia, amblyopia, and an endophthalmitis-like picture.

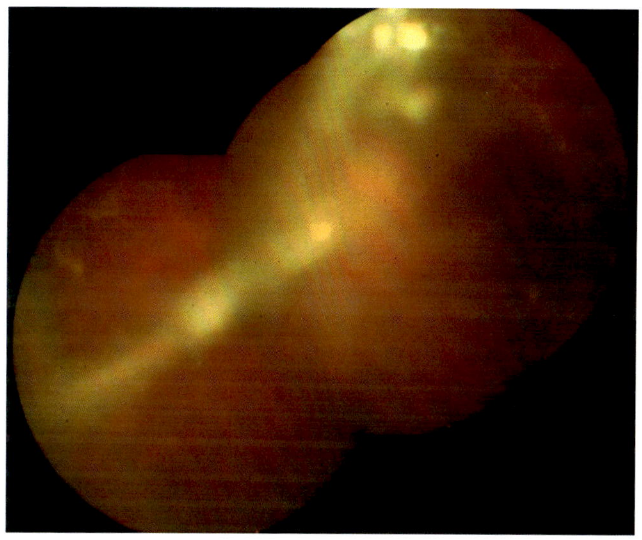

Fig. 6: Montage fundus photograph of an 11-year-old male showed presence of a granuloma with dense vitritis and fibrous proliferation suggestive of a toxocara granuloma.

The typical posterior pole lesion presents as a chorioretinitis lesion with overlying vitritis **(Fig. 6)**. Severe vitritis in some cases can present as an endophthalmitis like picture and may warrant pars plana vitrectomy (PPV). Surgical intervention is also required in patients who develop epiretinal membranes and tractional retinal detachments secondary to chronic inflammation. Investigations include enzyme-linked immunosorbent assay (ELISA) specific for toxocara antigen. Goldmann-Witmer coefficient, which shows specific antibodies in aqueous humor and confirms intraocular production of antibodies against toxocariasis, also aids in the diagnosis.

Treatment of ocular toxocariasis is controversial. While some clinicians do not recommend antihelminthic drugs, others advise them under cover of oral corticosteroids.

The most common class of drugs used in the treatment of systemic and ocular toxocariasis is benzimidazole derivatives. Albendazole is the most used and freely available drug. The aim of treatment is to keep the intraocular inflammation under control to prevent complications. The severe inflammatory response seen in this ocular condition has to be controlled to prevent complications like formation of epiretinal membrane and tractional retinal detachment. The oral corticosteroids are of paramount importance to control the inflammatory response and should be administered under the cover of oral antihelminthic drugs.

Acute Retinal Necrosis

Acute retinal necrosis (ARN) is a sight threatening, necrotizing retinitis that can affect healthy individuals. Due to the potentially blinding nature of the disease, its early diagnosis and treatment is of utmost importance. The viruses implicated in ARN are herpes simplex virus (HSV) and varicella zoster virus (VZV). As seen with other forms of infectious uveitis, the incidence of ARN in pediatric age group is lower than seen in adults.

The typical symptomology includes, decreased vision (acute or subacute), floaters, redness, and field loss. The typical triad seen in the disease is vitritis, occlusive-vasculitis, and retinitis. The anterior segment examination may reveal cells, flare, and KPs. Some patients may present with a raised IOP, due to associated trabeculitis. The vitritis is severe in most of the cases and foci of retinal necrosis are evident with a circumferential spread from the periphery toward posterior pole, producing typical "tongue-shaped" lesions **(Fig. 7)**. The vasculitis typically involves arteries more than the veins. Although the disease is diagnosed based on typical clinical features as described earlier, performing a PCR analysis for viruses (VZV and HSV) can add to the diagnosis. In about one-third of the cases, the fellow eye can get involved within 3 months of the onset of the disease. It is therefore imperative to start the treatment early and also observe the other eye meticulously.

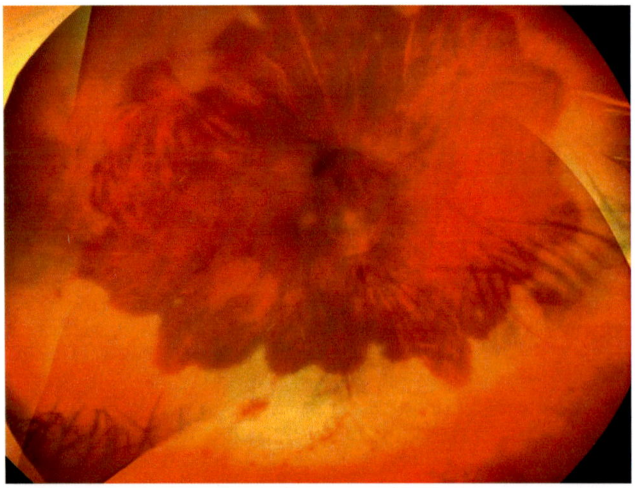

Fig. 7: Montage ultrawide field photograph of the right eye in a young patient showing vitritis, vasculitis, and typical tongue-shaped lesions suggestive of acute retinal necrosis.

The treatment regimen consists of administration of intravenous acyclovir at a recommended dosage of 15 mg/kg in three divided doses in the induction phase followed by oral acyclovir (800 mg five times a day), oral valacyclovir (1 g three times a day) for 6 weeks to 3 months duration. In cases of poor response to systemic acyclovir and valacyclovir, systemic ganciclovir can be administered. Oral corticosteroids are administered 24 hours after starting treatment with antiviral drugs. Aspirin (75 mg twice daily) can be started to prevent complications due to vascular occlusions.

About 75% of the patients develop a combination of rhegmatogenous and tractional retinal detachments due to development of retinal holes and tractional membranes as a sequela of intraocular inflammation. Management includes PPV with silicon oil tamponade. Although controversial, laser photocoagulation posterior to the areas of active retinitis (creating an artificial "ora serrata") has been advocated to reduce the risk of retinal detachment.

Ocular Tuberculosis

Intraocular tuberculosis is not an uncommon disease. It is seen frequently in the developing world where the disease is endemic. *Mycobacterium tuberculosis* infects almost one-third of the world population and causes significant morbidity and mortality world over. Eye involvement in tuberculosis can occur in form of an anterior, intermediate, posterior, or panuveitis. The finding in anterior segment includes granulomatous (mutton-fat) KPs, cellular reaction, flare, broad-based posterior synechiae, and iris nodules. Intraocular tuberculosis also presents as intermediate uveitis, mild-to-moderate vitritis, snowballs, snow banking, and vasculitis. *M. tuberculosis* involves the posterior segment and can have protean manifestations like tubercular serpiginous like choroiditis, tubercular choroidal granulomas, and subretinal abscesses **(Fig. 8)**. Choroidal granulomas and abscesses are associated with exudative retinal detachments and can cause severe visual loss. In severe cases, the subretinal abscesses can break into the vitreous cavity producing an endophthalmitis like picture.

The diagnosis of this condition is challenging. The validity of Mantoux test has a limited value in children due to its cross-reactivity to the Bacillus Calmette-Guérin (BCG) vaccination, especially in the developing world. Interferon-gamma release assays are more valid as chances of cross-reactivity to BCG vaccination are less commonly reported. Contrast-enhanced computed tomography (CECT) of chest is useful to find the infective foci (enlarged mediastinal and hilar lymph nodes). Tissue biopsies (Ultrasound guided transbronchial needle aspiration) can be obtained by a pulmonologist to confirm the diagnosis.

Treatment includes administration of antituberculosis drugs and oral corticosteroids. The Center for Disease

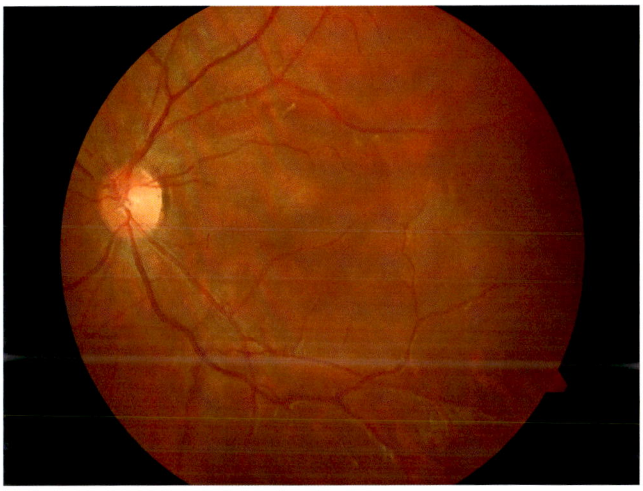

Fig. 8: Fundus photograph of left eye of a 14-year-old male showing presence of a tubercular granuloma with subretinal fluid at posterior pole.

Control (CDC, USA) recommends a regimen, which consists of isoniazid, rifampicin, pyrazinamide, and ethambutol for a total of 2 months, followed by 4–7 months of therapy with isoniazid and rifampicin.

Masquerade Syndromes

A child with uveitis not responding to standard anti-inflammatory therapy should raise suspicion of masquerade syndromes and the ophthalmologist should be cautious. The ophthalmologist can help in establishing the diagnosis in such serious systemic conditions and prompt treatment can be life-saving. Retinoblastoma, leukemias, medulloepitheliomas, and Coat's disease can masquerade as uveitis.

Uveitis in children with leukemias can be the presenting manifestation or can present in children already diagnosed with the disease. Masquerades can also involve the posterior segment and present as retinal hemorrhages, cotton-wool spots, and retinal infiltrates. A "white eye" with hypopyon uveitis (pseudohypopyon) can be a red-flag sign and caution the ophthalmologist. A diagnostic anterior chamber paracentesis and cytology can aid in the establishing the diagnosis.

Children <2 years of age can present with non-neoplastic histiocytosis proliferation, yellowish-orange skin lesions, and uveitis known as juvenile xanthogranuloma. The disease is associated with yellowish-white creamy lesions on iris, which can bleed spontaneously, presenting as hyphemia and hypopyon.

CHALLENGES SPECIFIC TO PEDIATRIC UVEITIS

The smaller children (<7 years old) may not cooperate while recording the visual acuity and examining on a slit lamp. However, providing a wooden block, on which the child can stand, may facilitate the examination. The children can also sit comfortably in the lap of parents, for a satisfactory slit-lamp examination. The +90 D lens examination may be difficult, but when properly explained, the children may cooperate resulting in posterior segment examination on a slit-lamp. Older children (>7 years) may cooperate for fundus fluorescein angiography, ultrasonography, ultrasound biomicroscopy, and optical coherence tomography when properly counseled.

Children, who may not cooperate, require examinations under general anesthesia. Special consideration should be given to management of amblyopia as it can lead to lifelong visual disability. The parents should be explained about the importance and proper technique of occlusion therapy.

COMPLICATIONS IN PEDIATRIC UVEITIS

A large proportion of children may develop ocular complication despite best management strategies. The most common complication in pediatric uveitis is cataract formation, which occurs due to persistent inflammation and use of corticosteroids. The other complications seen are BSK, anterior and posterior synechiae, secondary glaucoma, iris bombe, hypotony, cyclitic membrane formation, cystoid macular edema, tractional retinal detachment, and phthisis bulbi. Systemic adverse effects seen in children on oral corticosteroids include, weight gain, adrenal suppression, hyperglycemia, hirsutism, stunted growth, moon facies, osteoporosis, poor wound healing, and psychosis.

OVERVIEW OF TREATMENT IN PEDIATRIC UVEITIS

The infectious form of pediatric uveitis constitutes about 13% of all the cases. This form of pediatric uveitis is treated with specific antibiotics and topical corticosteroids. The management of noninfectious uveitis includes a "step-ladder approach". The core of treatment and management strategies in pediatric uveitis is achieving quiescence and following up these children regularly. The therapy includes corticosteroids (topical, periocular, and oral) and immunomodulator drugs.

Corticosteroids

Topical corticosteroids are the most used drugs for the management of anterior segment inflammation. Periocular steroids are used in the treatment of intermediate uveitis and oral corticosteroids are commonly indicated in bilateral posterior and panuveitis after ruling out infectious causes. High-dose intravenous steroids are commonly indicated in severe flare ups/recurrences and sight threatening lesions.

Immunomodulatory Therapy

The key to successful management in noninfectious uveitis is early initiation of immunomodulatory therapy. Oral corticosteroids have severe adverse effects and cannot be administered for long periods. The immunomodulator drugs commonly used in children are methotrexate, AZA, CYC, mycophenolate mofetil, TNF-α inhibitors, and monoclonal antibodies. Methotrexate is the most used drug in the treatment of pediatric uveitis due to its better safety, efficacy profile, and ease of administration. However, liver dysfunction is a common adverse effect and needs monitoring.

Biologicals have now recommended as the first-line therapy for treatment of pediatric uveitis. Biologicals are monoclonal antibodies that inhibit the proinflammatory cytokines. Infliximab and adalimumab are TNF-α inhibitors and are most effective in control of intraocular inflammation. Adalimumab is easy to administer and has a good safety profile. Infliximab and rituximab are now more commonly used. These drugs can have serious side effects and need to be administered under care of an experienced pediatric rheumatologist.

CONCLUSION

To manage pediatric uveitis is a diagnostic and therapeutic challenge. Timely detection of disease and aggressive treatment is the cornerstone in its management. A multidisciplinary approach, teamwork involving the parents, pediatric rheumatologist, pediatric ophthalmologist, and uveitis specialist are paramount to successful management.

SUGGESTED READING

1. Ahn SJ, Ryoo NK, Woo SJ. Ocular toxocariasis: clinical features, diagnosis, treatment, and prevention. Asia Pac Allergy. 2014;4(3): 134-41.
2. Andreoli CM, Foster CS. Vogt-Koyanagi-Harada disease. Int Ophthalmol Clin. 2006;46:111-22.
3. Ang M, Vasconcelos-Santos DV, Sharma K, Accorinti M, Sharma A, Gupta A, et al. Diagnosis of ocular tuberculosis. Ocul Immunol Inflamm. 2018;26:208-16.
4. Bansal R, Gupta A, Agarwal R, Dogra M, Bhutani G, Gupta V, et al. Role of CT chest and cytology in differentiating tuberculosis from presumed sarcoidosis in uveitis. Ocul Immunol Inflamm. 2019;27(7):1041-8.
5. Biester S, Deuter C, Michels H, Haefner R, Kuemmerle-Deschner J, Doycheva D, et al. Adalimumab in the therapy of uveitis in childhood. Br J Ophthalmol. 2007;91:319-24.
6. Chan NSW, Choi J, Cheung CMG. Pediatric Uveitis. Asia-Pac J Ophthalmol. 2018;7:192-9.
7. Citirik M, Berker N, Songur MS, Soykan E, Zilelioglu O. Ocular findings in childhood-onset Behçet disease. JAAPOS. 2009;13:391-5.
8. Dana MR, Merayo-Lloves J, Schaumberg DA, Foster CS. Visual outcomes prognosticators in juvenile rheumatoid arthritis-associated uveitis. Ophthalmology. 1997;104:236-44.
9. de Boer J, Berendschot TT, van der Does P, Rothova A. Long-term follow-up of intermediate uveitis in children. Am J Ophthalmol. 2006;141:616-21.
10. de Jong PT. Ocular toxoplasmosis; common and rare symptoms and signs. Int Ophthalmol. 1989;13:391-7.
11. Evereklioglu C. Current concepts in the etiology and treatment of Behçet's disease. Surv Ophthalmol. 2005;50:297-300.
12. Gordon KB, Rugo HS, Duncan JL, Irvine AR, Howes EL Jr, O'Brien JM, et al. Ocular manifestations of leukemia: leukemic infiltration versus infectious process. Ophthalmology. 2001;108:2293-300.
13. Gregory AC 2nd, Kempen JH, Daniel E, Kaçmaz RO, Foster CS, Jabs DA, et al. Risk factors for loss of visual acuity among patients with uveitis associated with juvenile idiopathic arthritis: the Systemic Immunosuppressive Therapy for Eye Diseases Study. Ophthalmology. 2013;120:186-92.
14. Guest S, Funkhouser E, Lightman S. Pars planitis: a comparison of childhood onset and adult onset disease. Clin Experiment Ophthalmol. 2001;29:81-8.
15. Gupta A, Bansal R, Gupta V, Sharma A, Bambery P. Ocular signs predictive of tubercular uveitis. Am J Ophthalmol. 2010;149(4): 562-70.
16. Gupta V, Gupta A, Rao NA. Intraocular tuberculosis—an update. Surv Ophthalmol. 2007;52:561-87.
17. Gupta V, Shoughy SS, Mahajan S, Khairallah M, Rosenbaum JT, Curi A, et al. Clinics of ocular tuberculosis. Ocul Immunol Inflamm. 2015;23:14-24.
18. Jahnukainen T, Ala-Houhala M, Karikoski R, Kataja J, Saarela V, Nuutinen M. Clinical outcome and occurrence of uveitis in children with idiopathic tubulointerstitial nephritis. Pediatr Nephrol. 2011; 26:291-9.
19. Kawaguchi T, Hanada A, Horie S, Sugamoto Y, Sugita S, Mochizuki M. Evaluation of characteristic ocular signs and systemic investigations in ocular sarcoidosis. Jpn J Ophthalmol. 2007;51:121-6.
20. Kishore K, Conway MD, Peyman GA. Intravitreal clindamycin and dexamethasone for toxoplasmic retinochoroiditis. Ophthalmic Surg Lasers. 2001;32(3):183-92.
21. Kumar K, Mathai A, Murthy SI, Jalali S, Sangwan V, Pappuru RR, et al. Sympathetic ophthalmia in pediatric age group: clinical features and challenges in management in a tertiary center in southern India. Ocul Immunol Inflamm. 2014;22:367-72.
22. Majumder PD, Biswas J. Pediatric uveitis: an update. Oman J Ophthalmol. 2013;6:140-50.
23. Morelle G, Gueudry J, Uettwiller F, Wouters C, Bader-Meunier B, Robert MP, et al. Chronic and recurrent non-infectious pediatric-onset uveitis: a French cohort. RMD Open. 2019;5:e000933.
24. Ohno S, Nakamura S, Hori S, Shimakawa M, Kawashima H, Mochizuki M, et al. Efficacy, safety, and pharmacokinetics of multiple administration of infliximab in Behcet's disease with refractory uveoretinitis. J Rheumatol. 2004;31:1362-8.
25. Petty RE, Smith JR, Rosenbaum JT. Arthritis and uveitis in children: a pediatric rheumatology perspective. Am J Ophthalmol. 2003;135:879-84.
26. Pinon JM, Dumon H, Chemla C, Franck J, Petersen E, Lebech M, et al. Strategy for diagnosis of congenital toxoplasmosis: evaluation of methods comparing mothers and newborns and standard methods for postnatal detection of immunoglobulin G, M, and A antibodies. J Clin Microbiol. 2001;39:2267-71.
27. Ravelli A, Moretti C, Temporini F, Rossi F, Magni-Manzoni S, Pistorio A, et al. Combination therapy with methotrexate and cyclosporine A in juvenile idiopathic arthritis. Clin Exp Rheumatol. 2002;20:569-72.
28. Rosenberg AM. Uveitis associated with childhood rheumatic diseases. Curr Opin Rheumatol. 2002;14:542-54.
29. Rosenberg KD, Feuer WJ, Davis JL. Ocular complications of pediatric uveitis. Ophthalmology. 2004;111:2299-306.
30. Samson CM, Ekong A, Foster CS. Uveitis in children: diagnosis and management. Intern Ophthalmol Clin. 2001;41:199-216.
31. Schoenberger SD, Kim SJ, Thorne JE, Mruthyunjaya P, Yeh S, Bakri SJ, et al. Diagnosis and treatment of acute retinal necrosis: a report by the American Academy of Ophthalmology. Ophthalmology. 2017;124:382-92.
32. Shetty AK, Gedalia A. Childhood sarcoidosis: a rare but fascinating disorder. Pediatr Rheumatol Online J. 2008;6:16.
33. Silveira C, Belfort RJ, Muccioli C, Holland GN, Victora CG, Horta BL, et al. The effect of long term intermittent trimethoprim/sulfamethoxazole treatment on recurrences of toxoplasmic retinochoroiditis. Am J Ophthalmol. 2002;134:41-6.
34. Simonini G, Paudyal P, Jones GT, Cimaz R, Macfarlane GJ. Current evidence of methotrexate efficacy in childhood chronic uveitis: a systematic review and meta-analysis approach. Rheumatology. 2013;52:825-31.
35. Soheilian M , Sadoughi MM, Ghajarnia M, Dehghan MH, Yazdani S, Behboudi H, et al. Prospective randomized trial of trimethoprim/sulfamethoxazole versus pyrimethamine and sulfadiazine in the treatment of ocular toxoplasmosis. Ophthalmology. 2005;112:1876-82.
36. Tugal-Tutkun I. Pediatric Uveitis. J Ophthalmic Vis Res. 2011;6: 259-69.
37. Vitale AT, Foster CS. Uveitis affecting infants and children: infectious causes. In: Hartnett ME, Trese M, Capone AJ (Eds). Pedatric Retina. Philadelphia: Lippincott, Williams and Wilkins; 2005. pp. 249-89.

9

CHAPTER

Pediatric Cataract

Abhay R Vasavada, Vaishali Vasavada

INTRODUCTION

Pediatric cataract is the most common cause of treatable childhood blindness, accounting for 5–20% of blindness in children worldwide. Cataracts in children may be congenital or developmental in nature. Further, they may occur in isolation, or may be associated with systemic diseases of the urinary tract, skeletal system, or even the nervous system. However, there are several aspects of pediatric cataracts and these growing eyes that make the behavior and therefore, management of these cases very different from adult eyes. This chapter aims at giving a broad overview of pediatric cataracts. In particular, it focusses on the following aspects:

- Lens embryology
- Morphology of pediatric cataracts
- Examination and diagnosis
- Surgical treatment, including timing of surgery and nuances of surgical technique
- Intraocular lens (IOL) implantation—timing, techniques, controversies, challenges, and calculations
- Postoperative management in pediatric cataracts
- Visual rehabilitation following pediatric cataract surgery
- Dealing with postoperative complications of pediatric cataract surgery.

LENS EMBRYOLOGY

Primary lens fibers expel their intracellular contents and form an optically clear embryonic nucleus about 0.35 mm in diameter during the 6th week of gestation. Equatorial, secondary lens fibers migrate anteriorly and posteriorly to meet each other at the sutures (anterior upright Y and posterior inverted Y sutures). These sutures demarcate the embryonic and fetal nucleus. The secondary lens fibers continue to form the fetal nucleus up to the 8th month of gestation. Fetal and embryonic nuclei both are present at birth. After birth, the equatorial fibers grow and elongate to form the cortex. The developing lens requires nutrition that is obtained through the tunica vasculosa lentis. This gradually starts regressing after the 85th day of gestation and completely regresses by the 7th month. At term, only wispy remnants of the pupillary membrane are left, and a vestigial hyaloid artery (Mittendorf's dot) may often be attached to the axial posterior surface of the lens.

Pediatric cataracts can be classified based on their etiology, morphology, and anatomic location of lens opacities **(Table 1)**. These cataracts may be isolated or part of a systemic condition.

TABLE 1: Congenital cataract classification.

Opacification	
Anatomical type	*Subtypes*
Anterior capsular cataract	Anterior polar
	Anterior capsular
	Anterior capsular plaque
Cortical cataract	Anterior cortical
	Posterior cortical
	Membranous
Nuclear cataract	Isolated nuclear
	Lamellar
	Sutural
	Punctate
Posterior capsular cataracts	Posterior polar cataract
	Posterior subcapsular
	Posterior lenticonus
Total cataract	
Mixed cataract	
Cataract with pre-existing posterior capsule defect	
Cataract with persistent fetal vasculature	
Size	Microspherophakia
Shape	Spherophakia
	Coloboma disciform
Location	Subluxated
	Dislocated
Developmental association	Persistent fetal vasculature
	(PFV or PHPV)

(PFV: persistence of fetal vasculature; PHPV: persistent hyperplastic primary vitreous)

ANATOMICAL CLASSIFICATION OF PEDIATRIC CATARACTS

Classification of lenticular opacities based on their anatomic location **(*see* Table 1)** facilitates precise localization of the lens opacities. Using the location of the opacities, meaningful information can be derived on the visual prognosis, timing and nature of the insult, and progression. It can also aid in the identification of associated ocular and systemic anomalies as well as helps the surgeon to plan appropriate management strategies.

Other methods to classify are:
- Unilateral or bilateral
- Congenital or acquired
- Partial or complete
- Stable or progressive
- Inherited or sporadic
- With or without systemic anomalies.

Anterior Cataracts

- *Anterior polar cataract:* Anterior polar cataract presents as a dot-like axial opacification on the anterior capsule **(Figs. 1A and B)**. It may sometimes project into the anterior chamber (pyramidal cataract). It is usually bilateral and symmetrical in both eyes. It represents anomalies of lens vesicle detachment or an abnormal growth of the primary lens fibers before closure of the lens vesicle. It is hereditary and transmitted as an autosomal dominant trait. As the nucleus is clear, this cataract develops relatively late in fetal life, not before the 4th month of gestation. It has been suggested that the progressive cortical opacification involved in certain types of anterior polar cataract is due to epithelial cell dysfunction. The depth of extension indicates the point at which the changes have taken place. They are usually stationary and not visually significant, but may be associated with astigmatism, thereby leading to amblyopia, or may be found along with corneal guttata or aniridia. This kind of cataract could be associated with small strands of the pupillary membrane between the polar opacity and the pupillary border. Association with corneal opacity and other signs of keratitis could indicate an intrauterine inflammation or a healed corneal ulcer. Pyramidal cataract has a greater impact on vision. Most cases do not warrant surgery. It is important to keep in mind that during surgery, anterior capsulorhexis is liable to tear out.
- *Anterior capsular cataract*: These opacities are plaques which are generally confined to the anterior capsule, sometimes extending into the underlying cortex. They are axial, and may be unilateral or bilateral. When bilateral, they are usually symmetrical. They are generally visible even without a microscope. This is why they are often diagnosed soon after birth. They remain static, and if not situated axially are visually insignificant. However, constant monitoring is required for any deterioration in vision. They are associated with persistent tags of the pupillary membrane when situated in the pupillary area. They are frequently hereditary, and the patient's offsprings are at high risk of incurring this form of cataract. Acquired cataract can be associated with severe skin disease.
- *Anterior capsular plaque:* These are axial opacities in the capsular epithelium **(Fig. 2)**. They are often associated with total white cataract but because of lack of contrast the diagnosis is often missed preoperatively. They occur either as multiple plaques distributed throughout the anterior lens epithelium or as a single large plaque which may be located centrally or eccentrically. They are commonly associated with persistent pupillary membrane and/or microcornea. They represent an abnormality in the regression of the pupillary membrane and require surgery only when they interfere with the development of vision.

Cortical Cataract

- *Anterior and posterior cortical cataract:* Isolated cortical cataract is less common in infants and young children

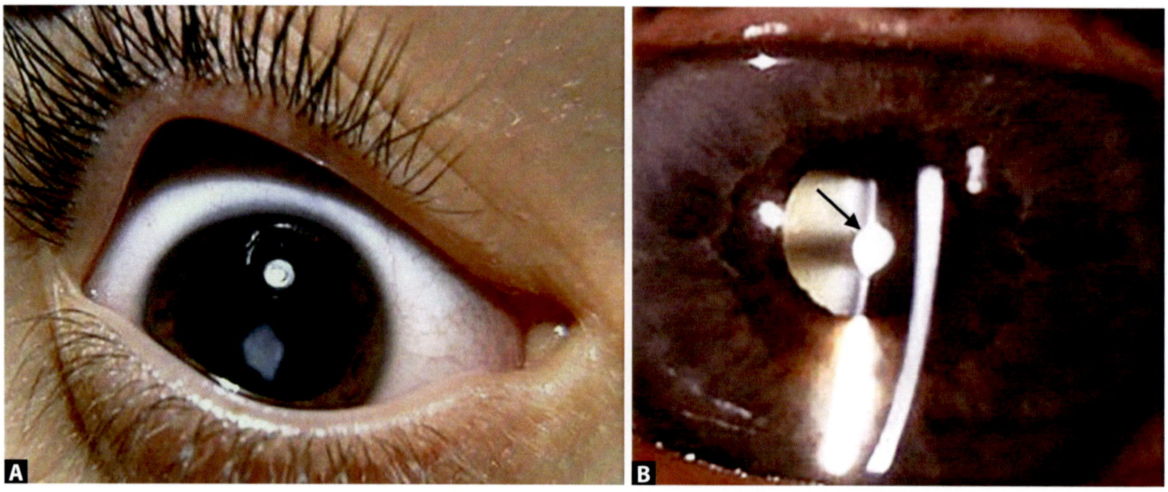

Figs. 1A and B: Anterior polar cataract.

(Figs. 3 and 4). Posterior cortical cataract is more common than anterior cortical cataract. Cortical cataract is usually present as club-shaped opacities in the periphery of the lens cortex, which does not interfere with vision. Diabetes mellitus in children can infrequently cause cortical opacities in teenage children. The classically described "coronary cataract" is a type of deep cortical cataract. It is bilateral and stationary. Usually sporadic, this is a developmental cataract that is diagnosed around puberty and is not visually significant in most cases.

- *Membranous cataract:* It is an advanced form of cortical cataract where the entire lens substance is absorbed, leaving a thin gray-white capsular membrane which replaces the cortex. It is frequently bilateral and visual prognosis is poor. It is often associated with aniridia and congenital rubella as a consequence of intrauterine iridocyclitis that remains active after birth, leading to persistent fetal vasculature (PFV) or microphthalmos. It has been described in Lowe's syndrome. Most cases are sporadic and a familial or dominant transmission is rare. The surgical outcome is variable, and it is very difficult to carry out in-the-bag IOL implantation in these cases.

Nuclear Cataract

- *Isolated nuclear cataract*: This has been classically described as the "central pulverulent cataract". The opacity involves the embryonic nucleus and is caused by an insult occurring during the first 3 months of development. It is always bilateral and nonprogressive. The white, discrete dots appear as a granular disk in the center of the lens and sometimes the dot-like opacities may extend into the overlying cortex. It is also known as the "blue-dot cataract". This form of cataract is visually insignificant. It is usually diagnosed on routine slit-lamp examination. Frequently, it may present as a dense chalky-white central cataract occupying the fetal nucleus and sometimes the embryonic and infantile nucleus. Bilateral dense nuclear cataracts have been described with congenital rubella.
- *Rubella cataract:* This cataract accounts for 4–5% of all congenital cataracts in developing countries **(Figs. 5 and 6)**. The infection is contracted by the mother during the first 3 months of pregnancy. This form of cataract is bilateral, progressive and may be associated with microphthalmos. It may present as dense nuclear

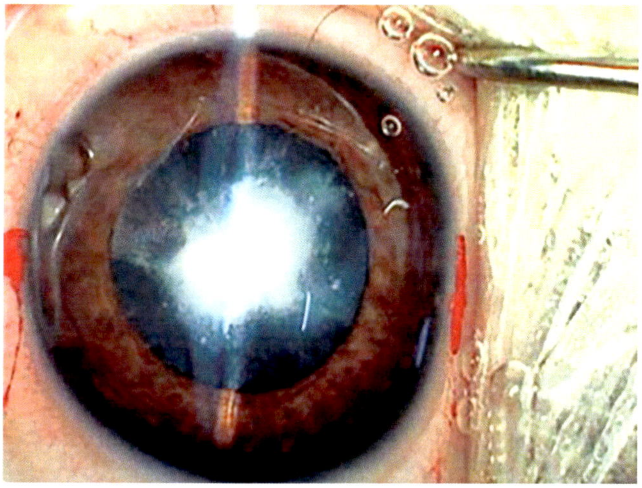

Fig. 2: Anterior capsular plaque.

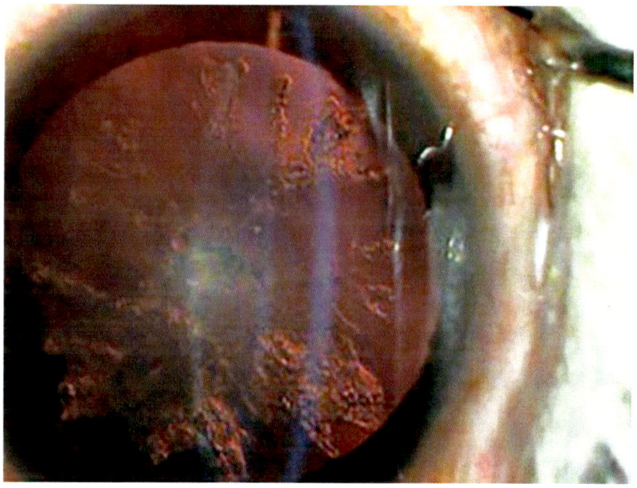

Fig. 4: Posterior cortical cataract.

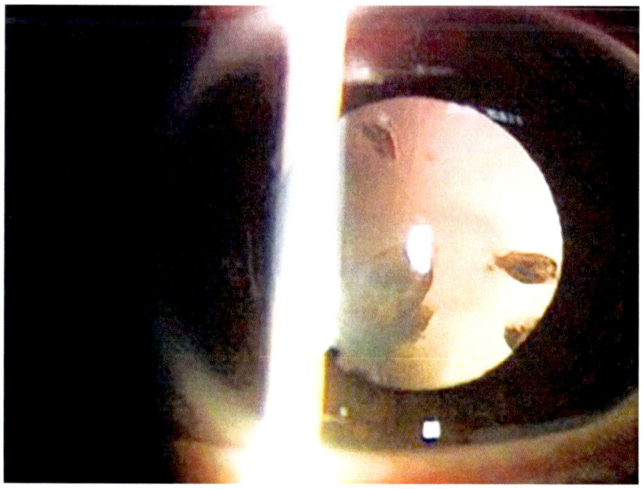

Fig. 3: Anterior cortical cataract.

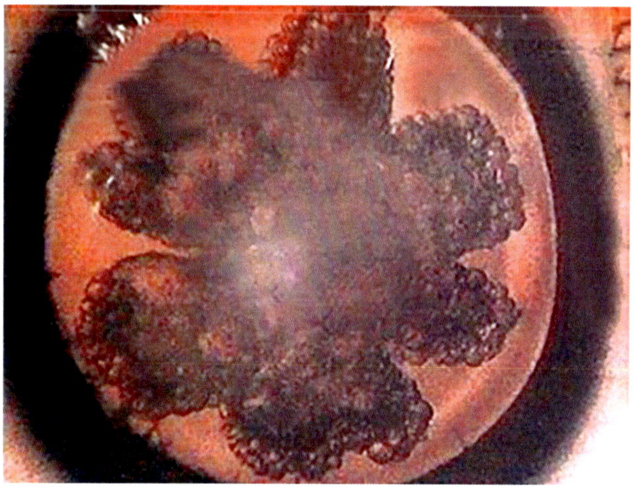

Fig. 5: Typical rubella cataract.

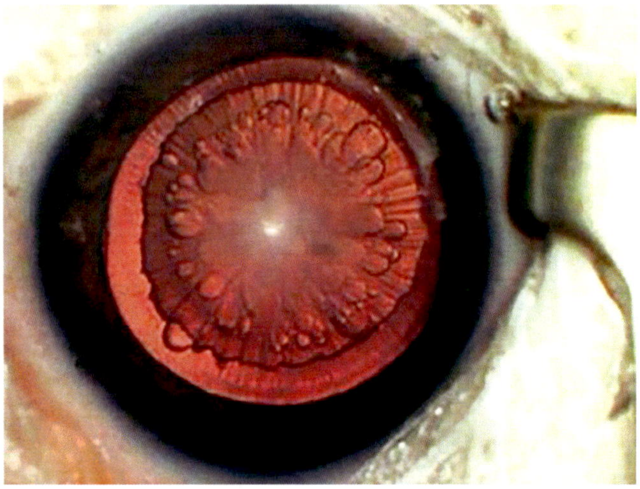

Fig. 6: Another case of a rubella cataract.

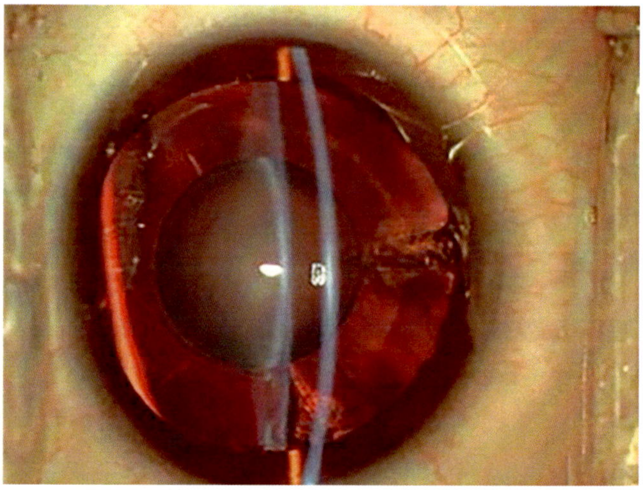

Fig. 7: Lamellar cataract. The cataract does not involve the entire nucleus.

cataract or as total cataract soon after birth. Membranous cataract is also commonly found in these eyes. A typical appearance is noted with clusters of vacuolar opacities in the cortex. These discrete clusters of opacities may represent pockets of viral replication. Early surgical intervention is mandatory in these cases. This cataract has demonstrated a strong autosomal dominant inheritance. Vaccination against rubella can prevent development of this cataract.

- *Lamellar cataract*: This form of cataract has been classically described as "zonular" or "perinuclear" cataract **(Figs. 7 and 8)**. It accounts for about 40% of congenital cataract and is predominant in males. It occurs bilaterally, and is symmetrical and stationary. It can either be congenital or developmental.

In the congenital form, the opacity is concentric, often occurring within the fetal nucleus and the embryonic nucleus is clear. The surrounding cortex also remains clear. The insult is caused after the first 3 months of embryonic development. More commonly, the opacity lies outside the fetal nucleus and represents an insult to the lens fibers later in intrauterine life or after birth. These are evident at birth.

In the developmental form, lamellar opacities occur due to an insult inflicted in early infancy or even in adolescent life. The opacity lies in the periphery of the lens. Associated "riders" (radial cataractous extensions into the clear overlying cortex) imply that the abnormality of fiber formation persisted beyond that particular time.

Lamellar opacities range from translucent, visually insignificant cataract to dense cataract, requiring early surgical intervention. Visual prognosis is better than in many other morphological types.

They are usually inherited as an autosomal dominant trait. In sporadic cases of the congenital form, parathyroid deficiency resulting in hypocalcemia and hypovitaminosis D in the mother during the last trimester of pregnancy in the fetus could be a cause. In such cases, cataract is frequently associated with imperfect calcification of the enamel of the teeth.

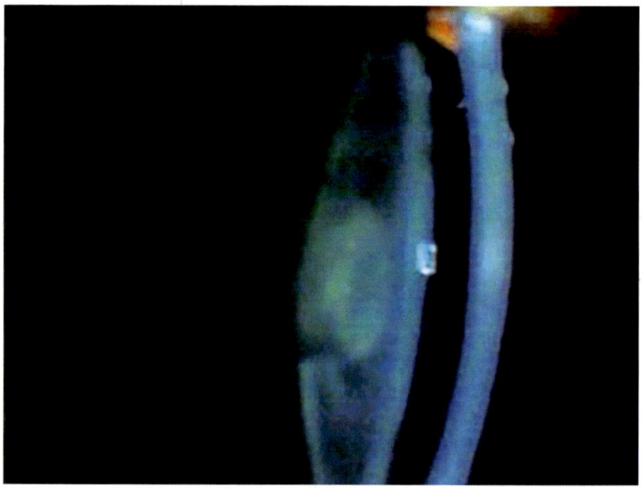

Fig. 8: Lamellar cataract. Slit view.

The developmental form could be associated with infantile tetany (carpopedal spasm, general convulsions, and laryngismus stridulus) and rickets. Untreated galactosemia classically causes an oil droplet **(Fig. 9)** or a lamellar cataract in infancy. A developmental (postnatal) lamellar cataract can develop in premature infants.

- *Sutural cataract:* It is a Y-shaped opacity affecting one or both the sutures of the fetal nucleus **(Fig. 10)**. The opacity is either around the suture or involves the sutures, more posterior than anterior. Opacification of both anterior and posterior sutures is called stellate cataract. They are stationary, bilateral, and visually insignificant. Occasionally, they may progress to form nuclear or central cataracts. This form of cataract is frequently associated with punctuate opacities elsewhere in the lens. They are usually noted as an incidental finding. It is transmitted as a dominant trait. This could be present in obligate carriers

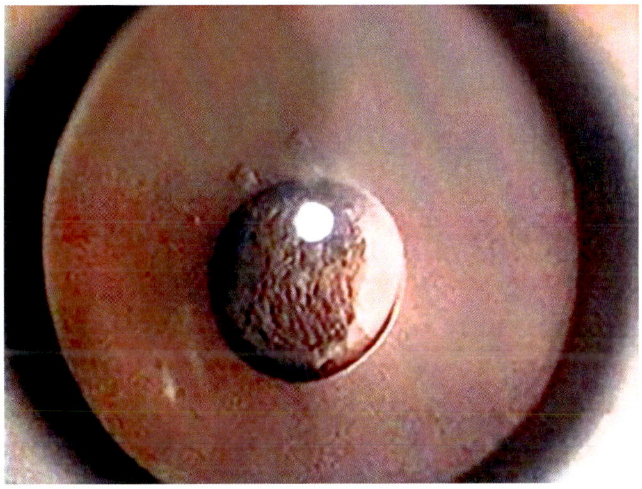

Fig. 9: Oil droplet cataract in galactosemia.

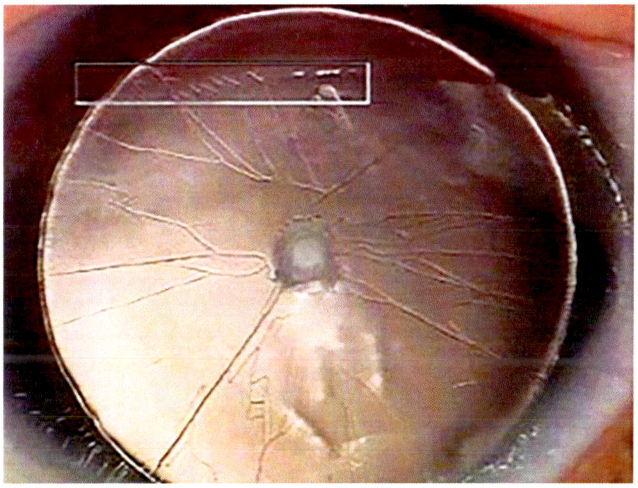

Fig. 11: Mittendorf's dot with persistent fetal vasculature.

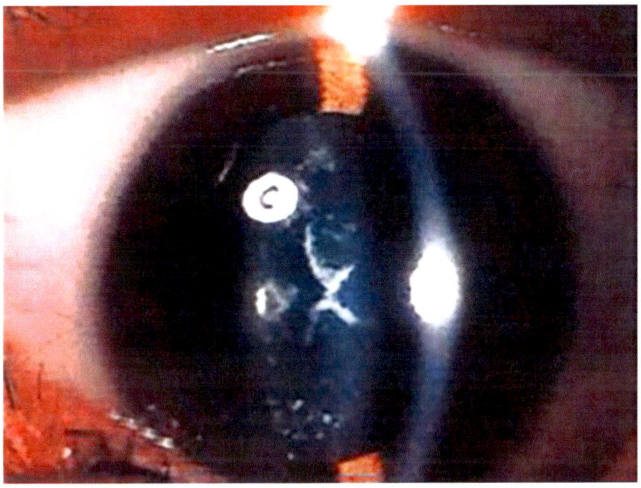

Fig. 10: Sutural cataract with punctuate cortical opacities.

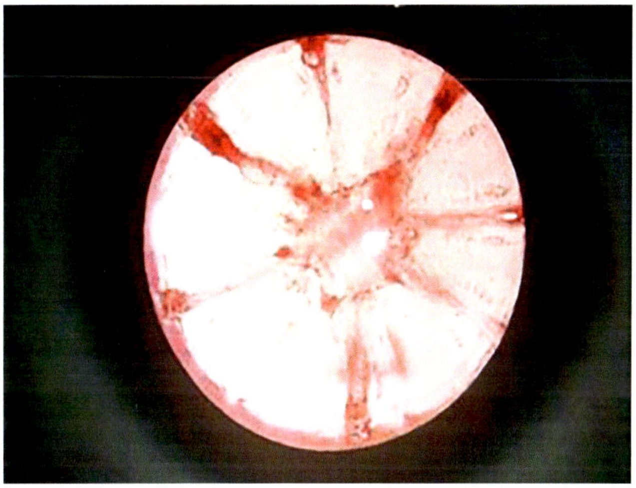

Fig. 12: Posterior subcapsular cataract.

of the Nance-Horan Syndrome (supernumerary teeth, prominent teeth and ears, and developmental delay).

- *Punctate cataract:* The floriform and coralliform cataracts are types of nuclear cataract. In floriform cataract, clusters of opacities are present around the fetal sutures. Sometimes they extend into the cortex which indicates their development after birth. They are transmitted as a dominant trait and could be associated with camptodactyly. Coralliform cataract has large crystals accumulated in the center of the lens without reference to the sutures. They radiate out without reaching the capsule. They are bilateral, axial, and stationary and can impede vision. They follow an autosomal dominant inheritance pattern.

Posterior Capsular Cataract

- *Posterior polar cataract:* In the stationary form, classically, a dense, saucer-shaped opacity covers the posterior pole of the lens. In the progressive form, radiating or punctate opacities appear in the overlying posterior cortex after birth at ages ranging from 3 to 28 years. The nuclear layers remain clear. This form of cataract is frequently bilateral. It is thought to represent a remnant of the vascular sheath of the lens, as a mild form of persistent primary hyperplastic vitreous. It has a marked visual effect because of its proximity to the nodal point. Some posterior cataracts such as Mittendorf's dots **(Fig. 11)** and posterior lenticonus (lentiglobus) may have a good visual prognosis. Posterior cataracts, especially if they are of congenital onset, may be associated with a poor visual prognosis. There is a strong hereditary tendency that is almost always dominant. During surgery, a breach in the posterior capsule should be anticipated.
- *Posterior subcapsular cataract:* This form of cataract is seen as vacuolar or plaque-like opacities close to the posterior capsule **(Fig. 12)**. Typically, it is seen in older children following trauma, uveitis or after prolonged use of steroids and radiation. Plaque-like opacities may be seen in congenital cataract, myotonic dystrophies, and Turner's syndrome. Being close to the nodal point, they are visually significant but progress very slowly. During surgery, in cases of thick plaque, posterior capsulorhexis may be required.

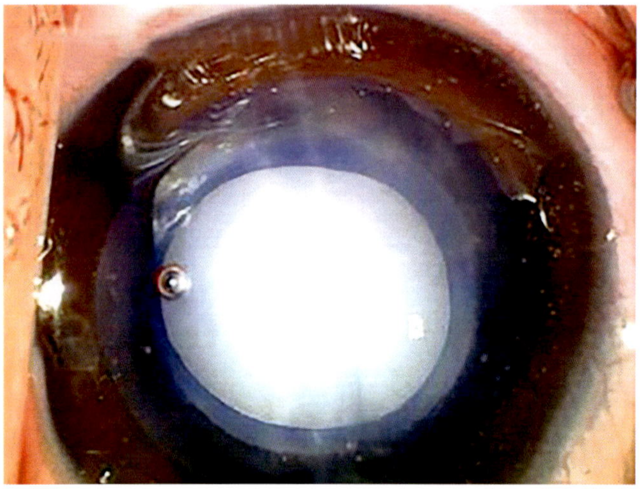

Fig. 13: Total cataract.

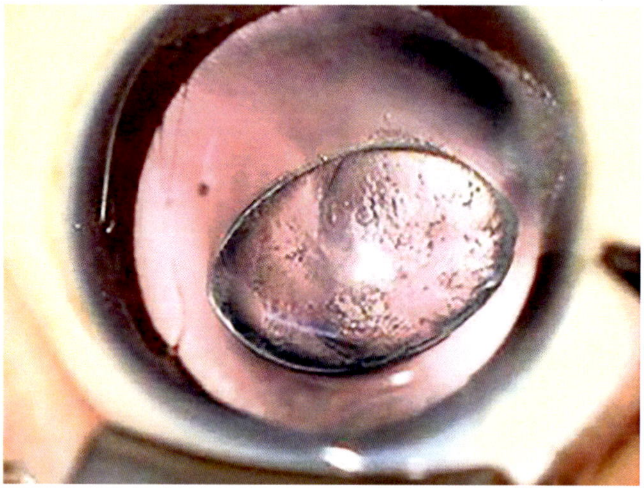

Fig. 14: Classical pre-existing posterior capsule defect.

- *Posterior lenticonus (lentiglobus):* It is a conoid protrusion of the posterior lens substance. It may be unilateral or bilateral, and if bilateral, is asymmetric. There is variable opacification of the overlying cortex. Amblyopia is frequently present, because of astigmatism, but vision may improve after postoperative amblyopia. Pathogenesis is believed to be due to progressive thinning of the posterior capsule, which may eventually lead to a posterior capsule defect (PCD). Posterior lentiglobus is associated with Lowe's syndrome. It is inherited as an X-linked condition.

Total Cataract

It presents as a general opacity of all the lens fibers **(Fig. 13)**. This occurs due to insult acting throughout the period of development or a severe insult late in fetal life. Some lenses are completely opaque when first diagnosed; in other cases they develop from lamellar or nuclear cataracts. They are frequently bilateral. In cases of early onset, they have a profound effect on visual development and may often mask underlying PCDs or posterior segment pathologies. Total cataract is frequently reported with congenital rubella syndrome, Down's syndrome, acute metabolic, or even sporadic cataracts. Aggressive surgical management is mandatory for good visual prognosis.

Mixed Cataract

Instead of isolated opacities, often, more than one anatomic types of cataract coexist in the same eye. Depending on the type and severity of opacities, vision may be affected.

Preexisting Posterior Capsule Defect (PCD)

It has been reported that preexisting PCD occurs in about 6.75% of Indian eyes. It is recognized by the presence of well-demarcated, thick defect margins and white dots on the posterior capsule and in the vitreous **(Fig. 14)**. When the globe is moved with forceps, the dots in the anterior vitreous move like a fish tail (fish-tail sign). These are frequently camouflaged by a mature cataract. They present bilaterally and are progressive. Unilateral PCDs perhaps begin as a posterior lentiglobus. It is important to recognize this entity, to avoid any surprises during surgery, and to anticipate and plan a suitable safe surgical strategy.

ETIOLOGICAL CLASSIFICATION OF CONGENITAL CATARACT

Numerous individual causes of cataract exist, and often, multiple factors act together, with plenty of scope for overlap between the groups. Some causes predispose to a specific morphological variety of cataract. Moreover, a given cause may produce more than one morphological form of cataract. The etiological classification of congenital cataract is elaborated in **Box 1**.

SPECIAL SITUATIONS

Ectopia Lentis

Ectopia lentis of the crystalline lens is a condition, where the crystalline lens is either partially or completely displaced from its original position **(Fig. 15)**, due to the absence or weakness of the zonules. In children, this has been associated with several ocular and systemic conditions **(Box 2)**.

Marfan's Syndrome

It is an autosomal dominant inherited systemic disease, with variable penetrance. It is the disease most commonly associated with sublauxated lenses. The syndrome consists of abnormalities of the cardiovascular, musculoskeletal, and ocular systems. It is caused by mutations in the fibrillin gene on chromosome. Physical characteristics of affected individuals have tall stature, arachnodactyly, loose, flexible joints, scoliosis, and chest deformities. Coexisting cardio-vascular abnormalities of aorta and heart are frequently present. Ocular abnormalities occur in 80% patients,

BOX 1: Etiological classification of congenital cataracts.

- Isolated findings
- Hereditary
  - Autosomal dominant autosomal recessive X linked
- Sporadic (one-third of all congenital cataracts)
- Part of syndrome or systemic disease
- Hereditary
  - *With renal disease*:
    - Lowe oculocerebrorenal syndrome and Alport syndrome (autosomal dominant)
  - *With central nervous system disease*:
    - Marinesco-Sjögren syndrome (autonomic recessive) and Sjögren syndrome (autonomic recessive)
    - Smith-Lemli-Opitz syndrome
    - Laurence-Moon-Bardet-Biedl syndrome with skeletal disease
    - Conradi syndrome (presence of cataract indicates worse prognosis)
    - Marfan's syndrome—stippled epiphysis
  - With abnormalities of the head and face Hallermann-Streiff syndrome, Francois dyscephalic syndrome, Pierre-Robin syndrome, and oxycephaly
    - Crouzon's disease
    - Acrocephalosyndactyly (Apert's syndrome) with polydactyly
    - Rubinstein-Taybi syndrome with skin disease
    - Bloch-Sulzberger syndrome
    - Congenital ectodermal dysplasia of the anhidrotic type and Rothmund-Thomson syndrome
    - Schaefer's syndrome, Siemen's syndrome, and incontinentia pigmenti
    - Atopic dermatitis, Cockayne's syndrome, and Marshall syndrome
  - *With chromosomal disorders*:
    - Trisomy 13 (usually die within 1 year), Trisomy 18: Edward's syndrome
    - Trisomy 21: Down's syndrome (often cataract formation delayed until approximate age of 10 years)
    - Turner's syndrome with metabolic disease
    - Galactosemia (autosomal recessive) and Galactokinase deficiency
    - Congenital hemolytic jaundice and Fabry's disease
    - Refsum's disease and mannosidosis
  - With miscellaneous hereditary syndromes, and Norrie's disease
    - Hereditary spherocytosis and myotonic dystrophy
- Nonhereditary
  - *Prenatal causes*:
    - Rubella syndrome, toxoplasmosis, varicella, cytomegalovirus, herpes simplex virus, and measles
    - Vaccinia
    - *Intrauterine hypoxia or malnutrition and postnatal causes*:
      - » Retinopathy of prematurely, hypoglycemia, and hypocalcemia
      - » Radiation, trauma, chronic uveitis
      - » Diabetes mellitus, Wilson's disease, renal insufficiency, drug induced
      - » High-voltage electric shock
  - Associated with another ocular abnormality, persistence of fetal vasculature (PFV), microphthalmos
    - Aniridia
    - Retinitis pigmentosa, Norrie's disease, and colobomas lenticonus

BOX 2: Conditions associated with ectopia lentis.

Systemic conditions:
- Marfan's syndrome
- Homocystinuria
- Weill-Marchesani syndrome
- Ehlers-Danlos syndrome
- Hyperlysinemia
- Sulfite-oxidase deficiency

Ocular conditions:
- Aniridia
- Iris coloboma
- Trauma
- Hereditary ectopia lentis

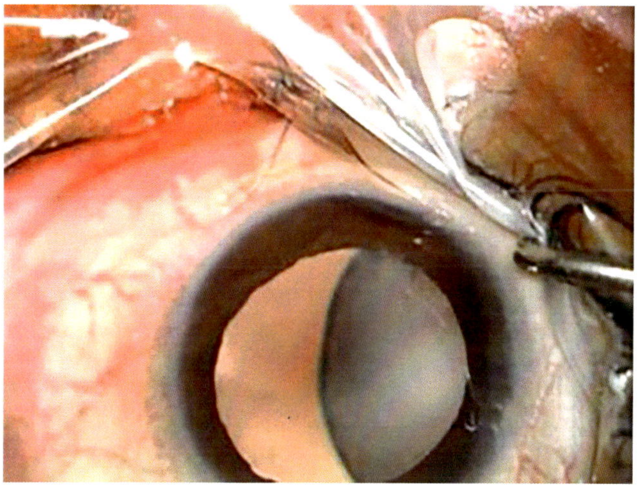

Fig. 15: Subluxated cataract in a child with loss of zonules.

including ectopia lentis, myopia, and greater risk of retinal detachment (RD). Typically, the lens is subluxated superotemporally. The zonules are often visible and unbroken. On examination, there is iridodonesis, phacodonesis, deep anterior chamber, and small and nondilating pupils. Myopia and RD are common in the second and third decades of life.

Homocystinuria

It is a rare, inherited, autosomal recessive disorder of metabolism of amino acid methionine due to deficiency of methionine synthase. Homocysteine is an intermediate amino acid formed by the conversion of methionine to cysteine. Due to deficiency of further conversion, there is raised concentration of homocysteine in urine and plasma. Clinical features are variable, affecting the eye, skeletal system, central nervous system, and vascular system. Ocular findings primarily consist of subluxated lenses (frequently downward and nasally). Systemically, vascular complications are common and secondary to thrombotic disease affecting large or medium-sized arteries and veins all over the body. Patients are usually tall, with osteoporosis, scoliosis, and chest deformities.

Ectopia Lentis et Pupillae

Ectopia lentis et pupillae is a rare autosomal recessive condition. It is manifested by bilateral displacement of the pupil, usually inferotemporally, with lens dislocation in the opposite direction. Patients have microspherophakia, meiosis, and poor pupillary dilatation with mydriatics.

Complicated Cataracts

Complicated cataracts occur commonly as a result of uveitis, often occurring in conjunction with arthritis (juvenile rheumatoid arthritis—JRA) or as a result of posterior or intermediate uveitis of any cause. Cataract may be the direct result of inflammation within the eye or can result from steroid use to treat the condition. Cataracts caused by steroid ingestion are usually posterior subcapsular. Children with JRA-associated cataracts also characteristically develop band keratopathy and posterior synechiae.

Secondary Cataracts

Less frequently, a cataract may be seen secondary to an intraocular tumor, a foreign body, or a chronic RD. Cataracts have also been known to occur after laser treatment for threshold retinopathy of prematurity.

Persistent Fetal Vasculature

Persistent fetal vasculature is a developmental ocular anomaly in which the embryonic hyaloid vasculature fails to regress normally. The disease entity has a wide spectrum with varying degrees of persistent components of the fetal hyaloid system. This may present as mild pupillary strands and a small central/paracentral posterior capsular opacification [Mittendorf's dot **(*see* Fig. 11)**] or as severe as retrolenticular membrane, retinal dysplasia, and RD. PFV is described as being anterior, posterior, or both depending on which ocular structures are involved.

Persistent fetal vasculature is typically known as an idiopathic congenital malformation that has no obvious cause and that is usually unilateral. The affected eye is often microphthalmic when compared with the unaffected eye. If the eye with PFV is not shorter than the normal fellow eye, then glaucoma should be suspected. The characteristic features of PFV include white vascularized retrolental tissue with or without a persistent hyaloid artery, centrally dragged ciliary processes, an anteriorly shifted and/or swollen lens and varying degrees of lenticular opacification. Over a period of time, the retrolenticular membrane can progressively contract, leading to RD. If left untreated, it can frequently lead to recurrent secondary glaucoma and eventual phthisis bulbi. Posterior PFV predominantly affects the posterior segment of the eye and is associated with poor visual outcome.

Traumatic Cataracts

They are a common cause of unilateral loss of vision in children. Penetrating injuries are usually more common than blunt injuries. Cataracts caused by blunt trauma classically form stellate or rosette-shaped posterior axial opacities, which may be stable or progressive, whereas, penetrating trauma with disruption of the lens capsule forms cortical changes that may remain focal if small or may progress rapidly to total opacification.

MANAGEMENT OF PEDIATRIC CATARACTS

The incidence of congenital cataracts has been reported as 2.5/10,000 by the age of 1 year, increasing to 3.5/10,000 by age 15. It is estimated that over 200,000 children are blind from disorders of the lenses. Although blindness in most cases can be principally attributed to unoperated cataract; dense amblyopia following delayed surgery, complications of surgery, or associated ocular abnormalities may also be other causes of blindness.

Visually significant cataract in children calls for prompt surgical intervention to clear the ocular media and provide a focused retinal image. Indications for cataract surgery include visually significant central cataracts, dense nuclear cataracts, cataracts obstructing the examiner's view of the fundus, and cataracts associated with strabismus. The timing of treatment is crucial to visual development and successful rehabilitation of children, especially during early infancy. In general, the first 6 weeks of life is reported to be the critical period during which the infant's eye may be relatively resistant to develop amblyopia since the vision is subcortically mediated. Surgery for unilateral cataracts should be performed within the first 6 weeks of life and that for bilateral cataracts within the first 8–10 weeks of life to prevent development of stimulus deprivation amblyopia. With bilateral cataracts, it is also important that the second eye should be operated as early as possible, often within a week so as to avoid deprivation amblyopia. In a recent study, it was reported that children undergoing surgery for unilateral cataracts between 28 and 48 days of birth had better recognition visual acuity (VA) outcomes at 4.5 years follow-up as compared to children who had surgery after 48 days.

Pediatric cataract surgery is a complex issue, best left to surgeons, who are familiar with its long-term complications and prolonged follow-ups. Cataract surgery in children is the first stepping stone in the long road to visual rehabilitation. Treatment is often difficult and tedious requiring a dedicated team effort, the most important members of the team being the parents. It is very important to counsel parents appropriately. Parents need to come for regular follow-up visits and see that the child wears glasses or contact lenses and complies with medication and occlusion therapy following surgery. Maintaining a clear visual axis while correcting the eye for a changing residual refractive error requires careful observation, sound judgment, and diligent follow-up.

Anesthesia: Pediatric cataract surgery is unique in that, preoperatively, intraoperatively, and postoperatively, the child requires multiple examinations under anesthesia. Prior to surgery, a detailed history and thorough pre-anesthetic check-up is mandatory.

Preoperative Evaluation

Preoperative examination includes detection of strabismus and nystagmus, a thorough anterior and posterior segment examination, and visual function by relevant age-matched vision acuity tests. In infants, fixation and fixation preference should be assessed.

Preoperative examination with fully dilated pupils, if necessary under anesthesia, is mandatory in both eyes. It includes examination under the operating microscope or slit-lamp biomicroscope to assess the cataract and tonometry to rule out any association of glaucoma. The examination also includes measurement of corneal diameter, posterior segment evaluation, keratometry, biometry, and gonioscopy. During the examination, the surgeon must look for the type and severity of cataract including preexisting PCD.

A complete preoperative checkup by anesthetist/physician/cardiologist should be performed to rule out any systemic disorder. Laboratory tests should include complete hemogram, blood sugar, TORCH test, hepatitis-B test and any special investigation if metabolic disorder is suspected.

Biometry: Intraocular Lens Power Calculation

Despite all efforts, predicting the axial growth of the eye and therefore, selecting an IOL of appropriate power for the eye is one of the biggest enigmas in pediatric cataract surgery. Accurate keratometry and biometry are essential to determine the IOL power for each eye. Most often, a handheld keratometry needs to be performed under general anesthesia **(Fig. 16)**. Ultrasound biometry is performed using the contact/immersion technique for axial length measurement **(Fig. 17)**. It is now quite well accepted that immersion ultrasound biometry is more accurate than contact biometry for children. Whether to aim for emmetropia or undercorrect the child anticipating a future myopic shift is still not clear. The general consensus, particularly for young children is to perform varying degrees of undercorrection, based on empirical guidelines and personal preferences. In general, younger the child, more should be the undercorrection. There are varying reports on the axial growth in children following cataract surgery, with some studies reporting retardation of growth and others reporting rapid elongation of the eyes. Several formulae, including the SRK-II, SRK-T, Hoffer Q, Holladay 1, Holladay 2, as well as Pediatric IOL Power calculator have been shown to be effective in IOL power calculation. However, the target of achieving targeted refraction still remains an enigma. Thus, it appears that all modern IOL power calculation formulae give some prediction error in pediatric eyes, more so in children <2 years of age.

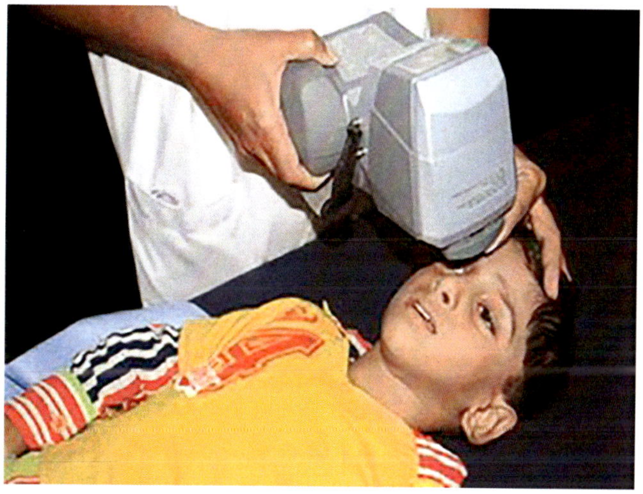

Fig. 16: Handheld keratometry being performed.

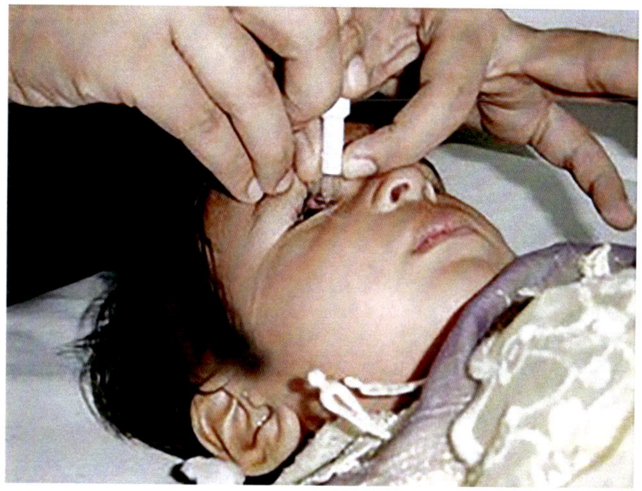

Fig. 17: Immersion ultrasound biometry being performed.

Several nomograms on IOL power selection have been published in literature. However, these tables are only meant to help as a starting point toward appropriate IOL power selection, which is a multifactorial decision customized for each child based on many variables [including age, laterality (one eye or both), amblyopia status (dense or mild), compliance with glasses, and family history of myopia]. The axial length increases faster in the first few years of life. If the decision regarding IOL implantation needs to be changed, e.g., in cases of ciliary sulcus implantation, appropriate adjustment may need to be done. The residual refractive error needs to be corrected with spectacles or contact lens that are adjusted throughout the growing period according to refractive development.

The approach of the authors for undercorrection depending upon the age at the time of surgery is given in **Table 2**.

As an example, in a 7-month old child, if the IOL power is calculated at +36.0D, it is undercorrected by 25%. So IOL power to be implanted would be 36 – 9 = + 27.0D.

TABLE 2: Undercorrection depending upon the age at the time of surgery.

Age	Undercorrection (%)
0–3 months	35%
3–6 months	30%
6–12 months	25%
1–2 years	20%
2–4 years	15%
4–6 years	10%
>6 years	5%

Surgical Technique

Pediatric cataract needs a special surgical strategy as these eyes have greater elasticity of the capsule, lower scleral rigidity, higher incidence of inflammation and posterior capsule opacification (PCO), a thick vitreous gel, and it is a small, growing eye. The surgeon should strictly adhere to the principles of the closed chamber technique, such as valvular incision, injection of ophthalmic viscosurgical devices (OVD) before removing any instrument from the eye, and bimanual irrigation/aspiration.

Two surgical approaches exist for lens removal in pediatric eyes:

1. *Pars plana lensectomy*: In children where aphakia is the chosen means of visual rehabilitation, lensectomy may be performed through a pars plana incision with an automated vitrector. The irrigation may be introduced through a scleral port or even through a corneal/limbal paracentesis incision. The disadvantage of this approach is that since the capsular bag is not preserved, it does not allow for in-the-bag IOL implantation either primarily or later in life.
2. *Limbal approach:*
   a. *The incision*: Pediatric cataract can be removed through a relatively small incision, as there is no hard nucleus. If no IOL implantation is planned, two paracentesis incisions at or near the limbus will suffice for performing bimanual irrigation/aspiration. When an IOL is being implanted a self-sealing valvular corneal/scleral incision should be made. The incisions are sutured due to the low scleral rigidity and because children have a tendency to rub their eyes.
   b. *Anterior capsule management*: The anterior capsule in children is very elastic, and therefore it may be difficult to perform a controlled manual continuous curvilinear capsulorhexis (CCC). However, a manual CCC is the gold standard in terms of maintaining the integrity of the capsular edge. The shape, size, and edge integrity of anterior capsulotomy are very important for long-term centration of the IOL. Alternatives to manual CCC currently available include vitrectorhexis, radiofrequency diathermy, Fugo plasma blade, the two incision push pull technique, and the four incision technique.
   c. High viscosity OVD and capsular staining with trypan blue or indocyanine green is a useful adjunct, especially in cases where there is poor glow. Care is taken to frequently grasp and regrasp the capsule to avoid peripheral extension of the CCC.
   d. Recently, the femtosecond laser capsulotomy, which has the promise of precision and automation in performing a desired size and centration of anterior capsulotomy has shown encouraging results in pediatric cataract surgery. While this technology continues to evolve, current limitations include the difficulty in docking the patient's eye while under general anesthesia, as well as the added cost of two patient interfaces. Newer advances such as the precision pulse capsulotomy also may make anterior capsulotomy more predictable and less skill dependent in the times to come.
   e. *Cortical cleaving hydrodissection*: Multiquadrant hydrodissection can be performed in all cases except in eyes with a total cataract or when a preexisting PCD is suspected. It is documented that multiquadrant cortical-cleaving hydrodissection in pediatric cataract surgery facilitates lens substance removal and reduces removal time.
   f. *Lens removal*: The lens material is usually aspirated bimanually using separate irrigation and aspiration ports. Since visual axis obscuration (VAO) is one of the most frequent complications in pediatric cataract surgery, meticulous removal of the lens fibers and lens epithelial cells is crucial. A bimanual approach minimizes anterior chamber fluctuations and aids in thorough removal of the cortex, especially in the sub incisional area.

Management of the Posterior Capsule and Anterior Vitreous in Children

The most frequent and significant problem following pediatric cataract surgery is VAO, with the incidence being almost 100% in younger children, if the posterior capsule is intact. Maintenance of a clear visual axis remains a high priority when planning management of the posterior capsule in the amblyogenic age range. Posterior capsulotomy can be performed with various approaches including manual posterior continuous curvilinear capsulorhexis (PCCC), vitrectorhexis, radiofrequency diathermy, and Fugo plasma blade. Manual PCCC is performed before IOL implantation, whereas a pars plana vitrectorhexis is performed after the IOL is implanted. The size of the posterior capsulorhexis should be large enough to provide a clear central visual axis, but smaller than the IOL optic, to allow stable in-the-bag IOL fixation. Manual PCCC offers the advantage of a controlled size and strong edges but is more difficult to perform **(Fig. 18)**.

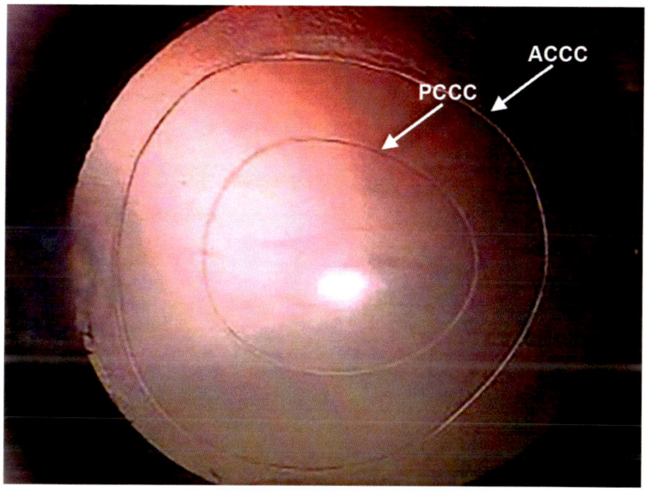

Fig. 18: Ideal size of a posterior capsulorhexis.
(PCCC: posterior continuous curvilinear capsulorrhexis; ACCC: anterior continuous curvilinear capsulorrhexis)

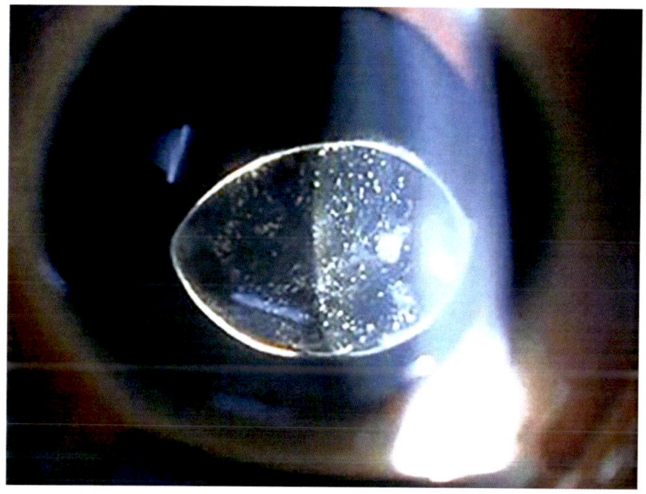

Fig. 19: "Fish tail" appearance of posterior capsule defects.

Posterior continuous curvilinear capsulorhexis alone may delay the onset of VAO but cannot eliminate it completely. The anterior vitreous face (AVF) may act as a scaffold for the proliferating lens epithelial cells. Moreover, since the inflammatory response in small children is severe, fibrous membranes may form on the intact AVF, resulting in VAO. Hence, anterior vitrectomy along with posterior capsulotomy is advocated in infants and children <6–7 years of age. Most surgeons prefer limbal anterior vitrectomy over pars plana vitrectomy. However, pars plana vitrectomy has the advantage that it tackles the vitreous through its natural origin in the posterior segment. Further, performing a pars plana vitrectomy along with vitrectorhexis, following IOL implantation allows the surgeon to perform an in the bag IOL implantation in the desired site without worrying about the size and centration of a manual PCCC. This is especially true for infant eyes where performing a desired size centration and size of PCCC may not be possible every time. With newer phacoemulsification machines, vitrectomy cutters have good cut rates and are usually compatible with 23-gauge instrumentation. The adequacy of anterior vitrectomy may be confirmed by injecting 0.1–0.2 mL of preservative free triamcinolone (4 mg/0.1 mL) to aid visualization of the vitreous.

Our strategy is to perform PCCC and anterior vitrectomy in all children up to 4 years of age, and older children who are not amenable to Nd:YAG capsulotomy. Children between 4 and 6 years are subjected to PCCC but no vitrectomy. In children over 6 years, PCCC is not performed as a rule.

Preexisting Posterior Capsule Defect (PCD)

Congenital cataract in infants and children sometimes presents with a preexisting defect in the PCO. Many theories have been proposed to explain the development of PCD. It is believed to begin as a posterior lentiglobus, which gradually progresses to a full blown PCD. In classic cases of PCD, the defect is hidden behind a seemingly "routine" pediatric cataract when viewed through a normal sized, undilated pupil. Maximum dilation is mandatory to unveil the important diagnostic signs.

Signs of preexisting PCD are ***(Fig. 19)***:

- Demarcated thick defect margins
- White dots on the posterior capsule and in the anterior vitreous
- Fish tail sign—a characteristic of PCD.

When the globe is moved with forceps, the white granules in the anterior vitreous move with the degenerated vitreous like a fish tail. It is important to recognize and suspect a preexisting PCD. The surgical strategy includes avoiding hydrodissection in such cases, as it might lead to a blowout of the posterior capsule.

Challenges in Intraocular Lens Implantation in Children

Early correction of aphakic refractive error is the most critical component in pediatric cataract surgery to prevent the development of amblyopia. Spectacles, contact lenses, and IOL implantation have been used for correction of surgical aphakia. However, usage of spectacles/contact lenses for young children is associated with practical problems of wearing, additional economic burden, and emotional turmoil for the child.

Primary IOL implantation has the advantage of providing at least a partial optical correction at all times. However, this benefit should be carefully weighed against the potential risks for intra- as well as postoperative complications. IOL implantation in children >2 years of age is now an accepted practice worldwide. Surgeons are still cautious about implanting an IOL in infants keeping in mind the severity of the intraoperative and postoperative complications including exaggerated inflammatory response, high rate of VAO, and secondary glaucoma. When surgeons choose IOL implantation in an infant eye at the time of congenital cataract surgery, they need to carefully weigh the benefits of surgery against the risks associated with the procedure.

Selecting the Appropriate Patient for Primary IOL Implantation

- Microcornea and microphthalmos are contraindications to *primary* IOL implantation, regardless of the age at surgery. Microcornea is usually defined as a horizontal corneal diameter of <9 mm, and microphthalmos is defined as an axial length (AL) which is <2 standard deviations of the reported normal AL for that age. PFV and juvenile/idiopathic arthritis, once considered as contraindications to IOL implantation are not absolute contraindications nowadays due to better techniques and technology. However, in both these conditions, presence of microphthalmos, microcornea, or severe, persistent, and intractable uveitis may cause additional complications and these patients are better left aphakic in primary surgery.
- Secondary implantation of customized IOLs may be considered in microphthalmic eyes and in eyes with uveitis once the disease is controlled. However, these cases should not be handled by occasional pediatric cataract surgeons.

Intraocular Lens Implantation in Unilateral Cataract

In the 1970s, it was believed by ophthalmologists that unilateral cataracts need not be operated upon since they are associated with poor visual prognosis. Subsequently, it was shown in studies that cataract surgery in unilateral cataracts yields good outcomes. Unilateral cataractous eyes may have comorbid conditions such as microphthalmos, PFV, microcornea, and colobomas. Further, the amblyogenic potential of unilateral cataracts is much more than bilateral cataracts, and therefore timely surgery followed by intensive amblyopia treatment and monitoring is required to prevent amblyopia and squint. Aphakic spectacles are practically not a viable option for these eyes due to their unilateral nature. Contact lenses are the only nonsurgical modality for optical correction of aphakia in these eyes. Advantages of contact lenses include the ability to change the contact lens power as needed to keep up with the rapidly growing eye's refractive needs and avoiding spectacle wear during the first few years of life. However, the use of contact lenses in infants has its own set of problems pertaining to difficulty in insertion and removal of the lens, the complications involved in fitting the lens onto the steep corneas of infants, as well as compliance issues. In developing countries, the repeated cost of replacing contact lenses due to frequent losses as well as change in refraction is often a limiting factor, along with parental education and hygiene levels that may prohibit effective contact lens usage.

In infants, there is still some controversy as to when primary IOL implantation can be performed. Recent studies in the United States of America and by British Isles Congenital Cataract Interest Group have found no added long-term visual benefit with primary IOL implantation in infants with added disadvantages of inflammatory sequelae, resurgeries, and anesthesia-related complications. However, it must be understood here that the control group (aphakic group) in these were compliant patients who used contact lenses. On the other hand, there have also been studies which report better VA with primary IOL implantation as compared to primary aphakia.

Therefore, the decision regarding IOL versus contact lens rehabilitation is a complex and multifactorial one, based on factors such as surgeon's experience, ability to perform regular and rigorous follow-ups, feasibility and safety of contact lens usage as well as availability of a dedicated team, including vision therapists and anesthesiologists.

Intraocular Lens Implantation in Bilateral Cataracts

Till a few years ago, it was believed that spectacles for bilateral aphakia were compatible with good vision and secondary IOL implantation could be performed once the child grew up. But now it has been well demonstrated by other researchers and authors that visual recovery is much faster when primary IOL implantation is performed, and the rates of serious postoperative complications are comparable after surgery in both groups (other group being children left aphakic). Thus, primary IOL implantation may be considered in infants with bilateral cataracts, wherever an in the bag IOL implantation can be performed. What is important is that the surgeon should have experience and expertise in implanting in-the-bag IOLs in children.

It is important to keep in mind that in pediatric eyes, the only safe place for IOL implantation is in the capsular bag. If the surgeon is unable to place an IOL within the capsular bag during surgery, ciliary sulcus IOL should be avoided, particularly in infants and young children.

Intraocular Lens Material, Type, and Size

Today, foldable hydrophobic acrylic IOLs have become the preferred IOL choice for most pediatric cataract surgeons instead of the polymethyl methacrylate (PMMA) IOLs which were once the IOLs of choice. Being foldable, these IOLs offer all the benefits of smaller incision cataract surgery. Further, the hydrophobic acrylic material has excellent biocompatibility and is reported to cause lesser and more delayed onset PCO. Recently, there have also been reports regarding the safety of hydrophilic IOLs in pediatric eyes. Another important issue is of IOL sizing. Most IOLs available today are designed for adult eyes and adult capsular bags. Infants and younger children have smaller ocular dimensions, and therefore, ideally would require IOLs with a smaller overall diameter. However, unfortunately, specially sized IOLs of the preferred biocompatible material are not very widely available for commercial use.

Optic Capture of Intraocular Lens

Visual axis obscuration is one of the biggest hurdles for successful visual rehabilitation following successful pediatric cataract surgery, particularly when surgery is performed at a young age. This is the reason why anterior vitrectomy has become an integral part of the surgical strategy for children <5–6 years of age. However, the technique of optic capture, which was first described for pediatric eyes by Dr Howard Gimbel offers a strategy whereby anterior vitrectomy can be avoided and yet VAO can be delayed or reduced. Here, an IOL is placed in the capsule bag following anterior and posterior capsulorhexes, and thereafter, the IOL optic is slid behind the PCCC margin, so as to "lock it" in position **(Figs. 20 and 21)**. This ensures both, IOL stability as well as retardation of VAO since the fusion of anterior and posterior capsulorhexis margins behind the IOL optic prevents central migration of proliferating lens epithelial cells. In a recent randomized study, we have shown that performing in the bag IOL implantation with anterior vitrectomy has similar safety and complication rates as performing optic capture of a three-piece foldable IOL without any anterior vitrectomy.

Toric and Multifocal Intraocular Lenses

Preexisting corneal astigmatism is a problem in both adult and pediatric cataract surgery. Further, astigmatism has the potential to cause meridional amblyopia in the pediatric population. Since toric IOLs have been largely successful in adult eyes, surgeons have started adopting the use of these IOLs to deal with preexisting corneal astigmatism even in pediatric eyes. Although, there are not many reports in literature, the technology appears promising by aiming to correct one of the amblyogenic factors in the growing population. However, it is important that only children above the age of 5 years and those who can cooperate for reliable biometry, keratometry and corneal topography measurements can be selected for toric IOL implantation. This is due to the fact that the corneal curvature only stabilizes by 5–6 years of age.

The use of multifocal IOLs is controversial in children, especially those below the age of 12 years. There are few reports suggesting good outcomes with multifocal IOLs, however, review of literature shows there is not enough evidence to suggest the use of these IOLs in pediatric eyes due to the several intraoperative and postoperative concerns. One of the primary concerns is that with currently available designs of multifocal IOLs, there is an inherent reduction in light sensitivity, which may lead to impaired contrast sensitivity and some disturbance in visual quality.

Primary Intraocular Lens Implantation below 2 years—What is the Verdict?

Primary in the bag IOL implantation is an accepted mode of visual rehabilitation in children >2 years of age. However, in younger children, there is some controversy. The Infant Aphakia Treatment Study (IATS) has cautioned against the use of IOL in unilateral cataract surgery under the age of 7 months. They report long-term results of a large randomized trial and report that reoperation rate and certain complications are higher when IOL is implanted in these specific groups of eyes. However, for bilateral cataracts, recent studies have shown that it is both safe and effective to implant IOLs in infants and children below 2 years.

Secondary Intraocular Lens Implantation

Often, children may be left aphakic during their primary surgery, either due to young age, surgeon's preference

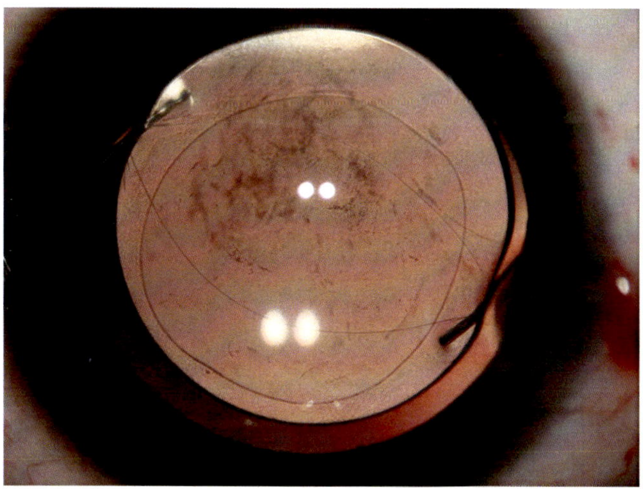

Fig. 20: Optic capture of IOL, intraoperative picture of ovalization of PCCC suggesting successful capture.
(IOL: intraocular lens; PCCC: posterior continuous curvilinear capsulorhexis)

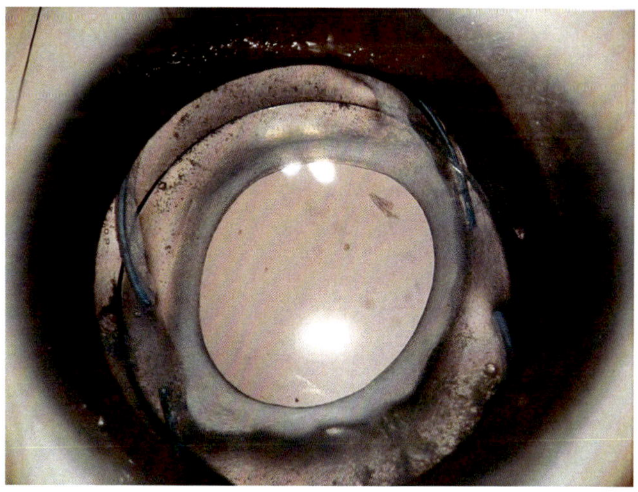

Fig. 21: 1.5 years follow-up of optic capture of intraocular lens (IOL), clear visual axis maintained.

or conditions that preclude primary IOL implantation. Secondary IOL implantation is a feasible option once the child grows up, and more importantly, the eye achieves an AL and corneal diameter suitable for IOL implantation. Most surgeons would prefer to perform secondary IOL implantation after the child achieves an age of at least 3 years. In case, a young child is being left aphakic, care should be taken during primary surgery to perform meticulously sized anterior and posterior capsulorhexes along with complete cortical removal, so that adequate capsular support is available for future IOL implantation.

As for the site of IOL placement, the IOL can be placed in the capsular bag or in the ciliary sulcus. In the bag, IOL placement requires the surgeon to open the fused capsules and create space in the capsular bag. Although ideal, this surgical strategy is challenging and may not be possible due to fused capsules. In this situation, a ciliary sulcus IOL should be placed, and the optic may be captured through the anterior capsulorhexis. It should be kept in mind that only three-piece foldable IOLs should be implanted in the ciliary sulcus. Single piece foldable IOLs, when implanted in the sulcus, are known to cause inflammation and/or glaucoma. There are reports in literature that suggest successful outcomes following secondary IOL implantation, both in the ciliary sulcus and in the capsular bag. Further, whenever secondary IOL implantation is performed, close follow-up should be maintained to watch for postoperative inflammation, glaucoma, and retinal complications.

Complications of Pediatric Cataract Surgery

Although there are several complications of pediatric cataract surgery, the most frequent complications, both in the short-term and long-term are discussed below:

Glaucoma

One of the most common complications after cataract surgery, it is reported in 10–20% of eyes following surgery. Some studies report that IOL implantation is protective against, whereas others say it may be a risk factor for development of glaucoma. Young age at surgery, particularly in the first few weeks of life has been reported by several studies, along with a smaller corneal diameter as two of the most important predictors for glaucoma. Further, glaucoma may develop several years after surgery, and therefore, a prolonged follow-up is essential to be able to diagnose this problem.

A large meta-analysis of studies in 470 infant eyes undergoing cataract surgery at 7 centers across the globe was recently published which investigated the effect of the following risk factors on development of glaucoma following cataract surgery in infant eyes (<1 year)—IOL implantation, age at surgery, additional surgeries, and unilateral versus bilateral cataracts. The following were identified as risk factors for development of glaucoma—age up to 4 weeks at the time of surgery, and additional intraocular procedures. Primary IOL implantation was found to be protective for glaucoma. Asrani and colleagues also reported that IOL implantation was protective against glaucoma. The recently published IATS reported a higher incidence of glaucoma in children <7 months of age undergoing unilateral cataract surgery when IOL was implanted (12%) compared to aphakia (5%), although the difference was not found to be statistically significant at 1 year follow-up. At 5 years follow-up in the same study, the incidence of glaucoma was 18% in IOL group versus 16% in the contact lens group, suggesting no protective effect of IOL on glaucoma.

Visual Axis Obscuration

Visual axis obscuration is undoubtedly the most frequent complication following pediatric cataract surgery, and can hamper functional visual outcomes despite a good anatomical outcome. Performing a primary posterior capsulotomy along with anterior vitrectomy has therefore become standard of care for infant eyes. Although primary posterior capsulorhexis, anterior vitrectomy, and in the bag placement of hydrophobic acrylic IOLs have helped to delay the onset or reduce the severity of VAO, it is still a major problem particularly in infantile eyes. Aggressive postoperative inflammation may lead to formation of membranes on the anterior/posterior surface of the IOL, which may obscure the visual axis. Therefore, intensive and prolonged anti-inflammatory treatment following surgery is very important. The IATS reported a much higher incidence of significant VAO in pseudophakic eyes compared to aphakic eyes. It is believed that the IOL in the bag prevents fusion of anterior and posterior capsule leaflets, thereby allowing proliferation and migration of lens epithelial cells into the visual axis. Not only does VAO obstruct vision in the crucial formative period, but it also necessitates additional surgical procedures under anesthesia, which may be a significant stress, both psychological and financial, to the parents/caregivers.

Several strategies to combat VAO are being used by surgeons, and ongoing research is being directed toward preventing or even delaying VAO, especially in very young children. Sealed capsule irrigation devices that use distilled water or 5-fluorouracil to irrigate the capsular bag and selectively destroy equatorial lens epithelial cells (LECs) seem like a promising modality to eliminate VAO. However, despite the idea being around for a long time, it has still not come into clinical use. Thus, both its efficacy as well as safety to surrounding structures, particularly the corneal endothelium needs to be established before it can be used. Two other ideas that promise to retard or delay VAO and yet avoid anterior vitrectomy are posterior optic capture of IOL and bag in the lens IOL implantation.

Professor Tassignon has designed a unique IOL where anterior and posterior capsulorhexes of identical size are performed manually, and a specially designed IOL is implanted, with the capsule leaflets being tucked into grooves of the IOL. The advantage of this approach is that the LECs are sequestered between the two leaflets and thereby VAO is avoided. Further, since there is no migration of the LECs behind the IOL optic, there is no need to perform anterior vitrectomy. Long-term studies with this IOL have shown very favorable results in pediatric eyes.

Management of Visual Axis Obscuration in Children

This depends on the age of the child, his or her cooperation, and on the density of the membrane.

- *Neodymium-doped yttrium aluminum garnet laser capsulotomy:* An Nd:YAG laser capsulotomy is preferred in children over 5 years as they can follow the instructions and cooperate during the procedure. This procedure has been shown to effectively maintain a clear axis in a significant proportion of children. However, a capsulotomy may have to be performed more than once in certain situations.
- *Secondary surgical membranectomy with vitrectomy*: In eyes in which the capsule is too thick and is not amenable to Nd:YAG capsulotomy, or, when the child is too young to cooperate for a laser procedure, a secondary surgical membranectomy/capsulotomy is done. The pars plana approach is preferred as it allows more direct and easier removal of the PCO.

Other Complications

Retinal detachment and cystoid macular edema are infrequent following aphakia in pediatric cataract surgery. The reasons for this low incidence of postoperative retinal complications are not very well known. Corneal astigmatism is recognized as a problem arising from cataract surgery. Postoperative astigmatism is more important in children than in adults because of its adverse effect on vision development and the risk of amblyopia.

MANAGEMENT OF SPECIAL SITUATIONS

Persistent Fetal Vasculature

The major surgical goal in eyes with PFV is to avoid the complications of the disease. The purpose of lens extraction is to restore a clear visual axis to release the traction on the ciliary body. However, with improved surgical techniques, successful visual rehabilitation is reported in most individuals with PFV, i.e., without disk or macular involvement. The presence of tenacious retrolenticular fibrovascular membranes can make surgery extremely difficult. The membrane itself and its treatment are associated with a high risk of intraoperative and postoperative complications including intraocular hemorrhage, pupillary block glaucoma, ciliary body and retinal traction, RD, and membrane recurrence.

Two surgical methods have been used to remove retrolenticular membranes, namely the anterior limbal approach and the posterior pars plana approach. This is described in conjunction with management of ectopia lentis.

Ectopia Lentis

Performing cataract surgery in eyes with no or minimal zonular support is technically challenging. There are two approaches in lens removal of dislocated/subluxated lenses:

1. *Limbal approach*: Here, capsulorhexis is performed through valvular incisions and attempts are made to keep the capsular bag intact. Special fixation devices, such as capsule tension ring (CTR) or Cionni modified CTR may be implanted in the bag in order to anchor the entire capsular bag to the scleral wall with the help of sutures. Thereafter, an IOL may be implanted in the capsular bag. In the absence of sufficient capsular support, however, a scleral fixated IOL may be sutured to the scleral wall.
2. *Pars plana approach*: This approach involves removal of the entire lens with its capsules with the help of a vitrector introduced through the pars plana route. A scleral fixated IOL can be sutured to the scleral wall. The limitation is that it does not maintain the capsular barrier and it does not allow for "in-the-bag" IOL implantation.

VISUAL REHABILITATION AND AMBLYOPIA MANAGEMENT

The visual rehabilitation of a child following cataract surgery is of utmost importance. If the child is left aphakic bilaterally, aphakic glasses or contact lenses may be prescribed. Contact lenses have the advantage of providing vision free of prismatic aberrations, a less magnified image and a wider field of vision. On the other hand, they are often difficult to fit in very young children, are expensive, have a potential risk of infection and high rate of loss.

In unilateral aphakia, contact lens fitting becomes mandatory. Even when primary IOL implantation is performed optical correction of residual refractive error should be performed with changing refraction. Bifocal glasses should be advised once the child approaches school going age.

In spite of successful cataract surgery, visual development may be limited by amblyopia. Untreated amblyopia in childhood may be a cause of permanent visual loss. Progression of amblyopia in early childhood is inversely proportional to the child's age; the younger the child, the faster the progression. Most cataractous patients are predisposed to all types of amblyopia. Even when optically corrected, these eyes are focused at a fixed distance and continue to optically defocus promoting amblyopia, especially if the other eye is normal.

Although, refractive correction alone can result in improved vision in anisometropic amblyopia, it is generally believed that most postcataract cases need amblyopia treatment. Amblyopia therapy requires a high-level of effort. First and foremost, any residual refractive error should be fully corrected with specks or contact lenses, even in eyes with IOL implantation. Amblyopia therapy should then be undertaken as per the standard guidelines.

Infants who have developed nystagmus before surgery and children, in whom such surgery has been delayed, may have amblyopia that is resistant even to aggressive occlusion treatment. Ideally, all cases of amblyopia should be treated, although the difficulties underlying treatment for both the patients and the parents should not be underestimated. The difficulties in treatment must be weighed against the potential lifetime benefit of successful treatment. The value of normal visual function and the effectiveness of treatment justify the difficulties and inconvenience of managing amblyopia in children.

CONCLUSION

Thus, as techniques, technology and surgeons' understanding of pediatric cataracts and their management has improved, there have been significant changes in the surgical treatment of pediatric cataracts. The cornerstones of pediatric cataract management are:

- Timely diagnosis of cataract and associated ocular anomalies
- Repeated examinations under anesthesia may be needed.
- Team approach, involving parents/caregivers, vision therapists, surgeons, and anesthesiologists
- Surgery to be performed by experienced surgeons. Start with older children, and with increasing experience, can tackle younger eyes.
- Adhering to the principles of a closed-chamber technique and microsurgical instrumentation during surgery will yield good results.
- Managing the posterior capsule and anterior vitreous is of paramount importance.
- Primary IOL implantation is now gaining more acceptances in pediatric cataract surgeons worldwide for younger children. However, it is in the infants that IOL implantation still poses some challenges. Future research as well as randomized, clinical trials from across the globe will hopefully pave the way to better and better anatomical and functional outcomes following pediatric cataract surgery.
- Finally, visual rehabilitation and management of strabismus/nystagmus as well as postoperative early detection of complications is extremely important.

SUGGESTED READING

1. Allen RJ, Speedwell L, Russell-Eggit I. Long-term visual outcome after extraction of unilateral congenital cataracts. Eye. 2010;24:1263-67.
2. Apple DJ, Solomon KD, Tetz MR, Assia EI, Holland EY, Legler UF, et al. Posterior capsule opacification. Surv Ophthalmol. 1992;37:73-116.
3. BenEzra D, Cohen E. Posterior capsulectomy in pediatric cataract surgery; the necessity of a choice. Ophthalmology. 1997;104:2168-74.
4. Birch EE, Cheng C, Stager DR Jr, Weakley DR Jr, Stager DR Sr. The critical period for treatment of dense, congenital bilateral cataracts. J AAPOS. 2009;13:67-71.
5. Birch EE, Stager D, Leffler J, Weakley D. Early treatment of congenital unilateral cataract minimizes unequal competition. Invest Ophthalmol Vis Sci. 1998;39:156-66.
6. Boger WP 3rd, Petersen RA, Robb RM. Spontaneous absorption of the lens in the congenital rubella syndrome. Arch Ophthalmol. 1981;99:433-4.
7. Bouzas AG. Anterior polar congenital cataract and corneal astigmatism. J Pediatr Ophthalmol Strabismus. 2000;29:210-2.
8. Brown SM, Graham WA, McCartney DL. Trypan blue in pediatric cataract surgery. J Cataract Refract Surg 2004; 30:2033.
9. Chougule P, Warkad V, Badakere A, Kekunnaya R. Precision pulse capsulotomy: an automated alternative to manual capsulorhexis in paediatric cataract. BMJ Open Ophthalmol. 2019;31(4):e000255.
10. Christensen GR. Pyramidal anterior polar cataracts. Ophthalmology. 2001;108:430-1.
11. Corredor-Ortega C, Gonzalez-Salinas R, Montero MJ, González-Flores R, Collura-Merlier A, Cervantes-Coste G, et al. Femtosecond laser-assisted cataract surgery in pediatric patients. J AAPOS. 2018;22:148-9.
12. Cross HE, Jensen AD. Ocular manifestations in the Marfan syndrome and homocystinuria. Am J Ophthalmol. 1973;75:405-20.
13. Elston JS, Timms C. Clinical evidence for the onset of the sensitive period in infancy. Br J Ophthalmol. 1992;76:327-28.
14. Fan DS, Rao SK, Yu CB, Wong CY, Lam DSC. Changes in refraction and ocular dimensions after cataract surgery and primary intraocular lens implantation in infants. J Cataract Refract Surg. 2006;32:1104-8.
15. Foster A, Gilbert C, Rahi J. Epidemiology of cataract in childhood: A global perspective. J Cataract Refract Surg. 1997;23:601-4.
16. Gimbel HV, Camoriano GD, Aman-Ullah M. Bilateral Implantation of Scleral-Fixated Cionni Endocapsular Rings and Toric Intraocular Lenses in a Pediatric Patient with Marfan's Syndrome. Case Rep Ophthalmol. 2012;3:16-23.
17. Gimbel HV. Posterior continuous curvilinear capsulorhexis and optic capture of the intraocular lens to prevent secondary opacification in pediatric cataract surgery. J Cataract Refract Surg. 1997;23:652-6.
18. Griener ED, Dahan E, Lambert SR. Effect of age at time at cataract surgery on subsequent axial length growth in infant eyes. J Cataract Refract Surg. 1999;25:1209-13.
19. Guo S, Wagner RS, Caputo A. Management of the anterior and posterior lens capsules and vitreous in pediatric cataract surgery. J Pediatr Ophthalmol Strabismus. 2004;41:330-7.
20. Gupta A, Kekunnaya R, Ramappa M, Vaddavalli PK. Safety profile of primary intraocular lens implantation in children below 2 years of age. Br J Ophthalmol. 2011;95:477-80.
21. Hartmann EE, Lynn MJ, Lambert SR, for the Infant Aphakia Treatment Study Group. Baseline characteristics of the Infant Aphakia Treatment Study Group. Invest Ophthalmol Vis Sci. 2005;56:388-95.
22. Jasman AA, Shaharuddin B, Noor RA, Ismail S, Ghani ZA, Embong Z. Prediction error and accuracy of intraocular lens power calculation in pediatric patient comparing SRK II and Pediatric IOL Calculator. BMC Ophthalmol. 2010;10:20.
23. Kekkunaya R, Gupta A, Sachdeva V, Rao HL, Vaddavalli PK, Prakash VO. Accuracy of intraocular lens power calculation formulae in children less than two years. Am J Ophthalmol. 2012;154:13-9.

24. Kugelberg M, Kugelberg U, Bobrova N, Tronina S, Zetterström C. After cataract in children having cataract surgery with or without anterior vitrectomy implanted with a single piece Acrysof intraocular lens. J Cataract Refract Surg. 2005;31:757-62.
25. Kumar P, Lambert SR. Evaluating the evidence for and against the use of IOLs in infants and young children. Expert Rev Med Devices. 2016;13:381-9.
26. Kuszak JR, Brown HG. Embryology and anatomy of the lens. In: Albert DM, Jacobeic FA (Eds). Principles and Practice of Ophthalmology. Philadelphia: Saunders; 1994. pp. 82-96.
27. Lambert SR, Buckley EG, Drews-Botsch CD, DuBois L, Hartmann E, Infant Aphakia Treatment Study Group, et al. The infant aphakia treatment study: design and clinical measures at enrolment. Arch Ophthalmol. 2010;128:21-7.
28. Lambert SR, Drack AV. Infantile cataracts. Surv Ophthalmol. 1996;40:427-58.
29. Lambert SR, Lynn M, Drews-Botsch C, DuBois L, Plager DA, Medow NB, et al. Optotype acuity and re-operation rate after unilateral cataract surgery within the first 6 months of life with or without IOL implantation. Br J Ophthalmol. 2004;88:1387-90.
30. Lewis TL, Maurer D, Brent HP. Development of grating acuity in children treated for unilateral or bilateral congenital cataract. Invest Ophthal Vis Sci. 1995;36:2080-95.
31. Magli A, Forte R, Carrelli R, Rombetto L, Magli G. Long-term outcomes of primary intraocular lens implantation for unilateral congenital cataracts. Semin ophthalmol. 2015;21:1-6.
32. Müllner-Eidenböck A, Amon M, Moser E, Klebermass N. Persistent fetal vasculature and minimal fetal vascular remnants: a frequent cause of unilateral congenital cataracts. Ophthalmology. 2004;111(5):906-13.
33. Neely DE, Plager DA, Borger SM. Accuracy of intraocular lens calculation in infants and children undergoing cataract surgery. J AAPOS. 2005;9:160-5.
34. Nischal KK. Two-incision push-pull capsulorrhexis for pediatric cataract surgery. J Cataract Refract Surg. 2002;28(4):593-55.
35. Plager D, Yang S, Neely D, Sprunger D, Sondhi N. Complications in the first year following cataract surgery with and without IOL in infants and older children. J AAPOS. 2002;6:9-14.
36. Ram J, Jain VK, Agarwal A, Kumar J. Hydrophobic acrylic versus polymethyl methacrylate intraocular lens implantation following cataract surgery in the first year of life. Graefes Arch Clin Exp Ophthalmol. 2014;252:1443-49.
37. Ram J, Singh R, Gupta R, Bhutani G, Gupta PC, Sukhija J. Toric intraocular lens implantation in children with developmental cataract and preexisting corneal astigmatism. Acta Ophthalmologica. 2017;95:e95-e100.
38. Ruth AL, Lambert SR. Amblyopia in the phakic eye after unilateral congenital cataract extraction. J AAPOS. 2006;10:587-88.
39. Solebo AL, Russell-Eggitt I, Cumberland PM, Rahi JS. British Isles Congenital Cataract interest group. Risks and outcomes associated with primary intraocular lens implantation in children under 2 years of age: the IoLunder2 cohort study. Br J Ophthalmol. 2015;99:1471-6.
40. Struck MC. Long-term results of pediatric cataract surgery and primary intraocular lens implantation from 7 to 22 months of life. JAMA Ophthalmol. 2015;133:1180-3.
41. Trivedi RH, Wilson ME Jr, Bartholomew LR, Lal G, Peterseim MM. Opacification of the visual axis after cataract surgery and single acrylic intraocular lens implantation in the first year of life. J AAPOS. 2004;8:156-64.
42. Trivedi RH, Wilson ME. Prediction error after pediatric cataract surgery with intraocular lens implantation: Contact versus immersion A-scan biometry. J Cataract Refract Surg. 2011;37:501-5.
43. Tuncer S, Gucukoglu A, Gozum N. Cataract extraction and primary hydrophobic acrylic intraocular lens implantation in infants. J AAPOS. 2005;9:250-56.
44. Vanderveen DK, Trivedi RH, Nizam A, Michael J Lynn, Scott R Lambert, Infant Aphakia Treatment Study Group. Predictability of intraocular lens power calculation formulae in infantile eyes with unilateral congenital cataract: Results from the Infant Aphakia Treatment Study. Am J Ophthalmol. 2013;156:1252-60.
45. Vasavada AR, Nath VC, Trivedi RH. Anterior vitreous face behavior with Acrysof in pediatric cataract surgery. J AAPOS. 2003;7:384-88.
46. Vasavada AR, Praveen MR, Nath V. Diagnosis and management of congenital cataract with pre-existing posterior capsule defect. J Cataract Refract Surg. 2004;30:403-8.
47. Vasavada AR, Trivedi RH, Apple DJ, Ram J, Werner L. Randomized, clinical trial of multiquadrant hydrodissection in pediatric cataract surgery. Am J Ophthalmol. 2003;135(1):84-8.
48. Vasavada AR, Vasavada V, Shah SK, Praveen MR, Vasavada VA, Trivedi RH, et al. Five-year postoperative outcomes of bilateral aphakia and pseudophakia in children up to 2 years of age: A Randomized Clinical Trial. Am J Ophthalmol 2018;193:33-44.
49. Vasavada AR, Vasavada V, Shah SK, Trivedi RH, Vasavada VA, Vasavada SA, et al. Postoperative outcomes of intraocular lens implantation in the bag versus posterior optic capture in pediatric cataract surgery. J Cataract Refract Surg. 2017;43:1177-83.
50. Vasavada V, Shah SK, Vasavada VA, Vasavada AR, Trivedi RH, Srivastava S, et al. Comparison of IOL power calculation formulae for pediatric eyes. Eye. 2016;30:1242-50.

10

CHAPTER

Congenital Glaucoma

Samiksha Fouzdar Jain, Mehmet C Mocan

OVERVIEW

Although a rare disorder in the western world, the incidence of congenital glaucoma is higher in the developing world. Congenital glaucoma is a devastating condition with life-long effects on the visual function and quality of a child's life.

Thus, timely diagnosis and management are imperative to control intraocular pressure (IOP) and limit visual loss in children. This chapter mainly deals with epidemiology, genetics, classification, clinical presentation, treatment, and the prognosis of primary congenital glaucoma (PCG).

INTRODUCTION

Primary congenital glaucoma is a heterogeneous group of diseases with significant visual morbidity if not diagnosed and treated early. The incidence of PCG in western countries is 1 per 10,000–20,000 live births. Its incidence is higher in the Middle Eastern countries. Most common in Saudi Arabia is 1 per 2,500 live births, the highest incidence of 1 per 1,250 live births in Slovakian Gypsies, respectively. Incidence is higher in populations with consanguinity.

Glaucoma is the second leading cause of vision loss, and childhood glaucoma is estimated to cause a significant percentage of blindness in children, ranging from 1.2% in Great Britain while 3 and 7% in Northern India and Southern India, respectively.

TERMINOLOGY AND CLASSIFICATION

Several classification systems have been used based on ocular anatomy, age of onset, and associated systemic disorders. Commonly they are described as primary and secondary glaucoma based on the etiology.

Congenital glaucoma refers to glaucoma present since birth. *Infantile glaucoma* presents between birth and 3 years of age, and *Juvenile glaucoma* refers to the age of 3 years through late teenage or early adulthood years.

The Childhood Glaucoma Research Network (CGRN) System for childhood glaucoma has recently unified the terminology which is pathologically and systematically approachable. The 9th World Glaucoma Association congress finalized the definitions of childhood glaucoma as given in **Box 1**.

BOX 1: Childhood Glaucoma Research Network (CGRN) definitions of disease.

Childhood: Based on national criteria, <18 years old (USA) or <16 years old (UK, Europe, UNICEF)

Childhood glaucoma: *Two or more* of the following are required:
- *Intraocular pressure (IOP)*: >21 mm Hg (investigator discretion on method of measurement and if EUA data alone is sufficient).
- *Visual fields*: Reproducible visual field defect that is consistent with glaucomatous optic neuropathy with no other observable reason for the visual field defect.
- *Axial length*: Progressive myopia or myopic shift with increased ocular dimensions that outpace normal growth.
- *Cornea*: Findings including Haab striae, corneal diameter >11 mm in newborns, >12 mm in children younger than 1 year old, and >13 mm in children older than 1 year old.
- *Optic nerve*: Progressive increase in cup-disk ratio, cup-disk asymmetry of ≥0.2 when optic disks are of similar size, and focal rim thinning.

Childhood glaucoma suspect: *At least one* of the following is required:
- *IOP*: >21 mm Hg on two separate occasions
- *Visual fields*: Suspicious visual field defect for glaucoma
- *Axial length*: Increased axial length in the setting of normal IOP
- *Cornea*: Increased corneal diameter in the setting of normal IOP
- *Optic nerve*: Suspicious optic disk appearance for glaucoma

GENETICS OF PRIMARY CONGENITAL GLAUCOMA

Primary congenital glaucoma is a genetic disease that can be sporadic or familial. Familial cases are about 10–40%, with an autosomal recessive inheritance pattern and varying penetrance ranging from 40 to 100%.

To date five genetic loci: GLC3A (located on chromosome 2p22-p21), GLC3B (1p36.2-p36.1), GLC3C (14q24.3), GLC3D (14q24.2-q24.3, not overlapping with GLC3C), and recent GLC3E (9p21) **(Box 2)**.

BOX 2: Classification of childhood glaucomas.

Primary congenital glaucoma and juvenile open-angle glaucoma:

Primary congenital glaucoma:
- The CGRN definition of childhood glaucoma is met.
- Ocular enlargement is usually seen (buphthalmos)
- Isolated angle anomalies (with or without mild congenital iris anomalies)
- Subcategories based on the age of onset:
  - Neonatal-onset (0–1 month)
  - Infantile-onset (>1–24 months)
  - Late-onset (>24 months)

Signs present with normal IOP and no progressive optic nerve changes: Spontaneously arrested PCG

Juvenile open-angle glaucoma:
- The CGRN definition of childhood glaucoma is met.
- No ocular enlargement
- Normal appearing angle (open-angle)

Glaucoma following cataract surgery:
- The CGRN definition of childhood glaucoma is met only after cataract surgery is performed.
- Supersedes conflicting classifications
- Includes all cataract etiologies:
  - Congenital idiopathic cataract
  - Congenital cataract associated with a systemic syndrome or ocular anomalies
  - Acquired cataract
- Categorized by gonioscopy findings:
  - Open-angle glaucoma (≥50% open)

Angle-closure glaucoma (<50% open or acute angle-closure)

Glaucoma associated with nonacquired systemic disease or syndrome:
- The CGRN definition of childhood glaucoma is met.
- Condition of predominately systemic disease/syndrome present at birth
- Ocular signs may or may not be present.

Examples of glaucoma associated with nonacquired systemic disease or syndrome:
- Chromosomal disorders:
  - Trisomy 21
- Connective tissue disorders:
  - Marfan syndrome
  - Weill-Marchesani syndrome
  - Stickler syndrome
- Metabolic disorders:
  - Homocystinuria
  - Lowe syndrome
  - Mucopolysaccharidoses
- Phacomatoses:
  - Neurofibromatosis
  - Sturge–Weber syndrome
- Rubinstein–Taybi:
  - Congenital rubella

Glaucoma associated with nonacquired ocular anomalies:
- The CGRN definition of childhood glaucoma is met.
- Condition of predominately ocular anomaly present at birth
- Systemic signs may or may not be present.

Examples of glaucoma associated with nonacquired ocular anomalies:
- Aniridia
- Axenfeld–Rieger spectrum
- Congenital ectropion uveae

Contd...

Contd...

- Iris hypoplasia
- Microphthalmia
- Oculodermal melanocytosis
- Peters anomaly
- Persistent fetal vasculature (before cataract surgery)
- Posterior polymorphous dystrophy
- Ectopia lentis

Glaucoma associated with acquired conditions:
- The CGRN definition of childhood glaucoma is met.
- Acquired conditions are those that are not present at birth but later develop (unless they develop over time due to a condition present at birth).
- Categorized by gonioscopy findings:
  - Open-angle glaucoma (≥50% open)
  - Angle-closure glaucoma (<50% open or acute angle-closure)
- Examples of glaucoma associated with acquired conditions:
  - Postsurgical (not including cataract surgery)
  - Retinopathy of prematurity
  - Steroid-induced
  - Trauma
  - Tumors
  - Uveitis

(CGRN: Childhood Glaucoma Research Network; EUA: examination under anesthesia)

Apart from conditions mentioned in **Table 1**, 5.5% of cases of PCG may be explained by the myocilin/trabecular meshwork-induced glucocorticoid response protein (*MYOC*) gene on chromosome 1q24, which is generally implicated in the pathogenesis of juvenile open-angle glaucoma and primary open-angle glaucoma.

PATHOPHYSIOLOGY

Primary congenital glaucoma arises secondary to abnormal development of the anterior chamber, which results in the obstruction of the outflow of aqueous humor. In 1949, Otto Barkan postulated a persistent fetal membrane overlying the trabecular meshwork, resulting in increased resistance to aqueous outflow.

Worst supported this hypothesis (1966) and termed it Barkan membrane. However, light and electron microscopic studies have failed to confirm this theory. The retention of primordial cell layer is another pathogenetic mechanism. This layer may obstruct the trabecular meshwork and be responsible for certain cases of congenital glaucoma.

In the third trimester, there is posterior sliding of the ciliary body and peripheral iris away from the cornea and sclera that contributes to the development of normal angle. However, in eyes with PCG, there is an interruption of this posterior movement of the ciliary body and peripheral iris due to excessive or premature accumulation of collagenous beams within the trabecular meshwork resulting in an anterior insertion of the iris root and ciliary muscle, which can, in turn, lead to obstruction of the trabecular meshwork, and narrow or completely compress the Schlemm.

TABLE 1: Various genetic loci associated/implicated with primary congenital glaucoma (PCG).

Locus	Chromosomal region	Gene product	Function	Clinical implication
GLC3A	2p21	CYP1B1	Endogenous steroid metabolism	15–20% of PCG cases in Japan and the United States, and all cases in Slovakia Roma
GLC3B	1p36	CDT6/ANGPTL7*	ECM organization and formation	AD inheritance with reduced penetrance
GLC3C	14q24	Unknown	Unknown	
GLC3D	14q24	*LTBP2*	ECM organization	AR, Romanian
GLC3E	9p21	TEK/Tie2	Formation and homeostasis of Schlemm's canal	AD with variable expressivity, reduced penetrance, accounts for 4% disease

*Implicated in PCG pathogenesis
(AD: autosomal dominant; AR: autosomal recessive; ECM: extracellular matrix)

Various genetic mutations have been implicated in trabecular dysgenesis that impairs normal trabecular meshwork development.

CLINICAL MANIFESTATIONS

Symptoms

Primary congenital glaucoma patients may present with one or more of the following symptoms such as epiphora, photophobia, and blepharospasm. These symptoms are secondary to raised IOP leading to corneal edema. Diagnosis of PCG is earlier in unilateral or asymmetric cases where differences in the size of the cornea can be perceived easily on gross examination. However, when the disease is bilateral and symmetric, increased corneal size may not be apparent and can cause a delay in diagnosis and management.

Signs

Buphthalmos (greek: bous-ox; ophthalmos-eye) refers to marked ocular enlargement occurring in response to raised IOP in children. Children with congenital/infantile glaucoma typically present with globe enlargement (buphthalmos), edema, and opacification of the cornea with horizontal or oblique rupture of Descemet membrane (Haab striae). Haab striae are present in 25% of eyes with PCG at birth, and at age 6 months, ≥60% of PCG eyes have it. Haab striae usually persist even after normalization of IOP and clearing of corneal edema **(Figs. 1A to C)**.

Additional clinical features include thinning of the anterior sclera and iris atrophy, anomalously deep anterior chamber, and structurally normal posterior segment except for progressive glaucomatous optic atrophy.

Corneal Findings

An average corneal diameter in newborn ranges between 9.5 and 10.5 mm in diameter and by age 1 year increases to 10.0–11.5 mm. A corneal diameter above 12.0 mm along with Haab striae is suggestive of congenital glaucoma.

Corneal diameter greater than 13 mm at any age is highly suspicious of glaucoma.

Cornea and sclera in kids are distensible; however, corneal enlargement halts approximately at age 3 years, though sclera remains distensible up to 10 years of age.

Patients present with the deep anterior chamber, axial myopia, astigmatism, anisometropia, and optic nerve cupping.

Optic Nerve Cupping

The optic nerve cupping may develop early and rapidly in infants and is primarily due to optic canal stretching and posterior bowing of the lamina cribrosa without a decrease in the neuroretinal rim.

Asymmetry of cupping from eye to eye also may be a sign of infantile glaucoma. Between-eye differences of >0.2 are seen in approximately two-thirds of infants with glaucoma and are very uncommon in healthy infants. In young children, the reversal of cupping may be noted with normalization of IOP. However, the retinal nerve fiber layer damage, if present, can be permanent.

Serial axial length measurements are instrumental in monitoring disease progression in an infant's eyes.

Diagnostic Examination

Generally, these infants frequently require an examination under anesthesia (EUA) for an accurate IOP determination. In the office, reliable IOP measurements cannot typically be obtained due to poor patient cooperation. Fixation and following behavior, the presence of nystagmus should be noted. Cycloplegic refraction must be attempted, which often reveals myopia and astigmatism.

Tonometry

Measurement of the IOP is vital for the diagnosis of glaucoma. IOP can be obtained in a cooperative child in the clinic setting with a Tono-pen (Reichert ophthalmic instruments, Depwe, NY) and/or Icare rebound tonometer (Icare Finland Oy, Helsinki, Finland) and a Perkins (Haag-Streit

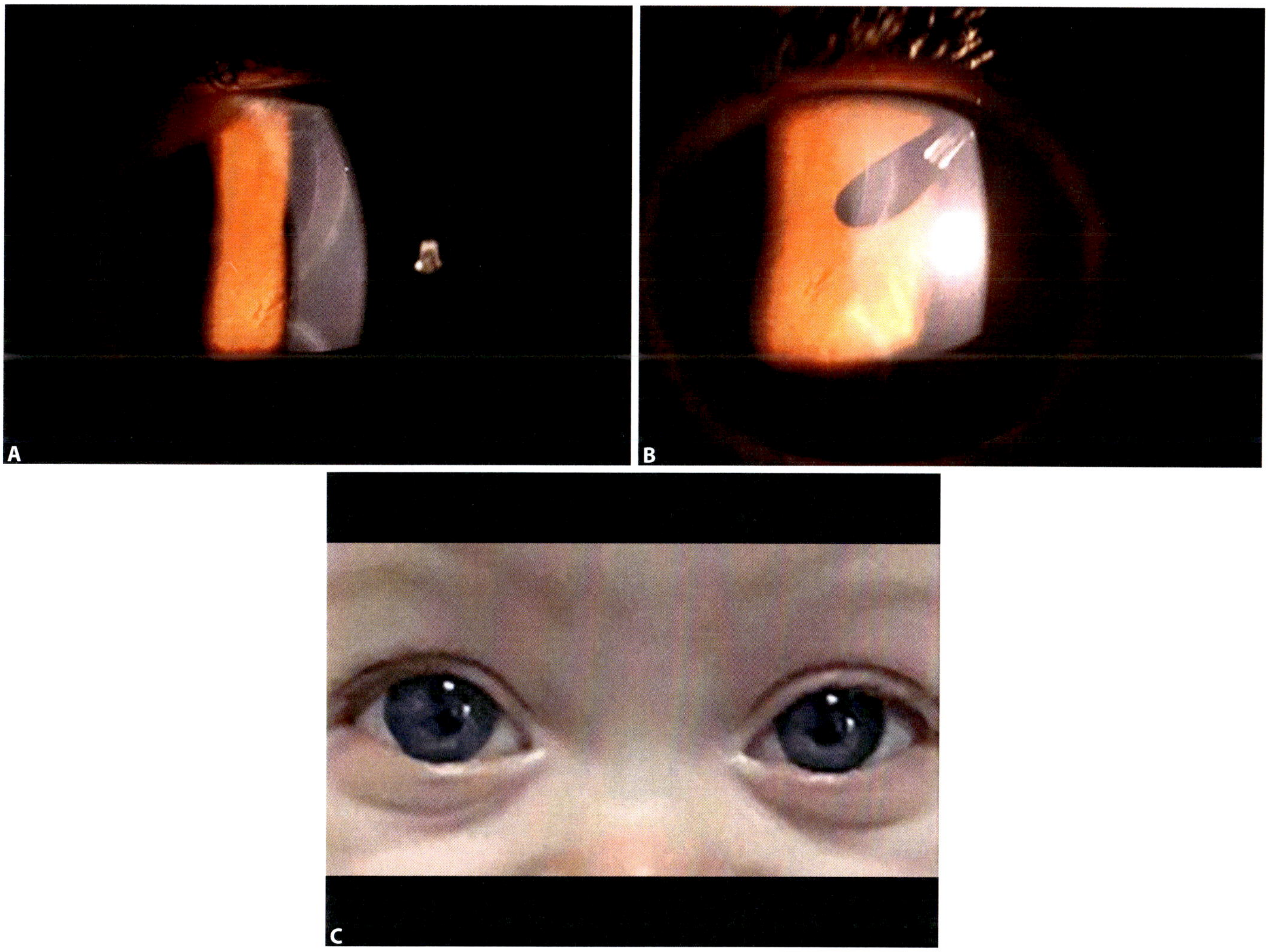

Figs. 1A to C: (A and B) Haab's striae in a 12-year-old boy; (C) Haab striae in a child.

USA, Mason, OH). In older cooperative patients, standard Goldmann applanation readings are preferred. A pneumotonometer may be less influenced by corneal abnormalities, which may be useful to confirm IOP during EUA. Anesthetic agents variably alter the IOP (usually lowered). IOP recordings should be performed after induction and before intubation during anesthesia. Ketamine has a moderate effect on IOP and may allow more accurate IOP measurements.

The IOP is lower in infants and young children as compared to adults. The average IOP of a normal newborn 10–12 mm Hg, by 7 or 8 years of age, increased to 14 mm Hg. In the presence of other clinical signs, an asymmetric measurement or an elevated IOP measurement should raise suspicion of glaucoma.

Corneal Evaluation

The corneal diameter measurement is crucial in the diagnosis of PCG. The cornea should be examined for clarity, size, and presence of Haab striae. Horizontal diameter can be measured by placing a millimeter ruler above the eyes, or a close-up digital photograph can be used to determine corneal diameter. Corneal thickness typically higher in infants with glaucoma can be measured using an ultrasonic pachymeter. Central corneal thickness is found to be thinner in children with congenital glaucoma, which may interfere with correct interpretation of IOP measurements.

A portable slit lamp, or a regular slit lamp, can be used to examine Haab striae depending on the child's age. Retro illumination in a dilated pupil can also be used to identify Haab striae.

Anterior Segment Examination

An abnormally deep anterior chamber and hypoplasia of the peripheral iris stroma are commonly present. A velvety smooth iris surface manifests iris hypoplasia. If the cornea is clear, a gonioscopic examination can be performed using a direct gonio lens (Koeppe) and a portable slit lamp or loupes. It provides information regarding the mechanism of glaucoma and surgical planning.

The angle of the anterior chamber in a normal infant differs from that of an adult. The trabecular meshwork is lightly pigmented, the Schwalbe line is often less distinct, and the uveal meshwork is translucent. There is an open-angle in infants with PCG, with flat and more anterior iris insertion on the trabecular meshwork. Scleral spur is not well-developed, and the peripheral iris may have scalloped edges and pale peripheral iris stroma in front of the angle, causing a "morning mist" appearance.

Posterior Segment Examination

Fundus examination can be performed using a direct or indirect ophthalmoscope. In the presence of a small pupil, a direct ophthalmoscope is used through a Koeppe gonioscopy lens to visualize the optic disk. Fundus photography is useful for documentation and future comparisons. Ultrasound B-scan helps rule out posterior segment pathology in the presence of opaque cornea that is frequently observed in severe cases of a neonatal form of PCG.

Diagnostic Imaging

Anterior segment optical coherence tomography (OCT) and ultrasound biomicroscopy (UBM) studies have been utilized in the evaluation of PCG, especially in the setting of corneal opacification, to evaluate accompanying anterior segment dysgenetic conditions. Recent UBM studies have reported a thin, stretched-out ciliary body and abnormal tissue at the iridocorneal angle seen in 90% of UBM scans.

The presence of peripheral anterior synechiae, posterior embryotoxon, or other abnormalities precludes the PCG diagnosis.

Visual field assessment is an integral part of adult glaucoma management. However, the reliability of visual field testing in children increases with age. In the absence of severe vision loss, nystagmus, and cognitive impairment, visual field testing can be attempted at age 7–8 years. Shorter testing algorithms such as SITA-Fast (Swedish Interactive Testing Algorithm) may permit children to perform the test more reliably.

Optical coherence tomography is a promising technology with great potential in diagnosing and monitoring pediatric glaucomas. Current machines have normative data from adults, which makes direct correlation in the pediatric population challenging. The handheld device can be utilized for younger kids with and without anesthesia.

Studies have shown increased nerve fiber layer thickness in children as compared to adults.

A-scan ultrasonography helps determine axial length, anterior chamber depth, and lens thickness and monitoring disease progression.

■ DIFFERENTIAL DIAGNOSIS

Epiphora

Congenital nasolacrimal duct obstruction, conjunctivitis, corneal abrasion, keratitis, and uveitis.

Corneal Clouding or Opacification

Birth trauma: Descemet vertical or oblique tears (unlike Haab striae, usually more horizontal or curvilinear).

Corneal Dystrophies

Congenital hereditary endothelial dystrophy, posterior polymorphous dystrophy, congenital or developmental abnormalities: Sclerocornea, Peters anomaly, and choristomas.

Keratitis

Herpetic infection, congenital syphilis, maternal rubella, and Riley-Day syndrome

Storage Diseases

Mucopolysaccharidoses, mucolipidoses, and cystinosis.

Corneal Enlargement

High axial myopia and megalocornea, unilateral high myopia, proptosis, lid retraction, microphthalmos, enophthalmos, or ptosis can give the appearance of an enlarged cornea because one eye is larger, more prominent, or more visible than the other.

■ NATURAL HISTORY

If left untreated, PCG invariably progresses to blindness. Many mechanisms can impair the visual function in children with congenital glaucoma: Severe myopia with fundus changes, scleral thinning, and spontaneous lens dislocation due to globe expansion, corneal vascularization, and opacification, optic nerve damage, and refractive amblyopia secondary to high irregular astigmatism due to Descemet membrane breaks or anisomyopia.

■ TREATMENT

The type of glaucoma determines therapy. Many secondary and almost all acquired glaucomas are initially treated medically similar to adult glaucomas. However, the primary treatment of PCG consists of performing an angle surgery such as goniotomy or trabeculotomy or trabeculectomy augmented with mitomycin C (MMC). Glaucoma drainage implants (Molteno, Baerveldt, or Ahmed implants) and cyclodestructive procedures, especially diode laser, are usually reserved for refractory cases. The principal aims of glaucoma treatment are to lower IOP to a safe level and treat any secondary complications such as refractive error and amblyopia.

Medical Therapy

Eye drops for PCG are typically used as a temporizing measure before surgery to clear the cornea, so a definitive surgical procedure can be performed or supplement to control IOP after surgery **(Table 2)**. Parents should

TABLE 2: Antiglaucoma medications used in the treatment of raised intraocular pressure (IOP) in children.

Medication type	*Indications*	*Side effects*	*Precautions*
Adrenergic agonists Epinephrine compounds	Rarely used, limited effectiveness	*Systemic effects:* Hypertension, tachycardia in small children	
α-agonists Apraclonidine 0.5% Brimonidine:	• Apraclonidine helps during and after angle surgery; useful in the short term in infants and after corneal transplantation • Use brimonidine only in older children; second or third-line therapy with JOAG, aphakia, and older children with other glaucoma types	• *Apraclonidine:* Tachyphylaxis, allergy, rarely red eye. • *Apraclonidine and brimonidine:* Hypotension, bradycardia, hypothermia central nervous system depression, and coma • Risks are greater for brimonidine	• Contraindicated in children <2 years of age • Caution in children <10 years of age or <20 kg • Use low dosage • Avoid in hepatic and renal impairment
β-blockers *Nonselective:* Timolol, levobunolol, and carteolol *$β_1$-selective:* Betaxolol	• First line of therapy • Start with lower concentrations in smaller children	*Systemic effects:* Bronchospasm and bradycardia	• Avoid in premature or tiny infants and children with a history of reactive airways • Add a use with caution in asthma or cardiac disease • Select lower concentrations • Use punctal occlusion • Cardioselective β-blockers to reduce risk of bronchospasm
Carbonic anhydrase inhibitors *Topical*: Dorzolamide, brinzolamide two to three-times a day *Oral*: Methazolamide (2–4 mg/kg/day) acetazolamide 10–20 mg/kg/day	First- or second-line in young children; Topical or in combination with oral	• Metabolic acidosis (rare) • Stevens–Johnson syndrome (SJS) • Cornea edema • Metabolic acidosis • SJS • Aplastic anemia • Headaches, nausea, dizziness, and paresthesia • Growth suppression, lethargy, decreased appetite, weight loss, gastrointestinal discomfort, diarrhea, failure to thrive, and bedwetting	• Contraindicated in renal insufficiency and sulfonamide hypersensitivity • Monitor infant feeding and weight gain • Caution in corneal disease • Contraindicated in renal insufficiency, • hypokalemia, hyponatremia, and • sulfonamide hypersensitivity • Monitor for metabolic acidosis • Monitor infant feeding and weight gain
Parasympathomimetic agents (miotics) Echothiophate iodide, pilocarpine	• Echothiophate is rarely used, sometimes in aphakia • Pilocarpine is used after angle surgery • Less effective at reducing IOP	• *Systemic effects mainly with echothiophate:* Diarrhea, urinary incontinence, cardiac arrhythmia, weakness, fatigue, headache, and iris cyst • Risk of pupillary block • Paradoxical rise in IOP • *Pilocarpine:* Headache, weakness; can induce myopic shift	• Avoid in uveitis • Caution in cardiac disease, asthma, and urinary tract obstruction • Limited dosage and use lower concentrations • *Echothiophate:* Avoid succinylcholine
Prostaglandins analogs • Latanoprost, travoprost, bimatoprost, and tafluprost • Latanoprostene bunod	• Used as second- or third-line after β-blockers and topical CAIs • However, first to third-line with JOAG	Systemically safe in children; long eyelashes, and redness.	• Avoid in patients with uveitis • Use caution following intraocular surgery

(JOAG: juvenile open-angle glaucoma)

perform punctal occlusion to minimize the systemic absorption of the drops.

β-blockers (β-adrenergic Antagonists)

Topical β-blockers play a great role in PCG treatment. They cause a 20–30% reduction in IOP. The major systemic side effects are respiratory distress caused by apnea or bronchospasm and bradycardia. β-blockers should be avoided in premature or small infants used cautiously in children with asthma and cardiac disease. A cardioselective β-blocker (betaxolol) can be used; however, it has a lower pressure lowering effect.

Carbonic Anhydrase Inhibitors

Both oral and topical forms are available, and they reduce IOP by suppressing aqueous production. Oral acetazolamide (diamox, dose 5–15 mg/kg/day divided into three or four doses) and methimazole neptazane, dose <2 mg/kg/day, divided into two doses. It reduces the IOP by about 20–35% compared to topical dorzolamide (27%). Systemic side effects with oral preparations are common and include lethargy, decreased appetite, weight loss, gastrointestinal discomfort, diarrhea, failure to thrive, and metabolic acidosis. Topical carbonic anhydrase inhibitors are less efficacious (about 25%) than oral carbonic anhydrase inhibitors and have fewer systemic side effects. Rarely, metabolic acidosis can occur, particularly in premature infants.

Topical carbonic anhydrase inhibitors should be used cautiously in children with a corneal transplant or pre-existing corneal disease due to the risk of corneal edema. Carbonic anhydrase inhibitors are contraindicated in renal insufficiency and sulfonamide hypersensitivity.

Topical α-2 Agonists

Topical α-2 agonists decrease aqueous production and enhance uveoscleral outflow. These medications can pass through the blood–brain barrier and cause hypotension, bradycardia, hypothermia, central nervous system depression, and coma, especially in neonates and infants; thus, it is strictly contraindicated in patients 2 years old or younger. Due to its hydrophilic nature, apraclonidine has fewer central nervous system side effects, which reduces its blood–brain barrier penetration than brimonidine and is used for short-term treatment. Long-term use is limited due to the high incidence of tachyphylaxis and ocular allergy.

Prostaglandin Analogs

Latanoprost effectively reduces the IOP in 15–20% of PCG patients. Side effects mainly include lash growth, conjunctival injection, and less commonly, iris pigmentation alteration, allergy, uveitis, and periocular hyperpigmentation. Children can develop prostaglandin-related periorbitopathy.

Parasympathomimetic Agents

Parasympathomimetic agents work by increasing trabecular flow by contraction of the ciliary muscle. They have a limited role in PCG due to angle anatomy and abnormal high ciliary muscle insertion into the trabecular meshwork. Common side effects include miosis, myopia, bronchospasm, hypertension, vomiting, diarrhea, dizziness, and weakness. These agents may be helpful in aphakic or pseudophakic glaucoma. Echothiophate causes prolonged paralysis, so avoid succinylcholine use.

Newer Agents

In late 2017, the Food and Drug Administration (FDA) approved latanoprostene bunod ophthalmic gel (Vyzulta, 0.024%; Bausch + Lomb) and netarsudil ophthalmic solution (Rhopressa, 0.02%; there is no safety data available for use in the pediatric population.

Surgery

Surgery is the treatment of choice for PCG. Angle surgery is performed first to open the trabecular meshwork allowing the adequate flow of aqueous from the anterior chamber.

Goniotomy

In the presence of a clear cornea, goniotomy can be performed, and it involves an incision across the trabecular meshwork under direct gonioscopic visualization. A goniotomy is performed using a goniotomy knife, MVR blade, 25-gauge needle, and goniotomy lens (Swan Jacob). Goniotomy for developmental glaucoma has a high success rate ranging from 70 to 93% in various studies.

Modified techniques such as gonioscopy-assisted transluminal trabeculotomy with suture or lighted microcatheter, or Omni and newer devices such as the Kahook dual blade, trabectome, are being used to perform goniotomy. Potential complications include hyphema, shallowing of the anterior chamber, peripheral anterior synechiae, occasionally cyclodialysis, iridodialysis, cataract, scleral perforation, epithelial ingrowth, and retinal detachment following trabeculotomy.

Trabeculotomy

Trabeculotomy can be performed even in the presence of cloudy cornea. A partial-thickness scleral flap is created to gain access to the Schlemm canal which is cannulated using a curved rigid pronged probe called a trabeculotome. A trabeculotome is gently rotated into the anterior chamber to incise the trabecular meshwork. A right- and left-handed trabeculotome are utilized to cut trabecular meshwork in opposite directions. In total, 100–200° of trabecular meshwork is incised **(Fig. 2)**.

A modification of this technique using a 6-0 polypropylene (Prolene) suture or an illuminated microcatheter to cannulate

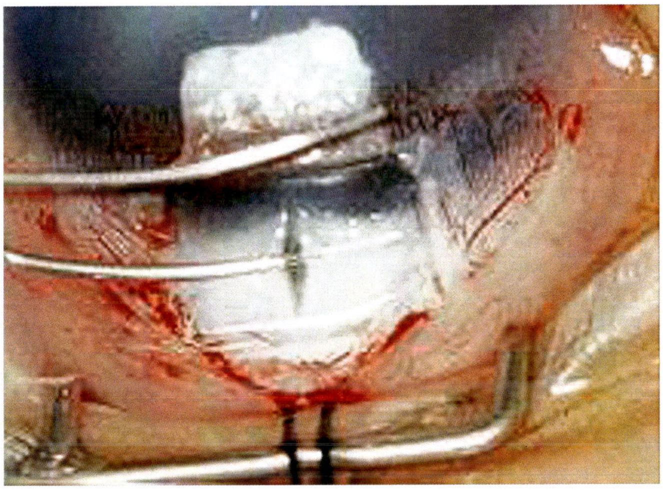

Fig. 2: Demonstrating use of Trabeculotome.

the entire Schlemm canal has been used, and 360-degree trabeculotomy is completed by pulling suture across the anterior chamber. Potential complications include iridodialysis, Descemet detachment, hyphema, unintentional filtering blebs, choroidal detachment, and lens damage.

The data from a Chinese retrospective study reported that lowering the IOP to ≤21 mm Hg after trabeculotomy was achieved in 91% and 87% among children aged 1 and 3 years, respectively. These results were comparable to the data from Western countries in the 1980s, which reported a 75–90% reduction of IOP after trabeculotomy.

Combined Trabeculotomy and Trabeculectomy

Combined trabeculotomy and trabeculectomy (CTT) are performed either as a primary or secondary procedure. Failure to cannulate the Schlemm canal during surgery or if prior trabeculotomy was unsuccessful, in that case, a trabeculectomy can be performed by removing a block of tissue underneath the scleral flap, surgical iridectomy is performed similarly as in traditional trabeculectomy. MMC CTT may be the procedure of choice in patients of Indian and Middle Eastern origin.

Trabeculectomy

Filtering surgery is considered in patients who have had one or more unsuccessful angle surgeries, or it is not suitable as in many cases of secondary glaucomas. Trabeculectomy with MMC has a 50% reported success rate; however, it carries a cumulative risk for bleb leaks and endophthalmitis. Glaucoma drainage device (GDD) implantation is generally offered once filtering procedures fail in pediatric patients.

Trabeculectomy for PCG has success rates ranging between 50 and 87%. The success rate of trabeculectomy shows a decline with time. Patients aged 1 year or less have a risk of failure that is 5.6 times higher than older infants and toddlers.

TABLE 3: The success rate for glaucoma drainage device (GDD) at 1 year and 5 years.

GDD	*At 1 year*	*At 5 years*
Molteno	56–95%	
Baerveldt	80–95%	<50%
Ahmed	87%	55%

Glaucoma Drainage Device

Glaucoma drainage devices or cyclodestructive procedures are offered to patients when trabeculectomy fails or is not feasible. All prototypes of GDDs (Molteno, Baerveldt, and Ahmed valve) have been utilized to control IOP, and they can be implanted safely in neonates with attention to eye and implant parameters **(Table 3)**. Using GDD has revealed a 28–49% reduction in the mean IOP and a success rate ranging from 63 to 97% after 1 year from surgery.

Complications from GDDs are many and include cornea-tube touch, tube erosion through the conjunctiva or cornea, implant migration, and cataracts. Infection rates are low.

Varying success rates for PCG and childhood glaucoma have been reported.

Beck et al. reported a cumulative probability of success of 87% in the Ahmed glaucoma valve (AGV) group versus 36% in the trabeculectomy with the MMC group after one year of follow-up.

Laser Cycloablation and Cyclocryotherapy

Laser cycloablation and cyclocryotherapy ablate ciliary epithelium and reduce aqueous production. They are helpful in patients with refractory PCG when all other options have failed to lower IOP. Laser cyclophotocoagulation (CPC) and cyclocryotherapy are the most commonly performed procedures. CPC using (semiconductor diode laser 810 nm) is currently preferred to cryotherapy with less postoperative inflammation and pain. The transscleral laser is performed under general anesthesia in the supine position in the pediatric population. Complications are rare, including post-operative inflammation, hypotony, retinal detachment, visual loss, and phthisis.

Studies have shown that success for transscleral CPC is low and ranges from 30 to 79%. Often repeat treatment is required. With retreatment, approximately ~70% of patients achieve adequate IOP control, and diode CPC and sequential tube shunt following primary tube shunt failure in childhood glaucoma showed similar efficacy and complication rates.

Endoscopic diode laser cyclophotocoagulation (ECP) is a reasonably effective procedure for controlling IOP in refractory pediatric glaucomas, especially in the setting of multiple failed tubes and/or trabeculectomies. Significant postoperative complications have been documented in aphakic patients, such as retinal detachment following ECP. Success for a single endo CCP ECP treatment at 1, 3, and

5 years was 64, 36, and 16%, respectively, with sequential ECP bringing the rate up to 81% at 1 year and 34% at 5 years.

PROGNOSIS AND FOLLOW-UP

Patients with PCG need to be monitored for their entire lives. These patients require frequent follow-ups in the early stages of the disease to monitor response to treatment and watch for complications secondary to the treatment itself. Patients may develop postoperative infection, hypotony, and inflammation. Even if there is adequate control of IOP from surgical intervention, regular life-long follow-up is needed (at least every 6 months). Stable congenital glaucoma may progress with sight-threatening complications even after many years of IOP stability.

Complications

Untreated disease can have grave consequences, complications, and significant visual impairment in addition to permanent optic nerve damage and glaucomatous visual field defects. Vision loss can be secondary to corneal scarring, axial elongation, cause abnormally high refractive errors, including myopia and astigmatism. However, the most common cause of poor outcome is amblyopia, secondary to corneal opacification and anisometropia.

Prognosis

The untreated disease frequently leads to buphthalmos and blindness, except in the rare case of spontaneously arrested PCG. Infantile-onset cases have a better prognosis as compared to patients with congenital onset and those with severe angle abnormalities. In general, with combined surgical and medical treatment modalities, adequate IOP control can be achieved in >80% of patients.

The treating physician should take stringent measures to control IOP, correct refractive errors, and manage amblyopia.

SUGGESTED READING

1. Anderson DR. The development of the trabecular meshwork and its abnormality in primary infantile glaucoma. Trans Am Ophthalmol Soc. 1981;79:458-85.
2. Autrata R, Rehurek J. Long-term results of transscleral cyclophotocoagulation in refractory pediatric glaucoma patients. Ophthalmologica. 2003;217(6):393-400.
3. Beck AD, Freedman S, Kammer J, Jin J. Aqueous shunt devices compared with trabeculectomy with Mitomycin-C for children in the first two years of life. Am J Ophthalmol. 2003;136(6):994-1000.
4. Bhattacharjee H, Das K, Borah RR, et al. Causes of childhood blindness in the northeastern states of India. Indian J Ophthalmol. 2008;56(6):495-9.
5. Capino AC, Dannaway DC, Miller JL. Metabolic acidosis with ophthalmic dorzolamide in a neonate. J Pediatr Pharmacol Ther. 2016;21(3):256-9.
6. Chouiter L, Nadifi S. Analysis of CYP1B1 Gene mutations in patients with primary congenital glaucoma. J Pediatr Genet. 2017;6(4):205-14.
7. deLuise VP, Anderson DR. Primary infantile glaucoma (congenital glaucoma). Surv Ophthalmol. 1983;28(1):1-19.
8. Donahue SP, Porter A. SITA visual field testing in children. J AAPOS. 2001;5:114.
9. Dorairaj SK, Bandrakalli P, Shetty C, et al Childhood blindness in a rural population of southern India: prevalence and etiology. Ophthalmic Epidemiol. 2008 May-Jun;15(3):176-82.
10. Eisenberg DL, Sherman BG, McKeown CA, Schuman JS. Tonometry in adults and children. A manometric evaluation of pneumatonometry, applanation, and TonoPen in vitro and in vivo. Ophthalmology. 1998;105(7):1173-81.
11. El Sayed Y, Esmael A, Mettias N, El Sanabary Z, Gawdat G. Factors influencing the outcome of goniotomy and trabeculotomy in primary congenital glaucoma. Br J Ophthalmol. 2021;105(9):1250-5.
12. Glaser, TS, Mulvihill, MS, Freedman SF. Endoscopic cyclophotocoagulation (ECP) for childhood glaucoma: a large single-center cohort experience. J AAPOS. 2019;23(2):84 e1- e7.
13. Gupta V, Jha R, Srinivasan G, Dada T, Sihota R. Ultrasound biomicroscopic characteristics of the anterior segment in primary congenital glaucoma. J AAPOS. 2007;11(6):546–50.
14. Ishida K, Mandal AK, Netland PA. Glaucoma drainage implants in pediatric patients. Ophthalmol Clin North Am. 2005;18:431-42.
15. Jayaram H, Scawn R, Pooley F, Chiang M, Bunce C, Strouthidis NG, et al. Long-Term outcomes of trabeculectomy augmented with mitomycin C undertaken within the first 2 years of Life. Ophthalmology. 2015;122(11):2216-22.
16. Kessing SV, Gregersen E. The distended disc in early stages of congenital glaucoma. Acta Ophthalmol (Copenh). 1977;55(3):431-5.
17. Khalil DH, Abdelhakim MA. Primary trabeculotomy compared to combined trabeculectomy-trabeculotomy in congenital glaucoma: 3-year study. Acta Ophthalmol. 2016;94(7):e550-e4.
18. Kim JS, Blizzard S, Woodward JA, Leyngold IM, Liss J, Freedman SF. Prostaglandin-associated periorbitopathy in children and young adults with glaucoma. Ophthalmol Glaucoma. In Press. Available online 3 April 2020
19. Kiskis AA, Markowitz SN, Morin JD. Corneal diameter and axial length in congenital glaucoma. Can J Ophthalmol. 1985;20:93.
20. Lewis CJ, Hedberg-Buenz A, DeLuca AP, Stone EM, Alward WLM, Fingert JH. Primary congenital and developmental glaucomas. Hum Mol Genet. 2017;26(R1):R28-R36.
21. Low S, Hamada S, Nischal KK. Antimetabolite and releasable suture augmented filtration surgery in refractory pediatric glaucomas. J Aapos. 2008;12(2):166-72.
22. Maida JM, Mathers K, Alley CL. Pediatric ophthalmology in the developing world. Curr Opin Ophthalmol. 2008;19(5):403-8.
23. Mandal AK, Gothwal VK, Nutheti R. Surgical outcome of primary developmental glaucoma: a single surgeon's long-term experience from a tertiary eye care centre in India. Eye. 2007;21(6):764-74.
24. Mandalos A, Tailor R, Parmar T, Sung V. The Long-term outcomes of glaucoma drainage device in pediatric glaucoma. J Glaucoma. 2016;25(3):e189-95.
25. Maumenee AE. Further observations on the pathogenesis of congenital glaucoma. Trans Am Ophthalmol Soc. 1962;60:140-6.
26. Mocan MC, Mehta AA, Aref AA. Update in genetics and surgical management of primary congenital glaucoma. Turk J Ophthalmol. 2019;49(6):347-55.
27. Pakravan M, Esfandiari H, Yazdani S, Doozandeh A, Dastborhan Z, Gerami E, et al. Clinical outcomes of Ahmed glaucoma valve implantation in pediatric glaucoma. Eur J Ophthalmol. 2019;29(1):44-51.
28. Pilat AV, Proudlock, FA, Shah, S. et al. Assessment of the anterior segment of patients with primary congenital glaucoma using handheld optical coherence tomography. Eye. 2019;33:1232-9.
29. Ricahrson KT, Shaffer TN. Optic-nerve cupping in congenital glaucoma Am J Ophthalmol.1977;84:358-70
30. Rodriques,MM, Spaeth GL, Weinreb, S. Juvenile glaucoma associated with goniodysgenesis. Am J Ophthalmol. 1976;81:786.
31. Ruiz-Villa, Joaquín O, Jaramillo-Rivera, Daniela A, Pineda-Gutierrez, Lina MA. Ketamine impact on intraocular pressure

of children: a systematic review and qualitative synthesis of evidence. Colombian Journal of Anesthesiology. 2019;47(4): 226-35.

32. Russell-Eggitt IM, Rice NS, Jay B, et al. Relapse following goniotomy for congenital glaucoma due to trabecular dysgenesis. Eye. 1992;6:197-200.
33. Sarfarazi M, Stoilov I, Schenkman JB. Genetics and biochemistry of primary congenital glaucoma. Ophthalmol Clin North Am. 2003;16(4):543-54.
34. Sood S, Beck AD. Cyclophotocoagulation versus sequential tube shunt as a secondary intervention following primary tube shunt failure in pediatric glaucoma. J Aapos. 2009;13(4):379-83.
35. Tawara, A, Inomata H. Developmental immaturity of the trabecular meshwork in congenital glaucoma. Am J Ophthalmol. 1981;92:508.
36. Thau A, Lloyd M, Freedman S, Beck A, Grajewski A, Levin AV. New classification system for pediatric glaucoma: implications for clinical care and a research registry. Curr Opin Ophthalmol. 2018; 29(5):385-94.
37. Wadia S, Bhola R, Lorenz D, Padmanabhan P, Gross J, Stevenson M. Ketamine and intraocular pressure in children. Ann Emerg Med. 2014;64(4):385-88.
38. Weinreb RN, Grajewski AL, Papadopoulos M, Grigg J, Freedman SF. Childhood Glaucoma: The 9th Consensus Report of the World Glaucoma Association. Netherlands: Kugler Publications, 2013.
39. Yanni SE, Wang J, Cheng CS, et al. Normative reference ranges for the retinal nerve fiber layer, macula, and retinal layer thicknesses in children. Am J Ophthalmol. 2013;155(2):354-60 e1.
40. Yassin SA. Long-term visual outcomes in children with primary congenital glaucoma. Eur J Ophthalmol. 2017;27(6):705-10.
41. Yu-Wai-Man C, Arno G, Brookes J, Garcia-Feijoo J, Khaw PT, Moosajee M. Primary congenital glaucoma including next-generation sequencing-based approaches: clinical utility gene card. Eur J Hum Genet. 2018;26(11):1713-18.
42. Zhang X, Du S, Fan Q, Peng S, Yu M, Ge J. Long-term surgical outcomes of primary congenital glaucoma in China. Clinics (Sao Paulo). 2009;64(6):543-51.

11

CHAPTER

Lid and Adnexal Anomalies in Children

Michael O'Rourke, Thomas Hardy

ANATOMY AND DEVELOPMENT

Embryology of the Eyelids, Orbit, and Lacrimal Apparatus

A critical event in craniofacial development occurs around day 22 of embryogenesis. As the neural folds fuse, the ectodermal neural crest tissues lose their epithelial affinity and form a middle layer between the neural tube and overlying surface ectoderm. Much of the facial tissues are derived from this ectodermal neural crest tissue. Merging and fusion of paired components of the first pharyngeal arch are important for most facial development. A single frontonasal and paired maxillary and mandibular prominences are the main building blocks of the developing face.

The cranial base and calvarium are derived from neural crest mesenchyme. Cartilage that gradually ossifies is important in the complex development of the skull base with numerous foramina for passage of nerves and vessels. Mesenchyme surrounding the developing brain subdivides into inner and outer layers. The inner layer forms the pia and arachnoid coverings while the outer forms the dura and cranial bones of the skull which ossify to form the cranial bones. The fontanelles allow for overlapping of neonatal bones in the birth canal and are all closed by 18 months postpartum. The skull continues to grow until midteenage years.

Orbital development depends on neural crest cells migrating around the evolving optic cup. The angle between the two developing orbits decreases as the bony walls and skull base develop.

The distal nasolacrimal system is formed by the fusion of the lateral nasal prominences and the maxillary prominence and starts as a nasolacrimal furrow with a double layer of epithelium centrally which canalizes near birth to form the nasolacrimal duct.

Anatomy

Eyelid

The eyelid skin is the thinnest of anywhere on the body measuring 0.6 mm. The eyelid functions to protect the eye and to distribute and maintain the tear film. The upper lid rests just below the superior limbus with its peak just nasal to the pupil. The lower lid rests at the inferior limbus with its the lowest point just temporal to the limbus, although racial variations exist, to a greater extent in the lower lid than the upper lid. The anterior lamella describes a surgical concept consisting of skin and preseptal and pretarsal orbicularis oculi muscle separated by the orbital septum from the posterior lamella, consisting of the tarsus and conjunctiva. The skin crease is formed by fibers of the levator aponeurosis extending anteriorly into the pretarsal orbicularis and skin and is usually located at the upper tarsal border in non-Asian eyelids.

Below the skin crease, the anterior lamella is firmly adherent to the tarsal plate. Above the skin crease, the anterior lamella is loose and freely mobile to allow for eyelid movement. The orbital septum originates from the superior orbital rim and inserts into the levator aponeurosis 3–5 mm above the upper border of the tarsus. The tarsus provides structural stability being a semilunar, malleable, fibrous plate. The upper tarsus is 1 mm in thickness, 22–25 mm in length and 9–10 mm in height. The posterior surface is lined with conjunctiva firmly adherent to the tarsus extending a further 8–10 mm above this with tight adhesion to Muller's muscle and then becomes loosely attached in the blind ending diverticulum of the fornix.

The upper lid skin crease represents the insertion of the levator aponeurosis fibers to the skin at the upper border of the tarsus. In Asian eyelids, this crease is often lower and related to the epicanthal tarsal fold. The lateral canthus is usually slightly higher than the medial canthus. A common variation in eyelid anatomy is the extra fold of upper lid tissue at the medial canthal area called an epicanthal fold and can be classified into four types: (1) supraciliaris (rare), (2) tarsalis (most common), (3) palpebralis, and (4) inversus [seen in blepharophimosis, ptosis, epicanthus inversus syndrome, blepharophimosis, ptosis and epicanthus inversus syndrome (BPES)].

The eyelid is divided into anterior and posterior lamellae with the gray line defining their interface. From anterior to posterior, the eyelid comprises of skin, orbicularis oculi, tarsal plate (or septum and eyelid retractors peripheral to the tarsi), and the conjunctiva which is reflected back on itself to form fornices. The orbicularis oculi muscle is supplied by the facial nerve and functions in closure of the eyelids and voluntary and involuntary blinking. The levator palpebrae superioris muscle is the main upper lid retractor and inserts via its aponeurosis to the upper border of the upper tarsal plate to elevate the upper eyelid with assistance from the Müller's muscle on its under surface. The inferior retractors are fibers from the inferior rectus which insert into the lower border of the lower tarsal plate and retract the lower lid on downgaze. The medial and lateral canthal tendons are condensations of the orbital septum and orbicularis oculi, with superficial and deep components. The medial canthal area is complete with splitting of the fascia to surround the lacrimal sac which aids in lacrimal pumping. Tears are produced by the lacrimal gland in the superotemporal anterior orbit. Meibomian glands at the base of each eyelash in the anterior eyelid lamella and accessory lacrimal glands throughout the conjunctiva contribute value components of the tear film to retain tears on the ocular surface.

Müller's muscle is a smooth muscle innervated by the sympathetic chain. The origin is the posterior layer of the levator palpebrae superioris inferior to Whitnall's ligament and inserts into the upper border of the tarsal plate. The levator palpebrae superioris is a striated muscle innervated by the superior division of the oculomotor nerve. It originates from the annulus of Zinn and fans out to divide into an anterior aponeurosis and a posterior portion that is continuous with Muller's muscle.

Lacrimal Drainage System

The nasolacrimal system provides a passageway from the ocular surface to the nasal cavity. A 0.3 mm diameter opening in the medial aspect of each eyelid (lacrimal punctum) opens to a 2 mm vertical canalicular segment which rotates to an 8 mm horizontal segment. Upper and lower canaliculi usually join to form a single common canaliculus which enters the lateral aspect of the lacrimal sac. The sac is located in the lacrimal fossa measuring 10–15 mm in length and opens to the nasolacrimal duct which exits to the inferior meatus of the nose. Valves within this system mark the points of entry into different tissue types. The valve of Rosenmuller is a fold of mucosal tissue preventing tear reflux from the lacrimal sac back into the common canaliculus. The valve of Hasner is a mucosal fold at the distal portion of the nasolacrimal duct at the opening to the nasal cavity. Failure of this valve to open is a common cause of congenital nasolacrimal duct obstruction. It usually opens during the first month of life. Spontaneous opening can occur for the first 12 months.

Children will have variation in the structures and relative measurements due to the system's immaturity in the early years of life. The inferior meatus is flat with little space between the floor of the nose, the lateral nasal wall and the inferior turbinate in the first year of life. The lacrimal crests are also flat with a shallow sac fossa and poorly developed lacrimal sac relative to adults. Such complexities related to anatomical immaturity make epiphora common in early childhood.

Orbit

This pear-shaped bony box houses the globe, extraocular muscles, fat, nerves, and blood vessels. The medial walls are parallel being separated by the ethmoidal and sphenoidal sinuses. It comprises of the ethmoid bone (the thinnest orbital bones referred to as the *lamina papyracea*), lacrimal bone, frontal process of the maxillary bone, and lesser wing of the sphenoid. The floor of the anterior cranial fossa is approximately at the level of the frontoethmoidal suture. The medial wall of the optic canal is formed by the lesser wing of the sphenoid/lateral wall of the sphenoidal sinus. The S-shaped optic nerve allows for free movement of the globe and exits via the optic canal posteriorly. The orbital floor is made up of the maxillary bone, palatine bone, and the orbital plate of the zygomatic bone. The floor ends posteriorly at the pterygopalatine fossa. The infraorbital groove and infraorbital canal transmit the infraorbital artery and maxillary division of the trigeminal nerve. The orbital roof is made up of the orbital plate of the frontal bone and the lesser wing of the sphenoid bone. It separates the orbit from the frontal sinus and anterior cranial fossa. The supraorbital notch transmits the supraorbital vessels and the supraorbital branch of the frontal nerve. The lateral wall is the thickest and is composed of the zygomatic bone and the greater wing of the sphenoid. The superior orbital fissure is located between the greater and lesser wings of the sphenoid bone and transmits many important structures to the cavernous sinus. The orbital contents are varied and complex, including a range of vascular, neural, skeletal and smooth muscular, glandular, adipose, and fibrous connective tissue structures. The detailed anatomy is beyond the scope of this chapter; further detail can be found in textbooks of anatomy by eminent authors such as JJ Dutton.

EYELID

Brow and Lash Disorders

Lashes

Eyelashes differentiate in association with their respective gland of Zeis which services each lash with the production of an oily substance. These and the meibomian glands form by invagination of surface ectoderm along the eyelid margin.

Distichiasis occurs when the pilosebaceous units differentiate into lashes instead of meibomian glands. This is due to a failure of epithelial germ cells to differentiate into meibomian glands, instead forming lash units. These extra lashes arising from the meibomian gland orifices may be present in both upper and lower lids. This may be congenital or acquired with acquired type being more symptomatic. *Lymphedema distichiasis syndrome* is a congenital autosomal dominant cause with incomplete penetrance with marked variability of expression. This is due to *FOXC2* mutations (16q24). De novo cases account for 20%. There are two parallel rows of cilia present at the eyelid margin from birth with symmetrical lymphedema of the extremities from puberty onward. Cardiac defects, varicose veins, ptosis, cleft palate, and spinal extradural cysts may also occur. Acquired causes are associated with conjunctival cicatrization such as ocular pemphigoid (OCP), blepharokeratoconjunctivitis, chemical burns, graft-versus-host disease, or Stevens-Johnston syndrome (SJS). The first presentation may be with ocular symptoms and the ophthalmologist should have a high clinical suspicion for associated autoimmune causes.

Trichiasis is an acquired lash disorder where the normal pilosebaceous units anterior to the meibomian glands become misdirected, growing toward the ocular surface. This results in corneal and conjunctival irritation and is usually secondary to chronic inflammation and cicatrization. Trachoma is the leading cause of preventable blindness world-wide. Chronic inflammation and scarring of the conjunctiva lead to the trichiasis and cicatricial entropion, abrading the cornea with subsequent scarring and vision loss. Mass antibiotic treatment with single dose oral azithromycin has been shown to prevent active trachoma. The most effective surgery being full-thickness incision of the tarsal plate and rotation of the terminal tarsal strap is often carried out in community-based surgery by nonphysician technicians in endemic areas.

Trichomegaly refers to abnormally large eyelashes. It is defined as increased length (>12 mm), curling, pigmentation or thickness of eyelashes. If congenital, it can be associated with some syndromes, e.g., Cornelia de Lange. Acquired associations are varied and include connective tissue disorders, allergic conditions, malnutrition, hypothyroidism, and medications including prostaglandin analogues.

It is best to take a stepwise approach to treatment of trichiasis and distichiasis. Lubricants will improve discomfort and discharge if there is conjunctival touch of the lashes. Corneal lash touch is associated with a risk of vision loss from corneal irregularity, infection, ulceration, and scarring. Electrolysis is the least destructive option and useful if only a few lashes. Selective follicle excision and trephination is another option. For more severe cases, lamellar split with cryotherapy (double freeze-thaw) may be considered or direct excision of the distal tarsus and replacing with a mucosal graft.

Eyebrow

Eyebrow anomalies are rare but can be noted as part of a wide range of syndromes. Sparse or absent brow hairs (and/or lashes) can occur in conditions such as ectodermal dysplasia, alopecia, progressive hemifacial atrophy, and trichotillomania. **Synophrys** refers to fusion of the eyebrows with the appearance of a single continuous long eyebrow ("unibrow" or "monobrow"). This is a recognized feature of Cornelia De Lange syndrome. **Prominent brow hair** can occur in conditions such as Rubinstein-Taybi syndrome. **Poliosis** (white or depigmented eyebrow hair) occurs in Waardenburg syndrome, Parry-Romberg syndrome, and VKH disease.

Epiblepharon

This describes an extra horizontal fold of skin and orbicularis muscle below and in front of the lashes. It occurs in all ethnicities but is more common in Asian children. The incidence is reported at 46% of infants in the Japanese population which decreases to 2% at 13–18 years. The overriding anterior lamella results in inward rotation of the lashes which can abrade the cornea. It is more common in the lower lids than the upper lids. Clinical signs are more obvious when the patient looks down as the extra skin fold pushes the lashes against the globe causing varying degrees of epithelial erosions and rarely infiltration, ulceration, and microbial keratitis. Most have minimal symptoms of watering or conjunctival injection. A definitive link with astigmatism has not been proven.

A key factor in the pathogenesis of epiblepharon is a deficiency of the attachment of the lower lid retractors to the skin via the capsulopalpebral fascia which is usually responsible for the eyelid crease. Therefore, the skin and orbicularis muscle roll upwards. Hypertrophy of the orbicularis muscle has not been proven. Adult onset epiblepharon has been associated with thyroid eye disease and increased BMI. As distinct from entropion, the eyelid margin is not rotated inwards. Epiblepharon can be managed conservatively with lubrication in most cases as children remain asymptomatic even with some degree of corneal punctate staining. As the midface grows, many cases of epiblepharon resolve spontaneously. Hyaluronic acid in the suborbicularis space at the valley of the epiblepharon skin fold has been described as a temporizing approach until self-correction occurs with age. The surgical approach described by Kim et al. involves a skin incision 1–2 mm below the lash line, debulking of pretarsal orbicularis, lash rotation anteriorly by anchoring subcutaneous tissue of the upper skin-muscle flap onto the tarsal plate (of inferior retractors if severe) and excision of a minimal amount of redundant skin and orbicularis muscle to avoid ectropion or retraction. We have found this technique superior to the Hotz procedure and everting sutures.

Entropion (Upper and Lower)

Congenital entropion is rare, often bilateral and mostly involves the medial lower lids. In contrast to epiblepharon, it does not improve with time and tends to worsen; surgical correction is almost always required. The tarsus may be developmentally absent with hypertrophy of the orbicularis muscle. Tarsal kink syndrome is a rare and severe form of upper lid entropion characterized by horizontal kink within the upper tarsal plate. Associated blepharospasm and absence of the upper eyelid fold with the folded edge of the tarsus or inturned lids and lashes lead to corneal ulceration. Unlike adults, children with isolated facial nerve palsy may be more prone to develop entropion rather than ectropion. Surgical correction involves Jones-type retractor plication in the lower lid, Quickert sutures or tarsal wedge resection in the upper or lower lids.

Acquired eyelid malposition in the setting of cicatricial conjunctival disease is complex to manage. Medically controlled or inactive cicatricial disease is optimal but not always practical if there is significant, sight-threatening exposure. A tarsorrhaphy can be performed as a temporary or permanent procedure. Fornix contraction will benefit from release of any symblepharon or ankyloblepharon and augmentation with autologous or donor mucosal grafts (buccal, hard palate, nasal or amniotic membrane). Eyelid malposition can be managed by addressing inferior retractor position and/or lid tightening. Keratinized conjunctiva can be replaced with amniotic or mucous membrane graft.

Ectropion and Eversion

Ectropion occurs due to vertical deficiency or shortening of the anterior lamella or elongation of the posterior lamella. Low orbicularis tone can contribute. Congenital ectropion is more often seen as part of a syndrome than an isolated condition, often associated with retraction and/or euryblepharon. Skin deficiency may result from trauma, burns or ichthyosis. Associated syndromes include BPES, trisomy 21, and facial dysostoses. Rarely, complete eversion of the eyelid may lead to a worsening cycle of orbicularis spasm, secondary edema and inability to reinvert the eyelid. Complete tarsal eversion may initially protect the cornea and timing of intervention will be guided by cornea and conjunctival health.

Spontaneous eversion may occur postpartum in the setting of a difficult delivery or Downs syndrome with spontaneous resolution often occurring in this context. Lubricants and eyelid taping will help. If there is skin shortage, this can be addressed with a flap preferable to a graft. Lower lid and midface support or augmentation may also be required with implants, bone grafts or fat transfer, either prior to or simultaneous with local skin flap augmentation. More advanced cases of ectropion associated with bony and/or soft tissue deficiency can require complex, multiple multidisciplinary procedures. Hyaluronic acid in the suborbicularis plane works as a tissue expander and may also act as a temporizing measure. Surgery is aimed at correcting the underlying cause - horizontal laxity is corrected by stabilization of canthal tendons, vertical height deficiency is replaced with a skin flap and any cicatrix is released.

Euryblepharon and Centurion syndrome may both result in lower lid ectropion. Euryblepharon refers to widening of the horizontal palpebral fissure with relative increase in the upper eyelid compared to the lower leading to lower lid ectropion. Surgical correction addresses laxity with lateral +/- medial tightening, soft tissue and skin augmentation with alloplasts, bone or fat grafts and skin flaps. Centurion syndrome refers to anterior displacement of the medial canthal tendon with punctal ectropion and a prominent nasal bridge. There may also be weakness in the posterior limb of the medial canthal tendon with loss of the posterior arching and some may have concomitant posterior globe displacement. Medial cantholysis allows better globe apposition and the necessity for a retro-punctal diamond and posterior plication suture is evaluated intraoperatively.

Upper Eyelid Retraction

Isolated congenital eyelid retraction is rare and may be transient and accounts for 13% of upper eyelid retraction. Anatomical causes included severe myopia and craniosynostosis/shallow orbits. A full evaluation for causes of proptosis should be considered. Acquired causes included thyroid eye disease (56%) and trauma (11%). Eyelid retraction in thyroid eye disease (Dalrymples sign) is the most common presenting sign of thyroid eye disease being present in up to 90%. Thyroid eye disease may occur in hyper-, hypo-, and euthyroid states and antibody testing should be included in a blood panel. Neurogenic causes included Marcus Gunn syndrome, congenital aberrant innervation of the oculomotor nerve, facial palsy, dissociated vertical deviation, dorsal midbrain syndrome, and benign transient conjugate downgaze in preterm infants. Scleral show may also occur post strabismus surgery with inferior or superior rectus recession. After orbital floor fracture, even subtle inferior rectus trauma can lead to unopposed action of the superior rectus/levator complex. Pseudoretraction from a contralateral ptosis is important to recognize and may likely resolve once the contralateral ptosis is corrected. In a series of 85 pediatric patients over a 35-year period with eyelid retraction, there were no cases of visual impairment. Tearing, ocular surface irritation and photophobia were noted in 45%. Nineteen (22%) underwent surgical correction. Lower eyelid retraction is very rare and is usually isolated or associated with motility defects (e.g., CFEOM or epiblepharon).

The need for intervention will be guided by the degree of lagophthalmos and corneal exposure risk for upper or lower eyelid retraction. Downward eyelid stretch may be trialed. Low dose botulinum toxin may be considered but the results can be unpredictable and of variable duration. Tarsorrhaphy (lateral +/- medial) will aid to protect the cornea. Muller's muscle recession (transconjunctival) offers up to 2 mm of upper eyelid lowering. Further recession targeting the levator aponeurosis is less predictable, with around 2–3 mm recession required to correct each 1 mm of upper eyelid retraction. A spacer graft above the tarsus may be required for bigger recessions. In the setting of acute corneal ulceration, a temporary tarsorrhaphy may be necessary.

Epicanthal folds are redundant semilunar folds of tissue in the medial canthal region and may be a normal facial finding or occur in conjunction with syndromes such as BPES. They are classified based on the origin and termination of the fold; supraciliaris (eyebrow to over lacrimal sac fossa), epicanthus tarsalis (upper eyelid crease to medial canthus), palpebralis (upper eyelid to lower eyelid) and inversus (lower eyelid to medial canthus). They are usually asymptomatic and nonamblyogenic and therefore surgical correction is generally for aesthetic reasons. Surgical repair includes a Y-V and Z-plasties and other variations, either alone or in combination.

Blepharophimosis, ptosis and epicanthus inversus syndrome (BPES) is an autosomal dominant inherited condition caused by mutation in the *FOXL2* gene (3q22.3). In addition to the typically poor levator function and severe ptosis, narrowed horizontal palpebral aperture (blepharophimosis) and pathognomonic epicanthus inversus, associations include hypertelorism, hypoplasia of the superior orbital rims, lower eyelid ectropion, and a poorly differentiated nasal bridge. Type I BPES is associated with premature ovarian failure whereas Type II BPES is not. The ophthalmologist may be the first to review such patients and a comprehensive genetic evaluation could be considered. It is the most common syndromic cause of ptosis in an ophthalmic clinic. Surgery is typically offered for correction of epicanthus inversus, ptosis and less commonly, lateral lower lid ectropion.

Telecanthus is an increased separation of the medial canthi (>2 SD above the mean) and occurs as part of BPES and many other conditions. It should be distinguished from **hypertelorism** which refers to increased separation of normal sized orbits. **Pseudohypertelorism** refers to increased separation of the medial but not lateral orbital walls and occurs due to conditions such as a midline encephalocele. **Hypotelorism** describes decreased separation (>2 SD below the mean) of the orbits.

Lateral Canthal Dystopias

Lateral canthal dystopias are associated with Treacher Collins syndrome, facial clefts and trauma and can be addressed with canthopexy, canthoplasty, and transposition flaps. Medial canthal dystopias are less common but more complex due to the proximity to the lacrimal drainage system. The medial canthal tendon is required for lacrimal pump function and may require a bony fixation (e.g., trans-nasal wire) and transposition flap for repair.

Ankyloblepharon

This refers to partial or complete fusion of the eyelids by strands of tissues. This may be congenital or acquired as a result of infection, trauma, Stevens-Johnson syndrome/toxic epidermal necrolysis and silicone tube intubation of the nasolacrimal system. Ankyloblepharon filiforme adnatum (AFA) occurs when multiple strands of tissue connect the upper and lower lids. This can be associated with iridogoniodysgenesis and juvenile glaucoma as well as cleft lip, cleft palate, hydrocephalus, meningomyelocele, imperforate anus, cardiac defects, and syndactyly. Surgical separation of the ankyloblepharon will restore normal architecture to prevent potential amblyopia.

Blepharoptosis

Classification and standardized assessment of blepharoptosis (or simply, "ptosis") helps guide treatment options and future interventions. Classifying by etiology is a reminder to the clinician of the importance of out ruling potentially concomitant medical conditions and appropriate investigations when necessary. The incidence of associated amblyopia is 18% in children with moderate to severe congenital ptosis and the best indicator of amblyopia is visual acuity and not lid height measurements. Ptosis is commonly associated with systemic disease and our understanding of the genetic basis of ptosis is evolving. A trend toward keratoconus-like changes in the corneas of congenital blepharoptosis, with the increase of ptosis severity is described.

Examination

Full ophthalmic examination includes visual acuity, refraction, cover test and ocular motility (in particular for SR weakness), and dilated ophthalmic examination. Comment on the severity, the levator function, the skin crease formation and height, laterality, and upper lid lag in downgaze. It may be difficult to measure accurately until the child is older and more cooperative. It is important to examine to such an extent so as to formulate a surgical plan from an early age. It may be difficult to assess eyelid closure or lagophthalmos in children but collateral history can be obtained from the parents as well as history of jaw-wink or other associated disorders. Treating any amblyopia and refractive error are crucial aspects of ptosis management; old photos and clinical photography are useful for complete documentation at each visit.

Ptosis Classification

Myogenic ptosis is the most common cause of congenital ptosis and can be unilateral or bilateral. It is also referred to as "simple (dysgenetic)" congenital ptosis. The levator muscle is dystrophic and replaced by fibrotic or fatty tissue with poor elevation on up gaze and lag on downgaze. There is likely failure of development of the neural branch to the levator muscle. A degree of lagophthalmos and "lid lag" (incomplete descent) on downgaze are commonly seen. Superior rectus weakness occurs in 5% and may be seen as double elevator palsy. Up to one-third may be bilateral and the condition may be asymmetrical. Strabismus is present in 10% and amblyopia in 14% of congenital ptosis patients. There is a broad range of severity of ptosis, which correlates positively with lid "lag" on downgaze and inversely with levator function and lid crease definition.

It may be associated with a number of syndromes. Congenital fibrosis of the extraocular muscles, esp. CFEOM 1 and 2, may also involve the levator muscle in addition to extraocular muscles. The degree of ptosis is worsened by enophthalmos. The child may compensate with a head posture and use of brows. Some myogenic ptoses are not present at birth and present later in life such as chronic progressive external ophthalmoplegia (CPEO). This mitochondrial disease results in bilateral, severe, and progressive ptosis. Kearns Sayre syndrome describes CPEO with the addition of heart block, retinal pigment degeneration, and foveal atrophy. Thyroid eye disease can rarely present with myogenic ptosis due to inflammation of the eyelid retractors.

Most cases of simple congenital ptosis are sporadic but up to one-third may have a family history (autosomal dominant in 18% and recessive in 14%). There are 3 identified ptosis genes associated with isolated familial ptosis: *PTOS1* (178300) (1p34.1-p32) is autosomal dominant, *PTOS2* (300245) (Xq24-q27.1) is X-linked dominant, and *ZFHX4* (606940) (8q21.13) is an autosomal dominant candidate gene for congenital bilateral ptosis. There is thought to be an abnormal development of the oculomotor nuclear and neural development. The condition is static and does not change over time with atrophy of Mullers muscle reported. It is important to check for synkinesis in muscles supplied by the trigeminal nerve (classically Marcus Gunn jaw wink syndrome and pterygoid muscles).

Aponeurotic ptosis refers to a defect in the tendon of the levator muscle. The skin crease is usually elevated due to dehiscence of the aponeurosis. The levator muscle itself is healthy and therefore levator function measures as normal. This is more common in elderly patients but can occur in children with developmental defect or forceps injury trauma at birth. Other causes of trauma leading to aponeurotic ptosis occur following surgery or trauma.

Neurogenic ptosis includes neuromuscular causes. Marcus Gunn jaw-winking (MGJW) ptosis accounts for up to 13% of congenital ptosis. There is synkinetic elevation of the eyelid caused by pterygoid (lateral > medial) muscle contraction e.g., sucking or chewing. It is usually unilateral and may improve with age – or the patient may learn better control of the movements.

Congenital CN III palsy is characterized by complete or partial ptosis, dilated nonreactive pupil and weak elevation, depression, and adduction of the eye. There is rarely aberrant regeneration with congenital CN III palsy compared to acquired palsies.

Horner syndrome presents as the triad of ptosis, miosis, and anhidrosis. Ptosis is usually mild and may be associated with 1–2 mm of inverse ptosis of the lower lid, causing "apparent enophthalmos." Additional signs include a small pupil that fails to dilate and a decrease in iris pigmentation on the involved side. Heterochromia is more characteristic of congenital Horner syndrome. Acquired Horner syndrome requires evaluation for a potential sympathetic pathway tumor.

Myasthenia gravis (MG) may be congenital or acquired, can be a great mimicker, and can present with ptosis. Fatigability and increased symptoms as the day progresses as characteristic. Varying and unusual motility patterns can occur. Weakness of orbicularis muscle on forced closure is a useful sign in children. The Cogan lid twitch is well described whereby the patient looks in downgaze, followed by up gaze resulting in the upper lid overshooting. The ice pack test is useful with a reversal of approximately 2 mm of ptosis temporarily with application of ice to the eyelid for 5 minutes. Serum anti-ACh receptor antibodies are present in 85–90% of systemic MG and 50% of ocular MG. Single fiber-electromyography and nerve conduction studies can be useful. The Tensilon test may be required in pediatric cases: edrophonium or neostigmine will reverse the ptosis.

Mechanical ptosis can be due to a mass, foreign body, post-traumatic scarring, or soft tissue swelling. The levator function may be normal or infiltrated by the disease process. Infantile hemangiomas and plexiform neurofibromas infiltrating muscle can make excision difficult.

Traumatic ptosis may occur in utero secondary to amniocentesis or during delivery with forceps. Accidental and nonaccidental trauma should be differentiated in the child presented with traumatic ptosis and may require a complete examination under anesthesia. Penetrating or blunt ocular and orbitocranial trauma is essential to exclude. A clue to involvement of the levator is the presence of orbital fat in the wound. Repair of lacerated muscle requires immediate attention and if not amblyogenic, a period of a few months allowed to restore function prior to any further surgical interventions.

Pseudoptosis may be apparent due to contralateral eyelid retraction, facial asymmetry, proptosis, enophthalmos, hypotropia, hypoglobus, eyelid inflammation, anisometropia or vertical strabismus; all these conditions may also coexist with true ptosis. Measuring globe position and performing a cover test is important to differentiate true from pseudoptosis.

Surgical Approach

Patients with poor levator function (with variable cut off of 4–6 mm of function) will undergo brow suspension. Brow suspension, or frontalis sling, is a mechanical sling suspending the upper eyelid to the frontalis muscle using alloplastic (e.g., silicone, "Supramid" suture, expanded polytetrafluoroethylene or mersilene mesh) or autogenous (fascia lata, plantaris, palmaris, temporalis fascia) materials. An alternative is the frontalis muscle flap, "supramaximal" levator resection or Whitnall's (internal) sling if the frontalis muscle is very weak. If good levator function (>6 mm) with a small degree of ptosis (1–2 mm e.g., Horner's syndrome) a Fasanella-Servat (tarsoconjunctival-Müllerectomy) or a Müller's muscle resection would be appropriate if the ptosis is responsive to phenylephrine. Typically, a levator resection (anterior or posterior approach) is performed for varying degrees of ptosis with moderate to good levator function. A Lemagne (levator transposition) procedure for MGJW ptosis will be described later.

Early surgery is indicated for patients who have failed amblyopia therapy or high risk of visual deprivation amblyopia. In these situations, a brow suspension with alloplastic material is undertaken, unless reliable measurements and donor site allows a definitive autogenous sling or levator resection. Later cases are typically delayed till just prior to school entry for psychosocial reasons and if fascia lata graft is required, the leg is usually long enough at this age. The surgery is largely dictated by the levator function and discussion with the parents regarding expectations. The phenylephrine test can be used as a guide if Müller's resection is considered.

Brow suspension is a static "sling" attached to frontalis muscle. Bilateral surgery may be offered to give the best chance of success in primary, up and down gaze in cases of unilateral ptosis. Weakening the normal levator muscle on the contralateral side may improve dynamic symmetry. Understandably, careful discussion with the parents or guardians is required before embarking on bilateral surgery for unilateral ptosis. Typically, a modified Fox pentagon procedure or a Crawford double triangle procedure is used for brow suspension. We perform the modified Fox procedure as a single pentagon with an open incision in the skin crease to suture the sling to the tarsal plate. The Crawford procedure involves a double triangle and 3 stab incisions in the eyelid and 2 separate pieces of sling material (classically, fascia lata) medially and laterally. The frontalis muscle flap can be of various formations, and is sutured to the tarsus directly. The conjunctival-Muller's resection can be performed as an open or closed (with a clamp, e.g., Putterman) procedure. The Fasanella-Servat procedure involves resection of a few mm of tarsus, Müller's muscle and conjunctiva. Anterior approach levator resection involves opening the skin crease, septum, and identifying the preaponeurotic fat pad which is retracted to exposure the levator. Cutting the medial and lateral horns is usually required, allowing the levator to be advanced the desired amount and sutured to the tarsal plate. Crowell Beard described an algorithm for the extent of resection based on the degree of ptosis and levator function. These guidelines are modified by each surgeon's personal experience. Generally, greater severity ptosis correlates with weaker levator function and more resection required. Raynold N Berke reported a similar algorithm based on intraoperative correction of eyelid position guided by levator function, with weaker levator function necessitating a higher position relative to the upper limbus at the end of surgery. A combination of both of these approaches is often utilized.

BEARD CONGENITAL PTOSIS TABLE

Degree of ptosis	*Levator function*	*Resection*
Mild (<2 mm)	>10 mm	Small (10–13 mm)
Moderate (3 mm)	>8 mm	Moderate (14–17 mm)
	<8 mm	Large (18–22 mm)
Severe (>4 mm)	<5 mm	Maximum (>23 mm)

PROCEDURE BASED ON LEVATOR FUNCTION

Levator function	*Procedure*
Excellent >13 mm	Aponeurosis advancement
Good (8–12 mm)	Aponeurosis advancement or moderate levator resection (14–17 mm)
Fair (5–7 mm)	Large levator resection (18–22 mm)
Poor (<4 mm)	Frontalis suspension or maximal/ supramaximal levator resection

PTOSIS: LID POSITION ON CORNEA

Levator function	*Lid position on cornea*	*Change in eyelid position post op*
>10 mm	3–4 mm below the limbus	Rise 2–3 mm
8–9 mm	3 mm below the limbus	Rise 1–2 mm
6–7 mm	2 mm below the limbus	Remain at same position
5–6 mm	1 mm below limbus	Remain at same position or drop 1–2 mm
0–4 mm	Frontalis suspension	

Marcus Gunn jaw winking syndrome is a synkinesis where the eyelid elevates with pterygoid muscle contraction, more commonly lateral than medial pterygoid. The degree of ptosis varies as does the size of the synkinetic "wink." Management is controversial. Some may opt to correct the ptosis alone in cases of minor synkinesis. To abolish the wink, a section of levator muscle must be resected followed by a unilateral or bilateral brow suspension or frontalis muscle flap. The levator transposition originally described by Lemagne involves is detaching levator in the posterior orbit and suturing this proximal end to the frontalis muscle. After several months, it is hoped that neurotization of the levator from the frontalis muscle (temporal branch of facial nerve) will occur. A secondary anterior levator resection is often required subsequently.

Successful outcomes from ptosis surgery include correction of lid height, natural lid contour, and symmetry of both lid height and supratarsal skin fold. Other important outcome factors include patient and family satisfaction, surgeon satisfaction. The patient and parents should be aware that the aim of surgical correction of ptosis is primarily to prevent amblyopia and improve vision but esthetic considerations and psychosocial well-being are also critical. Revision or primary procedures with primarily aesthetic intentions may yield better outcomes if addressed in adulthood, especially if the degree of ptosis is mild.

Complications

When consenting for ptosis surgery, the postoperative expectations include swelling, bruising (usually minor), and minimal or no pain. Lid "lag" on downward gaze and lagophthalmos during sleep are expected to some degree, and mild exposure symptoms may occur, typically in the first few weeks. Complications include asymmetry, under or over correction, unacceptable contour or lid fold/crease, severe exposure keratopathy, donor site morbidity (scar, hematoma), foreign body reaction to or extrusion of sutures or alloplastic sling material, infection, abnormal wound healing (scar, dehiscence), revision surgery, lash ptosis, or upper lid entropion (more common after brow suspension).

The difficulty in balancing corneal exposure with a functional and esthetically acceptable lid height and contour makes ptosis surgery difficult. Keratitis may lead to corneal scarring and corneal exposure related complications will usually require reversal of the ptosis correction. Ocular lubrication, particularly at night-time is recommended postoperatively. The slings may become eroded or exposed. The sleeve at the apex may erode and therefore layered closure is advised at this point. Exposure will require antibiotic prophylaxis and removal with deferred reinsertion is preferable. Permanent sutures in levator surgery can very rarely erode through tarsus and conjunctiva and abrade the cornea requiring removal.

PERIOCULAR DERMATOLOGY

Congenital Melanocytic Nevus

These can be divided into four groups: small (<1.5 cm diameter), intermediate (1.5–20 cm), large lesions (>20 cm diameter), and giant (greater than 50 cm). The potential for malignant change is 4–6% in a lifetime with 50% occurring before the age of 5. Congenital melanocytic nevi may arise on the eyelid and the conjunctiva. Indications for surgery include prevention of malignant change, mechanical ptosis, and cosmetic defect; ablative laser also has a role.

Nevus of Ota (Oculodermal Melanocytosis)

The presence of pigmentation within the dermis gives a characteristic blue-gray or blue-brown color. Most are unilateral and occur within the distribution of first and second divisions of the trigeminal nerve. The sclera is blue and conjunctiva brown in the affected eye. Pigmentation may also occur on eyelids, cornea, and optic disc, becoming progressively darker over time. There is increased risk of uveal melanoma and glaucoma in such cases.

Pilomatrixoma

These benign hair follicle tumors manifest as solitary, firm dermal or subcutaneous nodules with a pale or sometimes purple/blue color, commonly in the upper lid/brow area. The "teeter totter sign" refers to pressure on the lateral edge leading to elevation of the opposite side as the lesions is firm and calcified. Untreated lesions may ulcerate or extrude calcium contents. Malignant transformation is very rare. Prophylactic surgery is advised as they are unlikely to regress by themselves. Multiple pilomatrixomas are associated with Gardner syndrome, myotonic dystrophy, and Turner syndrome.

Pyogenic Granuloma

These rapidly growing lesions may present with recurrent bleeding. In the periocular area, they are thought to be a reactive lesion which can occur in sites of previous trauma including surgery. They have been reported in various parts of the eye. Topical beta blockers have been reported to successfully treat pyogenic granulomas as they express beta adrenergic receptors. Gentle cautery at the base is effective for excision and all should be sent for histopathology diagnosis as the differential diagnosis includes amelanotic melanoma, carcinoma, and sarcoma.

Syringoma

These benign tumors derive from eccrine duct structures. They are usually multiple, small skin-colored papules, found anywhere on the skin, and with increased prevalence in patients with Down syndrome. Treatment is for cosmetic reasons and includes topical retinoid therapy, cryotherapy, electrodesiccation, or excision.

Granuloma Annulare

This benign disorder is characterized by papules or nodules in a ring configuration with a clear center. These may occur at a site of previous trauma anywhere on the body, particularly hands and feet and are most common in children and young adults. The nodular or subcutaneous form is known as pseudorheumatoid nodules due to histological resemblance with rheumatoid arthritis. Localized lesions are more common in children; widespread lesions more common in adults. Adult type is also associated with diabetes which does not occur in children. A biopsy may be considered if multiple are present as the differential diagnosis is large. These lesions usually resolve spontaneously but topical steroids or calcineurin inhibitors (Tacrolimus) has been used successfully to hasten resolution.

Xeroderma Pigmentosum

This is a rare autosomal recessive disorder in which there is extreme sensitivity to ultraviolet (UV) light with resultant defective DNA repair. Patients may develop photophobia, conjunctivitis, keratitis symblepharon, corneal opacity, conjunctival nevi and epibulbar and lid neoplasms (BCC, SCC, and melanoma). These patients require avoidance of UV radiation (sunscreens and sunglasses), regular follow up, and early excision of suspicious lesions.

Ectodermal Dysplasia

This refers to a group of disorders characterized by abnormalities in two or more ectodermal derivatives including skin, hair, teeth, and sweat glands. The most common ocular findings are lacrimal drainage obstruction (including punctal agenesis, e.g., Hay-Wells syndrome), blepharoptosis, eyelash ptosis, refractive errors, and amblyopia. Possible genetic associations include *EDA1* gene and *TP63* gene variants.

Molluscum Contagiosum

This is a viral disorder of the skin and mucous membranes cause by the poxvirus family. The lesions are small, umbilicated papules that may be single or multiple. They appear on the face, trunk, or limbs. When occurring on the eyelids, they may lead to chronic conjunctivitis which rarely develops pannus. When associated with immune deficiency or immunosuppressive therapy they may be widespread and large. Molluscum is self-limiting lasting 6–18 months. They may be excised if troublesome such as recurrent conjunctivitis.

Warts

These are due to human papillomavirus (HPV). In the periocular region, they may cause a low-grade chronic papillary conjunctivitis. Multiple or recurrent warts require histological confirmation to exclude more sinister diseases such as epidermodysplasia verruciformis or basal cell nevus syndrome. Treatment includes excision, liquid-nitrogen cryotherapy, bichloracetic acid, trichloroacetic acid, and ablative laser.

Malignant Eyelid Tumors

Basal Cell Carcinoma

When encountered in the pediatric population, predisposing genetic conditions should be investigated such as xeroderma pigmentosum or basal cell nevus syndrome (BCNS), or a history of significant radiation exposure. BCNS is a rare autosomal dominant disorder caused by mutations in the hedgehog signaling pathway, mainly *PTCH1* which is involved in embryogenesis and tumorigenesis. Multidisciplinary team management is best with dermatology. A high clinical suspicion can be confirmed with genetic testing. Mohs micrographic surgery may be the most appropriate form of excision to minimize tissue loss and ensure precise tumor clearance. Radiotherapy is relatively contraindicated. Sun-protective measures are very important. Concomitant bone deformities, cardiac fibromas, medulloblastomas, ovarian fibromas, and mesenteric cysts can develop. While surgical excision is gold standard, photodynamic therapy, radiotherapy and smoothened (SMO) inhibitors (e.g., vismodegib) are potential options for advanced disease.

Squamous Cell Carcinoma

These lesions are extremely rare in children and predispositions to malignancies due to DNA repair disorders (xeroderma pigmentosum) or from severe photosensitivity related to medications (e.g., voriconazole) should be investigated. Mohs surgery is preferable for excision with clear margins.

LACRIMAL DRAINAGE SYSTEM DISORDERS

Epiphora is a common presentation in the early years of life. The causes are many and a thorough history and examination is important to guide interventions. The fully informed parents/guardians should understand that this condition can be complex and a step-wise approach to management based on the area of obstruction is necessary. There is still considerable variation in the management of pediatric epiphora. The skill set of pediatric ophthalmologists and those of lacrimal surgeons may differ. The child with epiphora is likely initially assessed and managed by the pediatric ophthalmologist, including primary lacrimal probing. Should this treatment fail, the lacrimal surgeon may provide further treatment including balloon dacryoplasty, intubation, and dacryocystorhinostomy.

Congenital nasolacrimal duct stenosis (CNLDS) or obstruction is usually a membranous block at the vale of Hasner. CNLDS is present in 70% at birth and is symptomatic in 6–20% of neonates and up to 6% of infants. Most open by 4–6 weeks of age and one third are bilateral. It is more common in premature births and Caucasians. Up to 90% resolve spontaneously by 6 months and 96% by 1 year. Nasolacrimal duct blockage can also be associated with clefting abnormalities involving the intranasal space. More proximal lacrimal drainage obstructions can occur as part of a syndrome [e.g., Lacrimo-auriculo-dento-digital (LADD)], an isolated finding (e.g., punctal agenesis or membranous obstruction), or acquired (e.g., following Stevens-Johnson syndrome, trauma, chemical burns). Duplications of the lacrimal drainage system may be asymptomatic or present with watering when associated with stenosis or obstruction locally or more distally (e.g., double punctum/canaliculus, congenital fistula).

Lacrimal Drainage System Anatomy

A comprehensive description of the lacrimal drainage system anatomy is beyond the scope of this chapter; however, some key points and normal measurements are as follows:

- The length of the canaliculi varies somewhat but measure approximately 2 mm in the vertical portion and 8 mm in the horizontal, joining to form a common canaliculus of 1-2 mm in most people.

- The sac measures 12-15 mm in length, with the "fundus" occupying 3-5 mm above the medical canthal tendon.
- The NLD measure 16-22 mm and is angulated slightly posteriorly, entering the nose 25-30 mm behind the lateral margin of the anterior nares, in the upper part of the inferior meatus.
- The inferior meatal space is often quite small in children, requiring inferior turbinate medialization or in fracture to be adequately visualized with the nasal endoscope.

Assessment

History

The onset of symptoms is important to differentiate congenital from acquired causes. There is often an assumption that children with watering have CNLDS, but a careful history including age of onset, progression, exacerbating and mitigating factors and associated symptoms such as discharge will narrow the differential diagnosis. Obstructive symptoms include persistent watering, discharge, recurrent low-grade conjunctivitis or even dacryocystitis. Reflex hypersecretion (e.g., secondary to blepharokeratoconjunctivitis, epiblepharon) is variable and may have concomitant ocular surface symptoms. A small dimple which may discharge tears suggests a congenital fistula. A swelling suggests a mucocele (which may be compressible) or amniotocele. A history of prior viral conjunctivitis and topical ocular medications may be associated with canalicular obstruction. Keratoconjunctivitis, herpes simplex blepharokeratoconjunctivitis, cicatrizing conjunctival disease, infiltrate, neoplastic disease, and trauma are all associated with pediatric acquired lacrimal drainage apparatus. Congenital glaucoma may also present as a watery eye.

Examination

In office tests used for adults may not be practical in the assessment of epiphora for most children. However, some clues can be obtained from a general inspection of the child for cyclid and lash position, facial asymmetry or suspected craniofacial abnormalities, the presence of a mucocele or any cause of reflex epiphora can be examined for. Swellings above the MCT may warrant radiological investigations for potential sinus mucoceles, encephaloceles, or malignancies.

Following instillation with fluorescein, an approximation of tear film height, asymmetry and any delay in fluorescein disappearance can be detected. The ocular surface can be difficult to assess in an uncooperative child, but a portable slit lamp can be very useful. Proceeding to further examination under anesthesia may be warranted - in which case initial intervention should also be consented for. Syringing and probing will often localize the blockage aided by nasal endoscopic confirmation of probe position in the inferior meatus. Dilated fundal exam, ocular motility, IOP, and cycloplegic refraction should be considered in addition to examination of the ocular adnexa in general. Functional epiphora is uncommon in children but may occur in facial palsy and Centurion syndrome.

LACRIMAL IMAGING

Dacryocystography (DCG) may aid localization of the site and degree of nasolacrimal obstruction. It may also identify fistulae, mucoceles, diverticula, neoplasms, and rarely dacryoliths. The lower punctum is cannulated and injected with radio-opaque contrast and sequential quasi dynamic images can be obtained. The test requires general anesthesia in most children. It provides anatomic information, with limited functional interpretation as the contrast injection pressure may artefactually open functionally significant stenoses. DCG is most commonly performed in the setting of failed primary probing.

Dacryoscintigraphy (DSG) gives a qualitative assessment of lacrimal outflow. The patient is positioned in front of a gamma camera so that both lateral canthus and the tip of the nose are in the camera's view. Ten microliters containing 100uCi of technetium-99 m pertechnetate is instilled to both eyes. Sequential analogue images are taken 4 times per minute for 20 minutes. Normative data suggest flow into the sac is seen within 1 minute and into the duct within 2-3 minutes. Maneuvers such as forceful blinking can simulate the lacrimal pump and help overcome any functional abnormality. The test can be carried out in children providing they are cooperative to stand in front of the camera or have their parents hold them (as young as 2 years). Sedation or anesthesia alters blinking and will decrease transit time affecting the usefulness of the test.

Other Imaging Modalities

CT alone or with DCG may be indicated in patients with trauma or craniofacial anomalies where nasoethmoid and skull base visualization are important. MRI may be useful in cases of midline or medial canthal masses (e.g., encephalocele).

Management

Meticulous preoperative examination of the lacrimal drainage system is critical in deciding on the appropriate intervention, and great care is required especially during closed interventions (probing, balloon dacryoplasty, intubation) to avoid damage to normal structures and creating 'false passages', particularly of the canaliculi.

Punctal/Canalicular Duplication

A failure of separation of the epithelial core from surface ectoderm leads to duplication of parts of the lacrimal drainage system such as puncta and canaliculi. If the opening is on the eyelid (double punctum), these are usually asymptomatic; medial canthal fistulae may be associated with discharge of tears or NLDS. Double puncta usually do not require specific treatment. Medial canthal fistulae may be excised; management of associated CNLDS seen in about a third is as per "standard" cases of CNLDS.

Punctal or Canalicular Blockage

A "cut down" membranectomy/punctoplasty with or without placement of a punctal plug or stent is highly effective. If there is true punctal agenesis which usually involves the canaliculus also, then a retrograde canaliculostomy and stenting is warranted, usually accompanied by DCR. A single punctum with NLDO usually requires a DCR. Complete punctal-canalicular agenesis may warrant a conjunctivo-DCR with insertion of a lacrimal bypass (e.g., Lester Jones) tube may be necessary at an appropriate time.

Dacryostenosis (CNLDS)

This may be partial or complete block of the nasolacrimal duct. Incomplete canalization of the duct at the valve of Hasner is the most common cause of dacryostenosis. This is usually managed without any surgical intervention since spontaneous resolution occurs in up to 95% at 1 year.

Crigler massage is the most important conservative intervention to initiate for CNLDS and is shown to be highly effective. It is important that a clear description be given to parents. The original description advised placing the adult's thumb over the sac in a way to shut off the return flow through the punctae. This is done by holding the thumb sidewise, with the thumbnail outward and forming an acute angle with the plane of the iris. The edge of the thumb is now pressed down over the puncta, compressing it against the rim of the orbit. With this point of pressure maintained the thumb is rotated, at the same time pressing downward abruptly over the sac. The fluid, now being compressed by the thumb, transmits the pressure to the walls of the sac which much give way at its weakest point, the nasolacrimal duct.

Topical antibiotic treatment may be used for recurrent conjunctivitis or low-grade dacryocystitis with chronic mucopurulent discharge.

Nasolacrimal duct probing with irrigation can be considered after 1 year of age. While some suggest probing at an earlier age, the general approach is to defer to allow for spontaneous resolution. Exceptions for earlier surgical intervention include dacrycystocoele, dacryocystitis/abscess or Down syndrome.

To perform NLD probing, a 0/00 Bowman probe to the lower punctum is usually adequate size although a 000/0000 probe may be required for the upper punctum. Cautious punctal dilatation may be required. Care is taken to maintain lateral traction on the eyelid when advancing the probe to avoid canalicular perforation and "false passage." Tactile feedback gives the experienced operator an idea of the nature and level of the stenosis or block. For example, a "pop" suggests a soft tissue block or stenosis has been overcome; a "tight, gritty" sensation indicates bony stenosis. Inferior turbinate in-fracture is often required for endoscopic visualization. Endoscopic photographs and recordings intraoperatively are useful for complete documentation, explanation to parents and planning for further invention if required. Endoscopy confirms patency with direct visualization of the probe endoscopically and Jones II testing with irrigation of fluorescein/saline.

The actual gestation age of premature babies should be considered. Success rates of primary probing have been described by age groups as follows: 77–89% success in children of age 13–18 months, 54–89% in children of age 18–24 months, 33–72% success in children of age 24–36 months. The success decreases with age, although this probably also reflects the persistence of watering in patients with significant pathology that is less likely to resolve spontaneously or with intervention. Factors predictive of probing failure include age greater than 36 months, bilateral involvement, failed conservative therapy, failed earlier probing, dilated lacrimal sac, and a tight bony canal.

Although some perform this as an in-office procedure, our preference is under general anesthesia for patient comfort and safety. Complications include damage to puncta, create a false passage or iatrogenic stenosis, and epistaxis (usually mild).

Failed Primary Probing

If initial probing fails, symptoms recur within 4–8 weeks and repeat probing may be an option although success rate in such instances is low. Repeat probing may be useful if the first procedure created a false passage. Considering the likelihood of success, proceeding to an alternative treatment may be better. If appropriate, a second closed intervention would be considered at the same time as repeat probing such as balloon dacryoplasty or lacrimal stenting ("intubation").

Balloon dacryoplasty involves intubation of the NLD with an inflatable catheter to dilate the NLD. Two such systems are in use – LacriCATH® [QuestMedical] and Ophtacath® [FCI Ophthalmic]. Success rate in those with initial failed probing is reported as 77–100%, with similar success rates to silicone stent intubation. Success rates may increase when combined with intubation. The cost of the device is a disadvantage; however, it avoids the risks of intubation and a second general anesthetic to remove a stent.

Silicone stent intubation can result in success rates of 69–100%; monocanalicular or bicanalicular systems have similar success rates. The stent is generally being left in place for a 2 3 months. The retention methods for stents can be intranasal (e.g., suture, silicone sleeve, hemostatic clip), punctal (self-retaining, e.g., Masterka), intranasal self-retaining by virtue of its wider diameter in the nose (e.g., Nunchaku, Bika) or intrasac (e.g., autostable bicanaliculus). Many different tubing options are available including pulled systems [Crawford, O'Donoghue, Ritleng system, Monoka] and pushed systems [monocanalicular (Masterka) and bicanalicular stents (Nunchaku)]. Self-retaining systems that do not require intranasal retrieval may be preferable because of easier removal in the clinic. Better outcomes have been achieved with monocanlicular stents and preferential use of the upper canaliculus protects the lower from any complications. Complications are rare but include premature loss or inadvertent removal, cheese wiring (bicanalicular stents), postoperative epistaxis, granuloma formation, infection, and stent dislocation leading to corneal irritation. In older children, the success rate is higher if stents are left in for longer than 3 months.

Dacryocystorhinostomy (DCR) may be indicated in cases of failed intubation or dilation or a major developmental anomaly (such as absent NLD). DCR has a comparable success rate to adults. Endoscopic surgery avoids scarring from external approach and has high reported success rates. Due to the compact anatomy in very young children, the assistance of rhinology colleagues may be useful if the endoscopic approach is undertaken; septoplasty if often required. Jones lacrimal bypass tubes can be used successfully in older children (around 10 years and older).

Congenital dacryocystocele/amniotocele This is a rare occurrence representing 0.1–0.3% of all congenital nasolacrimal duct obstructions. Around 90% are unilateral with is a female predisposition (64%) and mean age of presentation of 7 days. There is typically a tense blue medial canthal cystic swelling, watering, infection, and occasionally intranasal involvement which may present with nasal obstruction. The block occurs at the valves of Hasner and Rosenmuller where the canaliculi enter the sac. Amniotic fluid and mucus accumulate; this is initially sterile but may become infected. It should be differentiated from meningoencephalocele, dermoid cyst, and hemangioma. First line treatment is with massage, antibiotics and if no response then a probing procedure should be performed early. A nasal mucocele may need to be marsupialized or excised endoscopically.

Pediatric dacryocystitis requires prompt recognition, drainage and treatment with antibiotics to prevent preseptal and orbital cellulitis. Hospital admission for younger patients is more commonly advocated. Congenital NLDO is the main risk factor for developing dacryocystitis. When surgical intervention is indicated, microdebridement of an intranasal cyst and probing with possible stenting are helpful as initial procedures. Decompression of the infected sac externally will immediately relieve symptoms and also provide a specimen for microbiology culture to guide antibiotic use. Probing in the acute inflamed setting is at high risk of creating a false passage. Early, elective probing and endoscopic nasal exam aim to prevent recurrences which may require DCR surgery.

Acquired lacrimal obstruction and epiphora may be the presenting sign of conjunctival cicatricial disease and may occur following trauma and viral infections; dacryolithiasis is rare. The potential for intranasal and intrasac pathology should be investigated fully. Reversal of the inciting process may not be possible, and these cases are often treated as described above.

ORBIT

Obtaining a complete and thorough history is essential in patients presenting with suspected orbital disease. Basic information should include onset of symptoms, laterality, progression, discoloration, inflammatory features, changes with Valsalva maneuver (crying), systemic symptoms and old photos if available. Rapid progression of symptoms may suggest infection, malignancy, or hemorrhage, whereas slow progression is more typical of benign disease or structural malformations or cystic lesions.

Examination should include visual acuity, refraction, and full orthoptic and motility examination; forced duction test may occasionally be necessary. Optic nerve function and pupils should be assessed completely. Globe displacement can be measured using an exophthalmometer in older children. The globe should be palpated for pulsatility and the effect of the Valsalva maneuver assessed. The eyelid positions should be measured. Extra orbital examination may include trigeminal and facial nerve examination, lymph nodes, and general, craniofacial or ENT assessment as appropriate (e.g., stigmata of NF 1). Ophthalmic examination may identify Lisch nodules, a swollen optic nerve or choroidal folds.

Imaging is very important in investigating orbital disease. A plain film X-ray has limited use (e.g., metallic foreign body). Doppler ultrasound can have a role in assessing vascular lesions. The mainstay of imaging is CT and MRI. CT is quick and relatively cheap to perform and is ideal for assessing bony anatomy and some soft tissues, and is the modality of choice in the setting of trauma and suspected orbital infection. The potential risk of delayed malignancy due to radiation exposure should be considered. MRI takes longer to acquire, and poorly compliant patients may require sedation or general anesthesia to obtain a meaningful study, however, is the modality of choice in most pediatric orbital disease given the lack of radiation, and better characterization of soft tissues. Formal angiography may be required in arteriovenous malformations; CT or MRI with contrast angiography often provides adequate detail of vascular anatomy for most conditions.

Pediatric orbital surgery may often require opinion and input from a variety of specialists. Multidisciplinary approach will include the orbital surgeon, neurosurgery, otolaryngology, oral maxillofacial surgery, plastic surgery, and interventional radiology. The location of the lesion of interest and knowledge of the surrounding structures will minimize damage to the critical structures within the orbit - namely the globe and optic nerve. The endoscopic endonasal approach may be safest, particularly for the medial orbit. Computer-assisted surgery can be an extra tool in preoperative virtual surgical planning, intraoperative navigation, and postoperative assessment in complex cases.

This chapter will cover some of the more common and important pediatric orbital conditions excluding neoplasms, which are discussed in another chapter.

STRUCTURAL LESIONS AND CHORISTOMAS

Dermoid/Epidermoid

A choristoma describes a tumor-like mass of normal tissue in an abnormal location. Dermoid/epidermoid cysts develop from ectodermal rests that are pinched off at bony suture lines or within mesenchyme. The classic position is superolateral (zygomaticofrontal suture in 86%) or superonasal (frontonasal suture in 10%). Superficial dermoids (67%) will present early with mean age of presentation of 19 months. Deep dermoids (33%) occur within the orbit, intracranial or in the temporalis fossa and tend to have a larger diameter with mean age of presentation of 34 months. Conjunctival dermoids may be medial, lateral, or deep. Epidermoids contain squamous epithelium only whereas dermoids contain adnexal structures in addition. Generally, imaging is not required unless the location is deep or medial, or there are orbital signs as there may be components of the dermoid that cross over into other territories such as intracranial. Management of superficial lesions is complete excision prior to school age. More complex dermoids include the dumbbell shape with extension in the temporalis fossa and deep orbital or orbitocranial dermoids. If rupture occurs intraoperatively, persistent inflammation is uncommon (less than 4%) provided complete excision occurs; irrigation with saline or steroid may be required for complete removal of cyst contents. Spontaneous preoperative rupture of a dermoid cyst is more likely to lead to persistent inflammation. Older age and bony attachment are risk factors for cyst rupture.

DERMOLIPOMA

This choristoma represents skin sequestered within the conjunctiva most typically in the superolateral part of the orbit. The average age of presentation is 21.5 years but first symptoms are noted at 12.9 years. While some are asymptomatic, the most common symptoms are increasing size of a longstanding peribulbar lump, ocular irritation, episodic conjunctival injection, and mucoid discharge. Visible hairs may be present as well as widening of the lateral canthus and aberrant lacrimal gland ductules opening onto the skin and complex aberrant lateral canthal anatomy featuring external dermoid and internal dermolipoma. Excision of the visible portion with the integral subdermal fat lobule, in all cases the abnormal; nonwetting squamous epithelium is delineated and excised under microscopic control with the conjunctival defect directly or as a V-Y plasty for larger closure yields high success rate with low incidence of restrictive motility problems. It is important to avoid the lacrimal gland ductules, levator, and lateral rectus muscles nearby. The frequency of oculo-auriculo-vertebral spectrum in dermolipoma is estimated at 35% and features of hemifacial microsomia, Goldenhar's syndrome, and Duane's retraction syndrome should be specifically looked for.

DISORDERS OF THE EYE AS A WHOLE

Cryptophthalmos

This condition is also known as corneopalpebral adhesion and results from a failure of development of eyelid folds and manifests as a continuous fold of skin from the forehead to the cheek.

It can occur to varying degrees and is defined as such. Complete (total) is rare and there is no corneal or conjunctival epithelium. The eye underneath is abnormal with the globe being highly disorganized. The brow is absent or abnormal. Incomplete (partial) is more common whereby a skin fold, without tarsus, covers the medial palpebral aperture. The eye is also disorganized and there is significant adhesion between the lid and cornea and contracted socket. The abortive form (congenital symblepharon variant) describes when the lower lid is normal and there is absent or abnormal upper lid which is fused to a normal or phthisical eye.

Cryptophthalmos may occur sporadically or as part of an autosomal recessive syndrome, most commonly Fraser syndrome or Manitoba oculotrichoanal (MOTA) syndrome. Fraser syndrome (mutations in *FRAS1* and *FREM2*) is characterized by cryptophthalmos, syndactyly, genitourinary tract malformations, craniofacial dysmorphism, orofacial clefting, mental retardation and musculoskeletal anomalies. MOTA syndrome (mutation in *FREM1*) is characterized by cryptophthalmos, triangular growths of hair on the face, a bifid or broad nasal tip, and gastrointestinal anomalies. Underlying globe abnormalities may be difficult to assess clinically and ultrasound, electrophysiological testing and MRI may be necessary to ascertain the potential for vision prior to proceeding with any intervention. Reconstruction is multidisciplinary and challenging and involves restoring all functional components of the eyelids and corneal rehabilitation.

Microphthalmos, Anophthalmos, and Coloboma (MAC) Spectrum

The globe axial length at term is 17 mm reaching 22–25 mm in adulthood. Microphthalmos, anophthalmos and coloboma (MAC) refers to the range of failure of globe development. Microphthalmia refers to a globe with an axial length that is at least 2 standard deviations below the mean for age. Microphthalmos with cyst describes an associated cystic evagination of the abnormal eye. Anophthalmic refers to complete absence of the globe in the presence of ocular adnexa. Coloboma refers to the ocular malformations that result from failure of closure of the optic fissure. These will affect the orbital growth which is 90% formed at 5 years and 100% at 15 years and should be addressed to avoid underdevelopment of the orbit and ocular adnexa (micro-orbitism). A congenital cystic eye refers to the rare occurrence of an orbital cyst lined by neuroglia with no normal ocular structure present. Nanophthalmos refers to an axial length of <20 mm and usually has relatively thickened sclera. Cyclopia and synophthalmos are very rare and refer to complete or partial fusion of the eyes and is usually fatal.

They may be isolated or syndromic and may be unilateral or bilateral. Associated systemic anomalies occur in approximately 50% and often require extensive multidisciplinary team input. These can include hearing and intellectual disability and significant or even life-threatening cardiac, renal or CNS diseases. There may be an association with intrauterine infection, chromosomal anomaly or environmental insults. Genetics referral and counseling is important as there is a risk to future siblings. The unaffected eye in unilateral cases requires close monitoring with appropriate management of the visual potential in the affected side.

Examination under anesthesia may be required for a complete examination including the fellow eye which may have subtle anomalies. Parents and siblings should also be examined for any ocular anomalies. Electrodiagnostics can be useful to establish visual potential. MRI of the brain and orbits including midline structures is essential as well as a renal ultrasound, audiology, echocardiography, and other investigations to exclude coexisting abnormalities. A pediatric assessment including screening for intrauterine infections (rubella, VZV, HSV, CMV, *T. gondii*) and metabolic screen should be undertaken. Genetics referral should be sought. The most common mutations are *CHX10, GDF6, OTX2, RAX,* and *SOC2.* Antenatal ultrasound and amniocentesis can be offered to parents for future pregnancies.

Management aims to expand the socket by replacing or adding to achieve a normal volume equivalent. Ocular prostheses may be serially enlarged. A hemispheric hydrophilic expanding implant placed in the fornices or buried in the socket is useful for rapid expansion of the lids and orbit, although these are currently in short supply worldwide. An injectable implant can be inserted that will expand with serial saline injections. If a cyst or cystic eye is present, this should be left for volume purposes with excision occurring in later preschool years, unless growth is excessive. When the orbit is near maximal growth, solid implants (acrylic), or grafts (dermis-fat or micro-fat) can be employed. Dermis fat grafting has the potential benefit of continued growth and socket expansion with time and can also address the volume deficit of explanted exposed implants and contracted sockets, although excessive growth and cysts may require debulking.

There is currently no evidence for a superior type of socket expander. Soft tissue fillers are rarely used in children as they absorb more quickly in the orbit than in the dermis and are associated with orbital inflammation if repeat injections used. Socket contraction results in significant functional and psychological disability. The development of 3D printing and its potential use for socket reconstruction is topical and may add a further treatment option for such cases in the future.

Eyelid Colobomas

This is a full-thickness developmental defect of the eyelid margin. It is a form of facial cleft likely part of a spectrum of cryptophthalmos, coloboma, and symblepharon. They can be classified as isolated (complete, incomplete, symblepharon variant) or as part of a syndrome. Sporadic cases are more common and likely unilateral. Those associated with syndromes such as Fraser syndrome, Goldenhar syndrome, Treacher Collins syndrome, CHARGE syndrome, and MOTA syndrome may be bilateral. Therefore, a complete physical assessment by a pediatrician and referral to a geneticist for full evaluation should be undertaken. They occur most commonly in the upper eyelid and classically at the junction of the medial and middle thirds. Pseudocolobomas describe normal superficial ectoderm with the failure in development of underlying mesenchymal tissues such as orbicularis or bone. Lower eyelid colobomas are less common, and may occur as part of a clefting disorder.

The primary goal of management is corneal protection and amblyopia treatment. Repair of each coloboma requires a tailored approach depending on the size of the defect and the presence of corneal exposure. If there is no corneal exposure or obstruction of the visual axis then surgery can be delayed until 3 or 4 years of age. For small colobomas, direct appositional closure can be attempted. Larger colobomas require lateral canthotomy and cantholysis, or more complex repair with, generally, skin flaps and posterior lamellar grafts or flaps for large defects. These include Tenzel semicircular flap, or lid-sharing procedures such as Mustardé lid switch and Cutler-Beard reconstruction. Posterior lamellar reconstruction may require tarsal flap or graft or hard palate mucosa. Advancement of the levator aponeurosis in the upper eyelid will help avoid an upper eyelid ptosis.

NONINFECTIOUS ORBITAL INFLAMMATION

Orbital inflammatory disease is a nonspecific term encompassing a spectrum of pathologies and causes affecting many different structures within the orbit. Much of what we know is gained from adult inflammatory disease and is often associated with or may be a presenting sign of a systemic conditions. Our knowledge of the pathogenesis of autoimmune conditions has led to more tailored treatments with less steroid associated side effects. The spectrum of orbital inflammatory disease in children changes with age: infections are more common in the younger age group, with noninfectious disorders becoming more common in teenage years.

A complete systemic evaluation is warranted to identify specific causes of orbital inflammation. Baseline investigations include a full blood count with differential, C-reactive protein, erythrocyte sedimentation rate and urinalysis. Serum angiotensin converting enzyme (ACE) and chest CT may be positive in sarcoidosis (more common in teenage years, may be associated with ocular inflammation). T3, T4, thyroid-stimulating hormone levels, and thyroid antibodies can often confirm thyroid eye disease in the presence of subtle signs such as eyelid retraction, lid lag on downgaze and mild proptosis. Thyroid-associated orbitopathy rarely occurs before puberty, is more common in girls, and uncommonly presents with marked inflammatory features or motility problems; sight threatening disease is rare. Antineutrophil cytoplastic antibody (ANCA) if positive can be further tested for p-ANCA (MPO-ANCA) (e.g., microscopic polyangiitis) and c-ANCA (PR3-ANCA) in granulomatosis with polyangiitis (rare in children, typically bilateral, often associated with scleritis). Antinuclear antibody (ANA) positivity is indicative of systemic lupus erythematosus or Sjogren syndrome. Serum levels of IgG4 may be elevated in IgG4-related disease. The patient may have other systemic signs and symptoms to help guide diagnostic testing and offer alternative, less invasive sites of tissue biopsy if applicable, however there should be a low threshold for orbital biopsy to narrow the differential diagnoses.

Orbital inflammation may be categorized by the temporal nature of presentation (acute, subacute or chronic), by the histopathological diagnosis (granulomatous, sclerosing, or disease specific e.g., IgG4-related), or by the predominant tissue affected (e.g., dacryoadenitis, myositis). For example, classic orbital myositis is typically idiopathic, involving 1 or more extraocular muscles and responds rapidly and well to corticosteroids. Orbital myositis related to systemic autoimmune, inflammatory and infective conditions is more atypical with inflammatory bowel disease being the most associated.

Idiopathic orbital inflammation is a diagnosis of exclusion, and in the pediatric age group is mostly unilateral presenting with periorbital edema and ptosis and may be similar to orbital cellulitis. Constitutional signs are present in 40% and recurrent episodes occur in one-third and are more common in females. Classification can be on anatomical location (anterior, diffuse, apical) or tissue specific (e.g., myositis), with the anterior form being most common in childhood, often associated with uveitis. Orbital radiography may reveal dacryoadenitis in 40%, orbital mass in 40% and myositis in 33%. Ideally, a tissue biopsy should be obtained before initiation of steroid treatment to exclude serious systemic or malignant disease.

ORBITAL AND PERIOCULAR INFECTIONS

The prompt recognition and initiation of treatment is paramount in infections around the eye. These infections may have an obvious local cause such as trauma or may have spread from the nearby sinuses, dental area or hematogenous spread from distant location. The potential for orbital to spread to the intracranial space means these conditions can be both sight and life-threatening. Regular monitoring, recognition of clinical deterioration, and escalation of treatment are necessary as these conditions can have significant morbidity and mortality associated with them.

Preseptal Cellulitis

The orbital septum provides a biological barrier which aids to confine infection anteriorly. Predisposing factors to development of preseptal cellulitis include local trauma, upper respiratory tract infections, infected chalazion, conjunctivitis, dacryoadenitis, and dacryocystitis. There is usually a short history of eyelid edema and erythema. The child is usually well systemically. Preseptal cellulitis is mostly bacterial in origin and usually unilateral. The differential diagnosis includes allergic reactions, angioedema, renal disease, thyroid eye disease, and early orbital cellulitis.

Empirical antibiotic treatment is directed by local antimicrobial guidelines and can be later tailored to microbiological results from swabs (e.g., conjunctival, wound). Neonates and infants should be hospitalized and monitored. The immune system of children is less effective against encapsulated bacteria. Outpatient care may be appropriate after consultation with infectious disease and pediatric colleagues as needed. The most common pathogens are *Staphylococcus aureus* and *Streptococcus* species *Streptococcus pneumoniae* and *Haemophilus influenza* are decreasing in incidence due to vaccination. The possibility of an underlying foreign body or cutaneous abscess should be explored. There should be a low threshold for imaging in very young children.

Orbital Cellulitis

By definition, this denotes infection posterior to the orbital septum and constitutes an orbital emergency: high dose intravenous broad-spectrum antibiotics should be started promptly if there is any suspicion of orbital infection. Orbital cellulitis is more common in the pediatric age group. Clinical signs include proptosis, pain on eye movement, diplopia, restriction of eye movement, decreased vision (often from optic neuropathy), and chemosis. Ophthalmoplegia and proptosis are the most important distinguishing signs.

The degree of lid and conjunctival swelling may prohibit full ophthalmic examination, sometimes requiring examination under anesthesia. CT of the brain and orbits with bone and soft tissue windows should be acquired in all cases. Soft tissue infiltrative changes (e.g., "fat stranding") are typical; an intraorbital collection (abscess) may be present, typically subperiosteal. Sinusitis is the biggest risk factor for development of orbital cellulitis. Medially these are associated with ethmoidal sinusitis and superolaterally associated with frontal sinusitis. Drainage should be undertaken if these are large and impacting vision or if they are not responding to IV antibiotics, although smaller medial abscesses may resolve with antibiotics alone. Collaboration with ENT and sometimes neurosurgery is required, especially if surgical drainage of an abscess is planned as simultaneous sinus surgery may be appropriate. Sinus and abscess culture yield a high positivity rate to guide antibiotic treatment.

Streptococcus species are the most common pathogen in over half of cases with *anginosus* being the predominant species which is associated with requiring surgical drainage. Fungal cases are rare, but should be suspected in those with poor response to antibiotics and risk factors such as immunosuppression. The use of steroids concurrent with antibiotics may lead to reduced duration of hospital stay. There is significant variation in dose and delivery and a lack of randomized controlled trials for this intervention.

TRAUMA

Trauma is the most common cause for pediatric ophthalmic emergency visits. Of those admitted, globe rupture, eyelid laceration, and orbital fracture were the most common diagnosis with sporting activities being the biggest cause. The majority of lid and adnexal trauma is accidental and can be categorized as blunt or sharp trauma and burns.

A thorough history and exam is required to investigate beyond the obviously injured area. Adjacent structures and the potential for their involvement should always be considered – in particular the potential for acute or subacute intracranial injuries. The potential for systemic injuries should be assessed in the pediatric emergency room. One of the most important aims of the primary survey is to identify the possibility of a globe rupture. If suspected, further examination should be undertaken under anesthesia so as not to exacerbate the injury, seal the globe and minimize the risk of endophthalmitis and long-term vision loss.

Unfortunately, some injuries to children are nonaccidental. The clinician must always consider the potential for this possibility and the protection of the child is paramount in these situations. It is important to remain impartial in these situations and to involve child protection services from the outset should there be the slightest suspicion. A reliable history may not be possible from the patient. The injury may also have been unwitnessed.

Examination under anesthesia may be necessary for a complete evaluation including a dilated fundus exam. Documentation with photographs should form part of the clinical record. The potential for retained foreign bodies should be considered. There should be a low threshold for imaging in cases of periocular trauma. Radiopaque foreign bodies can be identified with CT imaging but organic foreign bodies can be more difficult to detect on CT and may require MRI. However, CT will often show soft tissue changes along the entry tract and the foreign body itself.

Lid Margin Lacerations

Trauma involving the lid margin requires specialist repair. Careful anatomic repair is necessary to avoid a notch, trichiasis and corneal abrasion. Particular attention should be paid to repair of the gray line and tarsus.

Nonmarginal Eyelid Lacerations

Careful exploration of eyelid lacerations is required to exclude a deeper foreign body and damage to deeper structures such as the globe, levator palpebrae superioris, and orbital vessels. Such wounds should be thoroughly washed out with saline +/- antiseptic. The presence of fat in a wound laceration points to a breach in the orbital septum and potential damage to deeper structures as outlined above. A secondary ptosis should be allowed at least 6 months to resolve spontaneously, however, this can be difficult in the amblyopic period, however this may be avoided with careful primary anatomic repair of any levator injury. The orbital septum should not be sutured as this can induce lid retraction and lagophthalmos.

Canalicular Trauma

Canalicular lacerations should be identified at the primary assessment and repaired promptly. The lower canaliculus is affected more commonly than the upper. The cut ends should be identified and the system intubated with silicone stent tubing (typically monocanlicular) and suturing end to end is the best chance to restore function. Identifying the distal end can be difficult as the trauma can extend medially up to the common canaliculus. Exploration of the area is best if bleeding can be avoided. Cautery to the area can confuse the anatomy further. A cotton bud soaked in local anesthetic can be used for gentle dissection. Syringing of the upper canaliculus with fluorescein can be useful to identify the lower end; careful use of a "pigtail" probe may be necessary. The operating microscope may be required in smaller children. Silicone stenting is removed at around 3 months to allow optimal time for an anastomosis of the canalicular epithelium to form.

Fractures

Trauma that causes ocular dysmotility should be considered as an orbital fracture until proven otherwise. Failure to recognize extraocular muscle compromise can lead to loss of binocular single vision and prolonged diplopia. Children less than 4 years old may manifest atypical orbital fractures from blunt trauma due to a high cranial-to-maxillofacial ratio in infants and the lack of pneumatized frontal sinuses. Orbital roof fractures are more likely before the age of 4 with the association of intracranial and orbital subperiosteal hemorrhages and CSF leak into the orbit.

The "white-eyed blowout fractures" refers to greenstick fractures of the orbital floor and medial wall in older children and teenagers. Imaging may reveal minimal or no bony displacement, however careful inspection will reveal soft tissue displacement with EOM abnormality varying from mild distortion to complete extraorbital entrapment. The "trapdoor" nature of the fracture means the bone snaps back into normal position after the injury with entrapment of orbital tissue - fat, connective tissue and extraocular muscle. The patient may exhibit vasovagal symptoms due to the oculocardiac reflex with bradycardia, hypotension, nausea, and vomiting. Failure to release the entrapped tissue can result in permanent ischemic muscle injury, therefore exploration, release of entrapped tissue, and fracture repair with a thin implant (e.g., porous polyethylene) should be undertaken as soon as possible - preferably within 24-48 hours. Interestingly, intraoperative time has also been shown to be associated with poorer outcomes suggesting manipulation of the entrapped muscle and complexity of the fracture are important considerations. Intraoperative forced-duction tests should be documented. Extraocular muscles may take weeks or months to recover function.

Traumatic Optic Neuropathy

Optic nerve injury may be subtle but clinical signs of optic nerve function deficit include decreased acuity or color vision, light brightness, red desaturation, relative afferent pupil defect, and visual field loss. This may be supported by imaging. The use of corticosteroids for traumatic optic neuropathy is controversial and inconclusive and may be contraindicated in cases of associated head injury. Surgical repair of optic canal fracture is also of unproven benefit and may carry significant risk.

SUGGESTED READING

1. Alaboudi A, Al-Shaikh O, Fatani D, Alsuhaibani AH. Acute dacryocystitis in pediatric patients and frequency of nasolacrimal duct patency. Orbit. 2021;40(1):18-23.
2. Alhammad F, Galindo-Ferreiro A, Khandekar R, Al-Sheikh O, Alzaher F, Schellini S. Management outcomes of canalicular laceration in children. Saudi J Ophthalmol. 2020;34(2):101-6.
3. Alsuhaibani AH, Bosley TM, Goldberg RA, Al-Faky YH. Entropion in children with isolated peripheral facial nerve paresis. Eye (Lond). 2012;26(8):109
4. Anderson RL, Nowinski TS. The five-flap technique for blepharophimosis. Arch Ophthalmol. 1989;107(3):448-52.
5. Baldwin HC, Manners RM. Congenital blepharoptosis: a literature review of the histology of levator palpebrae superioris muscle. Ophthalmic Plast Reconstr Surg. 2002;18(4):301-7.
6. Bansal O, Bothra N, Sharma A, Ali MJ. Congenital nasolacrimal duct obstruction update study (CUP study): paper II - profile and outcomes of complex CNLDO and masquerades. Int J Pediatr Otorhinolaryngol. 2020;139:110407.
7. Becker BB, Berry FD, Koller H. Balloon catheter dilatation for treatment of congenital nasolacrimal duct obstruction. Am J Ophthalmol. 1996;121(3):304-9.
8. Bladen JC, Malhotra R. Reporting outcomes of hyaluronic gel filler as a treatment for epiblepharon. Graefes Arch Clin Exp Ophthalmol. 2019;257(12):2769-73.
9. Campbell AA, Mahoney NR. Use of computer-assisted surgery in the orbit. Orbit. 2021:1-9..
10. Chan W, Wilcsek G, Ghabrial R, Goldberg RA, Dolman P, Selva D, et al. Pediatric endonasal dacryocystorhinostomy: a multicenter series of 116 cases. Orbit. 2017;36(5):311-6.
11. Chaung JQ, Sundar G, Ali MJ. Congenital lacrimal fistula: a major review. Orbit. 2016;35(4):212-20.
12. Chen L, Silverman N, Wu A, Shinder R. Intravenous steroids with antibiotics on admission for children with orbital cellulitis. Ophthalmic Plast Reconstr Surg. 2018;34(3):205-8.
13. Choi YM, Jang Y, Kim N, Choung HK, Khwarg SI. The effect of lacrimal drainage abnormality on the surgical outcomes of congenital lacrimal fistula and vice versa. Eur J Ophthalmol. 2021:1120672121994721.
14. Crawford JS. Repair of ptosis using frontalis muscle and fascia lata. Trans Am Acad Ophthalmol Otolaryngol. 1956;60(5):672-8.
15. Daniel P, Cogen M. Conservative management of congenital upper eyelid eversion. J AAPOS. 2020;24(1):46
16. Durrani J. Crigler massage for congenital blockade of nasolacrimal duct. J Coll Phys. Surg Pak. 2017;27(3):145-8.
17. Dutton J. Atlas of Clinical and Surgical Orbital Anatomy. Philadelphia: Elsevier/Saunders; 2011.
18. Ferraz LC, Meneghim RL, Galindo-Ferreiro A, Wanzeler AC, Saruwatari MM, Satto LH, et al. Outcomes of two surgical techniques for major trichiasis treatment. Orbit. 2018;37(1):36-40.
19. Gandhi NG, Rogers GM, Kardon RH, Allen RC. Periodic unilateral eyelid retraction in a pediatric patient. J Neuroophthalmol. 2011;31(4):350-2.
20. Golash V, Kaur H, Athwal S, Chakartash R, Laginaf M, Khandwala M. Management of congenital nasolacrimal duct obstruction: results of a national survey of paediatric and oculoplastic ophthalmologists. Eye (Lond). 2021;35(7):1930-6.
21. Goncalves R, Menezes C, Machado R, Ribeiro I, Lemos JA. Periorbital cellulitis in children: analysis of outcome of intravenous antibiotic therapy. Orbit. 2016;35(4):175-80.
22. Griepentrog GJ, Diehl N, Mohney BG. Amblyopia in childhood eyelid ptosis. Am J Ophthalmol. 2013;155(6):1125-8e1.
23. Gudeloglu E, Altan EV. Congenital total eversion of upper eyelids in a normal newborn. J Craniofac Surg. 2020;31(3):e239-e41.
24. Henriquez R, Noval S, Zafra B, De Manuel S, Contreras I. Ocular emergencies in children: demographics, origin, symptoms, and most frequent diagnoses. J Ophthalmol. 2020;2020:6820454.
25. Honavar SG, Prakash VE, Rao GN. Outcome of probing for congenital nasolacrimal duct obstruction in older children. Am J Ophthalmol. 2000;130(1):42-8.
26. Kaliki S, Jajapuram SD, Maniar A, Mishra DK. Ocular and periocular tumors in xeroderma pigmentosum: a study of 120 Asian Indian patients. Am J Ophthalmol. 2019;198:146-53.
27. Karademir S, Agaoglu G. Treatment of trichiasis by releasing follicle roots of eyelashes: a new technique. Plast Reconstr Surg Glob Open. 2021;9(3):e3480.
28. Kashkouli MB, Karimi N, Khademi B. Surgical management of congenital nasolacrimal duct obstruction; one procedure for all versus all procedures for one. Curr Opin Ophthalmol. 2019;30(5):364-71.
29. Katowitz JA, Welsh MG. Timing of initial probing and irrigation in congenital nasolacrimal duct obstruction. Ophthalmology. 1987;94(6):698-705.
30. Kaur S, Mahajan BB. Eyelash trichomegaly. Indian J Dermatol. 2015;60(4):378-80.
31. Kushner BJ. The management of nasolacrimal duct obstruction in children between 18 months and 4 years old. J AAPOS. 1998;2(1):57-60.

32. Lee MJ, Jin HC, Lee S, Choi YJ, Kim N, Choung HK, et al. Clinical characteristics and treatment outcomes of patients with congenital membranous punctal obstruction. J AAPOS. 2014;18(2):159-61.
33. Lemagne JM. Transposition of the levator muscle and its reinnervation. Eye (Lond). 1988;2 (Pt 2):189.
34. McElnea EM, Elder JE, Hardy TG, McNab AA. Acquired lacrimal drainage apparatus obstruction in children. J AAPOS. 2019;23(4):217e1-e5.
35. McMullan TF, Robinson DO, Tyers AG. Towards an understanding of congenital ptosis. Orbit. 2006;25(3):179-84.
36. McMullan TF, Tyers AG. X linked dominant congenital isolated bilateral ptosis: the definition and characterisation of a new condition. Br J Ophthalmol. 2001;85(1):70-72.
37. Mohney BG, Sathiamoorthi S, Frank RD. Spontaneous resolution rates in congenital nasolacrimal duct obstruction managed with massage or topical antibiotics compared with observation alone. Br J Ophthalmol. 2021.
38. Mombaerts I, Witters E. Jones lacrimal bypass tubes in children and adults. Br J Ophthalmol. 2019;103(9):1248-52.
39. Napier ML, Armstrong DJ, McLoone SF, McLoone EM. Congenital nasolacrimal duct obstruction: comparison of two different treatment algorithms. J Pediatr Ophthalmol Strabismus. 2016;53(5):285-91.
40. Olayanju JA, Griepentrog GJ, Mohney BG. Incidence and clinical characteristics of pediatric eyelid retraction. J AAPOS. 2019;23(4):213e1-e4.
41. Pediatric Eye Disease Investigator G, Repka MX, Chandler DL, Bremer DL, Collins ML, Lee DH. Repeat probing for treatment of persistent nasolacrimal duct obstruction. J AAPOS. 2009;13(3):306-7.
42. Pediatric Eye Disease Investigator G, Repka MX, Melia BM, Beck RW, Atkinson CS, Chandler DL, et al. Primary treatment of nasolacrimal duct obstruction with nasolacrimal duct intubation in children younger than 4 years of age. J AAPOS. 2008;12(5):445-50.
43. Prat D, Magoon K, Karen R, Katowitz JA, Katowitz WR. Management of pediatric acute dacryocystitis. Ophthalmic Plast Reconstr Surg. 2021.
44. Quaranta-Leoni FM, Fiorino MG, Quaranta-Leoni F, Di Marino M. Anophthalmic socket syndrome: prevalence, impact and management strategies. Clin Ophthalmol. 2021;15:3267-81.
45. Rosner M, Zloto O. Periocular molluscum contagiosum: six different clinical presentations. Acta Ophthalmol. 2018;96(5):e600-e5.
46. Sa HS, Lee JH, Woo KI, Kim YD. A new method of medial epicanthoplasty for patients with blepharophimosis-ptosis-epicanthus inversus syndrome. Ophthalmology. 2012;119(11):2402-7.
47. Seidman DJ, Nelson LB, Calhoun JH, Spaeth GL, Harley RD. Signs and symptoms in the presentation of primary infantile glaucoma. Pediatrics. 1986;77(3):399-404.
48. Sheth T, Attzs M, Tambe K. A new perspective in oculoplastic surgical management of symptomatic distichiasis in lymphedema-distichiasis syndrome. Orbit. 2019;38(5):424-7.
49. Siah WF, Al-Muhaylib AA, Rajak S, Ziahosseini K, Selva D, Malhotra R, et al. Clinical outcomes of ruptured periorbital and orbital dermoid cysts. Ophthalmic Plast Reconstr Surg. 2017;33(4):264-7.
50. Singh S, Ali MJ. Congenital dacryocystocele: a major review. Ophthalmic Plast Reconstr Surg. 2019;35(4):309-17.

12

CHAPTER

Neuro-ophthalmological Disorders in Children

Sangeeta Khanna, Joseph Conway, Swati Phuljhele

INTRODUCTION

Pediatric neuro-ophthalmology constitutes diagnoses, which are seen in adult patients, however, it is essential to understand it is not same as adult neuro-ophthalmology since the clinical presentation, course of the disease, prognosis, and treatment are different in both groups. This chapter aims to provide the distinct features of the common neuro-ophthalmological diseases in the pediatric age group. Details about a comprehensive neuro-ophthalmic examination including field changes secondary to intracranial lesions can be referenced from a standard textbook of neuro-ophthalmology.

CONGENITAL OPTIC DISK ANOMALIES

Congenital optic disk anomalies are often associated with subnormal vision in infancy. Associated central nervous system anomalies are common in these patients. It is important to be aware of these conditions since they can be easily misjudged as disk edema and may lead to patients being subjected to unnecessary investigations.

Optic Disk Drusen

Optic disk drusen (ODD) is the most common differential diagnosis of disk edema. These are benign deposits in the optic nerve head secondary to axoplasmic stasis. Unlike adults, ODD, in children, is most commonly buried in the substance of the optic nerve head. Most of the cases are asymptomatic and are generally diagnosed on incidental examination. The drusen becomes more superficial with the age and hence generally appears in adults. The most common symptoms are transient visual obscuration and visual field defect. The nasal steps, arcuate defects, enlarged blind spots, and generalized constriction are the commonly seen visual field defects.

Investigations such as ultrasonic B scan, fundus fluorescein angiography, and optical coherence tomography (OCT) may help in early detection of buried disk drusen **(Figs. 1A to D)**.

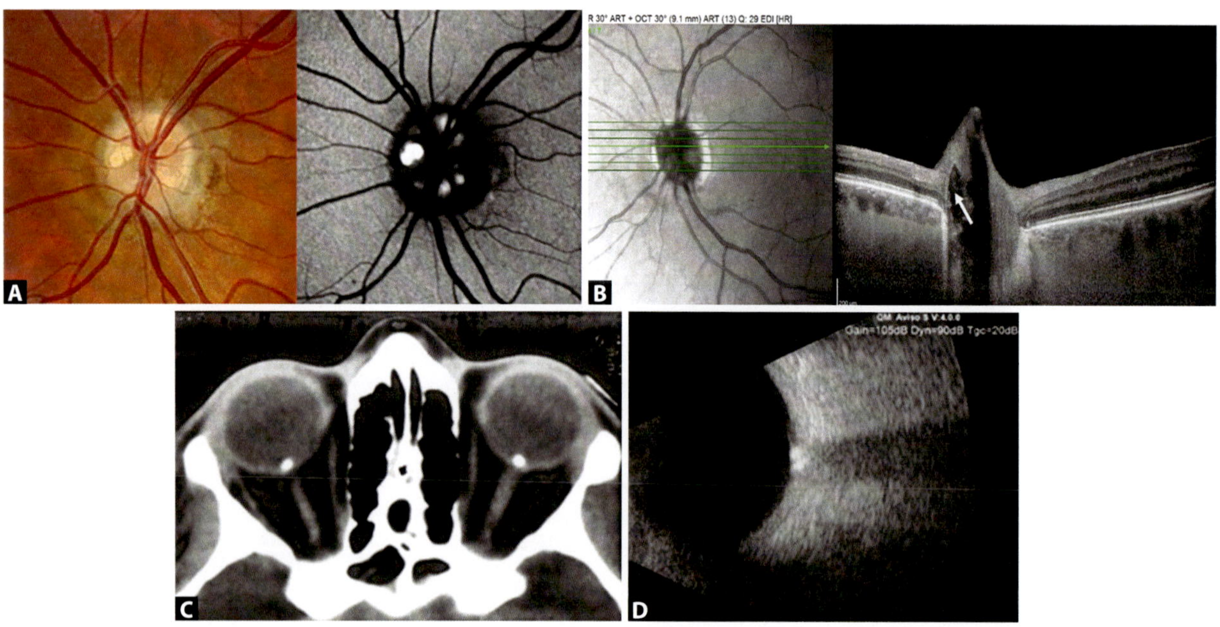

Figs. 1A to D: (A) Optic disk drusen with autofluorescence; (B) Optical coherence tomography (OCT) of optic disk with drusen: A hyporeflective ovid lesion with hyper-reflective margins; (C) Optic disk drusen on computed tomography (CT); (D) Optic disk drusen on ultrasonography (USG). (*Courtesy:* University of Michigan, Kellogg Eye Center)

Optic Nerve Hypoplasia

Optic nerve hypoplasia (ONH) is the most common congenital optic disk anomaly. It is associated with numerous gene mutations (e.g., *HESX1, PAX6, SOX2, NR2F1, OTX2, VAX1, ATOH7,* and *KANSL1*). There are several epigenetic factors that increase the risk of developing ONH as well: Drug and alcohol abuse being the primary one. ONH is often associated with hypothalamic and pituitary dysfunction. Therefore, patients commonly present with various hormonal defects such as growth hormone deficiency (most commonly), elevated prolactin levels, hypothyroidism, adrenocorticotropic hormone (ACTH) deficiency, elevated cortisol levels, and diabetes insipidus. ONH may be associated in some cases with a congenital absence of the septum pellucidum and agenesis of the corpus callosum, known as septo-optic dysplasia (De Morsier syndrome). Hypopituitarism is present in 62–80% of these septo-optic dysplasia patients.

The typical patient with ONH will present with visual acuity of 20/200 or worse. On examination, a relative afferent pupillary defect can be seen in unilateral cases. Fundus examination reveals a small and pale/gray disk and the classic "double-ring sign" can be seen as a yellow ring around the disk bordered by a ring of either hyperpigmentation or hypopigmentation. The major retinal vessels are often tortuous **(Fig. 2)**.

Investigations

Magnetic resonance imaging (MRI) should be obtained to assess for associated cranial nerve abnormalities such as abnormal septum pellucidum and/or corpus callosum anatomy; additionally, it may show reduced dimensions of the optic nerve and the optic chiasm, associated with ONH. OCT reveals thinning of the retinal nerve fiber layer (RNFL) and ganglion cell layer (GCL). Investigations in form of visual field may reveal nasal or inferior field defects. Serologic studies to assess endocrine function should be obtained to assess for hypothalamic and/or pituitary dysfunction.

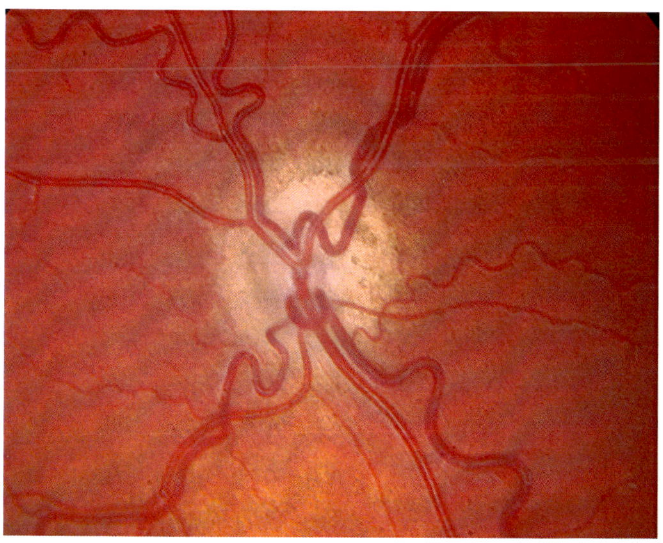

Fig. 2: Optic disk hypoplasia. Note the pigmentary changes around the disk. Also note the anomalous tortuosity of the retinal blood vessels.

(*Courtesy:* University of Michigan, Kellogg Eye Center)

Management

Treating associated amblyopia and correcting for refractive errors is the most important intervention. Long-term follow-up with a multidisciplinary team is recommended to follow the patient's visual development and systemic status.

Congenital Titled Disk Syndrome

This is a sporadic noninherited bilateral condition in which the superotemporal pole is elevated and the inferonasal pole is posteriorly displaced and the long axis is oblique. Patients with tilted disks may present with high myopia, astigmatism, bitemporal superior visual field defects, and partial achromatopsia. Retinal examination may show inferior or inferonasal crescent, situs inversus of the retinal vessels, and ectasia of the nasal fundus or posterior staphyloma. The bitemporal hemianopias are typically superior and incomplete representing a refractive scotoma secondary to ectasia of the inferonasal retina.

EXCAVATED DISKS

Morning glory anomaly, optic disk coloboma, pits, and peripapillary staphyloma are examples of excavated optic disk anomalies.

Morning Glory Anomaly

The morning glory disk anomaly is a funnel-shaped excavation of the optic disk. Most cases of morning glory defects are sporadic and unilateral. With rare exceptions, morning glory disk anomalies are not part of multisystem genetic disorder but do have association with basal encephalocele and ipsilateral carotid artery anomalies.

The morning glory defect is named for its characteristic appearance on examination of the fundus; the optic nerve appears enlarged and funnel-shaped, and the vessels originating from the disk spread in a radial pattern making it appear like the morning glory flower; the central retinal vasculature is ophthalmoscopically absent in the morning glory disk anomaly. The disk is excavated and filled with glial tissue, which gives the disk a white coloration. There is often abnormal pigmentation surrounding the disk. There tends to be increased vascularity, and the vessels run in a straight course from the disk margin **(Fig. 3)**. An afferent pupillary defect is often associated since most cases are unilateral. Patients can present with visual acuity ranging from mildly subnormal to very poor.

Optic Disk Coloboma and Pits

Optic disk colobomas may arise as a sporadic defect, as the result of an autosomal dominant genetic mutation

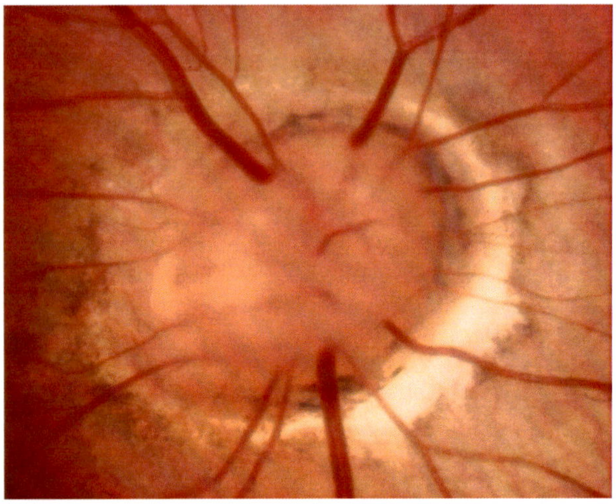

Fig. 3: Morning glory syndrome: Note the center of the disk filled with glial changes, pigmentary changes around the disk and abnormal vasculature radiating from the disk.
(*Courtesy:* University of Michigan, Kellogg Eye Center)

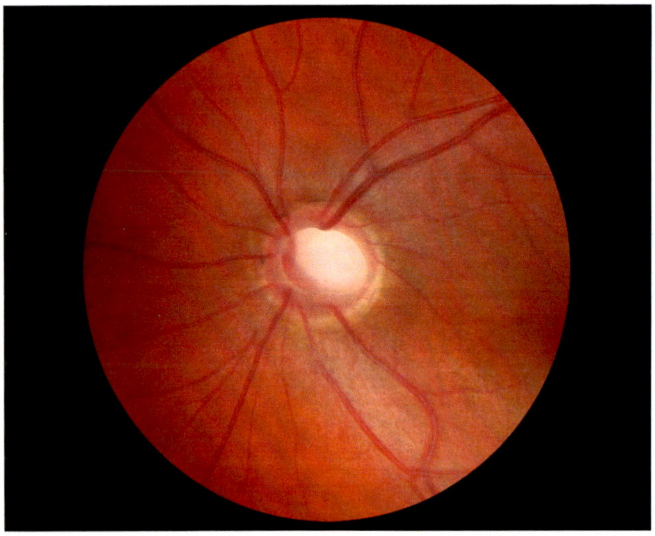

Fig. 4: Optic disk coloboma: Note the excavation in the center of the disk.
(*Courtesy:* University of Michigan, Kellogg Eye Center)

(e.g., PAX6), in association with a systemic syndrome (e.g., CHARGE syndrome), or intrauterine insults (e.g., thalidomide). Optic disk colobomas are thought to result from incomplete closure of the posterior (proximal) portion of the fetal fissure, whereas optic pits are associated with incomplete closure of the superior aspect. These may be unilateral or bilateral. Fundus examination for patients with coloboma of the optic nerve reveals bowl-shaped excavation of the inferior aspect of the disk **(Fig. 4)**.

Visual acuity is variably affected depending on how severely the fovea is involved. Microphthalmia may be associated. Coloboma of the optic nerve also commonly presents as one of many defects that result from an underlying syndrome (e.g., CHARGE syndrome, Walker-Warburg syndrome, Aicardi syndrome, Goldenhar syndrome, and renal coloboma syndrome).

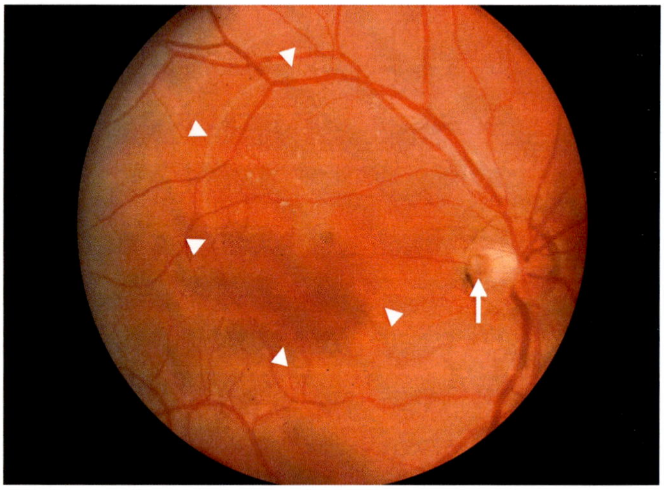

Fig. 5: Optic disk pit with serous maculopathy*:* Note a well defined small excavation in the inferotemporal of the disk. Also note the sub-macular fluid, often the most common complication of the lesion.
(*Courtesy:* University of Michigan, Kellogg Eye Center)

Optic pits seem to be primarily sporadic but some reports suggest they may result from autosomal dominant inheritance. The pits are commonly observed as a round excavation of the disk with abnormal coloration in the inferotemporal aspect of the optic disk. Optic pits often do not cause any symptoms, and therefore are discovered incidentally on routine eye examinations. When they do cause symptoms, it is due to leakage of fluid into subretinal space **(Fig. 5)** and patients may complain of metamorphopsia, impaired acuity, or blind spots.

Investigations

Basic workup for any type of disk excavation should include a comprehensive examination with visual fields. Visual field defects should be typically nonprogressive. Monitor intraocular pressure to rule out glaucoma-associated cupping. Every patient should receive neuroimaging as well to rule out associated brain anomalies.

Management

Treatment for most forms of disk excavation is supportive. Ophthalmologists should attempt to optimize the patient's visual acuity and prevent amblyopia with a trial of occlusion in young patients. Low vision aids may also be helpful. Patients with any form of optic disk excavation may be at increased risk of retinal detachment, therefore regular fundoscopic examinations should be performed to assess for this. If there is central nervous system (CNS) involvement, the patient should be referred to the appropriate specialist team.

PEDIATRIC OPTIC NEURITIS

Pediatric optic neuritis has differences from adult optic neuritis in the clinical presentation, etiology, and outcome and is considered as a distinct entity though with some overlap. The fundamental differences that have been demonstrated in case series and most recently in a prospective pediatric optic neuritis outcomes trial are that children more often present with optic disk edema (75 vs. 35% in adults) and 50% or more children with optic neuritis at presentation can have associated neurological syndrome.

Clinical Features

Optic neuritis typically presents with subacute decline in vision with pain on eye movements. Other complaints may include defective color vision or visual field defect. Young children may not report or notice unilateral vision loss, but bilateral vision loss is picked up sooner by change in behavior. A history of flu-like illness or vaccination preceding optic neuritis by days to weeks may be elicited. It may be unilateral or bilateral, bilateral involvement is more common in younger children (72% <10 years) than in older children (30%). Children often present with severe vision loss with 60% of children presenting with VA worse than 20/200 compared to adults (30%). Optic nerve head edema **(Figs. 6A and B)** is more common in children than adults and is seen in 40–70% of cases. The visual prognosis of optic neuritis in children is generally good and >90% recover to better than 20/40 at 1 year.

The etiology of optic neuritis in children is same as that in adults but more have associated neurological syndromes such as acute disseminated encephalomyelitis (ADEM), myelin oligodendrocyte (MOG), neuromyelitis optica spectrum disorder (NMOSD) multiple sclerosis (MS). A viral illness may present as ADEM, which is a multifocal acute demyelinating disease characterized by encephalopathy, fever, and meningeal signs. Optic neuritis may present at the time of ADEM or following it.

The risk of development of MS after optic neuritis has not been well documented in the pediatric population. Optic neuritis is the presenting feature of MS in 10–20% of pediatric MS cases. Age at presentation and abnormalities on brain MRI have been found to be the strongest predictors of the progression to MS. Around 13–36% of pediatric patients presenting with optic neuritis may develop MS depending on the age at presentation and the presence of white matter lesions on the baseline brain MRI.

Neuromyelitis optica (NMO) (also called Devic's disease) is traditionally characterized by optic neuritis and transverse myelitis with characteristic MRI findings of longitudinally extensive optic nerve and transverse myelitis lesions. The antibodies against aquaporin 4 receptor cause astrocytopathy that leads to the demyelination. Optic neuritis associated with NMO in children, as in adults, is often bilateral and visual loss is profound and is frequently associated with poorer visual outcomes.

Myelin oligodendrocyte is an NMOSD where antibodies are directed against the glycoprotein located on oligodendrocyte and myelin sheath. MOG-associated optic neuritis is more common in children than adults with neuroimmunological syndromes. It can present as recurrent isolated optic neuritis, ADEM with/without optic neuritis, NMOSD, or isolated myelitis.

Investigations

Workup of pediatric optic neuritis should be guided by thorough review of systems, but typically involves MRI of the brain and orbit with and without contrast.

Magnetic resonance imaging typically reveals contrast enhancement of the optic nerve, best seen with fat-suppressed T1 coronal images and/or bright signal on T2-weighted images best seen on fat suppressed fluid-attenuated inversion recovery (FLAIR) or STIR (short tau inversion recovery) sequences. Enhancement can be seen in 70–90% of patients if scanned within 20 days of visual loss. Additionally, the segment of optic nerve affected may appear swollen.

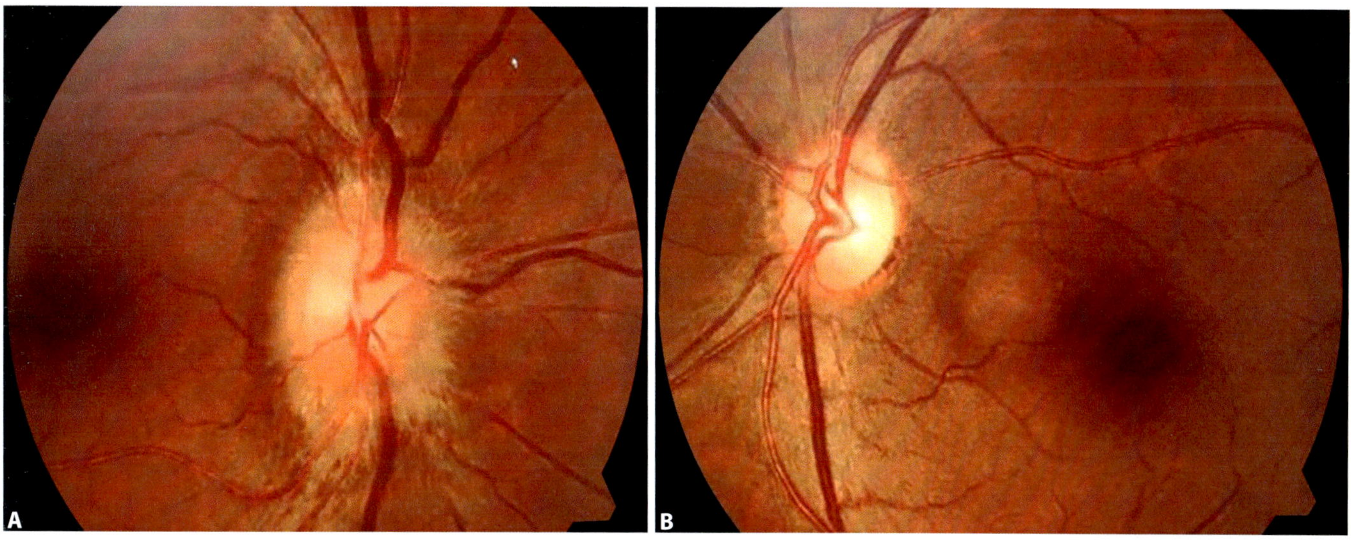

Figs. 6A and B: Bilateral disk edema in optic neuritis.

(*Courtesy:* Dr Rajendra Prasad Centre for Ophthalmic Sciences, All India Institute of Medical Sciences, New Delhi)

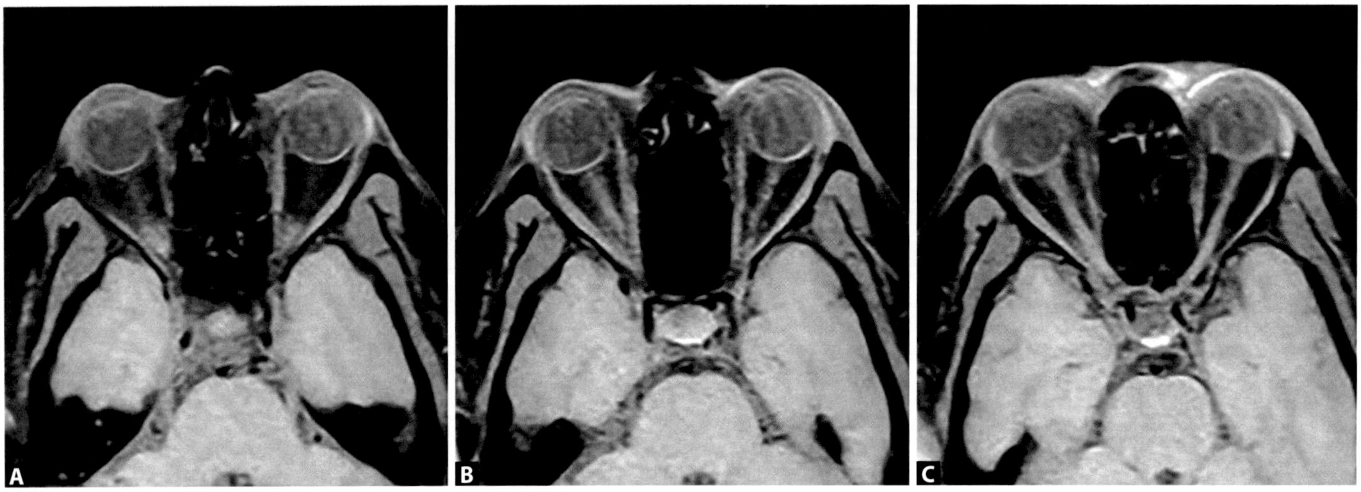

Figs. 7A to C: Magnetic resonance imaging (MRI) of the brain and orbits suggestive of bilateral optic neuritis. Right optic nerve thickened and edematous with bilateral enhancement of the optic nerves and fat stranding suggestive of bilateral optic neuritis.
(*Courtesy:* Dr Rajendra Prasad Centre for Ophthalmic Sciences, All India Institute of Medical Sciences, New Delhi)

The involvement of optic nerve in MS is unilateral, focal, and generally limited to retrobulbar part of the nerve, while in NMO and MOG associated optic neuritis, it is bilateral, longitudinally extensive (>50% of the nerve) with extension up to the intracranial compartment **(Figs. 7A to C)**.

Magnetic resonance imaging of the spine is indicated in cases where the clinical suspicion of NMOSD/MOG is high. Serum testing for anti-AQP4-IgG and anti-MOG IgG levels should be done in all cases. The live cell-based essays are more sensitive than ELISA (enzyme-linked immunoassay)-based tests or fixed cell-based tests. There is no role of adding cerebrospinal fluid (CSF) antibody testing since these antibodies are more sensitive when tested in serum. CSF analysis for pressure, protein, glucose, cells, and cultures may be required more frequently in children to rule out infective etiologies but is done based upon discretion of the treating physician. CSF analysis for oligoclonal bands, immunoglobulin G (IgG) index may be useful for supporting a diagnosis of MS.

Management

Due to the lack of clinical trials in children, treatment is extrapolated from the experience with adult optic neuritis. Recommendations are to treat an acute episode of optic neuritis with 3–5-day course of intravenous (IV) methylprednisolone (20–30 mg/kg/day; maximum dose of 1 g/day), followed by oral prednisone 1 mg/kg/day tapered over approximately 2–4 weeks. If the child does not show adequate response to IV methylprednisolone, intravenous immunoglobulin G (IVIg), and plasma exchange is recommended. At present, long treatment options for CNS demyelination are limited in children. The long-term implications of immunomodulatory drugs, which are recommended in adults, on the developing immune system of a child are still unknown though interferon-beta and glatiramer acetate have been used in pediatric MS.

In cases of NMOSD, early initiation of plasma exchange five to seven cycles is associated with better clinical outcome. Additional treatment may be indicated based upon the associated neuroinflammatory syndrome. For relapsing MOG disease, immune-modulation with agents such as rituximab or IVIg are used to reduce relapses. There are reports of use of immunosuppressive drugs such as azathioprine, cyclophosphamide, and mycophenolate mofetil to prevent relapses, though the effectiveness of these medications is not proven.

Even if it is an isolated optic neuritis at presentation, children will need follow-up for monitoring for multiple sclerosis if they have abnormal brain MRI. MS risk with optic neuritis increases with age. It has been reported that for every 1-year increase in age, there is a 32% increased risk of MS; and presence of lesion on brain MRI increased the odds ratio of an eventual diagnosis of MS to 28.0. However, the risk of MS also depends upon racial and geographic features.

PAPILLEDEMA

Papilledema is the term used for disk swelling due to raised intracranial pressure (ICP) **(Figs. 8A and B)**. Bilateral disk swelling without visual loss in a child with headaches, nausea, and vomiting is the typical presentation.

In children, raised ICP could be congenital due to congenital malformations. In very young children, this leads to hydrocephalus than papilledema. Infections still remain the common cause of raised ICP in this part of the world. Tuberculosis is one of the most common causes of meningitis in India; however, bacterial, viral, and fungal infections are also often diagnosed. It is important to rule out intracranial mass as a cause of raised ICP. Idiopathic intracranial hypertension (IIH) is an etiology that has shown increasing trend in children with rise in obesity but is a diagnosis of exclusion.

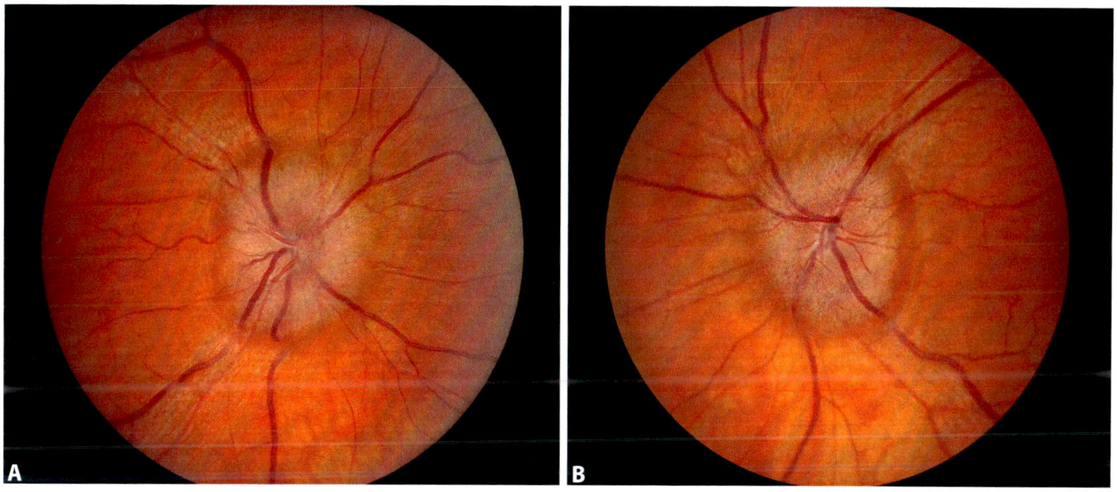

Figs. 8A and B: Established papilledema.
(*Courtesy:* University of Michigan, Kellogg Eye Center)

Pediatric Idiopathic Intracranial Hypertension

Incidence is about ~1/100,000, unlike in adults, prepubertal children who develop IIH may not be obese, and males are as likely to develop IIH as females in prepubertal presentation of IIH. (Prepubertal Obesity Rate: 43 vs. 90% adults); (female sex distribution in prepubertal: 50% 12–14: 88%).

Unlike adults, there is an underlying identifiable cause of IIH found in 55–73% of pediatric cases. The secondary causes of pediatric IIH include (1) endocrine disorders: Addison disease, hypoparathyroidism, and other endocrine disorders; (2) systemic disorders: Sleep apnea, hypercapnia (Pickwickian syndrome) anemia, renal failure, Turner syndrome, Down syndrome; (3) cerebral vascular disorder: Cerebral venous sinus thrombosis, bilateral jugular vein thrombosis or surgical ligation, middle ear or mastoid infection, increased right heart pressure, superior vena cava syndrome, arteriovenous fistulas; (4) decreased cerebrospinal fluid absorption from previous intracranial infection or subarachnoid hemorrhage; (5) medication related: Tetracycline antibiotics vitamin A, isotretinoin, growth hormone steroid use or withdrawal, lithium, and thyroid replacement therapy.

Children may present with nausea, vomiting, neck pain, in addition to the typical symptoms of headache (14% without headache), transient visual obscurations, pulsatile tinnitus, and diplopia. However, often they may present with vague symptoms such as irritability or change in behavior. Examination may reveal the presence of sixth nerve palsy.

In addition to careful history of medical disorders and medication and supplements, urgent neuroimaging-MRI being the preferred modality should be performed to exclude intracranial mass and inflammation. MRI signs of IIH include: Flattening of globe, enlarged optic nerve sheath, partially empty sella, narrowing of distal transverse sinus, and Chiari type 1. CSF opening pressure should be assessed in lateral decubitus position with legs extended. CSF analysis should be done to rule out infections and malignancy.

Diagnosis of IIH is based on modified Dandy criteria and these have been further elucidated by Rangwala and Liu for pediatric IIH as:

- Normal mental status
- Signs and symptoms of generalized intracranial hypertension or papilledema
- Alert and oriented patient
- No focal deficits (except sixth nerve palsy)
- If no other identifiable etiology found
- Improve with reduction in CSF pressure or with resolution of other signs and symptoms of ICH—sixth nerve palsy and seventh nerve palsy
- Normal neuroimaging (normal MRI, MR venogram—narrowing of transverse sinus allowed)
- Documented elevated ICP (lateral decubitus position), neonates: >7.8 cmH_2O, age 1–18 years: >28 cmH_2O; normal CSF composition.

Management

Acetazolamide is the first line of treatment to decrease ICP; 15–25 mg/kg/day in two to three divided doses is generally used. The alternative medications such as topiramate and furosemide can be considered where acetazolamide is not well tolerated. Severe vision loss due to IIH requires urgent optic nerve sheath fenestration and/or lumbar drain placement or permanent CSF diversion procedure such as ventriculoperitoneal shunt. Clinical evidence of the superiority of one approach over another in rescuing vision is not available.

HEREDITARY OPTIC NEUROPATHIES

Leber's Hereditary Optic Neuropathy

Leber's hereditary optic neuropathy (LHON) is the most common primary mitochondrial DNA disorder and the second most common inherited optic neuropathy. Most of cases are caused by three point mutations of mitochondrial DNA (11778G>A, 3460G>A, and 14484T>C), of which the m.11778G4A mutation is the most common (70–80%). These mutations result in impaired production of adenosine triphosphate (ATP) and increased oxidative stress on retinal ganglion cells (RGCs) via formation of reactive oxygen species. The presence of a pathogenic mtDNA LHON-causing mutation is necessary but not sufficient for the development of LHON since not all people with these pathogenic mutations, manifest disease. Triggering factors that contribute include toxins such as alcohol, tobacco, viral infections, and toxin exposure.

The classic presentation is unilateral subacute loss of vision, which often progresses to both eyes in the subacute period and may lead to permanent vision loss. It typically manifests in males in the second and third decade of life, but the age of onset may vary widely and female may also be affected. During and just prior to the acute stages, one may see a characteristic triad of findings of: Circumpapillary telangiectasias of the retinal arterioles, pseudoedema of the disk and surrounding nerve fiber layer and absence of leakage on fluorescein angiography. Eventually, the optic nerve becomes atrophic.

Leber's optic neuropathy still remains the diagnosis of exclusion. MRI of the brain and orbits is often obtained since presentation is often confused with optic neuritis. There is typically no enhancement of the optic nerves but signal change of the optic nerves and chiasm has been reported. Genetic testing is performed via targeted mutation analysis. The three most common mutations are 11778G>A, 3460G>A, and 14484T>C. However, in a certain proportion, patient's mitochondrial mutations responsible for LHON will be missed by screening of the three most common disease point mutations.

In 2017, an international consensus statement was released regarding the clinical and therapeutic management of LHON which described three stages of LHON based on the onset of vision loss: Subacute (<6 months), dynamic (6–12 months), and chronic (>12 months). It is important to identify LHON in the acute phase as early treatment may rescue suppressed RGCs from apoptosis. The best treatment for LHON at this time is idebenone—an analog of the mitochondrial electron transport protein, ubiquinone. Idebenone was shown to be efficacious in treating visual acuity loss secondary to LHON by controlled clinical trial and a large retrospective analysis published in 2011. It is currently recommended that treatment with high dose (300 mg three times daily) idebenone be started soon after diagnosis and continued indefinitely if well tolerated. A number of clinical trials are currently investigating and showing promise in the efficacy of viral-based gene therapy for patients harboring the m.11778G>A mtDNA mutation. Prognosis varies with mutation type, with the m.14484T>C mutation having the highest chance of improvement.

Autosomal Dominant Optic Atrophy

Dominant optic atrophy of Kjer is the most common hereditary optic atrophy; it has near complete penetrance and autosomal dominant pattern of inheritance but variable phenotype. Autosomal dominant optic atrophy (ADOA) is commonly associated with mutations in the nuclear OPA1 gene located on chromosome 3q28-q29. It manifests as insidious onset, binocularly symmetrical, mild-to-moderate decrease in vision within the first decade of life and affected children are often unaware of subnormal vision. It may be detected on routine screening as temporal pallor of both optic nerves and subnormal vision **(Figs. 9A and B)**.

The other causes of hereditary optic atrophy include; congenital recessive optic atrophy, an autosomal recessive

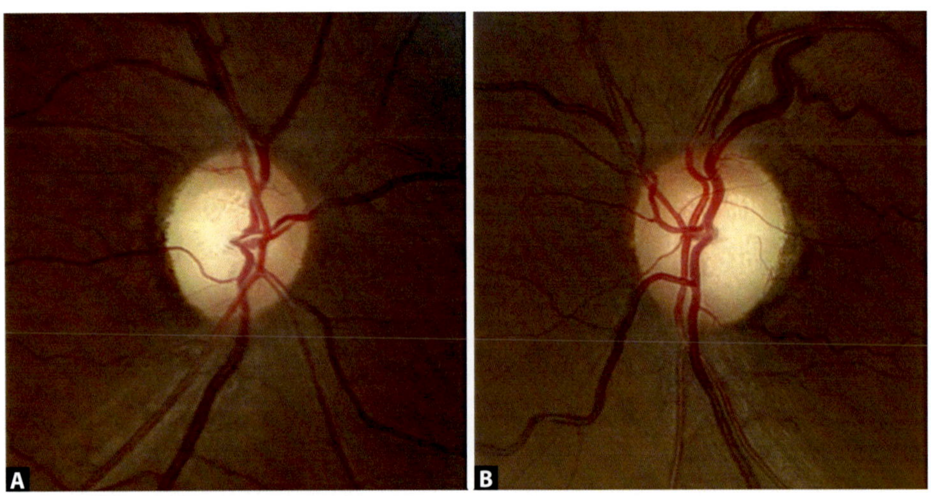

Figs. 9A and B: Dominant optic atrophy. Note the temporal pallor in both the eyes.
(*Courtesy:* University of Michigan, Kellogg Eye Center)

chiasmal optic neuropathy. Many of the hereditary syndromes are associated with deafness (hence important to ask for this in history). Additionally, there may be associated diabetes mellitus and diabetes insipidus as part of DIDMOAD (diabetes insipidus, diabetes mellitus, optic atrophy, and deafness—Wolfram syndrome). Genetic workup would be indicated for these cases and can be ordered as optic atrophy panel.

OCULAR MOTOR NERVE PALSIES

Ocular motor nerve palsies in children have different clinical concerns than adult since there is a relative preponderance of congenital palsies in children and rarity of vasculopathic disorders. When evaluating for cranial nerve palsy, rule out a masquerading restrictive disorder or neuromuscular disease.

Careful history should include: is this congenital or acquired (prior photographs can be of aid here), is there antecedent severe head trauma, are there associated neurological symptoms and signs? Cranial nerve palsy in childhood has impact in the visual development of the child, especially if congenital or acquired in early childhood. The common acquired causes include trauma, inflammation, and intracranial tumors.

Oculomotor Nerve Palsy

Most commonly in children, third nerve palsy is congenital. The developmental third can be isolated but often these children can have associated disease such as hemiparesis and developmental delay and other associated congenital abnormalities.

The most common cause of acquired third nerve palsy in children is trauma. Antecedent head trauma is often severe due to motor vehicle accidents and causes significant diffuse axonal injury, intracranial hemorrhage, basilar skull fracture, traumatic cavernous sinus thrombosis, or fistula. Minor trauma should not be taken as an explanation for acquired third nerve palsy and appropriate imaging for another cause should be undertaken.

Several types of compressive lesions can cause third nerve palsy in children. About 22% of third nerve palsies are related to tumors. In patients with neurofibromatosis type 2, schwannoma or meningioma of the third nerve can present in childhood. Aneurysmal compression can occur but is rare in children.

Various forms of infection such as basilar meningitis, acute bacterial, tuberculous, or fungal can affect the subarachnoid segment of the third nerve. This should be suspected if there are multiple cranial nerve palsies and if the patient is febrile. Septic cavernous sinus thrombosis is another cause of multiple ipsilateral or bilateral cranial nerve palsies.

Idiopathic third nerve palsy in children can be attributed to a postviral or postvaccination syndrome, so it is important to elicit this history.

Ophthalmoplegic migraine was once considered a cause of third nerve palsy in children, but this is considered a misnomer in modern practice and is now identified as recurrent painful cranial neuropathy. This is a diagnosis of exclusion as aneurysm, pituitary apoplexy, and Tolosa-Hunt syndrome should be excluded.

Aberrant regeneration/oculomotor synkinesis can occur a few weeks to months after injury of nerve. This is particularly seen in traumatic or compressive acquired causes and congenital causes.

Clinical Features

The clinical features of third nerve palsy include presence of ptosis, exotropia, hypotropia, or a large unreactive pupil in some combination depending upon whether it is partial or complete, pupil sparing or involved, or divisional if superior orbital fissure lesion **(Fig. 10)**.

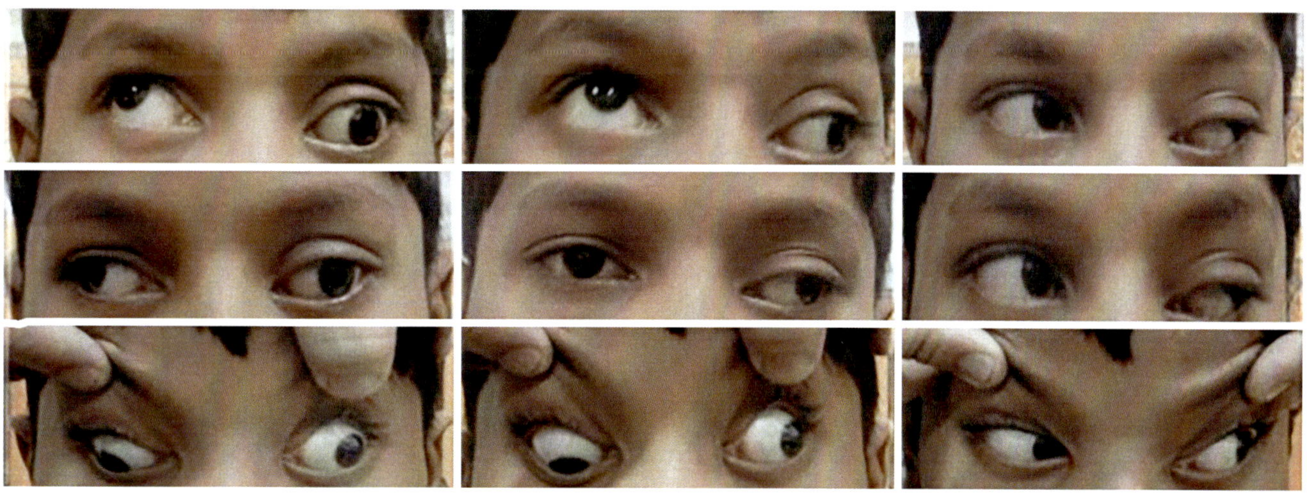

Fig. 10: Left oculomotor nerve palsy. Note left eye ptosis and limitation of movements in all directions except abduction. (*Courtesy:* Dr Rajendra Prasad Centre for Ophthalmic Sciences, All India Institute of Medical Sciences, New Delhi)

Congenital third nerve palsy may present with (1) complete ptosis and ophthalmoplegia or (2) a partial palsy. There is frequent presence of associated aberrant regeneration because of misrouting of regenerating III fibers in congenital palsy (83%). The pupil is frequently involved. The mydriatic pupil frequently becomes miotic over several years. Congenital partial or complete third nerve palsy can be associated with cyclic spasm of the affected muscles, known as cyclic oculomotor palsy. This palsy shows a pattern of the ptotic eyelid lifting every 1.5–2 minutes, the pupil constricts, the eye adducts, and myopic shift of refraction can occur.

Tumor-related third nerve palsy would present with progressive ptosis and exotropia and can have evidence of aberrant regeneration.

Whereas the presence of mydriasis in third nerve palsy suggests a compressive etiology in adults, this is not always the case in children.

The first attack of recurrent painful cranial neuropathy is usually seen in the first decade of life. A severe ipsilateral headache usually precedes the attack, but the headache may diminish before onset of ophthalmoplegia. The third cranial nerve is the most frequently involved followed by the sixth and fourth, respectively. The pupil may be affected. Complete resolution is common and may take up to 4 weeks.

Investigations

Magnetic resonance imaging and magnetic resonance angiogram (MRA) or computed tomography angiogram (CTA) are necessary to assess for compressive lesions both aneurysmal and tumor or signs of inflammation, unless history and examination clearly indicate a congenital etiology. If arterial imaging is negative by careful neuroradiologic evaluation for compressive/aneurysmal cause, there is typically no need for more invasive testing.

Differential Diagnoses

Consider myasthenia gravis, blowout fracture, congenital fibrosis syndrome, internuclear ophthalmoplegia and Duane syndrome type II.

Management

The main concern in children is development of amblyopia. Occlusion is recommended while waiting for recovery to avoid amblyopia due to ptosis. Crutch glasses can be prescribed along with the occlusion of the other eye. For the traumatic cases, observation with periodical examination is done till the deviation stabilizes for at least 6 months.

If recovery is incomplete and there is residual stable strabismus, surgical correction is undertaken but is most challenging for third nerve palsies due to the complexity and number of muscles affected. The goal of surgery should be: (1) To allow single binocular vision in primary position, (2) single binocular vision in primary and down gaze if possible, (3) get the best range of binocular single vision if more can be achieved, and (4) normalize the appearance. If medial rectus has some function and there is moderate exotropia, recession of lateral rectus, and resection of medial rectus may work. But if there is no function of medial rectus, transposition of the vertical muscles may be needed. Simultaneous surgery on >2 rectus muscles can lead to anterior segment ischemia so if needed this should be staged.

Sixth Nerve Palsy

Sixth nerve palsies are most often caused by elevated ICP, which can be due to trauma, tumors, or other space-occupying lesions or idiopathic intracranial hypertension. Elevated ICP can cause downward displacement and stretching of the nerve, which is tethered in Dorello's canal. This typically resolves with normalization of ICP.

Tumors causing sixth nerve palsy in children are most often posterior fossa tumors such as pontine gliomas, medulloblastomas, and cerebellar astrocytomas rather than skull base tumors in adults. Likewise, postoperative injury in tumor resection can cause nerve palsies. Significant head trauma can cause cranial nerve palsies, including sixth, but all cases should be imaged; mild head trauma may be false association and patient may harbor tumor.

Various sources of infection and inflammation can lead to a sixth nerve palsy in children. Meningitis can cause bilateral and multiple cranial nerve palsies via inflammatory processes affecting the cranial nerves. Painful sixth nerve palsy can be a result of Gradenigo syndrome, in which mastoiditis causes petrous bone inflammation. Benign recurrent sixth nerve palsy refers to a sudden onset, isolated, painless, severe unilateral abduction deficit episode that typically follows a viral illness or vaccination without signs of raised ICP, resolves occurs over 8–12 weeks and recurs in the same eye.

Clinical Features

Children may present with acute face turn and incomitant esotropia, greater at distance than near and greater when child fixates with paretic eye.

Duane's syndrome can mimic isolated abduction deficits but has other signs of synkinesis/misdirection-retraction or upshoot. These patients rarely complain of diplopia and the amount of esotropia is very small compared to the limitation of abduction.

Unless there is history of significant trauma to explain the nerve injury, MRI of the brain with and without contrast should always be obtained. Lumbar puncture can be performed as needed to assess for infectious and inflammatory etiologies and to assess for opening pressure for idiopathic intracranial hypertension.

Differential Diagnoses

Consider Duane syndrome, myasthenia gravis, spasm of near reflex, medial orbital fracture with entrapment, long-standing esotropia with medial rectus contracture.

Management

Once the systemic evaluation is addressed and the patient is stable, it is recommended to wait at least 6 months for resolution. Use part time occlusion of the fixating eye in the amblyogenic age group. Residual esodeviations can result from incomplete recovery or medial rectus contractures. Strabismus surgery is guided by the level of recovery of lateral rectus function.

Fourth Nerve Palsy

The most common cause of fourth nerve palsy is congenital or decompensated congenital. Additionally, this is the most common type of congenital cranial nerve palsy. Congenital absence of the superior oblique (SO) tendon has also been reported as an imitator of fourth nerve palsy.

In cases of nerve palsy resulting from trauma, the fourth nerve is the most commonly affected because of its slender shape and long course. Trauma can often cause bilateral fourth nerve palsies. Hence, it is important to inquire about a history of closed head trauma. Neurosurgical trauma from posterior fossa tumor surgery also causes fourth nerve palsy.

Hydrocephalus can cause unilateral or bilateral trochlear nerve palsies in children due to stretching of the superior medullary velum. Idiopathic fourth nerve palsy is rare in children.

Clinical Features

Congenital cases present with a history of long-standing head tilting, facial asymmetry due to head tilting, and large vertical fusional amplitudes (most easily checked in older children). In unilateral cases, there is hypertropia in primary position, and follows Park's three step test **(Figs. 11A to C)**. Additionally, cyclotorsion is typically <5° and there is no significant V pattern.

Excyclotorsion >10° is diagnostic of bilateral fourth nerve palsy. Additionally, bilateral cases will show right hypertropia in right head tilt, left hypertropia in left head tilt, and down gaze evokes a V pattern esotropia. Bilateral excyclotorsion is seen on fundus examination. Bilateral cases may be masked if the examination is highly asymmetric, therefore high suspicion is required.

Magnetic resonance imaging of the brain is indicated to assess for the presence of a tumor unless the etiology is clearly congenital or if there is a history of trauma. Lumbar puncture may be performed as indicated to assess for infectious and inflammatory etiologies.

Management

Acquired SO palsy should be observed for 6 months. Unlike other palsies, risk of amblyopia is lower since children can fuse with head posture. Surgical intervention is indicated to

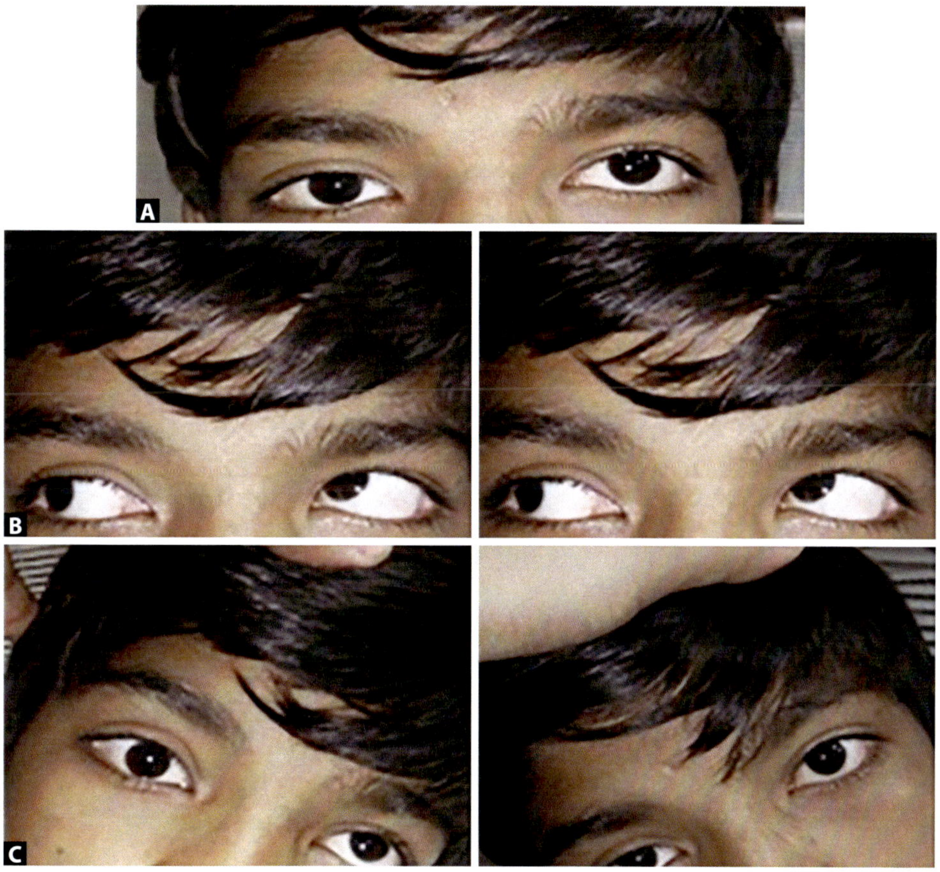

Figs. 11A to C: Left congenital trochlear palsy: Note the hypertropia increases on dextroversion and left head tilt. Note on Park's 3 step test; (A) The hypertropia in primary gaze; (B) Hypertropia increases on dextroversion; (C) Increase in left hypertropia on left head tilt.
(*Courtesy:* Dr Rajendra Prasad Centre for Ophthalmic Sciences, All India Institute of Medical Sciences, New Delhi)

normalize head posture and obtain a good range of binocular single vision. Since majority of SO palsy manifest as isolated overaction of ipsilateral inferior oblique muscle, these cases can be managed by weakening procedures of the inferior oblique muscle (recession or myectomy).

JUVENILE OR INFANTILE MYASTHENIA GRAVIS

This is an autoimmune disorder due to production of acetylcholine receptor antibody. About 30–50% of children with ocular myasthenia will generalize. About 40% of children with isolated ocular symptoms have positive antibody testing versus 70% if generalized. Neonatal myasthenia gravis is distinct from this and is a transient phenomenon seen in newborns of myasthenic mothers due to passive transfer of antibodies and this spontaneously improves over the first few weeks of life.

Clinical Features

As seen in adult cases, infantile myasthenia gravis presents with fatigue and weakness in a range of muscle groups including facial, bulbar, extraocular, and respiratory muscles. Depending on the severity of the case, the associated symptoms can range from drooling, ptosis, and diplopia to dysphagia, aspiration, and respiratory distress/failure. Symptoms generally worsen with activity and improve with rest.

Investigations

Bedside maneuvers such as the ice pack test or the edrophonium test may help support a diagnosis of infantile myasthenia gravis if clinical suspicion is high. The diagnosis is confirmed with serologic positivity of the acetylcholine receptor antibody or with an electrodiagnostic examination demonstrating progressive decline of compound motor action potentials on repetitive nerve stimulation.

Management

It is important to treat ocular myasthenia gravis in children due to risk of amblyopia with ptosis and strabismus. Treatment in the acute setting involves first stabilizing the patient's airway, and early intubation may be indicated if there are signs of respiratory distress. Acetylcholinesterase inhibitors may help for mild cases. More severe cases are treated with therapies with rapid onset, such as IVIg and plasma exchange. Glucocorticoids and/or other immunosuppressive therapies are used for acute and long-term management of ocular and generalized myasthenia. Thymectomy may be performed if indicated following initial stabilization during the same hospitalization or in the outpatient setting.

CEREBRAL VISUAL IMPAIRMENT

Cerebral visual impairment (CVI) is defined as vision loss resulting from damage to retrogeniculate pathway of visual system in the absence of any ocular pathology. With increased survival of preterm babies and better perinatal care, CVI has emerged as one of the leading causes of visual impairment. CVI is commonly defined as a loss in visual function in the absence of damage to the anterior afferent visual pathways or ocular structures. CVI has multiple causes but the most common is perinatal hypoxia.

Clinical Features

Visual impairment in CVI can be as severe as no light perception to normal visual acuity. Cognitive visual function may be impaired in most of these children leading to misinterpretation in relation to what objects are there and where they are. There is some evidence that dorsal stream magnocellular pathway deficits may be more common in children with CVI. Children with PVL frequently have accommodation dysfunction and resultant hypermetropic refractive error. Strabismus in the form of infantile exotropia and esotropia if often present in association with CVI. Optic atrophy is common and can be secondary either to hypoxia involving the optic nerves or retrograde atrophy. In cases of hydrocephalus, resulting papilledema may lead to secondary optic atrophy. Field defects in the form of bilateral inferior field defects are most common, homonymous hemianopia can also be present in association with hemiplegia and can be explained by interruption of axons of optic radiations and partly by the problems of simultaneous attention.

Cerebral visual impairment can typically be associated with neurological deficits including cerebral palsy, mental retardation and hemiparesis, microcephaly, hearing problems, abnormal mental development, behavioral problems, myelomeningocele, progressive degenerative disorders, and hypotonia indicating that the damage may not be limited to the visual pathways. Some patients may also have superimposed anterior afferent pathology from optic nerve-related disease.

Investigations

Diagnosis of this entity is suspected in the immediate neonatal period. Neuroimaging evidence of acute brain injury can be seen on brain MRI in children at risk.

Management

Some degree of visual recovery is seen in majority of children with cortical visual impairment, the improvement tends to be gradual over months, although exact mechanism is unclear. It has now been postulated that improvement of sight in patients of CVI is actually a form of delayed visual maturation. Addressing refractive error and initiating timely amblyopia therapy is crucial. Strabismus and motility evaluation is difficult owing to the behavioral aspects, yet has to be performed in multiple visits to know about stability of deviation, which helps decide optimal timing of surgical intervention.

The problems in patients of CVI are not just limited to vision, but are complex. A multidisciplinary approach is thus necessary not just for diagnosis but also for management. Rehabilitation services are much more needed, despite of progress in diagnostic methods, interventional treatments for CVI are still very limited. Rehabilitation support must include an approach that addresses psychosocial impact on patients and their families.

SUGGESTED READING

1. Akagi T, Miyamoto K, Kashii S, Yoshimura N. Cause and prognosis of neurologically isolated third, fourth, or sixth cranial nerve dysfunction in cases of oculomotor palsy. Jpn J Ophthalmol. 2008;52(1):32-5.
2. Brodsky MC. Congenital Optic Disc Anomalies in Pediatric Neuro-ophthalmology, 2nd edition. New York: Springer; 2010.
3. Carelli V, Carbonelli M, de Coo IF, Kawasaki A, Klopstock T, Lagrèze WA, et al. International Consensus Statement on the clinical and therapeutic management of Leber hereditary optic neuropathy. J Neuroophthalmol. 2017;37(4):371-81.
4. Chun BY, Rizzo JF 3rd. Dominant optic atrophy and Leber's hereditary optic neuropathy: update on clinical features and current therapeutic approaches. Semin Pediatr Neurol. 2017;24(2):129-34.
5. Dutton, G. Congenital disorders of the optic nerve: excavations and hypoplasia. Eye. 2004;18(11):1038-48.
6. Friedman NJ, Kaiser PK. Essentials of Ophthalmology. Philadelphia: Elsevier Health Sciences; 2007.
7. Good WV, Jan JE, deSa L, Barkovitch AJ, Groenveld M, Hoyt CS. Cortical visual impairment in children: a major review. Surv Ophthalmol. 1994;38(4):351-64.
8. Hoyt CS. Hydrocephalus, brain anomalies and cortical visual impairment. In: Taylor D, Hoyt CS, (Eds). Pediatric Ophthalmology and Strabismus. Philadelphia: Elsevier Saunders; 2005. pp. 675-86.
9. Jurkute N, Harvey J, Yu-Wai-Man P. Treatment strategies for Leber hereditary optic neuropathy. Curr Opin Neurol. 2019;32(1):99-104.
10. Klopstock T, Yu-Wai-Man P, Dimitriadis K, Rouleau J, Heck S, Bailie M, et al. A randomized placebo-controlled trial of idebenone in Leber's hereditary optic neuropathy. Brain. 2011;134 (Pt 9):2677-86.
11. Lucchinetti CF, Kiers L, O'Duffy A, Gomez MR, Cross S, Leavitt JA, et al. Risk factors for developing multiple sclerosis after childhood optic neuritis. Neurology. 1997;49(5):1413-8.
12. Newman NJ, Yu-Wai-Man P, Carelli V, Moster ML, Biousse V, Vignal-Clermont C, et al. Efficacy and safety of intravitreal gene therapy for Leber hereditary optic neuropathy treated within 6 months of disease onset. Ophthalmology. 2021;128(5):649-60.
13. Nielsen LS, Skov L, Jensen H. Visual dysfunctions and ocular disorders in children with developmental delay. 2nd Prevalence, diagnoses and actiology of visual impairment. Acta Ophthalmol Scand. 2007;85(2):149-55.
14. Olsen TW, Summers CG, Knobloch WH. Predicting visual acuity in children with colobomas involving the optic nerve. J Pediatr Ophthalmol Strabismus. 1996;33:47-51.
15. Phillips PH, Repka MX, Lambert SR. Pseudotumor cerebri in children. J AAPOS. 1998;2(1):33-8.
16. The NORDIC Idiopathic Intracranial Hypertension Study Group Writing Committee. Effect of acetazolamide on visual function in patients with idiopathic intracranial hypertension and mild visual loss: the Idiopathic Intracranial Hypertension Treatment Trial. JAMA. 2014;311(16):1641-51.
17. Wan MJ, Adebona O, Benson LA, Gorman MP, Heidary G. Visual outcomes in pediatric optic neuritis. Am J Ophthalmol. 2014;158(3):503-7.e2.
18. Witmer MT, Margo CE, Drucker M. Tilted optic disks. Surv Ophthalmol. 2010;55(5):403-28.
19. Writing Committee for the Pediatric Eye Disease Investigator Group (PEDIG); Pineles SL, Repka MX, Liu GT, Waldman AT, Borchert MS, et al. Assessment of pediatric optic neuritis visual acuity outcomes at 6 months. JAMA Ophthalmol. 2020; 138(12):1253-61.

13

CHAPTER

Pediatric Ocular Congenital Vasculopathies

Marina Roizenblatt, Emmanuel Y Chang, Kim Jiramongkolchai

INTRODUCTION

Ocular congenital vasculopathies are a varied group of diseases affecting the eye, particularly the retina. Some of them affect other parts of the body as well, and form a syndromic entity. Genetic abnormalities is the key to the origin of these vasculopathies in children, with number of genes identified with each disorder now, showing pleomorphic presentation and penetrance.

Retinal vascular disorders in children unlike those in adults, rarely represent the sequelae of chronic systemic diseases like diabetes or hypertension. They are more likely to suffer from congenital, developmental, infectious or traumatic vascular lesions.

Newer modalities and techniques of retinal imaging and vascular angiographies has enabled us to examine the disease process more precisely. Yet the ocular fundus examination offers the physician a unique opportunity of studying the living blood vessels.

The present chapter would highlight more prevalent congenital vasculopathies with particular focus on retina and choroid.

PERSISTENT FETAL VASCULATURE

Clinical Presentation

Persistent fetal vasculature (PFV) is a unilateral condition caused by failure of the fetal hyaloidal vessels to regress during embryogenesis. It is the second most common cause of acquired cataract during the first year of life. PFV is divided into three categories based on the amount of hyaloidal vessel involution: anterior, posterior, and combined anterior-posterior. Examples of anterior PFV are cataracts, retrolenticular membrane, posterior lenticonus, Mittendorf dot, elongated ciliary process, shallow anterior chamber, poor pupil dilation, microcornea, and iridohyaloid blood vessels.

Examples of posterior PFV are retinal detachment, retinal dysplasia, retinal folds, optic nerve hypoplasia, Bergmeister's papilla, macular anomalies, intravitreal hemorrhage, and vitreal membranes. The most common form of PFV, anterior-posterior accounts for 60% of all cases and is the most complicated. Combined PFV can lead to severe ocular malformation such as microphthalmos, buphthalmos, or phthisis bulbi.

Differential Diagnosis

The differential diagnosis for PFV should include causes of pediatric leukocoria such as retinoblastoma, advanced retinopathy of prematurity (ROP), familial exudative vitreoretinopathy (FEVR), Coats disease, Norrie disease, incontinentia pigmenti (IP), congenital cataract, ocular toxocariasis, retinal dysplasias, and severe intermediate uveitis. It is most important to rule out retinoblastoma, which can be a life-threatening disorder.

Several key characteristics can be helpful in differentiating retinoblastoma from PFV. Microphthalmos is suggestive of PFV as it is uncommon to see retinoblastoma in a microphthalmic eye. PFV is typically a unilateral condition, whereas retinoblastoma can be either unilateral or bilateral. Ancillary testing with radiologic findings and Doppler ultrasonography, computed tomography CT, and magnetic resonance imaging (MRI) can also be helpful in distinguishing PFV from retinoblastoma.

Diagnostic Examination

The presence of persistent congenital vessels extending from the optic disk to the lens is diagnostic of PFV. When visualization of the retina is poor, it is important to perform additional imaging tests to confirm the diagnosis. High-frequency ultrasonography, CT scan, MRI, and intravenous fluorescein angiography (FA) can be helpful adjunctive tests. Ultrasonography shows an echogenic inhomogeneous band extending from the lens posterior capsule to the optic disc **(Fig. 1)**. Color Doppler of this band will show arterial flow which represents the persistent hyaloid artery. CT and MRI will show enhancement of a linear structure suggestive of a hyaloid canal, shallow anterior chamber, irregular lens, and or a retinal detachment. It is important to confirm the absence of intraocular calcification with either CT or ultrasound to rule out retinoblastoma. FA will show a persistent anterior tunica vasculosa lentis extending to the margin of the iris.

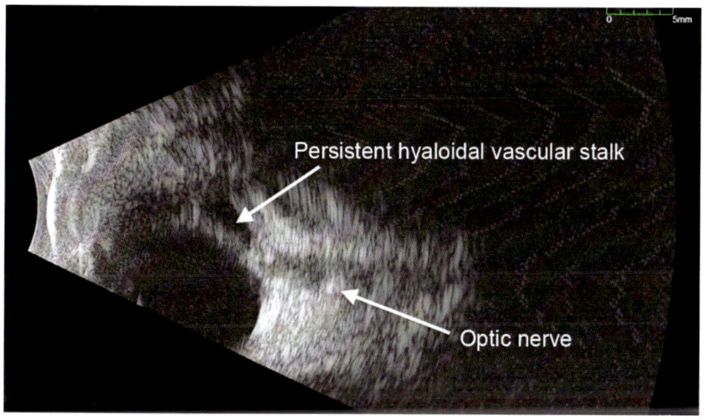

Fig. 1: A 2-month-old female with persistent fetal vasculature with the hyaloidal vascular stalk extending from the disk to the lens on B-scan ultrasound.

Treatment

Treatment depends on the severity of the disease and ranges from observation and treatment of amblyopia to surgery. Observation is indicated for isolated Mittendorf dot and Bergmeister's papilla in which there is minimal involvement from PFV.

Severe PFV requires surgery to prevent angle closure glaucoma, vitreous hemorrhage, retinal detachment, and phthisis bulbi. Indications for surgery are recurrent or severe intravitreal hemorrhage, progressive retinal detachment, progressive shallowing of the anterior chamber, or secondary glaucoma caused by closure of the anterior chamber angle. Surgery for anterior PFV associated with a visually significant cataract may require lensectomy and anterior vitrectomy with cautery of the tips of the hyaloid stalk. For PFV cases associated with elevated intraocular pressure, medical or surgical treatment for glaucoma is appropriate. For posterior PFV, the surgical approach may include release of traction with or without lens extraction. In the surgical approach of posterior PFV, it is important to visualize the pars plana prior to trocar cannula insertion as the peripheral retina may be abnormally inserted. If the pars plana cannot be visualized, a transpupillary or translimbal approach may be safer to prevent iatrogenic retinal breaks.

INCONTINENTIA PIGMENTI

Clinical Presentation

Incontinentia pigmenti is a rare inherited, X-linked dominant disorder, affecting multiple organ systems including the skin, teeth, hair, nails, eyes, and central nervous system (CNS). The key finding of IP is characteristic progressive skin lesions. The skin lesions begin with vesicular bullous lesions that progress to whorl-like pigmentary changes over four stages. The ocular findings and the CNS anomalies are less frequent than skin disorders and vary from mild to severe presentations.

The ocular findings in IP are present in 35% of cases and typically are unilateral. They are divided into retina and nonretinal findings, with the majority involving the retina. In untreated retinal disease, there is progressive retinal ischemia leading to neovascularization and retinal detachment. Macular findings include foveal hypoplasia. Nonretinal findings include nystagmus, strabismus, microphthalmos, pigmentation of the conjunctiva, anterior segment dysgenesis, and optic atrophy.

Dental abnormalities are the second most common finding and are seen in up to 80% of affected individuals. These dental abnormalities are missing, small, or abnormally peg-shaped teeth. Although CNS abnormalities are uncommon and are present in only 15% of cases, they are regarded as the most disabling conditions. Examples of CNS involvement are developmental delay, microcephaly, spasticity, and seizures.

Differential Diagnosis

The differential diagnosis for IP includes ROP, FEVR, Norrie disease, Eales disease, and sickle cell retinopathy. The skin findings are unique to IP and are not present with the above-mentioned conditions.

Diagnostic Examination

Landy and Donnai established the criteria for the diagnosis of IP. If there is a first-degree relative with IP, then only the features from **Box 1** are required. If there is no first-degree relative with IP and no genetic testing is available, then one major and at least two minor criteria from **Box 2** are required.

Although not a part of the diagnostic criterion, the identification of *IKBKG* gene mutation, also known as NEMO, is present in 80% of IP individuals and can be suggestive of IP. When IP is suspected, a genetics consult can be helpful for parental counseling regarding the risk of future affected offspring.

BOX 1: Criteria for diagnosis of incontinentia pigmenti (IP) in the presence of affected first-degree relative (Landy and Donnai, 1993).

1. History or evidence of typical skin rash
2. Pale, hairless, and atrophic linear skin streaks
3. Dental anomalies
4. Wooly hair
5. Retinal disease
6. Multiple abortions of male fetuses

BOX 2: Criteria for diagnosis of incontinentia pigmenti (IP) in the absence of affected first-degree relative (Landy and Donnai, 1993).

Major criteria:

1. Neonatal vesicular rash (erythema, vesicles, and eosinophilia)
2. Hyperpigmentation of the skin (especially on the trunk along the lines of Blaschko; disappears during adolescence)
3. Linear alopecia atrophic lesions

Minor criteria:

1. Abnormal dentition
2. Alopecia
3. Wooly hair and abnormalities of the nail
4. Retinal disease

Treatment

Treatment of IP is limited to management of symptoms. FA is required in all cases of IP as indirect ophthalmoscopy alone in inadequate to identify the extent of peripheral ischemia. Incomplete peripheral vascularization of the retina should be treated with laser photocoagulation. Intravitreal antivascular endothelial growth factor (VEGF) can be considered as adjunct treatment following laser if there is refractory disease following laser treatment. There should be a low threshold to bring the child for an examination under anesthesia for imaging and treatment.

NORRIE DISEASE

Clinical Presentation

Norrie disease is a rare X-linked bilateral disorder that is characterized by dysplastic retina caused by incomplete regression of the hyaloidal vessels and retinal vascularization. Systemic features with Norrie disease include hearing loss, mental retardation, and blindness. Unfortunately, most patients with Norrie disease usually present with little to no light perception at birth or shortly thereafter by 3 months of age.

Ocular findings of Norrie disease include cataract and retrolental fibroplasia, opaque cornea, iris atrophy, PFV, vitreous hemorrhage, dysplastic retina with a gray or grayish-yellow pseudoglioma appearance, retinal folds, and hemorrhagic retinal detachments **(Figs. 2A to C)**.

Differential Diagnosis

The differential diagnosis includes FEVR, PFV, Coats disease, ROP, retinoblastoma, and endophthalmitis. It can be difficult to distinguish Norrie disease from these other pediatric retinal vasculopathies, especially advanced stage 5 ROP. Helpful clues that favor the diagnosis of Norrie include family history of severe vision loss at or near birth in male family members. A birth history of prematurity and long hospitalization course can help distinguish between ROP and Norrie disease. Retinoblastoma can be distinguished often by clinical examination, but a CT or B-scan ultrasound may be necessary. Infants presenting with severe vision loss and retinal dysplasia should be genetically tested for Norrie disease.

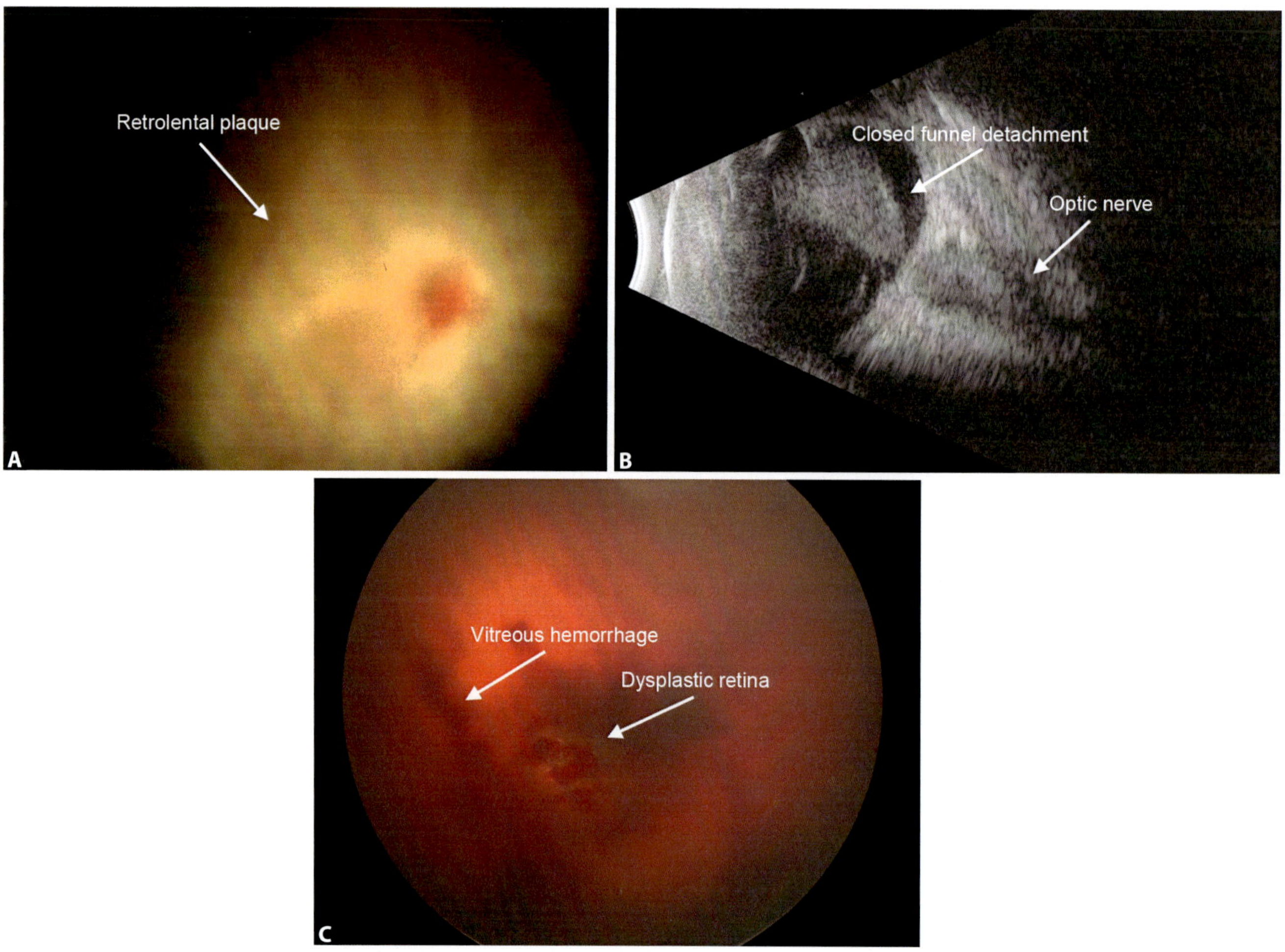

Figs. 2A to C: A 3-month-old presenting with Norrie disease with bilateral persistent fetal vasculature and vitreous hemorrhage. Retrolental plaque, right eye (A), closed funnel detachment on B-scan ultrasound, right eye (B), and retinal dysplasia, left eye (C).

Diagnostic Examination

The diagnosis of Norrie disease is based on birth and family history, ophthalmic findings, and systemic findings (one-third develops hearing loss and two-thirds have mental retardation). Mutation in the *NDP* gene can support the diagnosis of Norrie. Once the diagnosis of Norrie is made, audiologic and neurodevelopment evaluations are recommended. The gene expression is variable and the prenatal detection of the mutation in the *NDP* gene cannot predict the severity of the ocular phenotype. Prenatal ultrasound findings during late pregnancy can provide valuable information regarding the extent of the disease. Advanced disease on prenatal ultrasound will show calcification of the ocular wall, massive vitreous opacity, and retinal detachment.

Treatment

Historically, the management of Norrie disease was managing a blind and painful eye. The natural history of the disease is no light perception either at birth or by 3 months and development of phthisis bulbi in the first decade of life. Jacklin et al. reported that early vitrectomy and lensectomy can prevent phthisis bulbi at 2 years of by removing the anterior posterior traction and allowing eye growth and in some cases reattachment of the retina to the posterior pole. For this reason and the natural history of severe vision loss, vitrectomy and possible lensectomy are recommended as early as possible.

COATS DISEASE

Clinical Presentation

Coats disease is an idiopathic nonhereditary condition characterized by peripheral abnormal telangiectatic vessels and large macular subretinal and intraretinal exudates **(Fig. 3A)**. The telangiectatic vessels have a characteristic focal dilatation that resemble "light bulbs" **(Figs. 3B and C)**.

Common presentations for Coats disease are decreased vision, strabismus, and leukocoria.

Differential Diagnosis

The differential diagnosis for Coats disease includes causes of leukocoria such as retinal detachment, retinoblastoma,

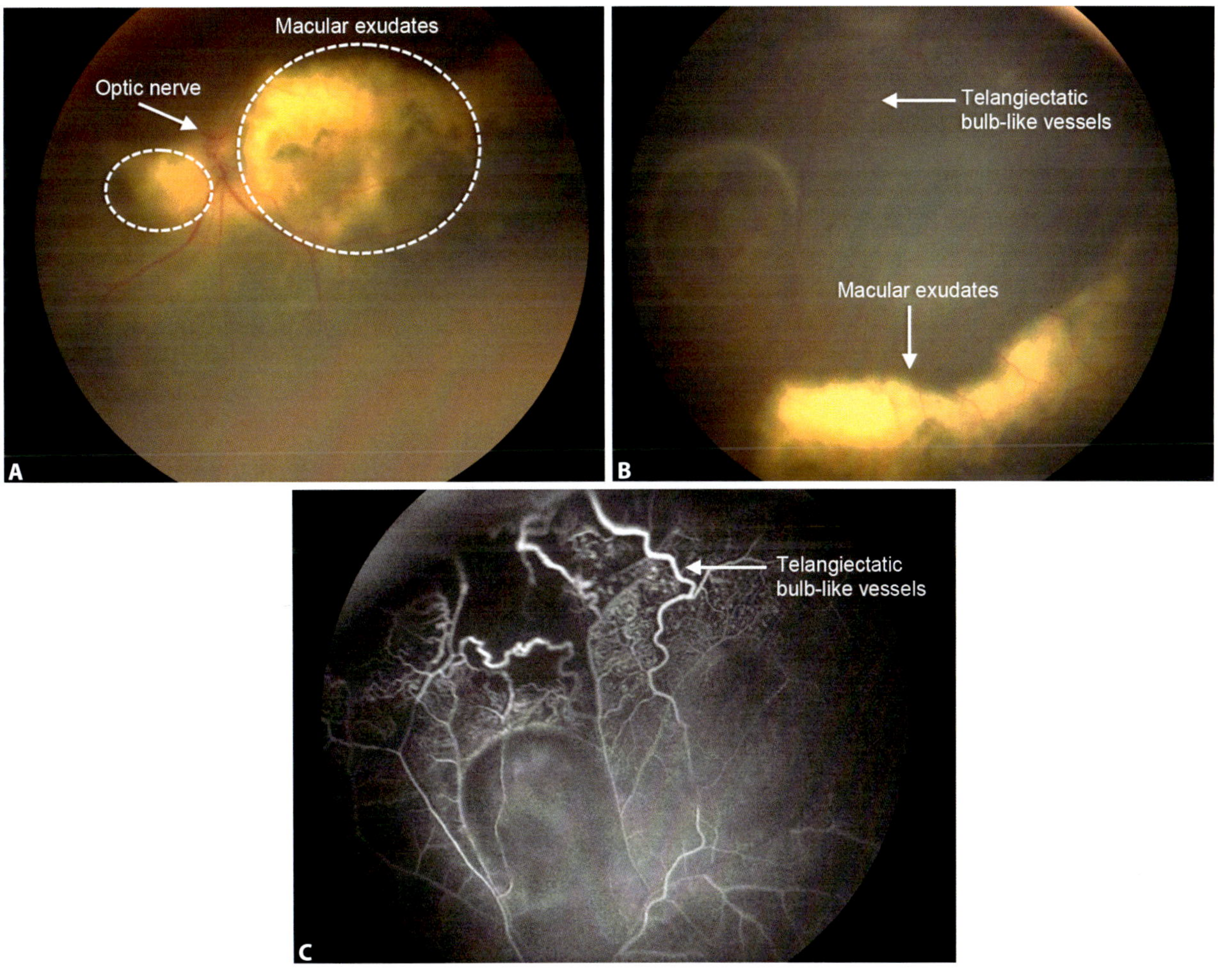

Figs. 3A to C: A 4-year-old with Coats disease in the left eye with macular exudates (dotted white circle) (A). Telangiectatic bulb-like vessels superior to the disk and macular exudates on fundus photograph (B) and fluorescein angiography (C).

PFV, ROP, congenital cataract, Norrie disease, toxocariasis, Eales disease, and FEVR. Approximately 50% of Coats disease are misdiagnosed, the common misdiagnosis being retinoblastoma.

Diagnostic Examination

The diagnosis can be made based on the patient's medical history, clinical findings, complete ophthalmologic examination, and auxiliary examination. In the presence of exudation, ancillary testing such as FA, ultrasound, computerized tomography, and MRI may be helpful.

Telangiectasia, aneurysms, beading of vessel walls, abnormal vascular termination, and vascular communicating channels are classic findings on FA. The absence of intraocular calcification on ultrasound is important to document in Coats disease. CT and MRI can also be used to differentiate Coats disease from retinoblastoma and from other leukocoric lesions.

Treatment

Treatment of Coats disease is dependent on the stage of disease. Observation may be reasonable for nonvision-threatening retinal telangiectasia without exudation. Patients with telangiectasia and exudation that threaten vision should be treated with laser photocoagulation or cryotherapy. Retinal detachment should be treated with surgery. Patients with advanced and asymptomatic disease may be left untreated. Combined therapy with anti-VEGF plus laser and cryotherapy may play a role in select severe Coats with exudation to reduce the amount of fluid to allow more effective ablative procedures.

FAMILIAL EXUDATIVE VITREORETINOPATHY

Clinical Presentation

Familial exudative vitreoretinopathy is a rare hereditary bilateral peripheral heterogeneous disorder characterized by peripheral abnormal retinal blood vessel development. FEVR can be inherited through an X-linked recessive, autosomal dominant, or autosomal recessive pattern due to mutations in one of the following genes: *NDP, FZD4, TSPAN12, LRP5, ZNF408, ATOH7, RCBTB1, and CTNNB1. NDP, LRP5, FZD4*, and *TSPAN12* account for 50% of cases. However, family history is positive in only 20–40% of cases and FEVR has variable expressivity and progression of disease even amongst family members **(Figs. 4A and B)**.

Mild cases of FEVR manifest with tenuous peripheral vascular abnormalities, such as a peripheral avascular zone, vitreoretinal adhesions, venous-venous anastomoses, and supernumerous vascular branching. Severe FEVR manifests with retinal neovascularization, subretinal and intraretinal exudates or hemorrhages, tractional retinal detachments, macula ectopia, epiretinal membranes, macular dragging, vascularized preretinal membranes that can lead to retinal folds, preretinal vitreous organization, and vitreous hemorrhage. The most widely used classification for FEVR was published in 1998 by Pendergast and Trese **(Table 1)**. It is important to note that FEVR does not necessarily progress in a stepwise fashion and careful monitoring at least every 6 months is recommended.

Differential Diagnosis

The differential diagnoses of FEVR are ROP, PFV, Norrie, IP, and Coats disease. A history of preterm delivery, low birth weight, and neonatal oxygen exposure is suggestive of ROP over FEVR whereas subretinal or intraretinal exudation is more suggestive of FEVR. The most relevant difference in terms of prognosis is that FEVR is a lifelong vascular active disease that tends to recur or reactivate and requires lifelong monitoring. Asymmetric FEVR can mimic PFV and widefield FA can be helpful to detect leakage that is not clinically apparent or suspected in eyes without exudation. The presence of microphthalmia, deafness, or mental retardation should raise the suspicion for Norrie disease. While FEVR has a more variable phenotype, Norrie disease

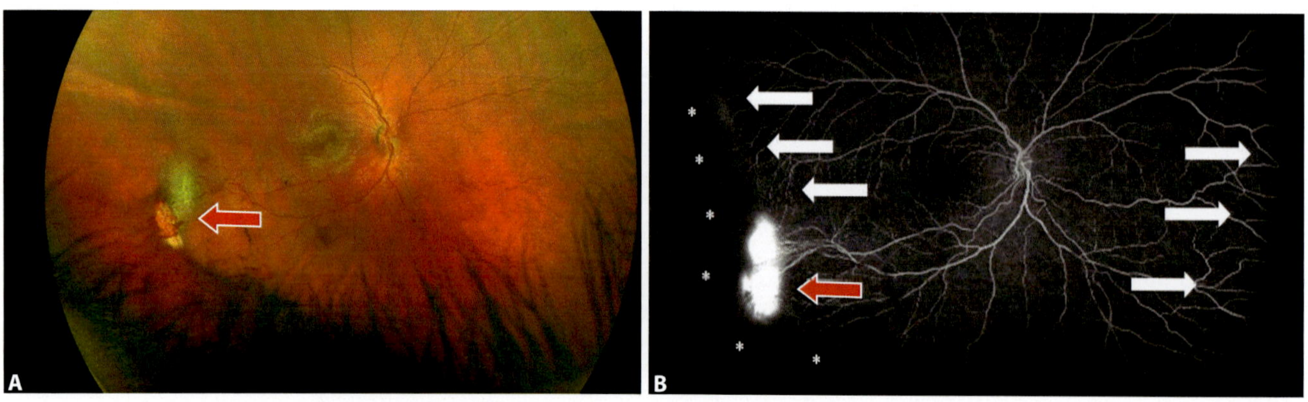

Figs. 4A and B: A 12-year-old boy with familial exudative vitreoretinopathy (FEVR) Optos widefield color fundus photograph showing peripheral retinal neovascularization (arrow) (A), fluorescein angiograph showing leakage from the peripheral retinal neovascularization (red arrow), supernumerous vascular branching (white arrows), and peripheral nonperfusion (*) (B).

TABLE 1: Update clinical classification of familial exudative vitreoretinopathy.

Stage	*Exudate**		
	Without	*With*	*Clinical features*
1	A	B	Avascular retinal periphery
2	A	B	Extraretinal neovascularization
3	A	B	Retinal detachment not involving macula
4	A	B	Retinal detachment involving macula
5	A (open funnel)	B (closed funnel)	Total retinal detachment

* For stages 1–4

clinically manifests as severe dysplastic retina with either a pseudoglioma appearance or total retinal detachment with dense retrolental fibrovascular tissue. Cutaneous skin lesion requires consideration of IP. Coats disease is typically unilateral, has male predilection, and is unlikely to present with tractional retinal pathology. Lastly, it is always important to rule out retinoblastoma.

Diagnostic Examination

Vascular changes in the early stages may be apparent only on widefield FA. Therefore, in the setting of positive family history it is recommended to combine clinical evaluation with a widefield fluorescein angiography screening examination. Findings on wide-angle FA are premature truncation of the peripheral vessels and subclinical neovascularization. FEVR requires lifelong follow-up with regular examinations, FA, and possibly treatment. Genetic testing can be helpful.

Treatment

Patients without exudation are generally observed. Laser photocoagulation is indicated when retinal ischemia or neovascularization in attached retina is detected on funduscopic or fluorescein angiographic examination. The aim of laser photocoagulation is to promote regression of neovascularization and clearing of exudation.

When retinal detachment is present, vitrectomy is a reasonable approach to release tractions. As a general guideline, vitrectomy with posterior traction release is essential in younger patients with vascularly active fibrovascular proliferation, while scleral buckling is indicated for cases with peripheral traction anterior to the equator.

According to Chen et al., surgical outcome are closely associated with the foveal dragging status. Scleral buckling procedures are suitable to treat patients with no or moderate foveal dragging without posteriorly located breaks, proliferative vitreoretinopathy, or vitreous opacities. Vitrectomy combined with scleral buckle may be necessary for patients with severe foveal dragging and peripheral pathology. The use of intravitreal anti-VEGF injection in treating FEVR remains controversial. It is important to remember that even with treatment, FEVR patients require lifelong treatment as the disease can reactivate at any time.

SUGGESTED READING

1. Atta H, Watson N. Echographic diagnosis of advanced Coats' disease. Eye (Lond). 1992;6(Pt 1):80-5.
2. Barañano D, Goldberg M. Incontinentia pigmenti. In: ME H (Ed). Pediatric Retina, 2nd edition. Philadelphia: Lippincott Williams & Wilkins; 2014. pp. 354-66.
3. Byrne SF, Green RL. Ultrasound of the Eye and Orbit, 2nd edition. Philadelphia, PA: Mosby; 2002.
4. Cernichiaro-Espinosa LA, Patel NA, Bauer MS, Negron CI, Fallas B, Pogrebniak A, et al. Revascularization after intravitreal bevacizumab and laser therapy of bilateral retinal vascular occlusions in incontinentia pigmenti (Bloch-Sulzberger Syndrome). Ophthalmic Surg Lasers Imaging Retina. 2019;50(2): e33-e37.
5. Chang-Godinich A, Paysse EA, Coats DK, Holz ER. Familial exudative vitreoretinopathy mimicking persistent hyperplastic primary vitreous. Am J Ophthalmol. 1999;127(4):469-71.
6. Chen C, Xiao H, Ding X. Persistent fetal vasculature. Asia Pac J Ophthalmol (Phila). 2019;8(1):86-95.
7. Chen SN, Hwang JF, Lin CJ. Clinical characteristics and surgical management of familial exudative vitreoretinopathy-associated rhegmatogenous retinal detachment. Retina. 2012;32(2):220-5.
8. Drenser KA. Norrie disease. In: Hartnett ME (Ed). Pediatric Retina, 2nd edition. Philadelphia: Lippincott Williams & Wilkins; 2014. pp. 351-6.
9. Fusco F, Pescatore A, Bal E, Ghoul A, Paciolla M, Lioi MB, et al. Alterations of the IKBKG locus and diseases: an update and a report of 13 novel mutations. Hum Mutat. 2008;29(5):595-604.
10. Ghorbanian S, Jaulim A, Chatziralli IP. Diagnosis and treatment of Coats' disease: a review of the literature. Ophthalmologica. 2012;227(4):175-82.
11. Goldberg MF. Persistent fetal vasculature (PFV): an integrated interpretation of signs and symptoms associated with persistent hyperplastic primary vitreous (PHPV). LIV Edward Jackson Memorial Lecture. Am J Ophthalmol. 1997;124(5):587-626.
12. Gologorsky D, Chang JS, Hess DJ, Berrocal AM. Familial exudative vitreoretinopathy in a premature child. Ophthalmic Surg Lasers Imaging Retina. 2013;44(6):603-5.
13. Greene-Roethke C. Incontinentia pigmenti: a summary review of this rare ectodermal dysplasia with neurologic manifestations, including treatment protocols. J Pediatr Health Care. 2017;31(6):e45-e52.
14. Haddad R, Font RL, Reeser F. Persistent hyperplastic primary vitreous. A clinicopathologic study of 62 cases and review of the literature. Surv Ophthalmol. 1978;23(2):123-34.
15. Ho M, Yip WWK, Chan VCK, Young AL. Successful treatment of refractory proliferative retinopathy of incontinentia pigmenti by intravitreal ranibizumab as adjunct therapy in a 4-years-old child. Retin Cases Brief Rep. 2017;11(4):352-5.

16. Hu A, Pei X, Ding X, Li J, Li Y, Liu F, et al. Combined persistent fetal vasculature: a classification based on high-resolution B-mode ultrasound and color Doppler imaging. Ophthalmology. 2016; 123(1):19-25.
17. Karjosukarso DW, van Gestel SHC, Qu J, Kouwenhoven EN, Duijkers L, Garanto A, et al. An FEVR-associated mutation in ZNF408 alters the expression of genes involved in the development of vasculature. Hum Mol Genet. 2018;27(20):3519-27.
18. Kartchner JZ, Hartnett ME. Familial exudative vitreoretinopathy presentation as persistent fetal vasculature. Am J Ophthalmol Case Rep. 2017;6:15-7.
19. Kashani AH, Brown KT, Chang E, Drenser KA, Capone A, Trese MT. Diversity of retinal vascular anomalies in patients with familial exudative vitreoretinopathy. Ophthalmology. 2014;121(11):2220-7.
20. Landy SJ, Donnai D. Incontinentia pigmenti (Bloch-Sulzberger syndrome). J Med Genet. 1993;30(1):53-9.
21. Liu J, Zhu J, Yang J, Zhang X, Zhang Q, Zhao P. Prenatal diagnosis of familial exudative vitreoretinopathy and Norrie disease. Mol Genet Genomic Med. 2019;7(1):e00503.
22. London NJS, Shields CL, Haller JA. Coats disease. In: Sadda A (Ed). Retina, 5th edition. London: WB Saunders; 2013. pp. 1058-70.
23. Mackeen LD, Nischal KK, Lam WC, Levin AV. High-frequency ultrasonography findings in persistent hyperplastic primary vitreous. J AAPOS. 2000;4(4):217-24.
24. Mafee MF, Mafee RF, Malik M, Pierce J. Medical imaging in pediatric ophthalmology. Pediatr Clin North Am. 2003;50(1):259-86.
25. Pendergast SD, Trese MT. Familial exudative vitreoretinopathy. Results of surgical management. Ophthalmology. 1998;105(6): 1015-23.
26. Pollard ZF. Persistent hyperplastic primary vitreous: diagnosis, treatment and results. Trans Am Ophthalmol Soc. 1997;95:487-549.
27. Ranchod TM, Ho LY, Drenser KA, Capone A Jr, Trese MT. Clinical presentation of familial exudative vitreoretinopathy. Ophthalmology. 2011;118(10):2070-5.
28. Ray R, Barañano DE, Hubbard GB. Treatment of Coats' disease with intravitreal bevacizumab. Br J Ophthalmol. 2013;97(3):272-7.
29. Sanghvi D, Sanghvi C, Purandare N. Bilateral persistent hyperplastic primary vitreous. Australas Radiol. 2005;49(1):72-4.
30. Shah PK, Bachu S, Narendran V, Kalpana N, David J, Srinivas CR. Intravitreal bevacizumab for incontinentia pigmenti. J Pediatr Ophthalmol Strabismus. 2013;50 Online:e52-4.
31. Shields JA, Shields CL, Honavar SG, Demirci H. Clinical variations and complications of Coats disease in 150 cases: the 2000 Sanford Gifford Memorial Lecture. Am J Ophthalmol. 2001;131(5):561-71.
32. Sims KB. NDP-related retinopathies. In: GeneReviews®[Internet]. Seattle: University of Washington; 2014.
33. Sisk RA, Berrocal AM, Feuer WJ, Murray TG. Visual and anatomic outcomes with or without surgery in persistent fetal vasculature. Ophthalmology. 2010;117(11):2178-83.e1-2.
34. Smith SE, Mullen TE, Graham D, Sims KB, Rehm HL. Norrie disease: extraocular clinical manifestations in 56 patients. Am J Med Genet A. 2012;158(8):1909-17.
35. Swinney CC, Han DP, Karth PA. Incontinentia pigmenti: a comprehensive review and update. Ophthalmic Surg Lasers Imaging Retina. 2015;46(6):650-7.
36. Tian T, Chen C, Zhang X, Zhang Q, Zhao P. Clinical and genetic features of familial exudative vitreoretinopathy with only-unilateral abnormalities in a Chinese cohort. JAMA Ophthalmol. 2019;137(9):1054-8.
37. Todorich B, Thanos A, Yonekawa Y, Capone A Jr. Repair of total tractional retinal detachment in norrie disease: report of technique and successful surgical outcome. Ophthalmic Surg Lasers Imaging Retina. 2017;48(3):260-2.
38. Trese MT, Capone Jr A. Diagnosis and management of persistent fetal vasculature syndrome. In: Hartnett ME (Ed). Pediatric Retina, 2nd edition. Philadelphia: Lippincott Williams & Wilkins; 2014. pp. 626-39.
39. Walsh MK, Drenser KA, Capone A Jr, Trese MT. Early vitrectomy effective for Norrie disease. Arch Ophthalmol. 2010;128(4):456-60.
40. Walsh MK, Drenser KA, Capone A Jr, Trese MT. Norrie disease vs familial exudative vitreoretinopathy. Arch Ophthalmol. 2011;129(6):819-20.
41. Walsh MK, Drenser KA, Capone A, Jr., Trese MT. Early vitrectomy effective for bilateral combined anterior and posterior persistent fetal vasculature syndrome. Retina. 2010;30(4 Suppl):S2-8.
42. Wood EH, Drenser KA, Capone A Jr. Diagnosis and management of familial exudative vitreoretinopathy: a lifelong, progressive, and often asymmetric disease. JAMA Ophthalmol. 2019;137(9): 1059-60.
43. Wu LH, Chen L-H, Xie H, Xie Y-J. Prenatal diagnosis of a case of norrie disease with late development of bilateral ocular malformation. Fetal Pediatr Pathol. 2017;36(3):240-5.
44. Wu WC, Drenser K, Trese M, Capone A Jr, Dailey W. Retinal phenotype-genotype correlation of pediatric patients expressing mutations in the Norrie disease gene. Arch Ophthalmol. 2007; 125(2):225-30.
45. Wycliffe ND, Mafee MF. Magnetic resonance imaging in ocular pathology. Top Magn Reson Imaging. 1999;10(6):384-400.
46. Yamane T, Yokoi T, Nakayama Y, Nishina S, Azuma N. Surgical outcomes of progressive tractional retinal detachment associated with familial exudative vitreoretinopathy. Am J Ophthalmol. 2014;158(5):1049-55. e1041.
47. Yang X, Wang C, Su G. Recent advances in the diagnosis and treatment of Coats' disease. Int Ophthalmol. 2019;39(4):957-70.
48. Zahavi A, Weinberger D, Snir M, Ron Y. Management of severe persistent fetal vasculature: case series and review of the literature. Int Ophthalmol. 2019;39(3):579-87.

14

CHAPTER

Retinopathy of Prematurity

Rajvardhan Azad, Sony Sinha, Prateek Nishant

INTRODUCTION

Retinopathy of prematurity (ROP; ICD-11 H35.1) is a vasoproliferative disorder affecting the immature, incompletely vascularized retina of premature infants. The spectrum of outcome findings ranges from the most minimal sequelae without affecting vision in mild cases to bilateral irreversible and total blindness. Low birth weight and prematurity are the main risk factors for the disease.

EPIDEMIOLOGY

The estimated global preterm birth rate for 2014 was 10.6% (uncertainty interval 9.0–12.0), equating to an estimated 14.84 million (12.65–16.73 million) live preterm births in 2014. 12.0 million (81.1%) of these preterm births occurred in Asia and sub-Saharan Africa. Approximately, 14% of all preterm infants are born with a gestational age of <32 weeks and are at particular risk of ROP. ROP is a leading cause of preventable childhood blindness, accounting for blindness or severe visual impairment in 20,000 (15,500–27,200) preterm births, and mild/moderate visual impairment in a further 12,300 (8,300–18,400) preterm infants worldwide, most of whom are born in low- to middle-income countries. In a study reporting data on infants with severe ROP, the mean birth weights from highly developed countries ranged from 737 to 763 g compared with values ranging from 903 to 1527 g in less developed countries. Mean gestational age of infants from highly developed countries ranged from 25.3 to 25.6 weeks compared with 26.3–33.5 weeks in less developed countries. In a recent study from the USA among 30–40 million live births, the total ROP incidence was 0.17% overall and 15.58% for premature infants.

India has the largest number of preterm births and accounts for 23.4% of all such births globally. An estimated 490,000 preterm infants are born with gestational age <32 weeks out of which 5,000 require treatment for ROP every year. According to 2016 estimates, approximately, 20% (3,200) of the surviving preterm infants are likely to develop any ROP and 5% (8,000) are at risk of blindness/visual impairment from sight threatening ROP. Additionally, infants with a gestational age of 32–36 weeks are also at the risk of sight threatening ROP particularly in settings where they receive less than optimal care. The incidence of ROP in India was reported earlier to vary between 38 and 51.9%. A recent study shows a declining trend over a period of 20 years, wherein the overall incidence of ROP has decreased to 26.6%. However, the comparison of epidemiological indicators of ROP from hospital or population-based studies is the biggest challenge because of substantial variability in screening criteria and study designs. Healthcare workers and their professional organizations today have a responsibility to improve data collection to track preterm births and measurements, such as consistent assessment of gestational age, birth weight, cause of death, data on impairment of vision, and ROP.

HISTORICAL PERSPECTIVE

Retinopathy of prematurity was first identified by Terry in 1942, designating the condition as retrolental fibroplasia based on his impression that the primary change involved a proliferation of the embryonic hyaloid system which incorporated the retina. Heath coined the term ROP in 1951 based on histopathological studies, which became the more accepted nomenclature.

In developed countries, two epidemics of ROP have been described. The "first epidemic" (of blindness) occurred in the 1940s and 1950s and principally affected premature babies in the USA and, to a lesser extent, Western Europe. At that time, unmonitored supplemental oxygen was the principal risk factor. Campbell in 1951 suggested that the toxic effects of oxygen in the neonates caused the disease. In 1953, studies proved that high concentrations of oxygen were causative. In 1954, Ashton hypothesized the release of vasoformative substances from the hypoxic retina. Thereafter, the practice of rigid curtailment of oxygen in the nurseries resulted in a sharp decline in the incidence of ROP. However, a comitant increase in morbidity and mortality led to discontinuation of this practice. Subsequently, decreased gestational age and low birth weight were recognized to be the most important risk factors, apart from administration of oxygen.

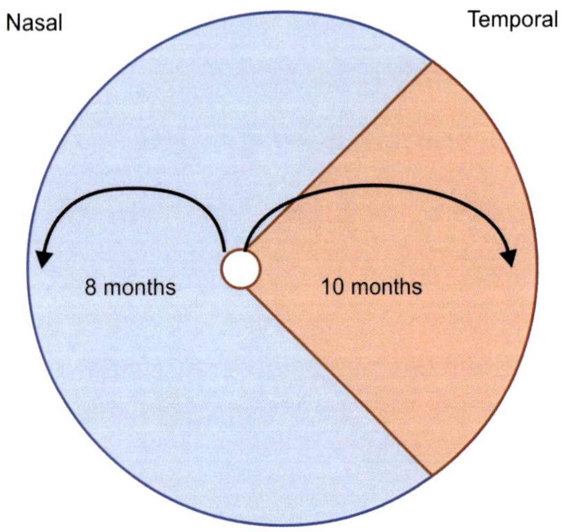

Fig. 1: Vascularization of the human retina. The white circle denotes the optic disk.

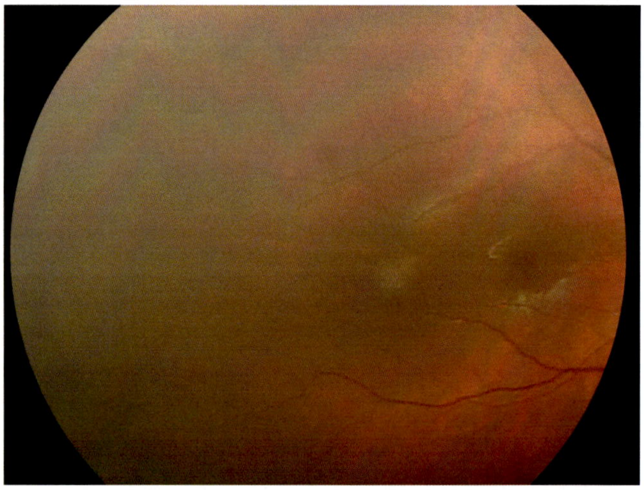

Fig. 2: Temporal avascular retina in a neonate born at 28 weeks of gestational age (33 weeks of postconceptional age).

The resultant policy of rigid curtailment gave way to monitored and controlled oxygen administration. A "second epidemic" (of acute ROP) in industrialized countries started in the 1970s, as a consequence of higher survival rates in extremely premature babies with advancements in neonatology. A similar situation now prevails in developing countries like India, which is now facing the "third epidemic" of ROP. Due to the escalation of services provided to the preterm infants in special newborn care units and intensive neonatal care units of Government and private sectors, there is an amplified risk of sight-threatening ROP(ST-ROP) in the Indian population. The risk of blindness due to ROP may be predicted on the basis of infant mortality rate (IMR) of a country.

- *Infant mortality rate ≤ 8/1,000*: Low risk due to good neonatal care and nursing.
- *Infant mortality rate = 9–60/1,000*: High risk due to inadequate screening and neonatal care.
- *Infant mortality rate ≥ 61/1,000*: Low risk due to poor survival of premature infants.

PATHOGENESIS

In the human embryo, the retinal fetal circulation begins to develop (*vasculogenesis phase*, 14th–21st week of gestation) from the disk at the 100 mm stage in the form of cords of mesenchymal spindle cells arising from the adventitia of the hyaloid artery that later canalize to transform into endothelial cells of the four major arcades of retinal vessels. After the 21st week, the retinal vascular development by budding of proliferating endothelial cells from existing blood vessels *(angiogenesis phase)*. The growth progresses at the rate of 0.1 mm/day until it reaches within one disk-diameter of the nasal ora serrata at the end of the 8th month gestational age and temporal ora serrata by the 10th month **(Fig. 1)**. Hence in later months of pregnancy, our main concern is of the advancing vascular network between equater and the ora

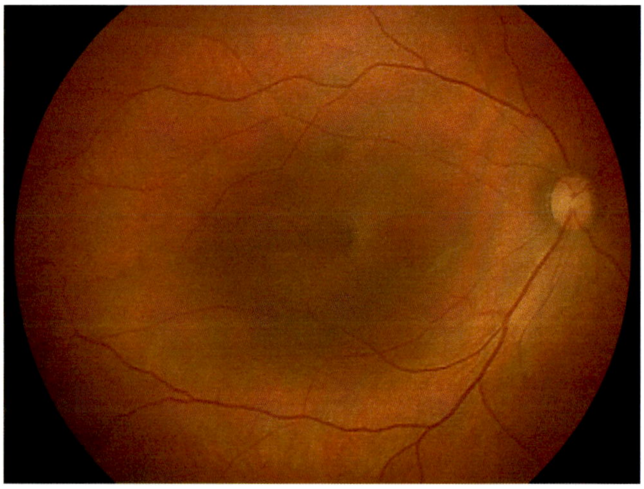

Fig. 3: Retinal vascularization is nearly complete at 40 weeks of postconceptional age.

(Fig. 2). Full retinal vascularization takes place in 90–100% infants by 40 weeks of conceptional age **(Fig. 3)**. Any retinal vascularization falling at least one-and-a-half disk diameters short of the ora has to be considered pathological.

The *classical theory* of pathogenesis of ROP proposed that elevated arterial perfusion pressure of oxygen causes retinal vasoconstriction, leading to vascular closure. If vasoconstriction is sustained, subsequent permanent vascular occlusion occurs. Thereafter, when the neonate returns to room air, endothelial cell proliferation adjacent to closed capillaries leads to neovascularization. The neovascularization may even reach the vitreous, producing hemorrhage, fibrosis, vitreous traction, and retinal detachment.

The *spindle cell theory* by Kretzer et al., postulated the induction of retinal and vitreal neovascularization by spindle cell insult. It proposed that after birth, spindle cells are exposed to hyperoxic environment because of increased oxygen diffusion from choroidal vasculature. Oxygen free radicals act as a cytotoxic agent and attack the compromised spindle cells which have poorly developed antioxidative defense mechanisms. Thus, abnormal spindle cells stop migration and canalization, and begin to release some angiogenic factor which leads to neovascularization.

Hellstrom in 2003, suggested role of insulin-like growth factor I (IGF-I) in the pathogenesis of ROP, as he observed that ROP is associated with low neonatal IGF-I serum concentrations and poor growth, however, recent work by Ley et al., treatment of preterm infants with recombinant human IGF-I/IGF binding protein-3 until 30 postmenstrual weeks showed no effect on ROP.

Our current understanding of ROP involves complex relationship between avascular retina, immature retinal vessels, oxygen levels, and angiogenic factors, especially vascular endothelial growth factor (VEGF). Vitreous levels of VEGF are elevated in ROP patients, as vitreous fluid samples for ROP eyes stimulate in-vitro growth of endothelial cells.

Physiologic expression of normal amounts of VEGF in the normal retina in utero likely helps to control vessel development and regression. However, ex utero, changes in oxygen tension may cause abnormal up or downregulation of VEGF expression, as occurs in the avascular retina of the preterm neonate with a larger avascular zone exposed to hyperoxic environment. Decreased VEGF expression leads to untimely vaso-obliteration, which, if sustained, causes ischemia and hypoxia in the nonperfused retina. This in turn, stimulates VEGF production and exaggerated vasoproliferation. Over time, if VEGF production decreases, ROP will regress, if VEGF production increases or persists, ROP progresses.

The *NDP* gene product "Norrin" is a ligand with conserved cysteine-knot residues. It activates the *Wnt* signaling pathway for early retinal development and vasculogenesis. There is clear evidence that *Norrin-Frizzled4* signaling is essential for vascularization beyond the early stages of vasculogenesis. Point mutations of the conserved cysteine residues result in improper protein folding. Patients with these mutations have severe retinal dysgenesis, whereas patients with noncysteine mutations have varying degrees of avascular peripheral retina, extraretinal vasculature, and subretinal exudate. This explains why the clinical features of ROP resemble familial exudative vitreoretinopathy (FEVR). In other studies, pathogenic variants of *FZD4, LRP5,* and *TSPAN12* genes were found to imply a role in the development of ROP.

PATHOLOGY

The pathology of ROP is divided into three zones, five stages, 12 clock hours, preplus disease, plus disease, and aggressive posterior (AP) ROP according to the revised International Classification of ROP (ICROP). The retina is divided into three zones by two concentric circles, each centered on the optic disk (**Fig. 4**):

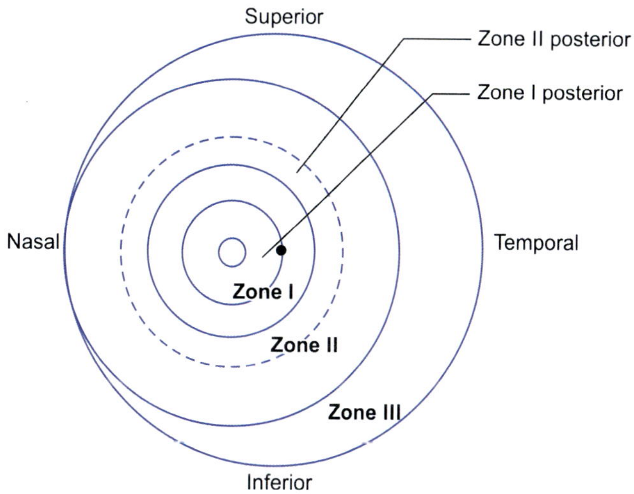

Fig. 4: Zones of ROP in right eye. The black dot denotes the center of the macula, and the central white circle is the optic disk.

1. *Zone 1*: Area within a circle with radius twice the distance from center of the optic disk to center of the fovea. By placing the nasal edge of the optic disk at one edge of the field of view, zone 1 is the temporal edge of the field of view with a +28 D lens. Zone I is further subdivided into anterior and posterior. Posterior zone I is a circular area defined by the radius from the disk to the center of the macula. ROP in this area is known as *zone half* ROP, which is seen in extremely premature infants wherein the macula is poorly developed.
2. *Zone 2*: Area outside zone 1, delimited by a circle with radius the distance from center of the optic disk to nasal margin of the retina (ora serrata). Zone II is also subdivided into anterior and posterior. The anterior boundary of posterior zone II is located one disk diameter peripheral to the anterior border of zone I. ROP should be considered zone II till it can be determined with confidence that the nasal-most 2 clock hours are vascularized to within one-disk diameter of the ora serrata.
3. *Zone 3*: The remaining crescent-shaped zone largely comprised of the temporal retina.

Histologically and clinically, the stages of ROP are:

- *Stage 1*: Presence of a white demarcation line (one-dimensional—length) at the junction of the vascular and avascular retina characterized by hyperplasia of vanguard mesenchymal tissue. (**Fig. 5**).
- *Stage 2*: Ridge formed by the transformation of demarcation line (three-dimensional—including height and width) due to further hyperplasia of the spindle cells, along with proliferation of the endothelial cells of the rear guard mesenchymal tissue (**Fig. 6**). Small isolated tufts of neovascular tissue lying on the surface of the retina called "popcorn" lesions may be seen separately posterior to the ridge.

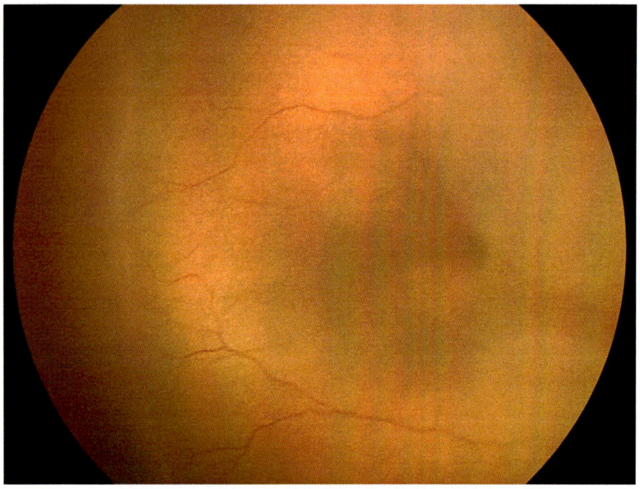

Fig. 5: Stage 1—demarcation line.

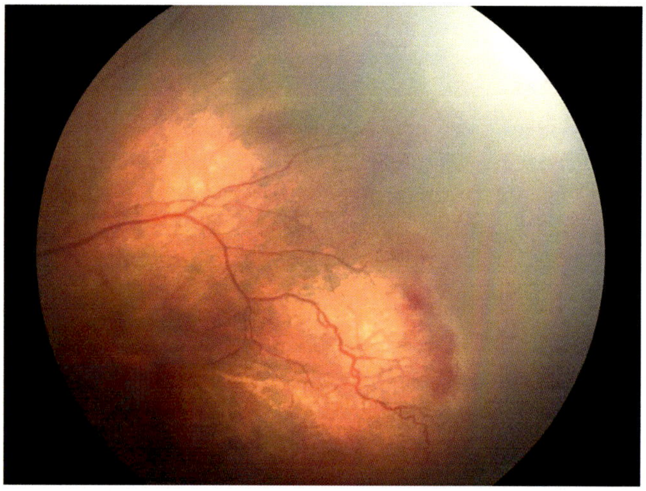

Fig. 7: Stage 3—Fibrovascular proliferation.

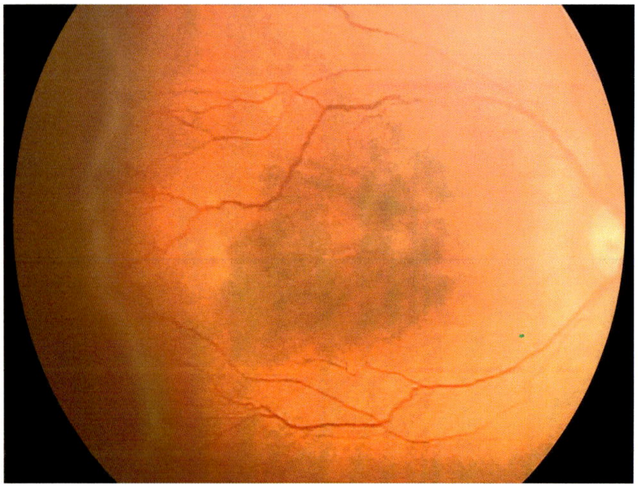

Fig. 6: Stage 2—ridge.

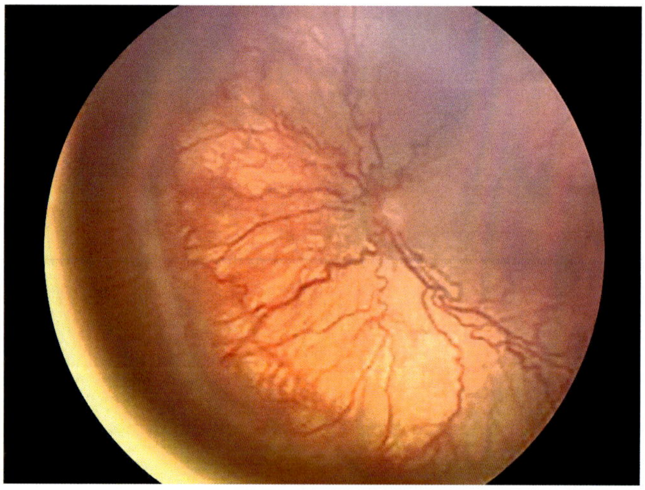

Fig. 8: Advanced fibrovascular proliferation (temporally) with plus disease. Note venous dilation and arterial tortuosity in the posterior pole with vitreous haze superiorly and nasally.

- *Stage 3*: Extraretinal fibrovascular tissue proliferates from the ridge due to abnormal angiogenesis of small, thin-walled vessels **(Fig. 7)**. The posterior aspect of the ridge appears irregular as the proliferation becomes more extensive **(Fig. 8)**.
- *Stage 4*: Subtotal retinal detachment occurs due to condensation of vitreous into sheets and strands oriented anteriorly toward the equator of the lens causing antero-posterior traction, and later by combined mechanism. They are generally concave and circumferential.
- *Stage 5*: Total retinal detachment, generally tractional but occasionally exudative. It occurs when the fibrovascular tissue at the ridge starts contracting. The vascularized posterior retina is progressively detached, while the avascular peripheral retina remains attached. This leads to a "peripheral trough" of variable width. Subsequently, the fibrosis spreads over the surface of the vascularized retina and extends across the trough up to the ciliary processes. Retinal detachments are usually funnel shaped, open, or closed anteriorly or posteriorly. Additionally, retrolental fibrovascular proliferation, acute angle closure, corneal edema, iris atrophy, posterior synechiae, ectropion uveae, and glaucoma can be present.

Plus Disease

Increased venous dilation centrally and peripherally, arterial tortuosity mainly centrally, associated with iris vascular engorgement, poorly dilating pupil and vitreous haze in at least two quadrants **(Fig. 8)**. Absence of plus disease is to be documented in clinical notes as "no plus" or "—" (minus).

Preplus Disease

Posterior pole tortuosity and dilatation to a lesser extent than plus disease that may not progress to the latter.

Aggressive Posterior Retinopathy of Prematurity ("Rush Disease")

Uncommon, severe form, can rapidly progress to retinal detachment without going through stages 1–3. This usually occurs in the smallest, most immature (<1,000 g and <30 weeks of gestational age) infants. There are prominent tortuous vessels at the posterior pole (zone I > zone II) forming arcades with otherwise innocuous looking retina sans ridge or extraretinal proliferation. Significant dilation of arterioles and venules makes it difficult to distinguish between them. There may be ill-defined, flat, mild-appearing, easily overlooked neovascularization at the junction between avascular and vascular retina circumferentially, often accompanied by a circumferential vessel or hemorrhages. The presence of annular or C-shaped hemorrhages and extraretinal fine vascular tangles without fibrosis is key findings that point to AP-ROP. This stage is better visualized with a +20 D than a +28 D lens.

Hybrid Retinopathy of Prematurity

Retinopathy of prematurity in which features of both AP-ROP and staged ROP are found, including saw-toothed shunts, tangled vasculature, closely packed multiple bridging shunts, anomalous circumferential vessels, retinal and preretinal hemorrhages, and ridge formation. Three patterns are described:

1. *Pattern I*: Ridge at the junction of vascular and avascular retina.
2. *Pattern II*: Ridge in the vascularized posterior retina.
3. *Pattern III*: Ill-defined ridge close to the optic disk, with mat-like fibrous proliferation into the vitreous. It may have worse prognosis.

Disease Extent

This is recorded as 1–12 clock hours of 30° sectors each. Total clock hours involved may be contiguous or noncontiguous and are recorded as such.

Regressed Retinopathy of Prematurity

Location of ROP changes to a more peripheral zone in serial examination, ridge color changes from salmon pink to white.

Peripheral vascular changes include failure of vascularization, abnormal, nondichotomous branching of retinal vessels, and vascular arcades with circumferential interconnection and telangiectatic vessels. Peripheral retina also shows pigmentary and vitreoretinal interface changes, thinning, peripheral folds, lattice-like degeneration, breaks, vitreous membranes, and traction-rhegmatogenous retinal detachment.

Posterior pole vasculature shows tortuosity, straightening of vessels in the temporal arcade and decrease in angle of insertion of major temporal arcade. Posterior pole also shows pigmentary changes, distortion and ectopia of macula, stretching and folding of retina leading to periphery, vitreoretinal interface changes, vitreous membranes, dragging of retina over optic disk, and traction-rhegmatogenous retinal detachment.

TABLE 1: Early Treatment of Retinopathy of Prematurity Cooperative Group (ET-ROP) classification of prethreshold disease, and action required.

	Zone	*Stage*	*Plus*	*Action required*
Type 1 prethreshold	I	Any	+	Treatment
	I	3	—	
	II	2/3	+	
Type 2 prethreshold	I	1/2	—	Follow-up
	II	3	—	

Cicatricial Retinopathy of Prematurity

Untreated or partially treated eyes can present with cicatricial ROP with sequelae as disk and macular dragging, peripheral vitreoretinal-lenticular adhesions, and subretinal pigmentation from reattached exudative detachments. These eyes have variable potential for vision and often benefit from low vision services.

The early treatment of retinopathy of prematurity (ET-ROP) study defined the terms "'prethreshold" and "threshold" ROP.

- *Threshold ROP*: Five contiguous or eight noncontiguous clock hours of stage 3 plus ROP in zone 1 or zone 2. In this stage, treatment is mandatory as chances of progression to retinal detachment are 50% if left untreated.
- *Prethreshold ROP*: Less than threshold ROP; subdivided into type 1 (high risk) and type 2 (low-risk, **Table 1**). However, the decision to treat is now based on the zone, stage, and presence of plus disease, rather than the number of clock hours. In addition to type 2 ROP, plus disease, stage 2, and retinal hemorrhages are independent predictors of ROP for which referral is warranted.

RISK FACTORS AND PREVENTION OF RETINOPATHY OF PREMATURITY

The risk factors for ROP can be summarized in the form of an epidemiological triad in order to explain the interaction between them (**Fig. 9**).

Age

Median age at detection of stage 1, ROP is 34 weeks, whereas threshold ROP appears at 34–38 weeks. Prevention of ROP is pivoted on early screening before 30 days of life. However, a baby born earlier than 28 weeks of gestation should be screened at 2–3 weeks. Atypically, ROP-like retinal findings

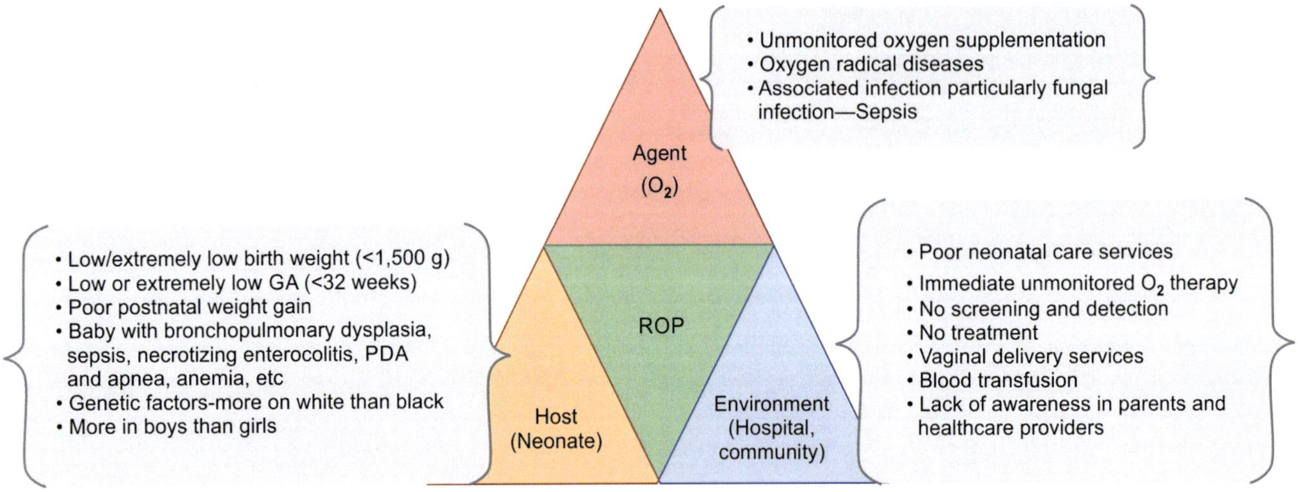

Fig. 9: Risk factors of retinopathy of prematurity.

Source: Senjam SS, Chandra P. Retinopathy of prematurity: addressing the emerging burden in developing countries. J Family Med Prim Care. 2020;9:2600.

may develop in near-term babies, and this may be related to retinal immaturity due to poorly understood causes.

Antenatal Steroid Use

Use of prenatal steroid is a well-known approach to prevent respiratory distress and intraventricular hemorrhage, two important risk factors of ROP. Antenatal steroids have not reduced occurrence of ROP, perhaps because smaller babies who are at higher risk of developing ROP are saved. Steroids improve lung maturity in preterm infants, and are likely to reduce need for oxygen therapy and thus reduce severe ROP.

Oxygen Therapy

Repeated hypoxic and hyperoxic episodes may be an important risk factor. Hence, strict management of oxygen delivery without fluctuations and with proper monitoring may be associated with decreased occurrence. If a preterm neonate <32 weeks of gestation needs resuscitation at birth, inhaled oxygen concentration (FiO_2) should be titrated to prevent hyperoxia and achieve gradual increase in oxygen saturation (70% at 3 minutes and 80% at 5 minutes after birth). Oxygen saturations in preterm neonates should be monitored with pulse oximetry and maintained between 90 and 95% to prevent infant death and severe ROP.

Blood Transfusion

The frequency of blood transfusions is an independent risk factor for development of ROP. This can be explained by the fact that adult RBCs are rich in 2,3-diphosphoglycerate and adult hemoglobin which binds less firmly to oxygen, thus releasing excess oxygen to the retinal tissue. It may also be related to iron overload due to repeated blood transfusions.

Postnatal Weight Gain

Poor postnatal weight gain implies <50% of birth weight by 6th week of life. WINROP®, an online monitoring system available at *www.winrop.com*, following weight gain, predicts development of ST-ROP. In a Swedish nation-based cohort of extremely preterm infants, WINROP correctly identified 96% of the infants who required treatment for ROP type 1. However, in the Indian scenario, initial experience has shown that population-specific tweaking of algorithm may improve the result and practical utility of WINROP.

Retinopathy of prematurity exhibits a predilection to start first in the nasal retina of the most immature neonate. The propensity to extend circumferentially is greatest when the site at onset is superior, followed by nasal and inferior retina.

SCREENING FOR RETINOPATHY OF PREMATURITY

The subject of screening for ROP is a matter of immense medicolegal importance, especially in India wherein failure to screen on the part of the neonatologists and ophthalmologists has resulted in heavy monetary penalty. The guidelines below are to be strictly followed by neonatologists and ophthalmologists for screening of ROP. An ROP diary should be maintained by all clinics supervising screening work and defaulters if any should be tracked. The minimum necessity is that all babies at risk of ST-ROP are screened and treated.

American Screening Guidelines

Babies ≤1,500 g birth weight or ≤30 weeks of gestational age, or selected infants with birth weight 1,500–2,000 g or gestational age >30 weeks may be screened at the discretion of the attending neonatologist.

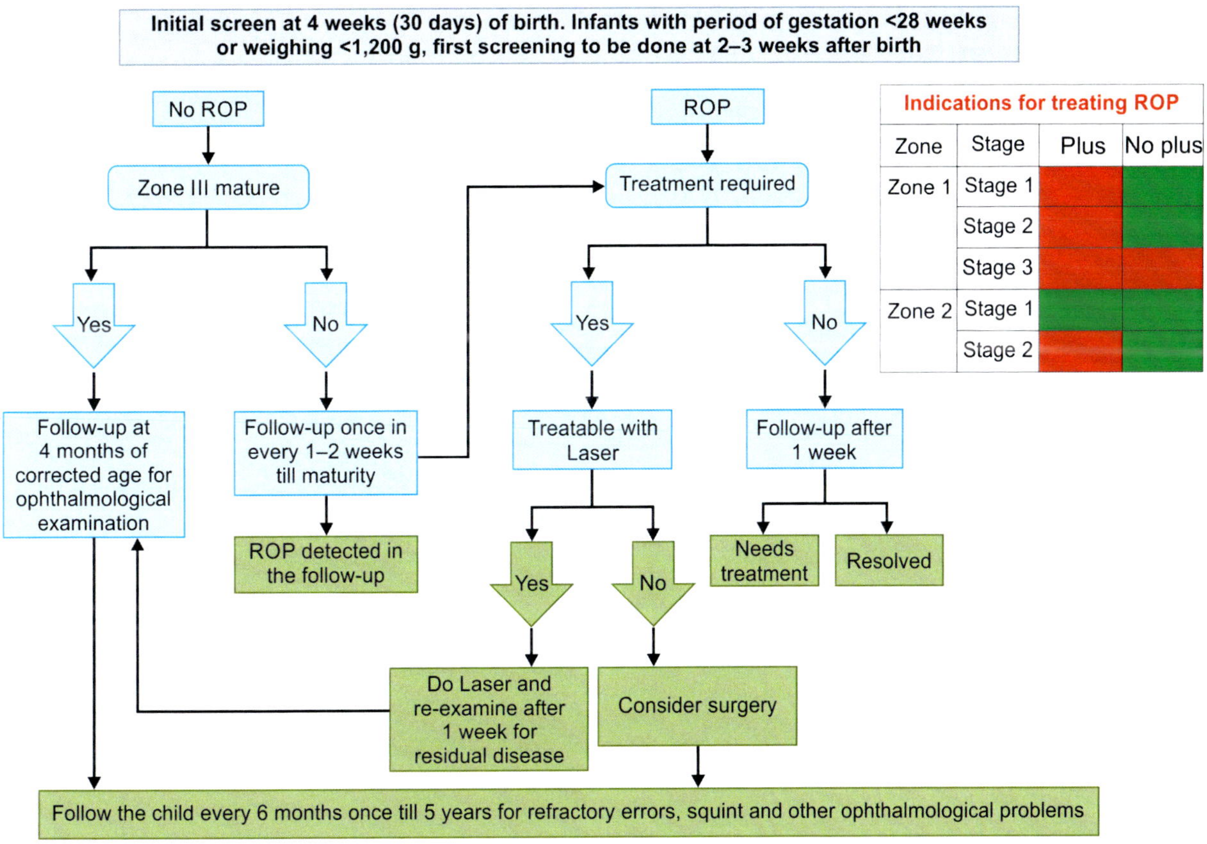

Fig. 10: Summary of screening, treatment, and follow-up protocol for ROP. In the chart on the top right, a red box implies that treatment is warranted.

Source: Rashtriya bal swasthya karyakram, Ministry of Health & Family Welfare, Government of India. (2017). Guidelines for Universal Eye Screening in Newborns including Retinopathy of Prematurity. [online] Available from: https://nhm.gov.in/images/pdf/programmes/RBSK/Resource_Documents/Revised_ROP_Guidelines-Web_Optimized.pdf [Last accessed August, 2021].

Indian Guidelines

Babies ≤2,000 g birth weight or ≤34 weeks of gestational age, gestational age 34–36 weeks with any of the above risk factors or any infant with an unstable clinical course may be screened, as determined by the neonatologist or pediatrician.

First screening should be at 4 weeks of birth, except for infants born at gestational age <28 weeks or <1,200 g who should be screened at 2–3 weeks after delivery **(Fig. 10)**.

EXAMINATION PROCEDURE

Neonates are best examined in the neonatal unit itself under supervision of attending pediatrician/neonatologist with all aseptic precautions. Stable and discharged babies can be reexamined as outpatients at ophthalmologist's office, however, basic resuscitation equipment should be readily available.

Pupils are dilated using a combination of 2.5% phenylephrine and 0.4–0.5% tropicamide. These eye drops, if not available commercially, are prepared by diluting available preparations with methylcellulose eye drops. Tropicamide 0.5% alone or cyclopentolate 0.5% alone may also be used. These drops should be instilled twice after a gap of 15 minutes. Care should be taken as phenylephrine has a propensity to raise the blood pressure of the neonate. Excess drops should be wiped from the medial canthus to avoid absorption and systemic toxicity.

If the pupil does not dilate, tunica vasculosa lentis, plus disease, or AP-ROP should be suspected. However, repeating drops should be avoided to prevent toxicity.

Care should be taken that the baby should have been fed no later than half an hour prior to examination, and is swaddled. Sterile sucrose solution 24-33% orally has been shown to reduce pain, followed by a pacifier. After instilling a topical anesthetic drop like proparacaine 0.5%, a neonatal wire speculum (alphonso speculum) is inserted to keep the eyelids apart. The room illumination is dimmed.

Screening of ROP involves indirect ophthalmoscopy (IO) using +20/28/30 D lens by an experienced ophthalmologist. First, the anterior segment of the eye is examined to look for tunica vasculosa lentis, pupillary dilation, and lens/media clarity followed by the posterior pole to look for plus disease. This is followed by sequential examination of all clock hours of the peripheral retina starting consistently with either the nasal or temporal retina, with scleral depression using schocket pediatric indenter or wire vectis. Oculocephalic reflex is used to aid the examination with the head being turned toward the side being examined. After examination, the child is given a mild antibiotic for a couple of days. A careful record of findings of anterior and posterior segment is then made.

The speculum and the scleral depressor are to be sterilized preferably by autoclave wherever available. If disinfection is needed between cases, it can be washed with povidone-iodine 10% solution, or soaked in 1:100 bleach solution for 10 minutes, followed by sterile water rinse. Rim of the fundus-viewing lens should be wiped with alcohol swab.

WIDEFIELD DIGITAL FUNDUS CAMERA SCREENING

Widefield retinal imaging has a sensitivity of 80–100% and specificity of 94.5–96% for ROP screening. RetCam®, RetCam Shuttle® (Clarity Medical Systems, Inc, Pleasanton, CA, USA; field of view 130°), Phoenix Icon (Phoenix Technology Group, LLC, Pleasanton, CA, USA; field of view 100°), 3nethra Neo® (Forus Health, Bangalore, India; field of view 120°), or smartphone-based portable retinal cameras can be an adjunct to document the status and explain to parents. It can also be used as a telescreening tool, remotely interpreting images to identify cases that require referral for immediate treatment or follow-up after treatment. For example, the Karnataka Internet Assisted Diagnosis of Retinopathy of Prematurity (KID-ROP) tele-ROP model demonstrates that ROP services can be delivered through using widefield imaging, telemedicine, nonphysician graders, and smart phone reporting to outreach despite lack of specialists. Automated analysis of fundus images is also possible, and newer computer programs such as ROP tool and artificial intelligence algorithms can measure tortuosity and dilation of posterior pole blood vessels in RetCam images. Retcam-assisted intravenous fluorescein angiography has also been found to be safe and helps in early diagnosis, prompt management, and monitoring regression. Optos® ultrawidefield scanning laser ophthalmoscope (Optos PLC, Dunfermline, UK; field of view 200°) has also been used for screening, however, reports suggest that it is stressful for the baby and may warrant SaO_2 monitoring.

DIFFERENTIAL DIAGNOSIS

Conditions that mimic acute ROP in infancy include FEVR, Norrie's disease, incontinentia pigmenti, and persistent fetal vasculature.

In advanced cases, the differential diagnosis of leukocoria includes exudative detachment in retinoblastoma, congenital cataract, persistent fetal vasculature syndrome (mostly unilateral, associated microphthalmos, and prominent ciliary processes), toxocariasis, toxoplasmosis, and coloboma of the optic disk or choroid. Differential diagnosis in case of vitreous hemorrhage must include shaken baby syndrome. Later in life, it is essential to rule out endogenous endophthalmitis, Coat's disease, diffuse choroidal hemangioma, and genetic syndromes such as trisomy 13, Norrie's disease, Warburg syndrome, and incontinentia pigmenti by genetic testing and/or characteristic systemic findings.

SUMMARY OF TRIALS IN RETINOPATHY OF PREMATURITY

CRYO-ROP (1983–2003)

In this multicenter trial of cryotherapy for retinopathy of prematurity (ROP), 4,099 infants weighing <1,251 g at birth underwent sequential ophthalmic examinations, beginning at age 4–6 weeks, to monitor the incidence and course of ROP. Overall 65.8% infants developed ROP to some degree and 81.6% infants of birth weight less than 1,000 g developed ROP. The timing of retinal vascular events correlated more closely with postconceptional age (PCA = gestational age + chronological age) than with postnatal age, implicating the level of maturity more than postnatal environmental influences in governing the timing of these vascular events. 492 infants developed threshold ROP. At 3 months, 49.3% reduction in unfavorable outcome in treated eyes versus controls occurred.

It provided evidence for the beneficial effect of cryotherapy to the avascular area anterior to the ridge in threshold ROP, as 62% untreated and 44% treated eyes with threshold ROP in zone II, and 90% untreated eyes in zone I went on to have unfavorable outcome. The benefit obtained was maintained across 15 years of follow-up. It additionally found that both treated and untreated eyes develop high myopia.

STOP-ROP (1999)

In a study of 649 premature infants with confirmed prethreshold ROP in at least 1 eye and median pulse oximetry <94% saturation, conversion from prethreshold ROP to threshold was 48.5% for the conventional oxygen group (89–94% saturation) and 40.9% for the supplemental oxygen group (96–99% saturation). This difference was not statistically significant, thus supplemental oxygen did not cause additional progression of prethreshold ROP but also did not significantly reduce the number of infants requiring peripheral ablative surgery. However, the risk of adverse pulmonary events increased.

ET-ROP (2003)

Infants with bilateral high-risk prethreshold ROP (n = 317) had one eye randomized retinal ablative treatment and the fellow eye managed conventionally (control eye). In asymmetric cases (n = 84), the eye with high-risk prethreshold ROP was randomized to early or to conventional management. It found early laser ablation of avascular retina in high-risk eyes (prethreshold type 1) to improve both structural picture and grating acuity outcomes. Low risk (prethreshold type 2) is to be observed weekly or twice weekly

TABLE 2: Early treatment of retinopathy of prematurity (ET-ROP) screening recommendations.

First examination	*Every 2 weeks*	*Every week*	*Every 2–4 days, till regression*
4–6 weeks 32 weeks postconception age Birth weight < 1,500g Gestational age < 32 weeks	Immature zone 2	Immature zone 1 Zone 2 stage 2	Zone 1 stage 1/2

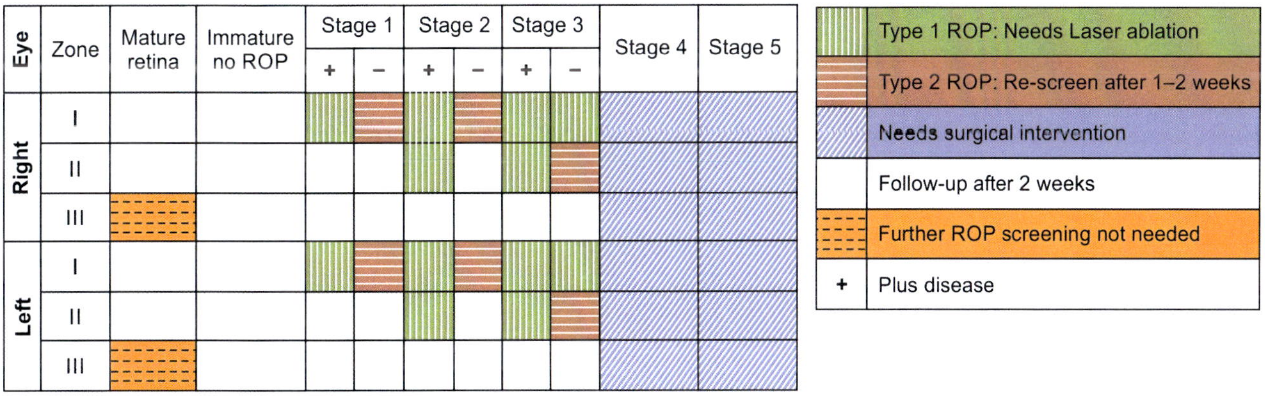

Fig. 11: Treatment protocol for ROP—suggested table to be included in screening documentation.

Source: Agarwal R, Deorari A, Paul V, Sankar M, Sachdeva A. Retinopathy of Prematurity: AIIMS Protocols in Neonatology. New Delhi: Noble Vision Publishers; 2019. pp. 468-81.

based on extent of ROP. It also recommended that infants with immature retina in zone II or III need to be reexamined every 2 weeks while those with immature zone I and zone II stage 2 need weekly follow-up. Infants with zone I, stage 1/2 needs to be followed up every 2–4 days **(Table 2 and Fig. 11)**.

PHOTO-ROP (2008)

This study evaluated the utility of remote digital fundus imaging as compared to IO to screen for ROP, and found that it is a useful adjunct to conventional bedside ROP screening, and highly unlikely that severe ROP would be missed when image quality was high. However, it is unlikely to supplant bedside ophthalmoscopic examination due to limitations in diagnostic sensitivity, specificity, and accuracy when image quality is poor.

BEAT-ROP (2011)

This study done on 150 infants with bilateral stage 3+ ROP zone 1 or posterior zone 2 compared bevacizumab monotherapy (0.625 mg in 0.025 mL) with conventional laser therapy. Primary outcome measure, recurrence of retinal vascularization by 54 weeks postconceptional age, was ascertained in 143 surviving infants. The rate of recurrence with zone 1 disease alone was significantly higher with conventional laser therapy (42%) than with intravitreal bevacizumab (IVB) (6%). The rate of recurrence with zone II posterior disease alone did not differ significantly between the two groups. Apparently, this trial seems to have given a green signal for the use of anti-VEGF monotherapy for zone I threshold disease. However, this study was too small to assess the safety profile in these babies. 71% of infant deaths occurred in those who had received bevacizumab. Moreover, the failure rate for laser treatment was unusually high as compared to ET-ROP study. Therefore, before accepting the veracity of results, one ought to study this trial and other reports critically. It also showed that eyes treated with anti-VEGF showed lowered risk of refractive errors (relative risk for very high myopia at 30 months of age = 0.06).

CARE-ROP (2016)

This pilot study among 19 infants between September 2014 and August 2016 demonstrated that ranibizumab was effective in controlling acute ROP and that 24% of the standard adult dose (0.12 mg) appeared equally effective as 40% (0.2 mg).

RAINBOW Trial (2017)

"Ranibizumab (0.2 mg and 0.1 mg per 0.02 mL) versus laser therapy for the treatment of very low birth weight infants (<1,500 g) with ROP" was an open-label multicentric superiority trial. It was conducted among 225 participants (214 assessed for primary outcomes at 24 weeks) in two regions, 26 countries, and 87 centers. It showed that ranibizumab seems to be superior to laser therapy associated with better eye outcomes and acceptable short-term safety profile, with unchanged systemic levels of VEGF among those with ROP zone I any stage, zone II stage 3+ or AP-ROP. Ranibizumab 0.2 mg (80%, odds ratio 2.19) was more effective than 0.1 mg (75%, odds ratio 1.57), which was more effective than laser (66%, p = 0.051). Lack of subgroup analysis between zone II stage 3+ and AP-ROP is a limitation of this trial.

The 5-year extension study of the RAINBOW trial is ongoing (available at: *https://clinicaltrials.gov/ct2/show/NCT02375971*).

MANAGEMENT

Ablation of Peripheral Avascular Retina

Timely treatment of ROP prevents retinal detachment and scarring and optimizes visual outcome.

Cryotherapy

In 1970s, Japanese physicians treated the ridge and adjacent avascular retina using cryotherapy. Hindle and Leyton in Canada treated the ridge and retina anterior and posterior to it. Kretzer et al., advocated the role of cryotherapy of the ridge and adjacent posterior avascular zone to destroy classified spindle cells, the presumed source of angiogenic factor. Ben-Sira and Nisssenkorn were the initial proponents of treating only the avascular zone and were supported by Topilov and Ackerman who also emphasized the width of the avascular zone as the prognostic factor. The procedure is difficult, time-consuming, and requires general anesthesia.

Complications are lid edema, conjunctival laceration, preretinal and vitreous hemorrhage as well as systemic complications such as bradycardia, cyanosis, and respiratory depression. Therefore, it is presently done only in cases with poor fundus visibility, lack of laser availability, or lack of training with indirect laser delivery techniques.

Laser Photocoagulation

Laser is the standard of care with indications for type I prethreshold ROP, threshold ROP, and AP-ROP. As compared to cryotherapy, there is less post-treatment pain, adnexal edema, exudative retinal detachment, vitreoretinal traction, and vitreous hemorrhage, due to reduced breakdown of the blood-retinal barrier. With infrared (810 nm) diode laser, favorable anatomic results have been reported in almost 85% eyes with zone I and posterior zone II disease, outcome is 86–93% for threshold ROP and nearly 100% for prethreshold ROP. Frequency-doubled neodymium-doped yttrium aluminum garnet (Nd:YAG) laser or 532 nm argon green laser can also be used. Presence of tunica vasculosa lentis is not a contraindication for laser.

Informed consent of parents is mandatory. Neonatology clearance for laser photocoagulation is mandatory in order to assess the general condition and oxygenation status, and discuss the need for intubation and concerns about apnea and/or bradycardia. Baby is fed an hour before and pupils are dilated.

Technique

Laser treatment is to be performed under supervision of neonatologist/anesthetist using laser indirect ophthalmoscope (LIO) delivery system and a +20/28 D lens. It is done either in the neonatal intensive care unit (NICU) or in an operating room equipped with suction apparatus and resuscitation and intubation equipment, but may have to be performed even when the neonate is inside the incubator with the laser projected through the wall of the incubator. The procedure is generally done under topical anesthesia with or without sedation. A neonatologist must monitor the swaddled baby continuously during the laser treatment. A neonatal lid speculum and scleral depressor/wire vectis are to be used to visualize the retina while frequent instillation of lubricant eye drops provides a clear view. An assistant holds the head while the surgeon stabilizes the chin between the fork formed by the little finger and ring finger, simultaneously holding the 20 D lens with the other three digits.

Grade II gray laser burns, 100 μm spot size, are applied in a near-confluent pattern half-burn-width apart. It is prudent to start by demarcating the posterior limit of ablation first, followed by burns in the avascular area closest to the most severe pathology first, thereupon proceeding to the entire avascular area up to but generally excluding the ridge. The burns may be titrated beginning from 300 mW to 300 ms, and areas requiring indentation should be treated last. A total of 1,500–1,800 spots may be required. Posterior retina requires more energy than anterior retina, and AP-ROP requires more spots, more intense and tightly spaced. Supplementary treatment to skip areas can be given. In recent studies, additional posterior barrage was found to be a safe technique that led to faster and more complete regression in eyes with zone 2 stage 3 advancing ROP. The most difficult areas to focus are the inferotemporal mid-periphery in each eye (7 o'clock in right eye and 5 o' clock in left). Residual new vessels arising from inadequate treatment are not uncommon in these areas.

The eyelids and conjunctiva generally have moderate edema, erythema, and subconjunctival hemorrhage for 3–4 days. NICU staff and parents must be told of these adnexal effects to avoid alarm. Postlaser, one drop of homatropine 2% is instilled once- or twice-a-day in both eyes for 5 days. Topical steroids are prescribed thrice a day to reduce any inflammation and to decrease the risk of postlaser posterior synechiae. With weekly follow-up, signs of regression are noted which are characterized by the following **(Figs. 12A and B)**:

- Media clears
- Pupil dilates fully and readily
- No new vessels in the iris
- No new vessels in the retina
- All retinal/preretinal and vitreous hemorrhages clear
- Regression of dilatation and tortuosity of retinal vessels
- No increase in retinal traction manifested by disk/macula/arcade drag
- No elevation of retina/ridge at or posterior to area of laser
- Feeder vessels to area of active new vessels/hemorrhages/elevated ridge and so on, achieve normal caliber

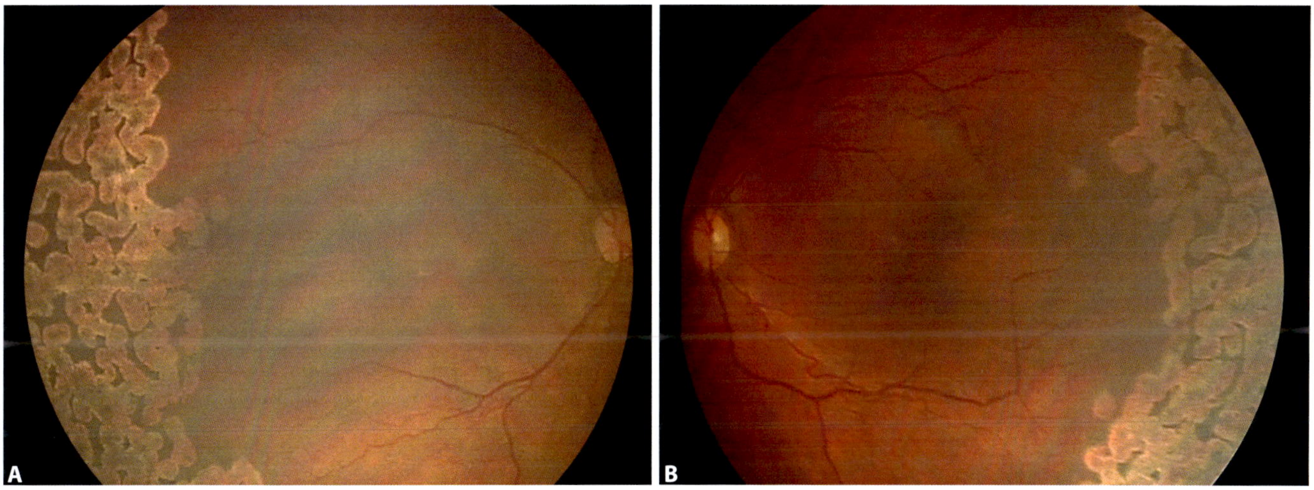

Figs. 12A and B: Laser photocoagulation was performed in this patient for stage 3+ ROP at a gestational age of 26 weeks and birth weight of 980 g. 4 weeks later, the eyes show complete regression of ROP with no plus disease.

- Demarcation between laser-treated and normal retina is quiet and flat in terms of vasculature, with adequate scar effect of the laser.

The treatment of AP-ROP may be undertaken in a single session with laser spots delivered to the avascular periphery, including the retina underlying flat neovascularization. It may also be undertaken in stages wherein in the first sitting, the laser spots are delivered to the avascular periphery up to the flat neovascularization, with a second sitting 5–10 days later, when the neovascular frond involutes, to treat the residual retina under direct visualization. Eyes with AP-ROP may follow an atypical course after laser ablation. Such eyes may still fare poorly, even when plus disease wanes. Additional laser to avascular retina may be necessary after the overlying flat stage 3 neovascularization regresses. The absence of obvious fibrosis at the time of laser should provide no reassurance as to reduced probability of progression to retinal detachment. A gestational age of <29.5 weeks, posterior zone 1 disease, preretinal hemorrhages, and need for repeat laser treatment are the significant risk factors for progression to retinal detachment despite confluent laser.

Complications include corneal, iris or ciliary body burns, cataract, Bruch's membrane rupture, retina and vitreous hemorrhage, ocular ischemic syndrome, angle closure glaucoma and inadvertent damage to the vascularized retina including macula.

Surgery for Retinopathy of Prematurity

Indications

Less than three clock hours of stage 4A detachment can be observed because often the fibrovascular membrane spontaneously separates into the vitreous cavity causing release of traction on the retina. Laser and/or intravitreal ranibizumab (IVR) treatment may be effective as a nonsurgical treatment for selected cases of stage 4A ROP (specially stage 4A ROP <6 clock hours). Surgery is indicated for retinal detachments (stage 4A, stage 4B, and stage 5 ROP), dense vitreous hemorrhage, and bilateral cases. Apart from B-scan ultrasonography to assess funnel configuration, ultrasound biomicroscopy (UBM) performed preoperatively is an effective tool to assess anterior surgical space in eyes with stage 5 ROP.

A trained anesthesiologist and preferably a neonatologist as well should be involved in administering anesthesia to the baby.

Scleral Buckling

In Stage 4a and b, an encircling band of 2.5 mm is applied with or without external drainage; a paracentesis should be performed in the latter case. Success rates of 60–75% have been reported. The band needs to be divided after 3–6 months to permit growth of the eye.

Lens-sparing Vitrectomy

The aim of surgery is to sequentially remove as much proliferation as possible, taking care not to cause iatrogenic tears in the retina and to avoid touching the lens. Trocar sclerotomies are made 0.75–1.25 mm posterior to the limbus through the pars plicata or plana with trocars and instruments angled toward the center of the eye. Ports are placed in areas with minimum fibrovascular proliferation, even if it requires an "all-nasal" approach. Surgical planes of dissection are in the following order:

- Ridge/retina to lens/anterior hyaloid face
- Ridge to ridge
- Ridge to optic nerve
- Ridge to vitreous base and
- Circumferentially along the ridge

The posterior hyaloid often cannot be removed due to its firm attachment. There is poor prognosis for reattachment, if iatrogenic retinal tears occur. The anatomic success of lens-sparing vitrectomy (LSV) for stage 4A ROP has been reported to be up to 100%, and 4B up to 75%. LSV in stage 4B ROP achieves greater success than lensectomy and vitrectomy. It has been seen that the lens remains clear for several years after LSV.

Lensectomy and Vitrectomy

In surgery for stage 5 ROP, ports are made 0.5 mm posterior to the limbus creating a cleavage plane in the retrolenticular tissues using two bent 26-gauge needles in a cruciate fashion. These membranes are then dissected from the center to the periphery. Viscoelastic injection into the funnel opens it up. Iris retractors may be used for better visualization of the periphery. An effort is made to relieve all traction and settle the posterior pole completely. No drainage is done, and extreme care is taken to avoid iatrogenic tears. Air-fluid exchange is performed at the end. After surgery, the child is placed face-down to tamponade the posterior pole and displace the subretinal fluid. The bulk of subretinal fluid absorbs in 2–4 months. This is followed by amblyopia therapy. Outcomes have been reported to be complete posterior pole attachment (macula attached) in 28% **(Figs. 13A and B)** and partial posterior pole attachment (macula detached) in 5%. Only a minority of eyes achieve visual acuity better than 5/200, and some successfully attached retinas later redetach.

Late identification of disease, lack of prior treatment, narrow-narrow funnel, and lensectomy and vitrectomy in the other eye are predictors for poor surgical outcome. Vascularly active stage 5, ROP detachments have poor prognosis. The use of intravitreal triamcinolone acetonide as a postoperative adjunct may improve the likelihood of retinal reattachment in select cases.

Intravitreal Anti-VEGF Therapy

Bevacizumab (Avastin®; Genetech, South San Francisco, CA, USA) was first found to be useful in 2007. In three cases of AP-ROP, the worse eye was treated with a single injection of 0.75 mg of IVB as monotherapy or complementary to laser therapy. In 24 hours, all injected eyes showed regression of the tunica vasculosa lentis and iris vessel engorgement and disappearance of iris rigidity. In the same year, Shah et al., also reported bevacizumab salvage treatment for postlaser anterior segment ischemia in a case of AP-ROP. Later, BEAT-ROP study advocated use of bevacizumab in stage 3 zone 1 or posterior zone 2 ROP in a dose of 0.75 mg, however, recently, half-adult dose i.e., 0.62 mg/0.025 mL has been found to be effective and safer. Ranibizumab (Accentrix®; Genetech, South San Francisco, CA, USA) 0.25 mg/0.025 mL and (1 mg/0.025 mL) of aflibercept (Eylea®, Regeneron Pharmaceuticals Inc., Tarrytown, NY, USA) have also been used for the same purpose.

The pharmacokinetics of anti-VEGF intravitreal injection in premature infants is not fully understood. Blood-retinal barrier is well developed in the adult eye, whereas it is compromised in the immature eyes of a premature baby. About two-thirds of pediatrics and retina specialists report lack of certainty in the systemic effects of intravitreal anti-VEGF agents to treat ROP. However, recent studies have found no reduction in circulating VEGF levels in neonates treated with IVR. The ongoing extended arm of the RAINBOW study will answer questions about the long-term safety and sequelae of this intervention.

Anti-VEGF agents have been used as monotherapy, combination therapy with laser or as an adjunct prior to vitrectomy.

Monotherapy

Several demerits of monotherapy with anti-VEGF in ROP have been reported. The peripheral retina remains avascular in about one-third to half of the cases. There can be atypical neovascularization and traction bands. In a study of 264 eyes with type 1 ROP, recurrence after treatment with ranibizumab

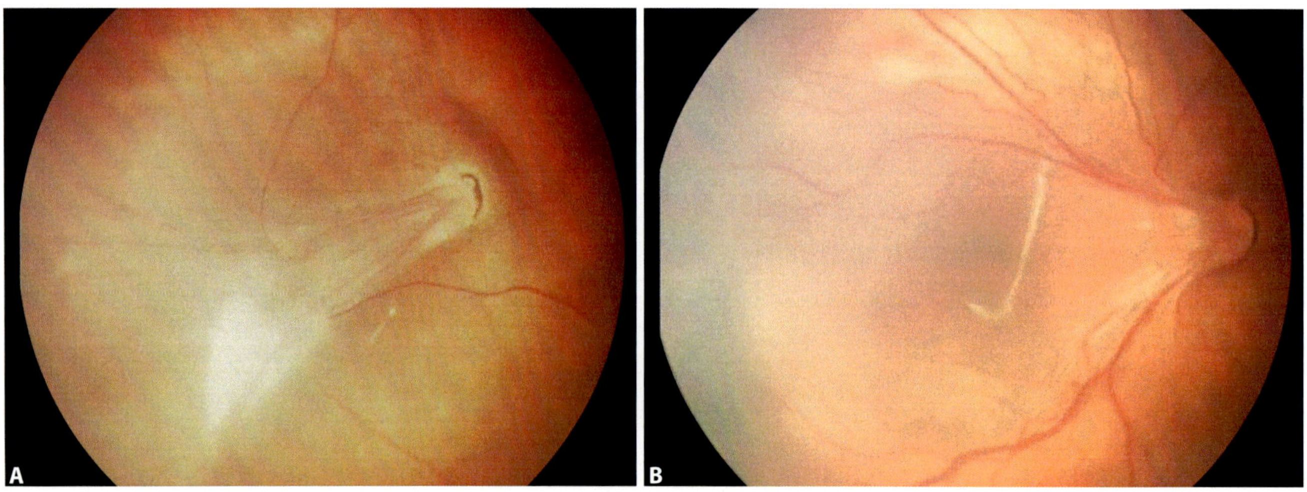

Figs. 13A and B: Fundus pictures showing anteriorly open—posteriorly closed funnel retinal detachment (stage 5 ROP, A) and its postoperative outcome after lensectomy and vitrectomy (B).

occurred at about 6 weeks earlier than with bevacizumab, which may be related to shorter half-life of ranibizumab.

A recent meta-analysis evaluated the efficacy and safety of anti-VEGF drugs when used either as monotherapy, or in combination with planned cryo/laser therapy in preterm infants with type 1 ROP. Monotherapy with IVB/IVR did not improve short-term structural outcomes (partial or complete retinal detachment and recurrence of ROP) but significantly reduced the risk of refractive errors at 30 months of age. While IVB/IVR might reduce the risk of recurrence of ROP in infants with zone I ROP, it can potentially result in higher risk of recurrence requiring retreatment in those with zone II ROP (see below).

Combination Therapy

As these drugs have no effect on mature vessels once pericytes have been laid down, a combination of anti-VEGF therapy (which neutralizes the preexisting VEGF in the vitreous cavity) and laser (which reduces the hypoxic stimulus to VEGF production) appears to be a logical mode of treatment. There is low level evidence that risk of complete or partial retinal detachment is significantly lower in the eyes of preterm infants with stage 3+ ROP randomized to intravitreal pegaptanib plus laser therapy, as compared to cryo/laser alone. In a recent series, about 78.6% of eyes with zone half ROP had unfavorable outcome with laser alone; combination therapy is indicated in such cases. For posterior zone I ROP, laser ablation should be applied after anti-VEGF at a time when vascularization proceeds to zone 2 and before the expected recurrence of the disease, i.e., 4–5 weeks after ranibizumab and 6–8 weeks after bevacizumab. Early laser may be considered in cases where extensive neovascularization and hemorrhages are present. In some cases, anti-VEGF may be considered first when laser machine, or an ophthalmologist trained to deliver laser is not immediately available **(Figs. 14A to C)**.

However, in a recent series, complications of adjunctive treatment with anti-VEGF for severe stage 3 plus after failed laser (seven eyes), stage 4A plus (eight eyes), and stage 4B/5 plus (nine eyes), included macular hole and retinal breaks causing rhegmatogenous retinal detachment, bilateral, progressive vascular attenuation, perivascular exudation, and optic atrophy.

Indications

Anti-VEGFs are indicated in case of severe rubeosis iridis causing poor pupillary dilation, media opacities such as vitreous hemorrhage and zone 1 ROP that has poor outcome with laser. The optimal window for treatment with anti-VEGF therapy is at the first sign of plus disease or neovascularization but before the formation of extensive fibrovascular membranes. If the latter is treated, fibrous contraction of the proliferative membrane, the most common local adverse effect, will cause tractional retinal detachment.

Technique

At the average age of 35–36 weeks, when the injection is given, infant eyes are small with 16 mm axial length and 12 mm posterior segment. By comparison, the lens, being adult-sized, occupies a large volume. The pars plana is poorly developed and the retina may be lifted in advanced stages. These anatomical differences have to be considered while administering the intravitreal injection. Despite this, there is no consensus regarding injection site in neonatal patients; a point of entry 0.75–1.5 mm behind the limbus may be safe, and transillumination of the sclera has been advocated for more accuracy. Entry is made parallel to the visual axis with a 30–32-gauge needle 4–8 mm in length. If bilateral injection is planned in the same sitting, both eyes can be cleaned with 10% povidone-iodine solution, draped with sterile plastic eye drape in a way that both eyes are exposed, both speculums

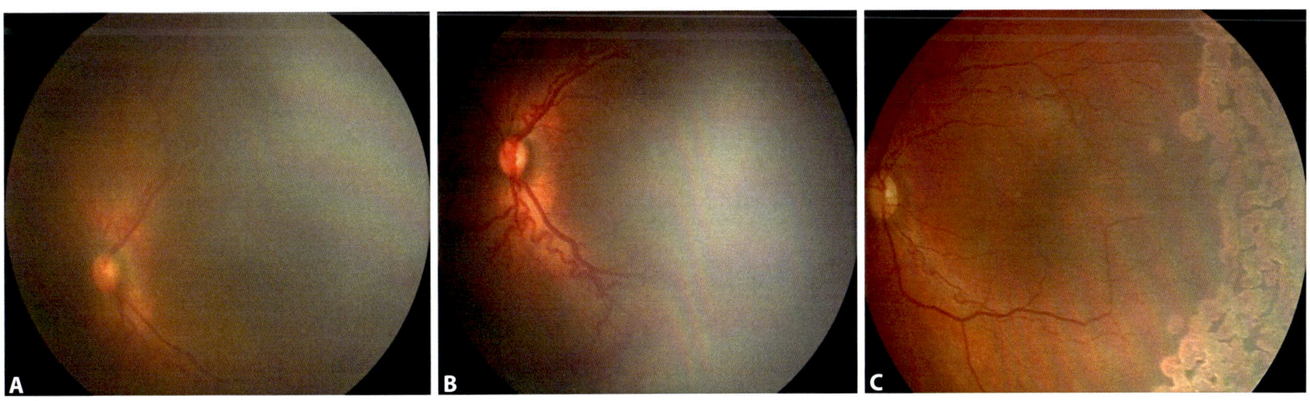

Figs. 14A to C: Sequential fundus photographs of the left eye of an infant of 30 weeks postconceptional age at presentation. The birth weight was 1,100 g and gestational age was 27 weeks. The patient had been on oxygen therapy for 16 days, and had a history of sepsis and blood transfusion. Examination showed a rigid pupil, tunica vasculosa lentis and extensive vitreous haze, with few tortuous vessels visible in the inferotemporal arcade (A). With a diagnosis of APROP, intravitreal bevacizumab was given. On day 3 postinjection, the vitreous haze had decreased and extensive dilated and tortuous vessels were visible throughout the retina (B). Thus, laser was done immediately. 14 days after laser, the fundus showed regressed ROP with no plus disease (C).

are placed together, and the surgeon changes gloves or scrubs again between successive injections in the two eyes. The surgeon's gloves should never touch the infant's skin or lashes. The conjunctival cul-de-sac is filled with a drop of 5% povidone-iodine solution before and after the injection. Postinjection topical antibiotics are given for a week.

Sequelae

Yetik et al., studied the effect of IVB for type-1 prethreshold, threshold, and AP-ROP. At least 1 week after in most of the cases, they observed that anterior segment becomes very silent, pupils can be fully dilated easily, vitreous clears and demarcation line with proliferations are replaced by a corkscrew-like communicating shunt-vessel between main branching retinal vessels like a filament in tungsten bulbs, the "tungsten filament sign". This condition is a sign of inactive disease and after a mean of 4.5–5 months of follow-up; the retina matures without any further treatment. However, persistence of avascular retina, loss of normal dichotomous branching, abnormal capillary tangles, and tungsten filament sign suggest persistent abnormal vasculogenesis after therapy.

After anti-VEGF for AP-ROP, at 6 weeks, sawtooth shunt (STS) vessels are seen at the junction of the vascular and avascular retina, with three morphological variations. Most commonly, these are thin, less curved, serrated STS bridging a large part of the entire circumference; second, a hybrid variant with part of the shunt as a multi-layered structure; and third, additional brush-border pattern fine vessels. Further, they persist for 1–14 weeks (mean 5–6 weeks) after which regression may occur either directly or after conversion to staged ROP, tanged vasculature, or anomalous circumferential vessels followed by staged ROP. It has been hypothesized that that the vascular changes following intravitreal anti-VEGF at half-adult doses could be classified into three major phases.

1. *Phase I*: Phase of rapid quietening that happens within a week of intravitreal injection secondary to rapid neutralization of the VEGFs already secreted into the vitreous.
2. *Phase II*: Slow vascular development that happens when the injected anti-VEGF is eliminated from vitreous with slow accumulation of new VEGF/other VEGF isoforms not blocked by the injected anti-VEGF.
3. *Phase III*: Regression of disease, similar to staged ROP.

Fundus fluorescein angiography with 1 mg/kg of 10% dye may be essential to detect recurrence during follow-up after laser or anti-VEGF. It can be done under general or topical anesthesia. The video camera of the wide field fundus camera should be kept on and recording started promptly after injection. Later on, stills of the various phases of FFA can be extracted for a permanent record.

Repeat Injection

Median time between treatment and retreatment was 55 days in ranibizumab 0.2 mg group and 57 days in ranibizumab 0.1 mg group in the RAINBOW trial.

Sequelae of Treated Retinopathy of Prematurity

Children with previously treated ROP may present with myopia—12–14% in prethreshold, 65–71% in severe ROP, and 21–100% in laser-treated ROP. In a study conducted by Katoch et al., among 69 eyes, the median refractive error was 0.75 D, 26.1% infants had myopia (SE > 0.25 D) and 1.4% had high myopia (SE > 5 D). Contributory factors are the smaller axial length and anterior chamber depth, more globular lens and a higher corneal refractive power. It has been found that myopia increases by -0.14 dioptres per 100 laser spots applied. Keratoconus associated with oculodigital sign has been described as a sequel of ROP. There is also risk of astigmatism, strabismus, cortical visual impairment, and anisometropia. Nearly half of all patients with treated ROP may develop strabismus. Cataract can occur from 2 months to 13 months after ROP, either spontaneously or after treatment with laser, LSV, or regressed ROP. Cataract surgery is made difficult by thick lens (pachyphakia), angle closure, and microcornea in these patients. Hence treated ROP should be followed up 3 monthly till 2 years of age, then 6 monthly till 6 years and annually thereafter.

Primary congenital glaucoma (rare), secondary closed or open angle or neovascular glaucoma may coexist with ROP, and the two have to be managed together.

CONCLUSION

The critical factors to ensure better outcomes in ROP are to screen early, follow-up closely, watch out for plus and/or new vessels, and treat such eyes vigorously for full avascular retina ablation. ROP is a continuous race against time with a very small window of opportunity of 7–10 days, where optimum treatment outcomes with least complications can be achieved. Safe and effective treatment techniques must be applied to achieve outcomes that are both optimal and satisfying in the long term.

ACKNOWLEDGMENTS

Prof Mangat Dogra, Dr Subhadra Jalali, Dr Deeksha Katoch, Dr Gaurav Sanghi, Dr Anand Vinekar, Dr Savleen Kaur, Dr Ramanuj Samanta, Dr Gitanjli Sood, Dr Devesh Kumawat.

SUGGESTED READING

1. Abdel HA, Mohamed GB, Othman MF. Retinopathy of prematurity: a study of incidence and risk factors in NICU of Al-Minya University Hospital in Egypt. J Clin Neonatol. 2012;1:76-81.
2. Agarwal K, Jalali S. Classification of retinopathy of prematurity: from then till now. Community Eye Health. 2018;31:S4-7.
3. Agarwal R, Deorari A, Paul V, Sankar M, Sachdeva A. Retinopathy of Prematurity: AIIMS Protocols in Neonatology. New Delhi: Noble Vision Publishers; 2019. pp. 468-81.
4. Ashton N, Ward B, Serpell G. Effect of oxygen on developing retinal vessels with particular reference to the problem of retrolental fibroplasia. Br J Ophthalmol. 1954;38:397-432.

5. Athikarisamy SE, Lam GC, Ross S, Rao SC, Chiffings D, Simmer K, et al. Comparison of wide field imaging by nurses with indirect ophthalmoscopy by ophthalmologists for retinopathy of prematurity: a diagnostic accuracy study. BMJ Open. 2020;10: e036483.
6. Axer-Siegel R, Maharshak I, Snir M, Friling R, Ehrlich R, Sherf I, et al. Diode laser treatment of retinopathy of prematurity: anatomical and refractive outcomes. Retina (Philadelphia, Pa.). 2008;28:839-46.
7. Axer-Siegel R, Snir M, Cotlear D, Maayan A, Frilling R, Rosenbaltt I, et al. Diode laser treatment of posterior retinopathy of prematurity. Br J Ophthalmol. 2000;84:1383-6.
8. Azad R, Chandra P, Khan MA, Darswal A. Role of intravenous fluorescein angiography in early detection and regression of retinopathy of prematurity. J Pediatr Ophthalmol Strabismus. 2008;45:36-9.
9. Azad R, Gilbert C, Gangwe AB, Zhao P, Wu WC, Sarbajna P, et al. Retinopathy of prematurity: how to prevent the third epidemics in developing countries. Asia Pac J Ophthalmol (Phila). 2020;9: 440-8.
10. Azad R, Khan M. Management of retinopathy of prematurity. In: Garg A, Prost ME, Azad R, Crouch ER, Mehta KR, Bovet JJ, Grover AK, Pajic B, Trivedi RH, Mehta CK (Eds). Surgical and Medical Management of Pediatric Ophthalmology. New Delhi: Jaypee Brothers Medical Publishers; 2007. pp. 1053-60.
11. Azad R, Mannan R, Chandra P. Role of ultrasound biomicroscopy in management of eyes with stage 5 retinopathy of prematurity. Ophthalmic Surg Lasers Imaging. 2010;41:196-200.
12. Azad R. Use of intravitreal anti-VEGF: Retinopathy of prematurity surgeons' in Hamlet's dilemma? Indian J Ophthalmol. 2011;59: 421-2.
13. Azad RV, Pal N, Chandra P. Enhanced mydriasis during indirect diode laser therapy for threshold retinopathy of prematurity. J Pediatr Ophthalmol Strabismus. 2006;43:54-5.
14. Azad RV, Pasumala L, Kumar H, Talwar D, Pal R, Paul VK, et al. Prospective randomized evaluation of diode-laser and cryotherapy in prethreshold retinopathy of prematurity. Clin Exp Ophthalmol. 2004;32:251-4.
15. Ben-Sira I, Nissenkorn I, Grunwald E, Yassur Y. Treatment of acute retrolental fibroplasia by cryopexy. Br J Ophthalmol. 1980;64:758-62.
16. Blair MP, Shapiro MJ, Hartnett ME. Fluorescein angiography to estimate normal peripheral retinal nonperfusion in children. J AAPOS. 2012;16:234-7.
17. Blencowe H, Lawn JE, Vazquez T, Fielder A, Gilbert C. Preterm-associated visual impairment and estimates of retinopathy of prematurity at regional and global levels for 2010. Pediatr Res. 2013;74:35-49.
18. Blencowe H, Moxon S, Gilbert C. Update on blindness due to retinopathy of prematurity globally and in India. Indian Pediatr. 2016;53(Suppl 2):S89-92.
19. Bron A, Tripathi R, Tripathi B. Wolff's Anatomy of the Eye and Orbit, 8th edition. London: Chapman and Hall; 1997.
20. Campbell K. Intensive oxygen therapy as a possible cause of retrolental fibroplasia; a clinical approach. Med J Aust. 1951;2:48-50.
21. Cernichiaro-Espinosa LA, Harper CA, Read SP, Wright LM, Scribbick FW, Young R, et al. Report of safety of the use of a short 32g needle for intravitreal anti-vascular endothelial growth factor injections for retinopathy of prematurity: a Multicenter Study. Retina (Philadelphia, Pa.). 2018;38:1251-5.
22. Chang TC, Tran KD, Cernichiaro-Espinosa LA, Leung EH, Grajewski AL, Hodapp EA, et al. Microcornea and thickened lens in angle closure following nonsurgical treatment of retinopathy of prematurity. J Ophthalmol. 2020;e7510903.
23. Charan R, Dogra MR, Gupta A, Narang A. The incidence of retinopathy of prematurity in a neonatal care unit. Indian J Ophthalmol. 1995;43:123-6.
24. Chawanpaiboon S, Vogel JP, Moller AB, Lumbiganon P, Petzold M, Hogan D, et al. Global, regional, and national estimates of levels of preterm birth in 2014: a systematic review and modelling analysis. Lancet Glob Health. 2019;7:e37-46.
25. Chawla D, Agarwal R, Deorari A, Paul VK, Chandra P, Azad RV. Retinopathy of prematurity. Indian J Pediatr. 2012;79:501-9.
26. Chow LC, Wright KW, Sola A, CSMC Oxygen Administration Study Group. Can changes in clinical practice decrease the incidence of severe retinopathy of prematurity in very low birth weight infants? Pediatrics. 2003;111:339-45.
27. Coats DK, Miller AM, Brady McCreery KM, Holz ER, Paysse EA. Involution of threshold retinopathy of prematurity after diode laser photocoagulation. Ophthalmology. 2004;111:1894-8.
28. Cusick M, Charles MK, Agrón E, Sangiovanni JP, Ferris FL, Charles S. Anatomical and visual results of vitreoretinal surgery for stage 5 retinopathy of prematurity. Retina (Philadelphia, Pa.). 2006;26:729-35.
29. Davitt BV, Christiansen SP, Hardy RJ, Tung B, Good WV. Incidence of cataract development by 6 months' corrected age in the early treatment for retinopathy of prematurity study. J AAPOS. 2013;17:49-53.
30. Dhingra D, Katoch D, Dutta S, Samanta R, Aggarwal K, Dogra MR. Change in the incidence and severity of Retinopathy of Prematurity (ROP) in a Neonatal Intensive Care Unit in Northern India after 20 years: Comparison of two similar prospective cohort studies. Ophthalmic Epidemiol. 2019;26:169-74.
31. Dogra MR, Katoch D, Dogra M. An update on retinopathy of prematurity (ROP). Indian J Pediatr. 2017;84:930-6.
32. Dogra MR, Katoch D. Current perspectives in the management of retinopathy of prematurity. Delhi J Ophthalmol. 2014;25:108-17.
33. Dogra MR, Singh SR, Katoch D, Dogra M, Moharana B, Jain S, et al. "All-nasal" approach for 25-gauge lens sparing vitrectomy in stage 4B retinopathy of prematurity. Retina (Philadelphia, Pa.). 2020.
34. Dogra MR, Vinekar A, Viswanathan K, Sangtam T, Das P, Gupta A, et al. Laser treatment for retinopathy of prematurity through the incubator wall. Ophthalmic Surg Lasers Imaging. 2008;39:350-2.
35. Drenser KA. Wnt signaling pathway in retinal vascularization. Eye Brain. 2016;8:141-6.
36. Early Treatment for Retinopathy of Prematurity Cooperative Group. Revised indications for the treatment of retinopathy of prematurity: results of the early treatment for retinopathy of prematurity randomized trial. Arch Ophthalmol. 2003;121:1684-94.
37. El Rayes EN, Vinekar A, Capone A. Three-year anatomic and visual outcomes after vitrectomy for stage 4B retinopathy of prematurity. Retina (Philadelphia, Pa.). 2008;28:568-72.
38. Ells AL, Gole GA, Lloyd Hildebrand P, Ingram A, Wilson CM, Geoff Williams R. Posterior to the ridge laser treatment for severe stage 3 retinopathy of prematurity. Eye (Lond). 2013;27:525-30.
39. Ells AL, Holmes JM, Astle WF, Williams G, Leske DA, Fielden M, et al. Telemedicine approach to screening for severe retinopathy of prematurity: a pilot study. Ophthalmology. 2003;110:2113-7.
40. Ezisi CN, Kekunnaya R, Jalali S, Balakrishnan D, Kumari PR, Mohamed A, et al. Cataract surgery in children with retinopathy of prematurity (ROP): surgical outcomes. Br J Ophthalmol. 2017;101:1128-31.
41. Fidler M, Fleck BW, Stahl A, Marlow N, Chastain JE, Li J, et al. Ranibizumab Population pharmacokinetics and free VEGF pharmacodynamics in preterm infants with retinopathy of prematurity in the RAINBOW Trial. Transl Vis Sci Technol. 2020;9(8):43.
42. Fielder AR, Shaw DE, Robinson J, Ng YK. Natural history of retinopathy of prematurity: a prospective study. Eye (Lond). 1992;6:233-42.

43. Fleming TN, Runge PE, Charles ST. Diode laser photocoagulation for prethreshold, posterior retinopathy of prematurity. Am J Ophthalmol. 1992;114:589-92.
44. Flynn JT, Chan-Ling T. Retinopathy of prematurity: two distinct mechanisms that underlie zone 1 and zone 2 disease. Am J Ophthalmol. 2006;142:46-59.
45. Fung THM, Abramson J, Ojha S, Holden R. Systemic effects of optos versus indirect ophthalmoscopy for retinopathy of prematurity screening. Ophthalmology. 2018;125:1829-32.
46. Gilbert C, Fielder A, Gordillo L, Quinn G, Semiglia R, Visintin P, et al. Characteristics of infants with severe retinopathy of prematurity in countries with low, moderate, and high levels of development: implications for screening programs. Pediatrics. 2005;115:e518-25.
47. Gilbert C, Rahi J, Eckstein M, O'Sullivan J, Foster A. Retinopathy of prematurity in middle-income countries. Lancet. 1997;350: 12-4.
48. Gilbert C. Retinopathy of prematurity: A global perspective of the epidemics, population of babies at risk and implications for control. Early Hum Dev. 2008;84:77-82.
49. Gohari M, Dastgheib SA, Noorishadkam M, Lookzadeh MH, Mirjalili SR, Akbarian-Bafghi MJ, et al. Association of eNOS and ACE polymorphisms with retinopathy of prematurity: A systematic review and meta-analysis. Fetal Pediatr Pathol. 2020;39:334-45.
50. Goktas A, Sener EC, Sanac AS. An assessment of ocular morbidities of children born prematurely in early childhood. J Pediatr Ophthalmol Strabismus. 2012;49:236-41.

15

CHAPTER

Ocular and Orbital Neoplastic Lesions in Children

Santosh G Honavar, Ankita Aishwarya, Raksha Rao

INTRODUCTION

The spectrum of ocular and orbital tumors in children differs from that of adults. Orbital cystic lesions constitute a unique entity seen commonly in children. Pediatric ocular tumors are challenging as they are often difficult to diagnose at the initial stages and a delay in diagnosis, even when benign, can have a grave visual prognosis and cause morbidity. While dermoids are the most common cystic lesions of the pediatric orbit, capillary hemangioma is the most common congenital tumor in the periocular region. Retinoblastoma (RB) is the most common intraocular malignancy and rhabdomyosarcoma is the most common extraocular orbital tumor. Leukemia, the most common overall malignancy of childhood, can cause leukemic deposits both in the orbit and retina. The objective of this article is to familiarize the reader with the common tumors, both benign and malignant, that affect the eye and orbit in the pediatric age group.

Tumors of the eye and orbit presenting in the pediatric age group are more commonly benign in nature, although malignant tumors can also occur rarely. Rapidly progressive tumors carry a potential risk for vision and eye loss, with malignant ones even carrying a risk to life. Hence, it is important to recognize them early and institute appropriate management. **Table 1** contains a list of ocular and orbital neoplastic lesions that can present in children. Only the more common tumors have been described in the following chapter.

EYELID TUMORS

Tumors of the eyelid in children are mostly benign and malignant eyelid lesions are generally associated with a systemic process that manifests itself in the eyelid or elsewhere in the body.

Capillary Hemangioma/ Strawberry Hemangioma

Overview

Congenital capillary hemangioma is the most common benign vascular tumor of the eyelid in children. They may have a systemic association with Kasabach–Merritt syndrome (hemangioma with thrombocytopenia) and PHACE syndrome (posterior fossa malformation, hemangiomas, arterial abnormalities, cardiac abnormalities, eye abnormalities, and sternal cleft and supraumbilical raphe syndrome).

Clinical Features

They generally present at birth or may develop a few weeks after birth and are generally unilateral. Depending upon the location, they can be classified into superficial, deep, and mixed. When superficial, they may be solitary presenting as a bright red, lobulated, soft, and compressible lesion **(Fig. 1A)**, or can be multifocal presenting as multiple cherry red lesions **(Fig. 1B)**; a deeper lesion appears purplish **(Fig. 2A)** which blanches on pressure and becomes more prominent on crying **(Fig. 2B)**. Some children may present with ptosis. These can have a conjunctival or orbital extension. Their growth pattern has been described in various phases; proliferative phase where the lesion grows rapidly in size for 6–12 months of age; this is followed by plateau phase in which the lesion is seen stable for 1–2 years and lastly, involutional phase where they slowly involute by 4–7 years of age. It has been estimated that about 30% of cutaneous capillary hemangioma regress completely by age 3 years and 75–90% by age 7 years. They have a potential risk for strabismus and amblyopia.

Treatment

Since the lesion regresses spontaneously, it is mostly observed and amblyopia treatment is initiated when necessary. Active treatment depends on the location, its severity, and any association with vision problems. The various treatment options are corticosteroids, cryosurgery, intralesional interferon α-2a, interferon α-2b, and laser treatment with pulsed dye laser (PDL), neodymium-doped yttrium aluminum garnet (Nd:YAG) laser, carbon dioxide laser, or argon laser. However, oral propranolol (2–3 mg/kg per day) and topical propranolol (1% ointment), a nonselective β-blocker, has been described as the first line of a drug. Topical administration may be indicated in small superficial lesions or PHACE syndrome due to a high risk of cerebral ischemia with systemic administration. Recently topical timolol maleate (0.5%) solution has been used for superficial ones.

TABLE 1: Classification of ocular and orbital neoplastic lesions in children.

Group	Benign	Malignant
Eyelid tumors		
Epidermal tumors	Eyelid papilloma	Xeroderma pigmentosum
	Sebaceous nevus	Basal cell carcinoma
Fibrous tumors	Juvenile fibromatosis	
	Eyelid nodular fasciitis	
Histiocytic tumors	Juvenile xanthogranuloma	
	Angiofibroma	
Pigmented tumors	Eyelid nevus	Melanoma of eyelid
	Oculodermal melanocytosis	
Neural tumors	Eyelid neurofibroma	
	Eyelid schwannoma	
Vascular tumors	Capillary hemangioma	
	Cavernous hemangioma	
	Eyelid lymphangioma	
	Varix	
	Eyelid nevus flammeus	
Others	Molluscum contagiosum	
	Pilomatrixoma	
Ocular surface tumors		
Choristoma	Dermoid	
	Dermolipoma	
	Complex choristoma	
	Epibulbar osseous choristoma	
Epithelial tumors	Papilloma	Conjunctival squamous cell carcinoma
	Hereditary benign intraepithelial dyskeratosis	
	Conjunctival dacryoadenoma	
Pigmented tumors	Conjunctival nevus	Conjunctival melanoma
	Ocular melanocytosis	
	Primary acquired melanosis	
Vascular tumors	Lymphangioma	
	Pyogenic granuloma	
	Conjunctival glomangiomas	
	Conjunctival capillary hemangioma	

Contd...

Contd...

Group	Benign	Malignant
Neural tumors	Conjunctival neurofibroma	
	Epibulbar schwannoma	
Fibrous tumor	Conjunctival nodular fasciitis	
	Fibrous histiocytoma	
Histiocytic tumors	Juvenile xanthogranuloma	
Intraocular tumors		
Iris tumors		
Cystic lesion	Iris pigment epithelial cyst	
	Congenital iris stromal cyst	
	Iris choristoma	
Pigmented tumors	Iris nevus	Iris melanoma
Vascular tumors	Iris capillary hemangioma	
Histiocytic tumors	Iris juvenile xanthogranuloma	
Others		Iris rhabdomyosarcoma
		Metastatic iris tumor
Choroidal and ciliary body tumors		
	Choroidal nevus	Choroidal melanoma
	Choroidal osteoma	Metastatic leukemia
	Choroidal hemangioma	Ciliary body rhabdomyosarcoma
	Ciliary body medulloepithelioma	
Retinal and optic nerve tumors		
	Melanocytoma of the optic nerve	Retinoblastoma
	Congenital hypertrophy of retinal pigment epithelium	
	Combined hamartoma of retina and retinal pigment epithelium	
	Astrocytic hamartoma of the retina	
	Retinal capillary hemangioma	
	Retinal cavernous hemangioma	
	Racemose hemangioma	

Contd...

Contd...

Group	Benign	Malignant
Orbital tumors		
Orbital cystic lesions	Dermoid cyst	
	Teratoma	
	Colobomatous cyst	
	Congenital cystic eye	
	Orbital cephalocele	
	Orbital mucocele	
	Congenital choristomatous respiratory cyst	
Orbital vascular lesions	Orbital capillary hemangioma	
	Orbital lymphangioma	
Orbital neural tumors	Schwannoma	Orbital alveolar soft part sarcoma
	Orbital neurofibroma	
	Orbital paraganglioma	
	Juvenile pilocytic astrocytoma	
	Optic nerve meningioma	
	Primitive neuroectodermal tumor	
Orbital myogenic tumors	Orbital leiomyoma	Rhabdomyosarcoma
Orbital fibrous tumors	Orbital nodular fasciitis	Orbital fibrosarcoma
	Orbital infantile myofibromatosis	
	Orbital solitary fibrous tumor	

Contd...

Group	Benign	Malignant
Orbital osseous tumors	Orbital fibrous dysplasia	Orbital osteosarcoma
	Orbital ossifying fibroma	
	Orbital giant cell reparative granuloma	
	Orbital cartilaginous chondroma	
Orbital lipomatous and myxomatous tumors	Dermolipomas	Orbital liposarcoma
	Orbital lipoma	
Orbital histiocytic tumors	Langerhans cell histiocytosis	
	Juvenile xanthogranuloma	
Orbital primary melanocytic tumors	Rosai–Dorfman disease Melanocytic hamartoma	
Lacrimal gland tumors	Pleomorphic adenoma	
Orbital metastatic cancer		Metastatic neuroblastoma
		Metastatic Wilms' tumor
		Metastatic Ewing tumor
Orbital lymphoma and leukemia		Non-African Burkitt lymphoma
		Post-transplantation lymphoproliferative disorder
		Granulocytic sarcoma ("chloroma")

Contd...

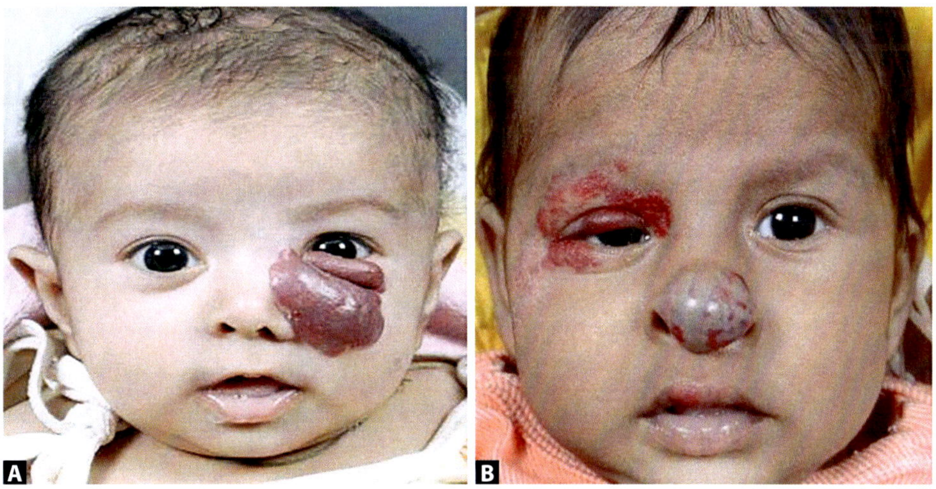

Figs. 1A and B: (A) Superficial capillary hemangioma arising from the lower eyelid and cheek. Note the bright red color and lobulation; (B) Multifocal superficial hemangioma involving upper and lower eyelid, forehead, nose, temporal scalp, and upper lip.

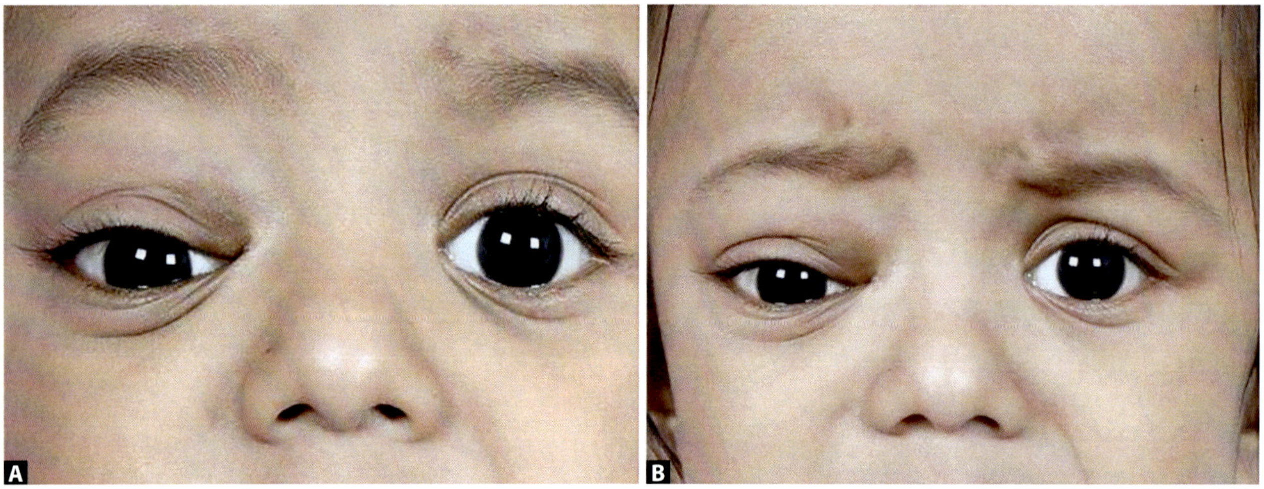

Figs. 2A and B: (A) Deep capillary hemangioma above the right upper eyelid imparting blue color to the skin; (B) Becomes more prominent when the child cries.

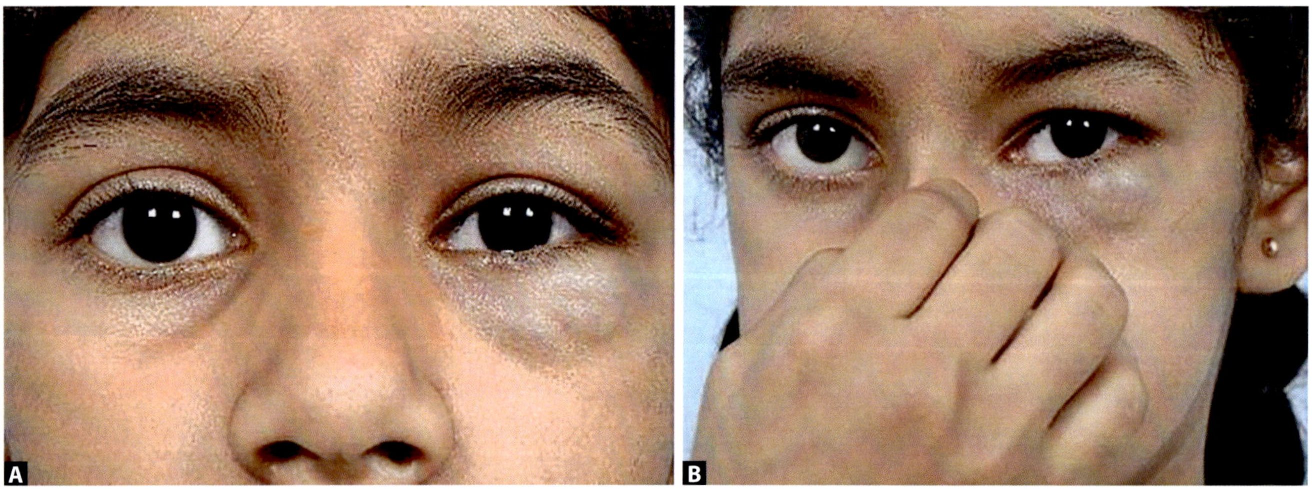

Figs. 3A and B: (A) Lymphangioma in the left lower eyelid with a bluish hue and an irregular surface; (B) Enlarges in size during Valsalva suggestive of associated venous malformation.

Lymphangioma

Overview

Eyelid lymphangioma is a hamartomatous growth of the lymphatic vessels that usually appears in the first decade of life. It mostly represents a superficial component of an orbital lymphangioma.

Clinical Features

It generally appears as a unilateral bluish soft compressible mass **(Fig. 3A)** which may increases on Valsalva if associated with lymphaticovenous malformation **(Fig. 3B)**. They may contain clear fluid, but often some of them contain blood and are called "chocolate cysts". Lymphangioma is associated with upper airway and palate lesions which increase during the viral illness.

Treatment

Various modalities have been tried for the treatment of lymphangioma but none of them is definite. Surgical excision is difficult due to excessive bleeding and radiotherapy usually does not eradicate the tumor. Injection bleomycin, a chemotherapeutic agent derived from *Streptomyces verticillus*, has been used with success due to its sclerosing effect on the endothelium of the abnormal vasculature when injected intralesionally. It is given at a dose of 0.5 mg/kg body weight and a maximum dose of 6 mg/mL can be injected. Other sclerosing agents such as sodium tetradecyl sulfate, OK-432 (Picibanil), and sodium morrhuate has been used. Repeat injections can be given in case of recurrence. Carbon dioxide laser and brachytherapy have been used to treat conjunctival lymphangioma with partial success.

Nevus Flammeus (Port-wine Stain)

Overview

This is a capillary malformation of vessels of the skin affecting the eyelid and periorbital region. About 10% have associated Sturge-Weber (congenital glaucoma, diffuse choroidal hemangioma, leptomeningeal hemangiomatosis, and seizures). Bilateral port-wine stains of the eyelids have a higher likelihood of being associated with Sturge-Weber syndrome. Sometimes they may have an association with Klippel-Trenaunay-Weber syndrome (nevus flammeus and hypertrophy of soft tissues and bone in the extremities).

Clinical Features

It manifests clinically as a sharply demarcated pink to purple patch that does not blanch with pressure **(Fig. 4A)**. The lesion is typically located along the trigeminal nerve but sometimes can be bilateral **(Fig. 4B)**. They may be associated with a higher incidence of ipsilateral glaucoma, diffuse choroidal hemangioma, and secondary retinal detachment.

Treatment

The port-wine stain does not regress, unlike eyelid capillary hemangioma. The child should be kept on close observation for glaucoma, choroidal hemangioma, and seizures. Various types of lasers have been used for cosmetic correction with carbon dioxide, argon laser, and PDL and they are effective in permanently closing the dilated blood vessels and improving the cosmetic appearance.

Eyelid Neurofibroma

Overview

Cutaneous neurofibromas are benign nerve tumors that can be solitary or diffuse; the latter one is associated with neurofibromatosis type 1. Based on the extent of tissue involvement, neurofibromas can be classified as cutaneous or subcutaneous, nodular plexiform, or diffuse plexiform. It is inherited as an autosomal dominant disease caused by a mutation in a gene located on chromosome 17.

Clinical Features

They generally appear towards the end of the first decade of life. Subcutaneous neurofibroma is usually a well-circumscribed solitary nodular lesion that is often confused with the chalazion **(Fig. 5A)**. They have a typical S-shaped deformity of the upper eyelid. In plexiform neurofibroma, the eyelid becomes very thick starting as an S-shaped deformity of the upper eyelid to contiguous involvement of the deeper tissues of the orbit leading to complete ptosis **(Fig. 5B)**. On palpation, it may demonstrate the classic "bag of worms" texture. This is also considered as the pathognomonic of type 1 neurofibromatosis (von Recklinghausen's disease). Evaluation of first-degree relatives should be done.

Treatment

If it single well-defined lesion then the treatment of choice is simple excision or even observation. If it is diffuse or plexiform then surgical resection is difficult because of its ill-defined nature and profuse bleeding at the time of surgical resection so debulking is attempted whenever cosmesis is needed.

Xanthogranuloma of the Eyelid

Overview

Eyelid xanthogranuloma (XG) is a benign self-limited cutaneous disorder of early childhood. Eyelid lesions are exceedingly rare. Cutaneous XG can be seen in both Langerhans cell histiocytosis (LCH) and juvenile xanthogranuloma (JXG), although very rare in the latter.

Clinical Features

It appears as placoid or elevated orange to yellow to the red lesion which is well demarcated as solitary or multiple

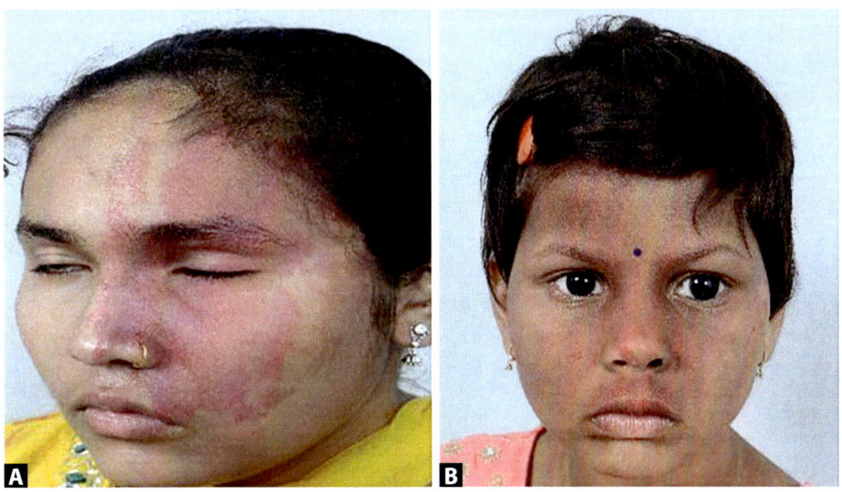

Figs. 4A and B: (A) Nevus flammeus involving left side of the face along V1 and V2 respecting midline on forehead and nose; (B) Bilateral nevus flammeus involving the forehead, eyelids, cheek, and chin of a 4-year-old girl.

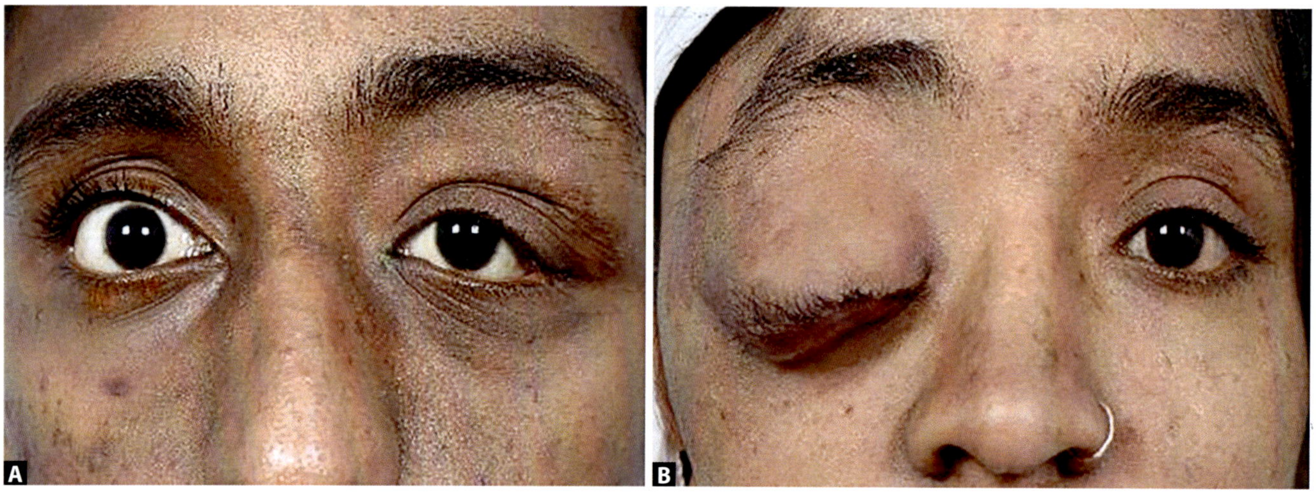

Figs. 5A and B: (A) Solitary nodular subcutaneous neurofibroma presenting as S-shaped lid deformity of the left upper eyelid; (B) Plexiform neurofibroma of the right upper eyelid in 16-year-old girl.

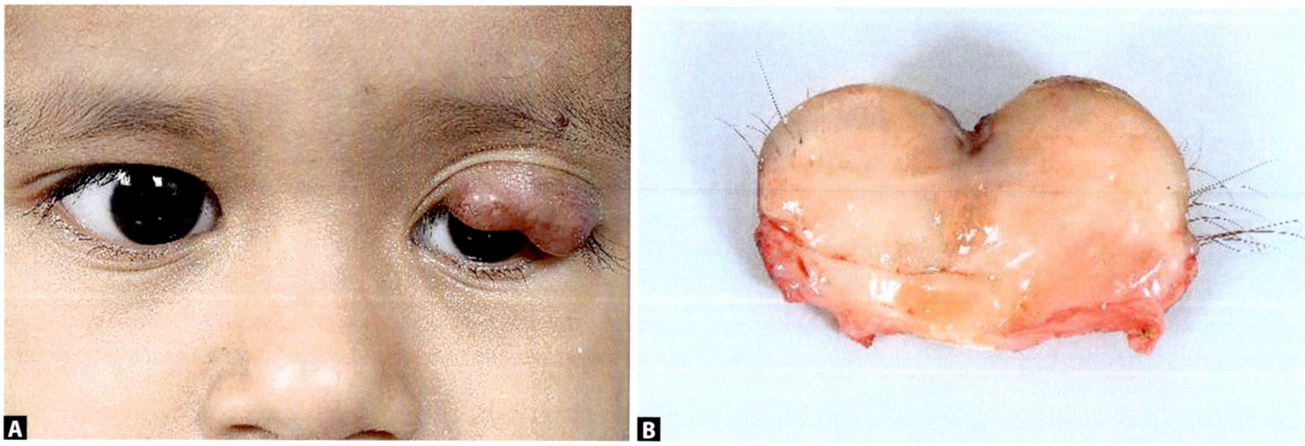

Figs. 6A and B: (A) Eyelid xanthogranuloma seen in the upper eyelid of the left eye; (B) Following excision biopsy.

nodules **(Figs. 6A and B)**. Regressed skin lesions often are flat and wrinkled in appearance and may leave atrophic hypopigmented scars.

Treatment

Since it is self-limited and resolves, observation is needed. Systemic or intralesional corticosteroids triamcinolone acetonide (40 mg/mL) can be given in recalcitrant cases and if no response surgical excision may be considered.

Molluscum Contagiosum

Overview

Molluscum contagiosum is an infection caused by a poxvirus which is a double-stranded deoxyribonucleic acid (DNA) virus. It is seen in children between 2 and 4 years of age. Single molluscum contagiosum lesion is more common in school-going children who are otherwise healthy while multiple lesions are seen in immunosuppressed patients. It can be transmitted via direct contact or indirectly via infected linens, swimming pools, or autoinoculation.

Clinical Features

They present as a single or multiple pale-pink-pearly elevated waxy smooth umbilicated lesion which is characteristic **(Fig. 7A)**. Lesions on the lid margin may have associated ipsilateral chronic follicular conjunctivitis **(Fig. 7B)**, epithelial keratitis, or pannus with mild discharge.

Treatment

It resolves spontaneously but shave excision, cauterization, chemical ablation, cryotherapy, and PDL may be needed in recalcitrant cases. Recently Perone LASIK forceps have been used for easy extraction of the eyelid margin lesions.

Eyelid Nevus

Overview

Congenital nevi are hamartomatous benign tumor seen in 2–3% of neonates. Based on the size they are classified into (1) small (<1–5 cm in diameter), (2) medium (1–5 cm to 20 cm in diameter), and (3) large (>20 cm in diameter). Sometimes, it may involve upper and lower eyelids of the same eye which

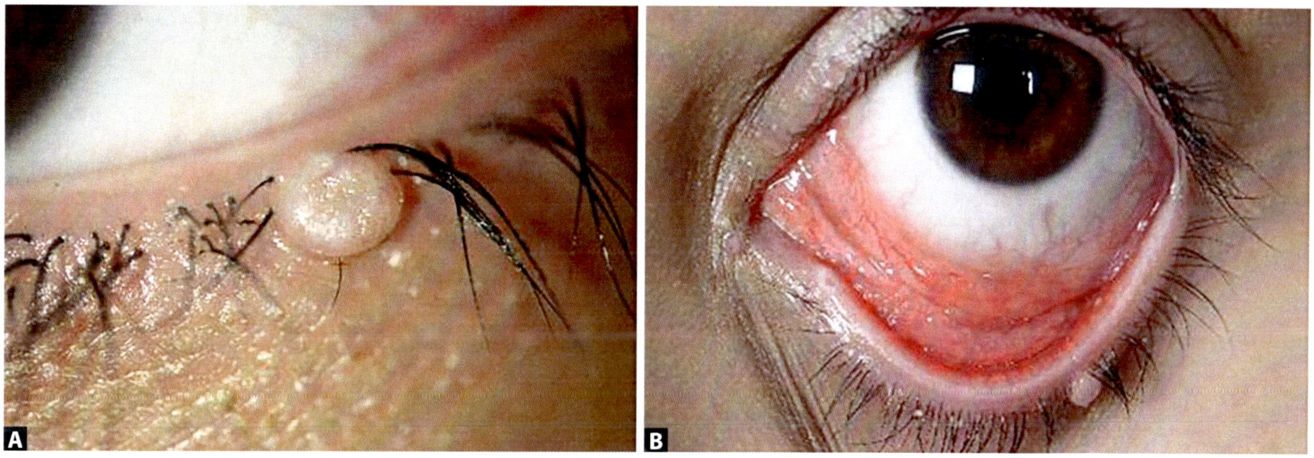

Figs. 7A and B: (A) A closer view of the left lower eyelid of the patient shows a waxy circumscribed papule with an umbilicated center; (B) Lower tarsal conjunctiva shows follicular conjunctivitis.

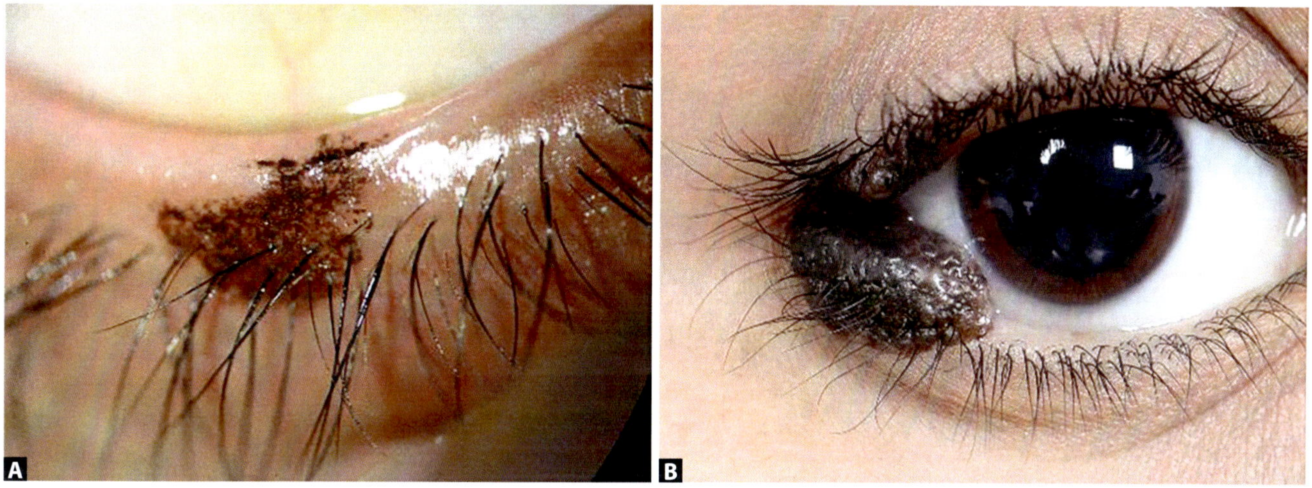

Figs. 8A and B: (A) Variably pigmented eyelid margin nevus with the upper palpebral conjunctival involvement of the left lower eyelid in a 14-year-old boy. Note that the cilia is intact; (B) Pigmented kissing nevus of upper and lower eyelids with micronodular elevated surface and excess hair.

is called kissing nevus or divided nevus. Larger elevated lesion with excess localized hair has a risk of malignant transformation in approximately 5% of the cases.

Clinical Features

It appears in the first decade of life as a flat variably pigmented lesion **(Fig. 8A)**, sometimes can be elevated or even hairs can be seen and may be associated with ptosis. It can involve any parts of the eyelid but involvement of the lid margin mandates careful examination of the tarsal, palpebral, and bulbar conjunctiva to be done as they may have a conjunctival extension. The kissing variant of the nevus may be elevated, thick, irregular surface, and associated with abnormal hair growth in a localized area **(Fig. 8B)**.

Treatment

Flat eyelid nevus is generally observed until there is an increase in size or associated loss or eyelash. Surgery is needed generally for the cosmesis or suspected malignant transformation. In the early years of life, the superficial lesion may be treated with dermabrasion. If deeper layers are involved, then the treatment consists of full-thickness excision followed by repair with skin graft is done.

OCULAR SURFACE TUMORS

Limbal Dermoid

Overview

A limbal dermoid is a choristoma (normal tissue in an abnormal location) and is the most common tumors of the corneal limbus. Choristomas makeup approximately 3% of conjunctival and corneal tumors. The growth rate of these masses is very slow or even stationary. Anatomically, they have been classified into three grades. Grade I limbal dermoid is a superficial lesion measuring <5 mm. Grade II limbal dermoids are larger and extend into the corneal stroma down to Descemet's membrane. Grade III limbal dermoids involve the whole cornea and structures of the anterior chamber.

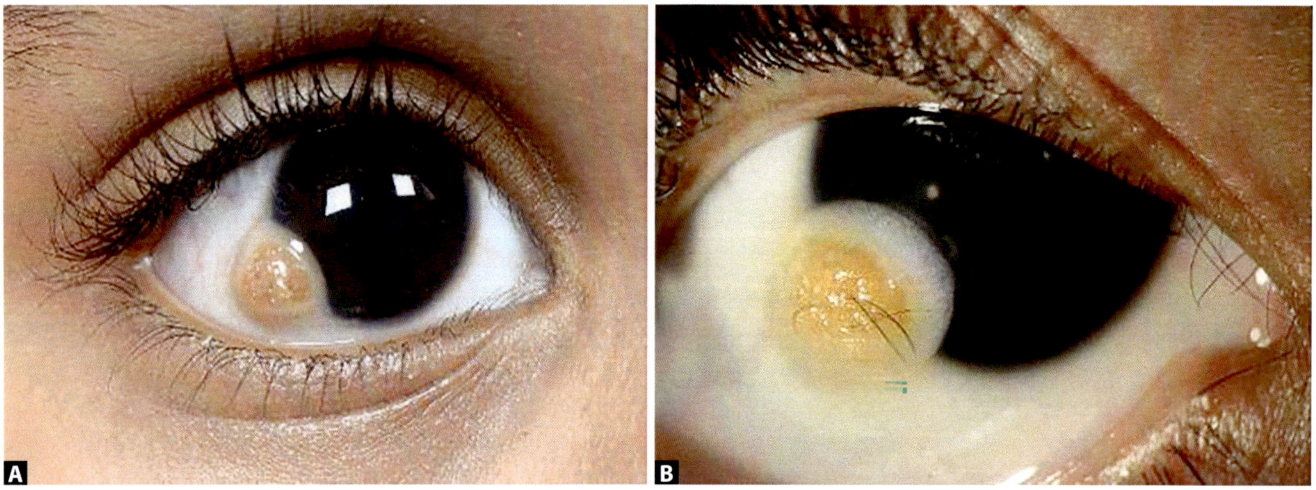

Figs. 9A and B: (A) Limbal dermoid with subtle corneal lipid line in the inferotemporal quadrant; (B) Inferotemporal limbal dermoid with a prominent hair in a 5-year-old child.

Clinical Features

It presents in childhood as a well-circumscribed solitary or multiple white to the yellow lesion, firm in consistency, and most commonly involving inferotemporal quadrant **(Fig. 9A)** with or without hair **(Fig. 9B)**. They are associated with Goldenhar syndrome (preauricular appendages, deafness, and vertebral anomalies), Treacher Collins syndrome (mandibulofacial dysostosis), and linear nevus sebaceous of Jadassohn (cosmetic deformity, alopecia, or malignant transformation). They have a risk for amblyopia, secondary astigmatism, chronic irritation, dellen formation, and cosmetic considerations.

Treatment

Treatment is indicated for amblyopia and cosmesis. Important concerns during the excision of the limbal dermoid are intraoperative perforation, postoperative epithelial defects, and peripheral vascularization of the cornea. In grade I limbal dermoid, treatment is generally observation or corneal tattooing with a sutureless limboconjunctival autograft after excision has been tried for cosmesis. In grades II and III, various surgeries in combination such as excision biopsy, lamellar keratoplasty, with the amniotic membrane, or limbal stem cell transplantation have been used. This has led to better and more stable long-term ocular surface cosmesis with fewer complications in comparison with traditional methods of excision and lamellar keratoplasty. The topical use of mitomycin C seems to have a protective effect in preventing the occurrence of a pseudopterygium.

Dermolipoma/Lipodermoid

Overview

Dermolipoma is a congenital solid choristoma that is derived from an ectopia of the ectoderm to the conjunctiva, probably due to sequestration at the time of embryonic development of the eyelid. It classically remains asymptomatic for years and might not be detected until adulthood. Rarely they may extend to orbit, lacrimal gland, and extraocular muscle. They may have an association with Goldenhar syndrome.

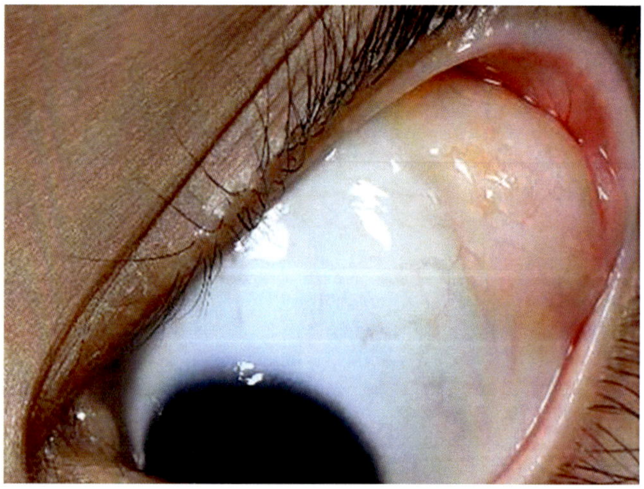

Fig. 10: Dermolipoma superotemporally in left eye in a 9-year-old child. Note that the curvature of the anterior margin is concave (curvature parallel to limbus).

Clinical Features

It becomes clinically apparent in the first to the second decade of life and presents as a unilateral soft or firm pinkish-white or yellow mass with a straight or slightly concave anterior margin subconjunctival mass seen mostly superotemporally **(Fig. 10)**. Fine hairs sometimes may be seen on the surface. It is not freely movable, cannot be repositioned into the orbit, and is not affected by retropulsion of the globe which are the features of subconjunctival fat prolapse that occurs mainly in the elderly.

Treatment

Most warrant observation only; symptomatic lesions with ocular irritation may require excision and reconstruction. One must carefully identify contiguous structures, especially the palpebral lobe of the lacrimal gland and lateral rectus muscle while dissection. Removal of only that portion of the dermolipoma which is anterior to the lateral orbital rim is generally done. The surgery of dermolipoma is fraught with dangers such as damage to the lacrimal secretory system, intractable diplopia, blepharoptosis, and even keratoconjunctivitis sicca.

Conjunctival Complex Choristoma

Overview

Complex choristoma of the conjunctiva is a congenital nonhereditary lesion that the complex choristomas contain more than two elements of ectopic tissues (lacrimal gland tissue, nerve bundles, cartilage, bone, etc.). The most common cause of complex choristoma is organoid nevus syndrome. The complex choristoma can be isolated or associated with linear nevus sebaceous of Jadassohn syndrome (a component of organoid nevus syndrome), which frequently affects the skin of the face, retroauricular area, and scalp and has a tendency to develop basal cell carcinoma, squamous cell carcinoma, or rarely sebaceous gland carcinoma.

Clinical Features

They may present as solitary or multiple smooth tan to gray or whitish conjunctival lesion with central vascularity. They may have multiple subcutaneous nodules. Nevus sebaceous of Jadassohn syndrome can present with linear placoid pigmented lesion on the face, eyelid coloboma with hypertrichosis and subcutaneous nodules along the edge of the coloboma **(Fig. 11A)**, distichiasis, trichiasis, complex choristoma which extends deeper into the stroma **(Fig. 11B)**, calcification or ossification of the ciliary body, and multifocal choroidal calcification. Systematically, there is linear pigmentation seen on the trunk, they have a bald patch **(Fig. 11C)**, as they grow older there is the development of curly hair over the bald patch and later can develop an ulcer or fleshy mass (indication for malignant transformation).

Treatment

Smaller nonamblyopic lesions can be observed. Surgery with surface reconstruction is needed in larger lesions which amblyogenic potential. Treatment should be planned

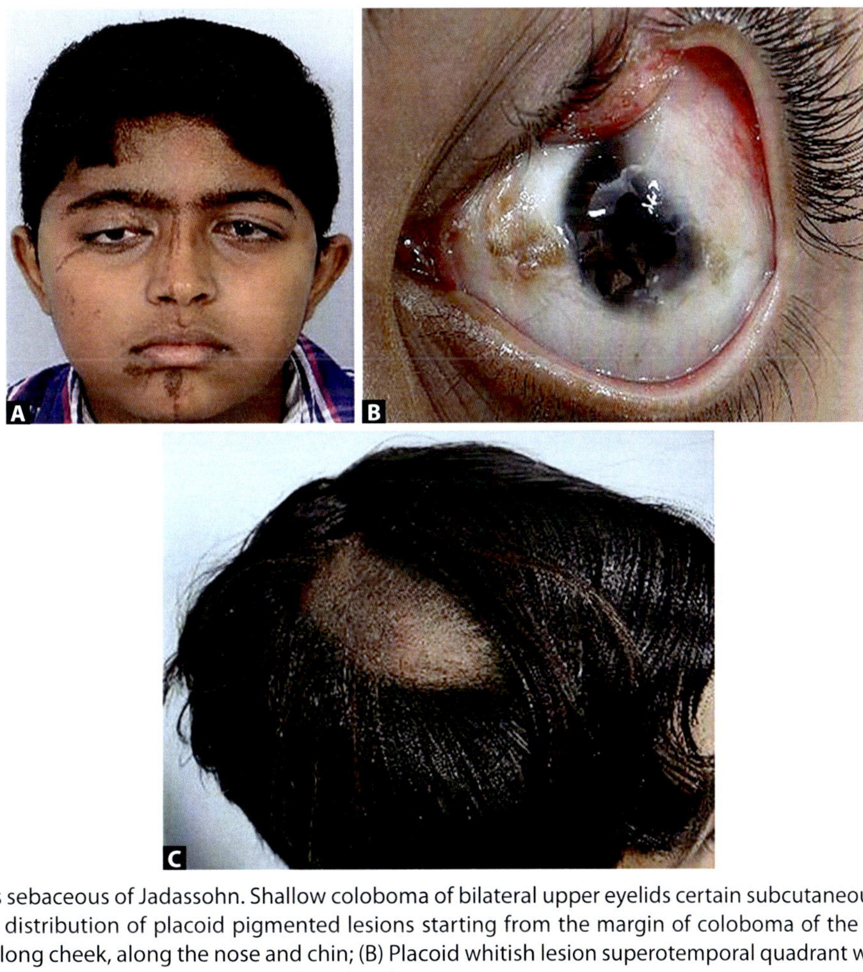

Figs. 11A to C: (A) Nevus sebaceous of Jadassohn. Shallow coloboma of bilateral upper eyelids certain subcutaneous nodules at medial edge of the coloboma. Linear distribution of placoid pigmented lesions starting from the margin of coloboma of the eyelid going towards the brow, inferotemporally along cheek, along the nose and chin; (B) Placoid whitish lesion superotemporal quadrant with corneal and epibulbar extension with the area of vascularization; (C) Bald patch on head.

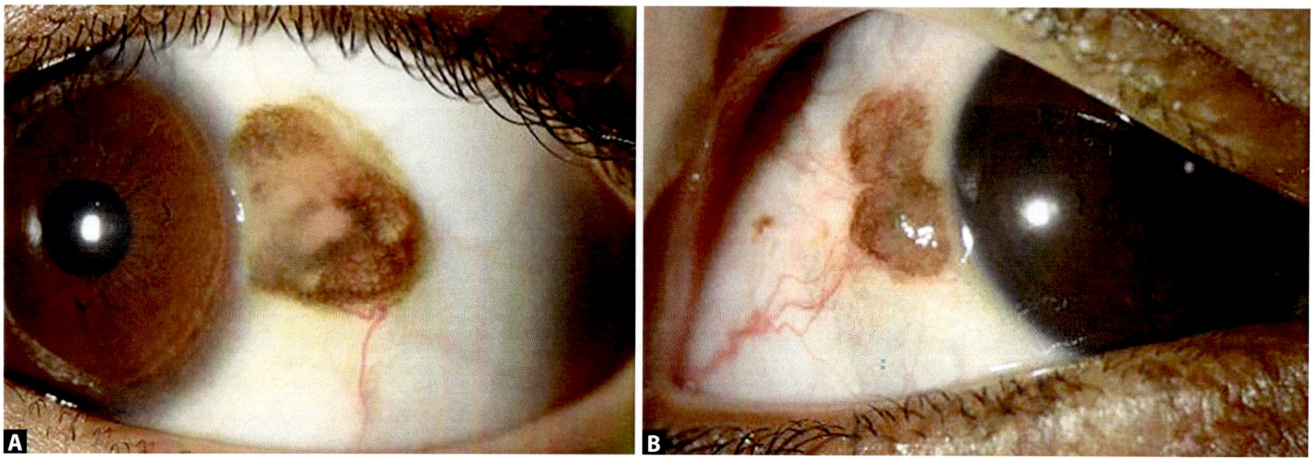

Figs. 12A and B: (A) Variably pigmented conjunctival nevus showing multiple clear cystic spaces and feeder vessel; (B) Bilobed variably pigmented nevus with multiple microcysts, feeder vessels, and satellite nevus temporally.

according to the depth, site, and size of the lesion, ranging from simple excision biopsy with surface reconstruction by amniotic membrane graft, lamellar keratoplasty, and penetrating keratoplasty to autologous limbal stem cell allograft. Rarely enucleation may be required in the extensive lesion.

Conjunctival Nevus

Overview

The most common pigmented conjunctival lesion is the nevus. They are typically noticed in the first decade of life and it increases in size during puberty, pregnancy, and sun exposure. Although most conjunctival nevi are pigmented (84%), some may be amelanotic or partially pigmented (16%).

Clinical Features

They appear as mildly elevated variable pigmented lesions with typical microcysts **(Fig. 12A)**. They may be single or multiple **(Fig. 12B)**, may or may not be associated with feeder vessels or intrinsic vascularity. There is no corneal epithelial invasion or episcleral fixity. They are most commonly located in the bulbar conjunctiva (72%), caruncle (15%), plica (11%), fornix and tarsus (1%), and cornea (<1%). Less than 1% can transform into malignant melanoma. A sudden increase in size, alteration in color, and increased thickness with prominent feeder vessels indicate malignant transformation.

Treatment

Management is generally periodic observation. If they are located in the fornix or palpebral conjunctiva, size >10 mm in diameter, exuberant feeder blood vessels or exuberant intrinsic vascularity and hemorrhage, lesions with no cysts and dark uniform pigmentation or cosmetic concern needs surgical excision with a clear margin by no-touch technique.

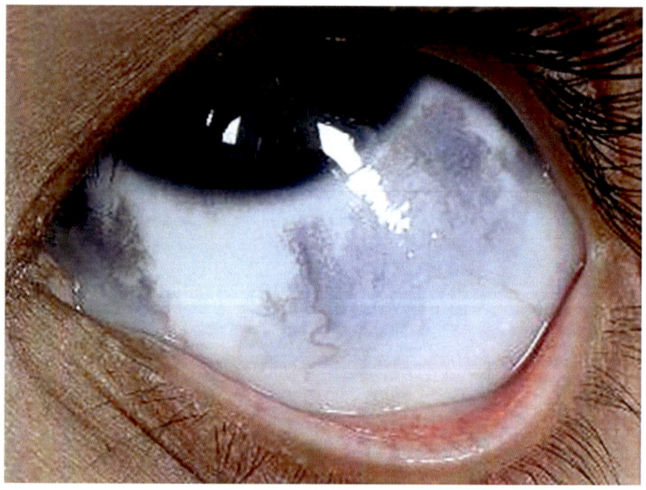

Fig. 13: Ocular melanocytosis showing a blue-gray discoloration of the sclera in a 6-year-old child.

Ocular Melanocytosis

Overview

Ocular melanocytosis is a congenital pigmentary condition of the periocular skin, sclera, orbit, meninges, and soft palate. Studies have shown that mutations in G proteins (GNAQ and GNA11) can lead to melanoma.

Clinical Features

There are flat brown to gray color irregular patches of scleral and episcleral pigmentation **(Fig. 13)**. The overlying conjunctiva is not involved and can be moved over the lesion. If they have associated hyperpigmentation of the eyelid, this is termed as nevus of Ota. One should look for the hairline pigmentation for meningeal melanoma or palatal pigmentation for esophageal melanoma, glaucoma, heterochromia iridis, and fundus examination for ipsilateral pigmentation of the fundus and to exclude uveal melanocytosis or melanoma.

Treatment

Only observation is needed to look for the development of glaucoma or malignant transformation.

INTRAOCULAR TUMORS

Retinoblastoma

Overview

It is the most common intraocular malignancy of childhood. It results from a mutation in the *Rb* gene (tumor suppressor gene) located at chromosome 13q14. 94% are sporadic while 6% are familial. Germline mutation patients are at risk for pinealoblastoma and second cancers like osteosarcoma. The average age at diagnosis is 18 months and 25–35% of cases are bilateral.

Clinical Features

Table 2 lists the common presenting features of RB. A child with suspected RB must undergo complete ophthalmic evaluation including a dilated fundus examination under anesthesia (EUA). The sequence of documentation is illustrated in **Table 3**. Ultrasonography B-scan shows an intraocular mass with calcification **(Fig. 14A)**. As the tumor grows, three patterns are usually seen. Endophytic, in which the tumor grows into the vitreous cavity and result in vitreous seeds **(Fig. 14B)**, where the retinal vessels are not seen on the tumor surface. The second is exophytic, in which the tumor grows towards the subretinal space. Retinal detachment usually occurs and retinal vessels are seen along with subretinal seeds **(Fig. 14C)**. The diffuse infiltrating tumor is the last type in which the tumor diffusely involves the retina without an obvious mass. This is generally seen in older children and usually, there is a delay in the diagnosis. A mixed pattern can also occur. Magnetic resonance imaging is specifically indicated if orbital extension, optic nerve invasion, or an intracranial extension is suspected and in bilateral RB to rule out pinealoblastoma. Grouping is a clinical system of prognosticating organ salvage **(Box 1)** while staging prognosticates survival **(Box 2)**.

Treatment

The aim of treatment is sequential goals of life salvage, eye salvage, and vision salvage. Management of RB is based on several factors—the age at presentation, laterality, tumor

TABLE 2: Common presenting features of retinoblastoma.

Leukocoria	56%
Strabismus	20%
Red painful eye	7%
Poor vision	5%
Asymptomatic	3%
Orbital cellulitis	3%
Unilateral mydriasis	2%
Heterochromia iridis	1%
Hyphema	1%

TABLE 3: Documentation of retinoblastoma during examination under anesthesia.

Parameter	***Right eye***	***Left eye***
Lymph nodes		
Corneal diameter		
IOP (Perkins)		
Anterior segment (neovascularization, seeds, hyphema, and signs of inflammation)		
Fundus examination (ora-to-ora 360° with indentation)		
Group		

(IOP: intraocular pressure)

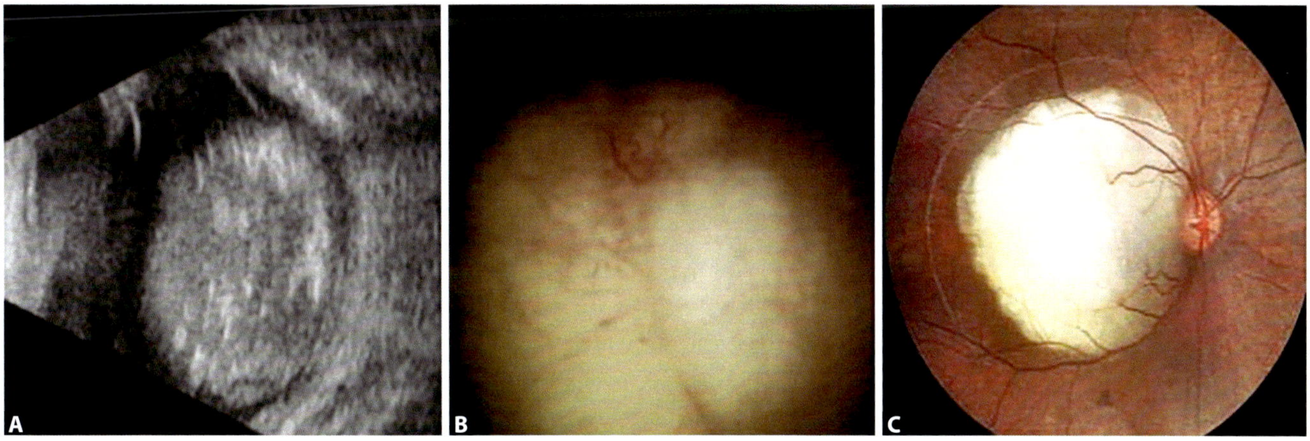

Figs. 14A to C: (A) Ultrasonography (USG) shows an intraocular mass with calcification; (B) Endophytic mass filling >50% of vitreous cavity; (C) Exophytic macular mass.

BOX 1: International Classification of Intraocular Retinoblastoma.

International Classification of Intraocular Retinoblastoma (Murphree)

Group A: Small intraretinal tumors away from foveola and disk
- All tumors are 3 mm or smaller in greatest dimension, confined to the retina
- All tumors are located further than 3 mm from the foveola and 1.5 mm from the optic disk

Group B: All remaining discrete tumors confined to the retina
- All other tumors confined to the retina not in Group A
- Tumor-associated subretinal fluid <3 mm from the tumor with no subretinal seeding

Group C: Discrete local disease with minimal subretinal or vitreous seeding
- Tumor(s) are discrete
- Subretinal fluid, present or past, without seeding involving up to one-fourth of the retina
- Local fine vitreous seeding may be present close to discrete tumor
- Local subretinal seeding <3 mm (2 DD) from the tumor

Group D: Diffuse disease with significant vitreous or subretinal seeding
- Tumor(s) may be massive or diffuse
- Subretinal fluid present or past without seeding, involving up to total retinal detachment
- Diffuse or massive vitreous disease may include "greasy" seeds or avascular tumor masses
- Diffuse subretinal seeding may include subretinal plaques or tumor nodules

Group E: Presence of any one or more of these poor prognosis features
- Tumor touching the lens
- Tumor anterior to anterior vitreous face involving ciliary body or anterior segment
- Diffuse infiltrating retinoblastoma
- Neovascular glaucoma
- Opaque media from hemorrhage
- Tumor necrosis with aseptic orbital cellulites
- Phthisis bulbi

BOX 2: International Staging System for Retinoblastoma.

Stage 0: No enucleation (one or both eyes may have intraocular disease)
Stage I: Enucleation, tumor completely resected
Stage II: Enucleation with microscopic residual tumor
Stage III: Regional extension
- A. Overt orbital disease
- B. Preauricular or cervical lymph node extension

Stage IV: Metastatic disease
- A. Hematogenous metastasis
    1. Single lesion
    2. Multiple lesions
- B. Central nervous system (CNS) extension
    1. Prechiasmatic lesion
    2. CNS mass
    3. Leptomeningeal disease

location, tumor grouping and staging, primary or recurrent tumor, the status of the other eye, visual status, and economic factors of the patient. Management options are discussed in **Box 3**. Genetic counseling is very important. The important differential diagnosis is discussed in **Table 4**.

BOX 3: Current suggested protocol for retinoblastoma.

A. Intraocular tumor, International Classification Group A to C
1. Focal therapy (cryotherapy or transpupillary thermotherapy) alone for smaller tumors (<3 mm in diameter and height) located in visually noncrucial areas
2. Intra-arterial chemotherapy (IAC) if unilateral or standard six cycles intravenous chemotherapy (IVC) with focal therapy for those located in visually crucial areas
3. For refractory vitreous seeds periocular or intravitreal chemotherapy
4. Plaque brachytherapy for residual tumor in the macular and juxtapapillary areas

B. Intraocular tumor, International Classification Group D
1. IAC, if unilateral or standard six cycles IVC with focal therapy
2. For refractory vitreous seeds periocular or intravitreal chemotherapy

C. Intraocular tumor, International Classification Group E
1. IAC, if unilateral or standard six cycles IVC with focal therapy
2. Primary enucleation
3. Evaluate histopathology for high-risk factors

D. High-risk factors on histopathology, International Staging, Stage 2
1. Baseline systemic evaluation for metastasis
2. Standard six cycles adjuvant chemotherapy
3. High dose adjuvant chemotherapy and orbital external beam radiotherapy in patients with scleral infiltration, extraocular extension, and optic nerve extension

E. Extraocular tumor, International Staging, Stage 3A
1. Baseline systemic evaluation for metastasis
2. High dose chemotherapy for three to six cycles, followed by enucleation or extended enucleation, external beam radiotherapy, and continued high dose chemotherapy for 12 cycles

F. Regional lymph node metastasis, International staging, Stage 3B
1. Baseline evaluation for systemic metastasis
2. Neck dissection, high dose chemotherapy for six cycles, followed by external beam radiotherapy, and continued high dose chemotherapy for 12 cycles

G. Hematogenous or central nervous system metastasis, International Staging, Stage 4
1. Palliative therapy in discussion with the family
2. High dose chemotherapy for hematogenous and intrathecal chemotherapy for central nervous system (CNS) metastasis

Retinal Capillary Hemangioma/ Retinal Hemangioblastoma

Overview

Retinal capillary hemangioma is a benign congenital vascular lesion that begins as a small vascular mass that slowly enlarges. It can be classified based on their growth as (endophytic, exophytic, and sessile), based on the area of involvement (peripheral and juxtapapillary), depending upon features (exudative form and tractional form), and

TABLE 4: Important differential diagnosis of retinoblastoma.

Condition	Features
Coats disease (most common)	• Xanthocoria • Subretinal exudation • Bullous retinal detachment almost touching lens • Feathery calcification • Peripheral retinal telangiectasia
Persistent hyperplastic primary vitreous	• Present at birth • Relative microphthalmos • Prominent ciliary process • Posterior subcapsular cataract with a frond till disk • Closed funnel retinal detachment
Toxocara	• Anterior uveitis with cataract • Falciform fold • Drag disk appearance
Ciliary body medulloepithelioma	• Maldevelopment of zonules of the lens • Lenticular or zonular coloboma • Displaced lens • *Hypopyon*: Sago grain-like seeds • Hyaline cartilage or bone can be seen

their relationship to von Hippel–Lindau (VHL) disease (with or without VHL disease). VHL is a multiorgan disorder characterized by retinal capillary hemangiomas, central nervous system (CNS) hemangioblastomas, and various solid and cystic visceral hamartomas and renal cell carcinoma. The mean age at diagnosis is 18 years for patients with VHL and 36 years for those without VHL. In a patient with a solitary hemangioblastoma, the risk of developing VHL is 45% if the patient is <10 years of age at diagnosis and 1% if >60 years of age.

Clinical Features

Clinically it appears as a reddish-pink-orange tumor in the peripheral retina **(Fig. 15)** or on the optic disk supplied by a feeder artery and a draining vein associated with exudates. They can lead to the formation of fibrotic bands, which can progress to tractional or rhegmatogenous retinal detachment, vitreous hemorrhage, secondary glaucoma, and phthisis bulbi. The diagnosis is made by the typical ophthalmoscopic features. Fluorescein angiography (FA) shows hyperfluorescence which may be associated with the leakage of dye into the vitreous.

Treatment

Management depends upon the size, location, and associated findings. Laser photocoagulation is done for smaller lesions. Cryotherapy and brachytherapy are done for larger peripheral lesions, especially those with exudative retinal detachment. Vitreoretinal surgery may be required for nonabsorbing vitreous hemorrhage, epiretinal fibrosis, or tractional retinal detachment. Photodynamic therapy (PDT) and antivascular

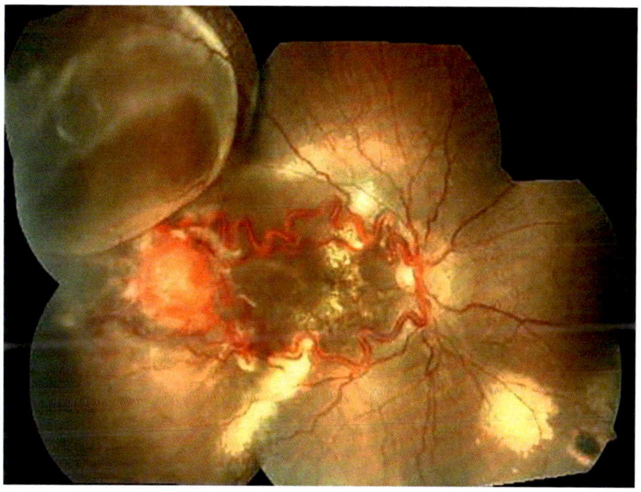

Fig. 15: Retinal hemangioblastoma at the periphery with a feeding artery and a draining venule from the disk in a patient with von Hippel–Lindau (VHL). Note the exudative reaction and traction retinal detachment.

TABLE 5: Differential diagnosis of retinal capillary hemangioma.

Condition	Features
Coats disease	• Unilateral young male • Retinal telangiectasia and retinal exudation
Retinal macroaneurysm	• Single lesion in the posterior pole within arteriole • Elderly • Associated more with hemorrhage rather exudates • Absent feeder vessels
Vasoproliferative tumor	• Absence of prominent feeder vessels • Extreme peripheral location • Nonfamilial

endothelial growth factor (VEGF) agents may be particularly appropriate for juxtapapillary tumors. The differential diagnosis is discussed in **Table 5**.

Astrocytic Hamartoma of Retina

Overview

Astrocytic hamartoma is a glial tumor of the retina and optic nerve. It is a benign condition associated with tuberous sclerosis (intracranial astrocytoma, cardiac rhabdomyoma, renal angiomyolipoma, pleural cysts, ash leaf spot, or hypomelanic macules, facial angiofibromas, shagreen patches, ungual fibromas, and dental pit) and NF-1.

Clinical Features

A yellowish or white semitransparent plaque, nodule, or mulberry-like lesion **(Fig. 16)**, often semitransparent in its periphery and calcified centrally. The calcification in an astrocytic hamartoma is a more glistening yellow, resembling fish eggs. The diagnosis of retinal astrocytic hamartoma can be made with indirect ophthalmoscopy and a physical evaluation looking for signs of tuberous sclerosis. FA of retinal astrocytic hamartoma shows a prominent superficial network of fine vessels in the arterial phase with leakage in the venous phase. The late phase shows homogeneous staining of the mass. Optical coherence tomography (OCT) of retinal astrocytic hamartoma reveals full-thickness replacement of the retinal anatomic layers with the tumor and shadowing corresponding to the intralesional calcification. The differential diagnosis is discussed in **Table 6**.

Treatment

Treatment includes annual observation for associated exudative retinal detachment. Other treatment modalities are combined bevacizumab and triamcinolone acetonide injections for macular edema in a patient with astrocytic hamartomas and tuberous sclerosis.

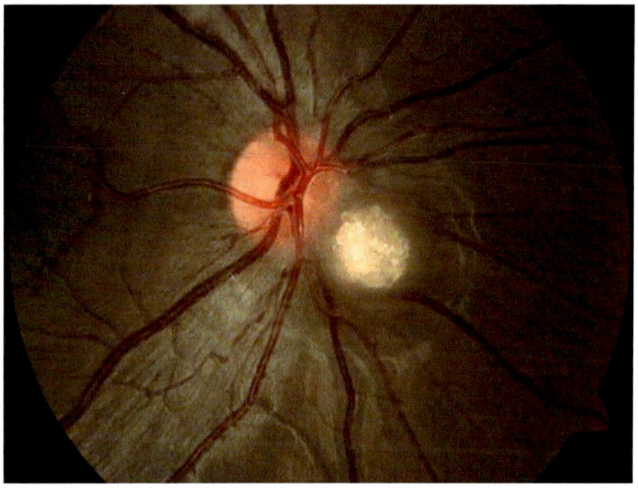

Fig. 16: Calcified mulberry-shaped astrocytic hamartoma inferonasal to the optic disk in the right eye.

TABLE 6: Differential diagnosis of retinal astrocytoma.

Condition	*Features*
Retinoblastoma	• White mass with white calcification • Feeder vessels • Grows if untreated
Myelinated nerve fibers	• White patch • No calcification • Vessels obscured • Absent exudation
Retinal capillary hemangioma	• Round red lesion • No calcification • Prominent feeder vessels • Exudation • Associated with von Hippel–Lindau (VHL) disease
Optic disk drusen	• White mass • Calcification • No vessels

Melanocytoma of the Optic Nerve/ Magnocellular Nevus

Overview

Melanocytoma is a congenital hamartoma which is a benign and heavily pigmented ocular tumor involving the optic disk. Unlike melanoma, it occurs more commonly in darkly pigmented individuals. Malignant transformation into melanoma occurred in 1–2%.

Clinical Features

Most cases are asymptomatic, detected incidentally. It appears as a unilateral dark brown or black, flat, or slightly elevated lesion with feathery edges **(Fig. 17)** (because of extensions into the nerve fiber layer) that may extend over the edge of the disk into the choroid or retina. FA shows dense hypofluorescence which persists through all phases of the angiogram. B-scan ultrasonography detects an acoustically solid optic disk mass. It should be differentiated from optic disk melanoma which is more of brownish color arising from the juxtapapillary choroid and extending over the optic nerve associated with visual symptoms. It does not usually infiltrate the nerve fiber layer, and may be associated with intrinsic vascularity.

Treatment

Mainly periodic observation is needed. Sometimes it can undergo spontaneous necrosis, which results in profound visual loss. A rapid increase in the size or vision loss may be a sign of malignant transformation and hence enucleation is considered. Other complications include optic nerve compression and retinal vein obstruction.

Diffuse Choroidal Hemangioma

Overview

Circumscribed choroidal hemangioma is seen in adults. Diffuse choroidal hemangioma is usually evident at birth and

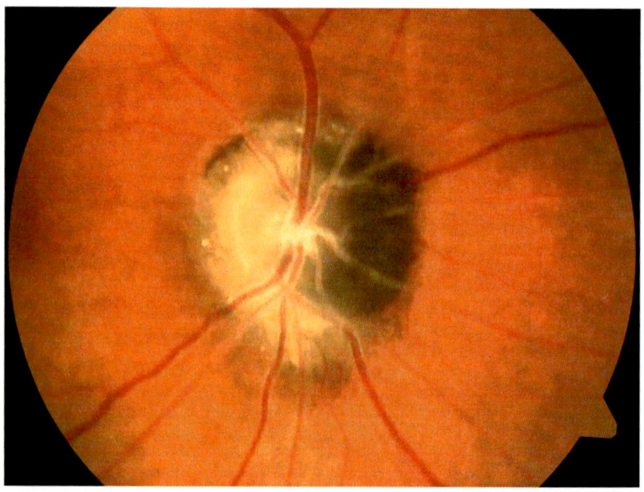

Fig. 17: Fundus photograph optic disk melanocytoma. Note the feathery margin of the lesion.

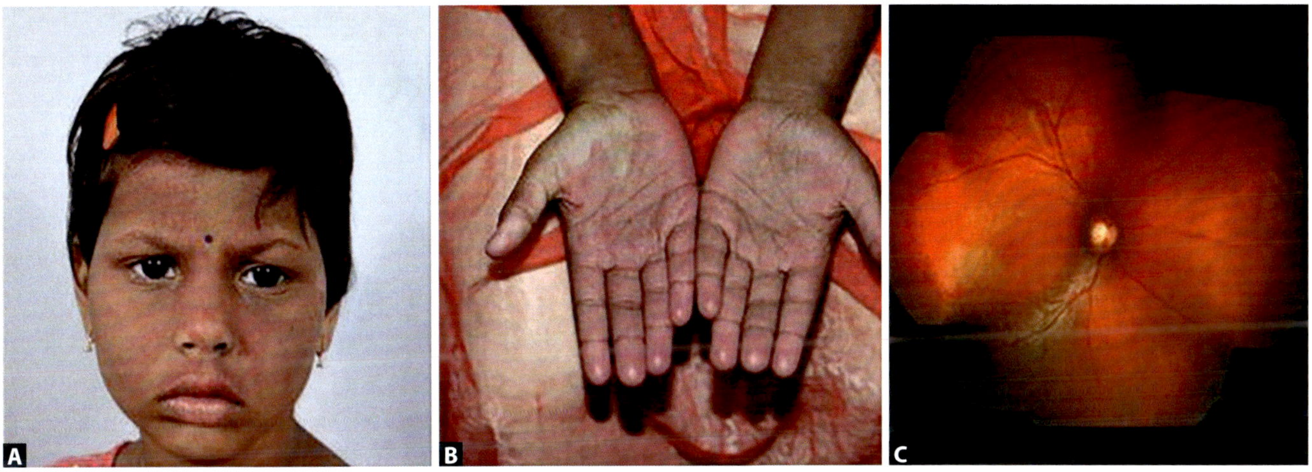

Figs. 18A to C: (A) Facial hemangioma of a 4-year-old girl with a variant of Sturge–Weber syndrome. In this case, both sides of the face are extensively involved; (B) Palm and hands are also involved; (C) Diffuse choroidal hemangioma.

is associated with Sturge-Weber syndrome (leptomeningeal hemangiomatosis and seizures).

Clinical Features

Externally they may have unilateral or bilateral facial nevus flammeus **(Figs. 18A and B)** and fundus examination shows a diffuse orange to red, choroidal thickening **(Fig. 18C)** giving "tomato catsup fundus" appearance. It is usually unilateral and ipsilateral to the nevus flammeus. They can present with vision loss due to refractive errors, foveal distortion, and exudative retinal detachment. They can produce a total retinal detachment and secondary neovascular glaucoma. Diffuse thickening of the choroid is seen in ultrasonography. FA shows diffuse leakage. OCT discloses the thickening of the choroid with expanded choroidal vessels and a smooth surface.

Treatment

Observation is done in asymptomatic cases. Radiotherapy, PDT, and oral propranolol may be used to regress the tumor or for the resolution of subretinal fluid.

Congenital Hypertrophy of Retinal Pigment Epithelium

Overview

It is an umbrella term encompassing solitary congenital hypertrophy of retinal pigment epithelium (CHRPE), grouped (multifocal) CHRPE, and atypical CHRPE. Although believed to be congenital, the median age at diagnosis is 45 years.

Clinical Features

Patients are asymptomatic, diagnosed incidentally. It is a well-circumscribed, round, flat, and pigmented lesion at the level of the retinal pigment epithelium **(Fig. 19)** surrounded by a hypopigmented halo that can occur anywhere in the fundus. They may have depigmented lacunae. The underlying retina and vessels appear normal. FA and indocyanine green angiography generally show blockage of fluorescence throughout most of the sequence.

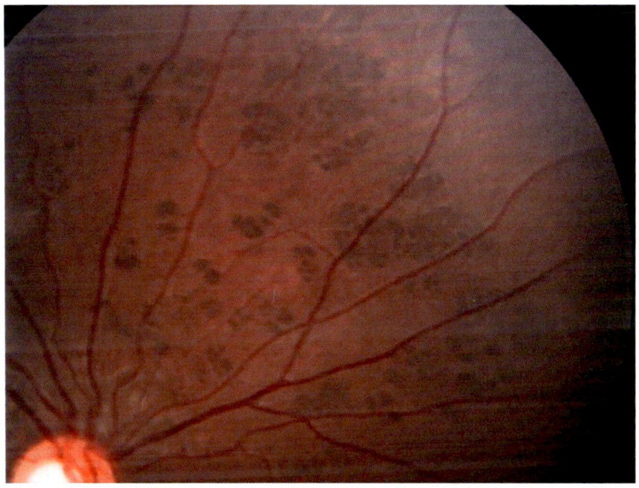

Fig. 19: Congenital hypertrophy of retinal pigment epithelium (CHRPE) seen as well-circumscribed multiple round, flat, and pigmented lesion at the level of the retinal pigment epithelium.

Treatment

These are generally observed periodically with documentation of fundus pictures. If it produces exudation or subretinal fluid, laser photocoagulation or cryotherapy can be considered.

Intraocular Leukemia

Overview

Intraocular leukemic infiltration occurs most often in children with acute lymphoblastic leukemia (ALL). There is a bimodal distribution, the first peak occurring between the age of 2 and 5 years, with the incidence rising again after the age of 50. Ocular involvement is usually a sign of severe disease.

Clinical Features

It can involve the iris, ciliary body, choroid, retina, vitreous, or optic nerve. Spontaneous hyphema, heterochromic iris, seeding of the anterior chamber may be the presenting sign. Anterior segment infiltration may be the initial and only sign of relapse. In the retina, they may present as leukemic retinopathy manifesting as white-centered hemorrhages **(Fig. 20)**, cotton wool spots, neovascularization, and serous retinal detachment. Choroidal involvement gives a "leopard skin" appearance on the fundus. The optic nerve involvement is more commonly seen in children with ALL. Optic disk edema may be there due to raised intracranial pressure. When the optic nerve is involved in a distinction between papilledema from increased intracranial pressure and direct cellular infiltration is urgently required.

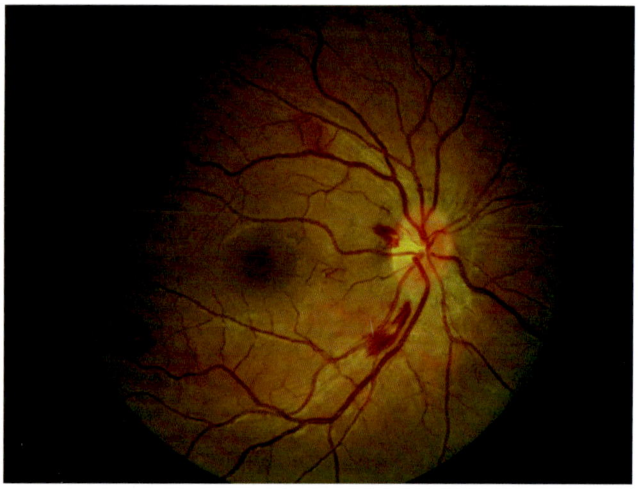

Fig. 20: Right eye showing multiple white-centered hemorrhages or Roth spot in a child with leukemia.

Treatment

Management is usually the treatment of systemic disease, especially in leukemic retinopathy. Whenever the optic nerve is involved immediate ocular irradiation may save the vision. Irradiation and chemotherapy are therefore required to eradicate any viable neoplastic cells in the eye.

Ciliary Body Medulloepithelioma/Diktyoma

Overview

Medulloepithelioma is an embryonal tumor of nonpigmented ciliary epithelium that arises from the inner layer of the optic cup. According to Zimmerman's classification, medulloepithelioma may be divided into nonteratoid (contains pure neuroepithelial structures) and teratoid types (contains cartilage, skeletal muscle, and brain tissue), and either may have benign or malignant cytologic features.

Clinical Features

It becomes clinically apparent during the first decade of life or may even manifest later with poor vision, pain, or leukocoria. Examination reveals a fleshy, irregular, variably sized white or pink to gray translucent mass arising from the ciliary body or intraocular mass appearing behind the pupillary area **(Fig. 21A)**. The presence of cysts within the tumor is a very typical feature. They may develop cyclitic membrane, iris neovascularization, and secondary angle-closure glaucoma, lens coloboma or displacement **(Fig. 21B)**, cataract, uveitis, hyphema, hypopyon (sago grain-like seeds), hyaline cartilage or bone can be seen, retinal detachment, and vitreous hemorrhage. Children with neovascularization of the iris of unknown cause should be evaluated to exclude underlying medulloepithelioma. It is mostly a clinical diagnosis. Early

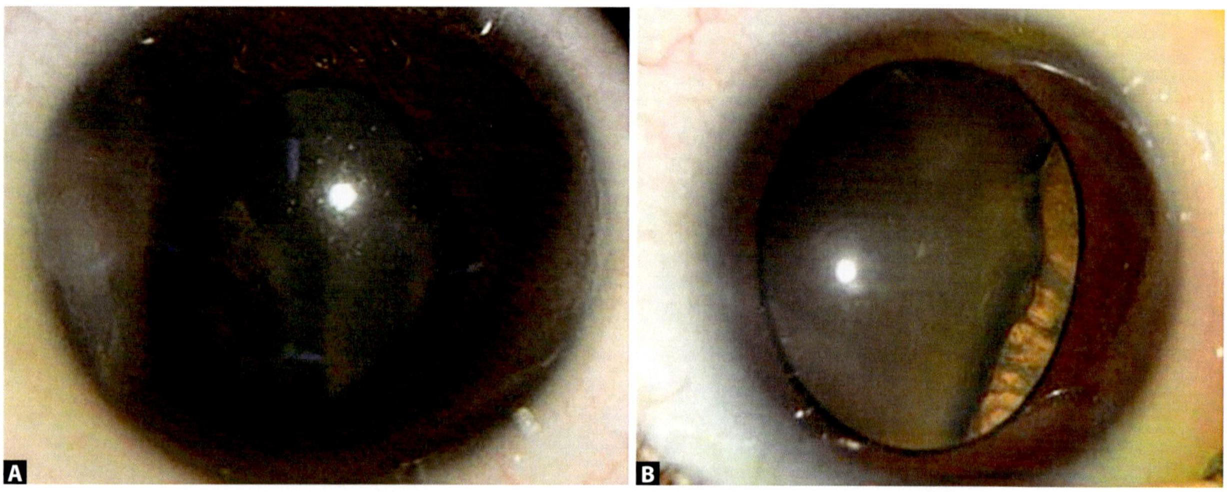

Figs. 21A and B: (A) Temporal medulloepithelioma in a 2-year-old boy. Note the fleshy-white lesion with a cyst, pigmented ciliary body mass displacing the lens nasally and posterior synechiae; (B) Typical lens notch, or "coloboma" with neovascularization in a 1-year-old boy with the enlarged ciliary process.

hyperfluorescence and late staining are noted on fundus FA. Ultrasonography may show a solid mass pattern with intratumoral cysts and can produce higher echoes similar to those with calcification seen in RB.

Treatment

Iridocyclectomy or plaque brachytherapy can be done in a small and circumscribed medulloepithelioma. Because of the invasive nature of these tumors and being mostly malignant, enucleation is preferred.

ORBITAL TUMORS

Dermoid Cyst

Overview

These are developmental choristomas arising from anomalously entrapped ectoderm within the suture lines and are the most common benign tumor of pediatric orbit. Classification is discussed in **Table 7**. Approximately 60% of all dermoids arise superotemporally **(Fig. 22A)** from the frontozygomatic suture; 25% arise superomedially **(Fig. 22B)** from the frontolacrimal suture. Others may arise from frontoethmoidal sutures, deep temporalis fossa, or sphenozygomatic suture.

Clinical Features

They present in childhood as subcutaneous nodules adjacent to the orbital rim or as unilateral proptosis or temporal drooping of the lid with a smooth, nontender, firm to the cystic lesion, usually tethered to the adjacent periosteum with palpable posterior margins. Dumbbell dermoid can have proptosis or change in the vision on mastication. If the cyst ruptures, a clinical picture resembling orbital cellulitis or fistula to the skin can occur.

TABLE 7: Classification of dermoid cyst based on location.

Ocular dermoid	***Orbital dermoid***	***Extraorbital dermoid/deep dermoid***
Limbal dermoid	Anterior orbital dermoid	Orbitocranial dermoid
Corneal dermoid	Posterior orbital dermoid	Sino-orbital dermoid
Conjunctival dermoid		Dumbbell dermoid
		Orbitotemporal dermoid

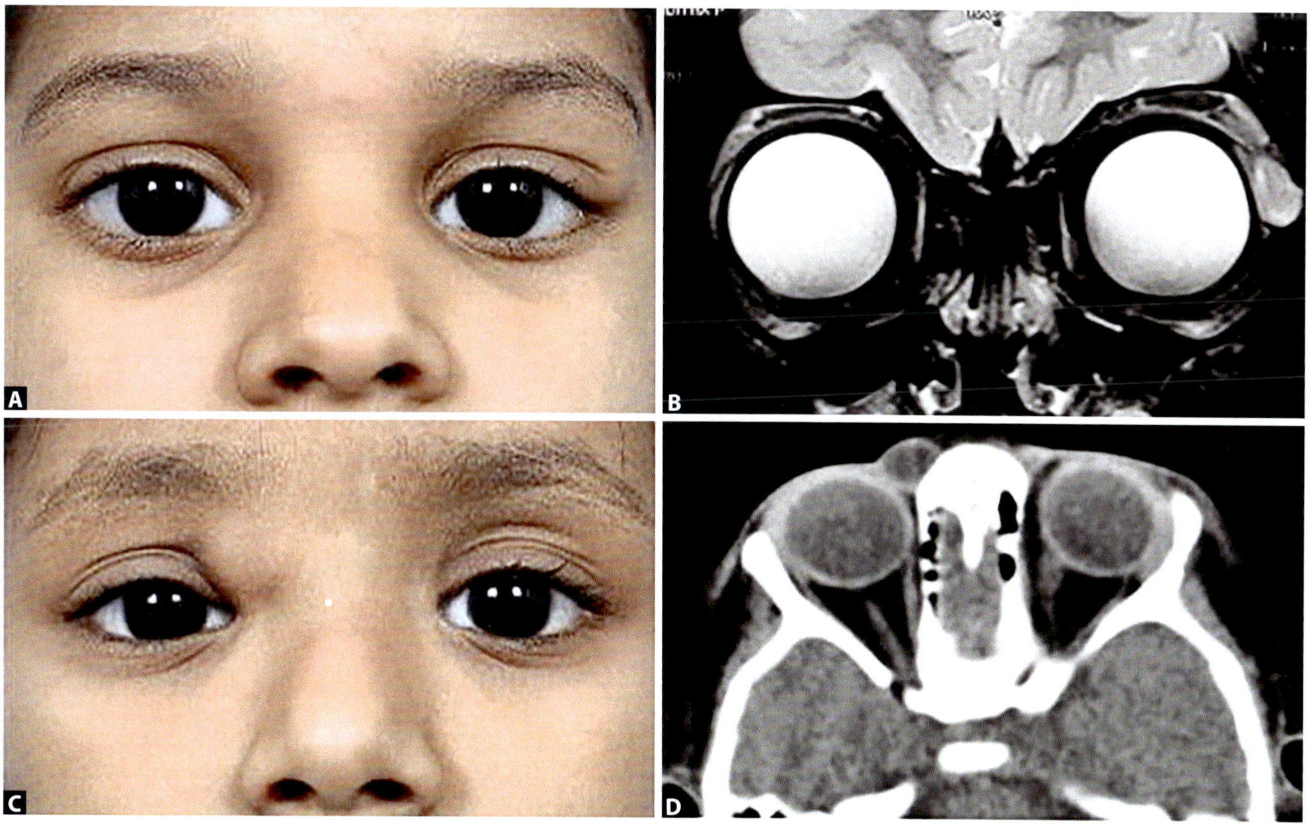

Figs. 22A to D: (A) Left superotemporal mass with mild temporal drooping of the upper eyelid; (B) Coronal magnetic resonance imaging in T2-weighted image shows left well-defined superotemporal cystic mass; (C) A 2-year-old girl with superonasal subcutaneous mass; (D) Axial CT showing cystic lesion medially. The lumen of the cyst is hypointense, similar to vitreous.

Diagnostic Evaluation

On MRI, fat suppression is the best way to see dermoid. Imaging features that suggest a dermoid include a cystic appearance, internal fat attenuation or signal intensity (T1 hyperintensity), and internal calcification **(Fig. 22C)**.

On a CT scan, a well-circumscribed heterogeneous cystic lesion **(Fig. 22D)** with the enhancement of the wall with or without calcification and fluid levels is seen. 85% are associated with bony fossa formation bone with thinning and scalloping of adjacent bone. In some instances, a dermoid cyst can have extraorbital and intraorbital components that are connected through a defect in bone (dumbbell dermoid).

Treatment

Treatment of choice is the complete surgical removal of the lesion. Superficial dermoid should be excised in toto to avoid traumatic rupture. Most can be safely removed via an anterior or anterolateral orbitotomy. If an inadvertent rupture of the cyst should occur, the area should be irrigated with an antibiotic solution or corticosteroids is advisable to prevent postoperative inflammation. The deeper cyst may require orbitotomy with bone removal. Dumbbell tumors with extension into the temporal fossa are removed first from the orbit. The temporal component and the bony canal are subsequently removed. The bony tunnel should be cored out to remove the connecting stalk in dumbbell tumors.

Orbital Teratoma

Overview

It is a very rare congenital multicystic mass derived from more than one germ layer and usually from all three. Most of them are benign but can be malignant.

Clinical Features

It presents with severe unilateral proptosis at birth which increases over the first few days or weeks. The globe is usually pushed forward and upward by the mass which is soft to firm in consistency with marked orbital distortion **(Fig. 23A)**. The tumor can extend to involve the temporal fossa. Mucus secretion from the embryonic intestinal tissue is responsible for the sudden increase in size.

Diagnostic Evaluation

The diagnosis of orbital teratoma should be considered in any child with a large mass present at birth. Computed tomography of the orbit shows a cystic, multiloculated soft tissue mass displacing the normal globe with the expansion of the orbit **(Fig. 23B)**.

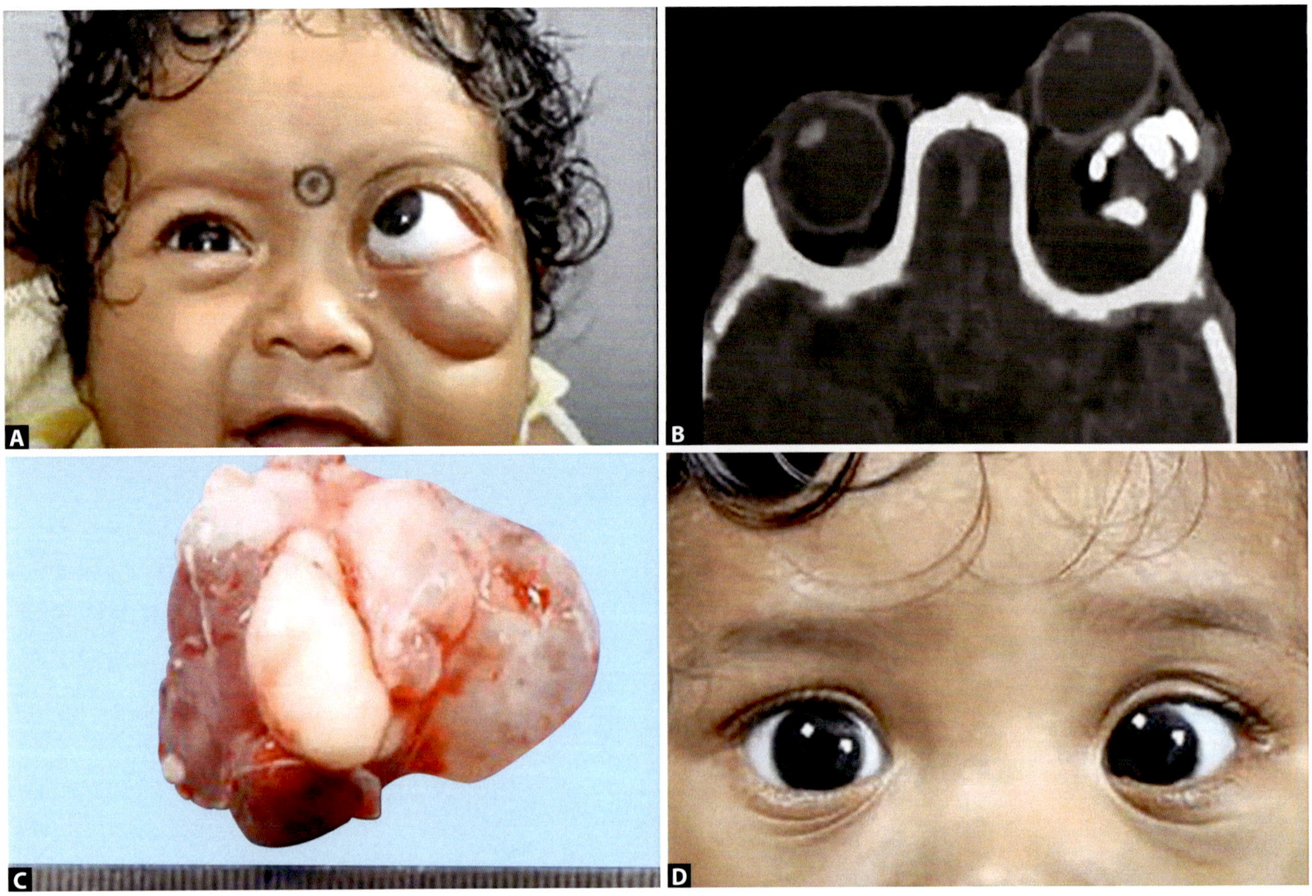

Figs. 23A to D: (A) A 3-month-old child with left inferotemporal teratoma displacing the eye superonasally; (B) CT scan shows an ill-defined mass with tooth inside both intra- and extraconally; (C) Tumor was taken out in toto via inferior transconjunctival orbitotomy procedure; (D) Postoperatively, there is residual esotropia but the vision is appropriate for the age.

Treatment

Recurrent teratomas may undergo malignant degeneration so a close follow-up is mandatory. It is best to do in toto removal of the lesion but if it is very large then first aspirate the fluid from a larger cyst to decrease the size of the mass and facilitate complete removal **(Figs. 23C and 23D)**.

Colobomatous Cyst/Microphthalmos with Cyst

Overview

Colobomatous cyst is a congenital abnormality that consists of a small, malformed eye with a coloboma through which a cystic herniation of glial tissue protrudes into the orbit. It is present at birth and is usually nonheritable, although familial cases have been documented. It has been observed in a patient with cleft lip and palate, Goldenhar syndrome, optic nerve glioma, polycystic kidney, trisomy 13, and Edward syndrome.

Clinical Features

They present with inferior orbital mass with a bluish hue pushing the eyeball superiorly **(Fig. 24A)**. The overlying skin is normal and there are no signs of inflammation. They have microphthalmos (abnormally small eyes with anatomic malformations) which may be difficult to see clinically **(Fig. 24B)**. Always look at another eye for microphthalmos and look for characteristic "triangulation sign of cornea". The site of triangulation is the site of coloboma through which neuroglial tissue protrudes. The coloboma almost always involves the optic disk, with or without uveal involvement.

Diagnostic Evaluation

B-scan ultrasonography shows the fluid level, microphthalmic eye, coloboma, and orbital cystic structure. Orbital CT is done to exactly locate the fluid-filled colobomatous cyst, to assess the size of the eye, and to find any communication between the cyst and the eye. If the other eye is normal, the differentials are capillary hemangioma, lymphangioma, teratoma, congenital cystic eye, and anteriorly located dermoid.

Treatment

The management depends upon visual potential. This is explained in **Flowchart 1**. If recurs repeat, aspiration may be needed **(Fig. 24C)**.

Orbital Capillary Hemangioma/Benign Hemangioendothelioma

Overview

Capillary hemangioma is the most common vascular orbital tumor in childhood. They are benign vasoproliferative tumors of vascular endothelial cells.

Clinical Features

They present with progressive unilateral swelling and proptosis after birth. It present as a bluish mass in the anterior orbit **(Fig. 25A)** which increases in size while crying or sucking

Flowchart 1: Management of colobomatous cyst.

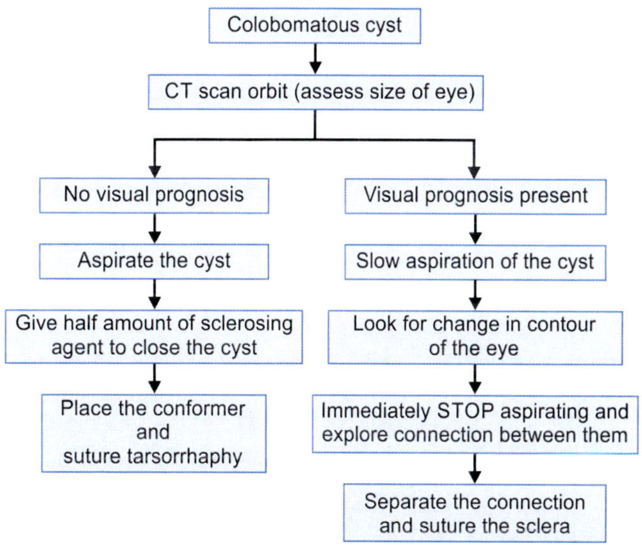

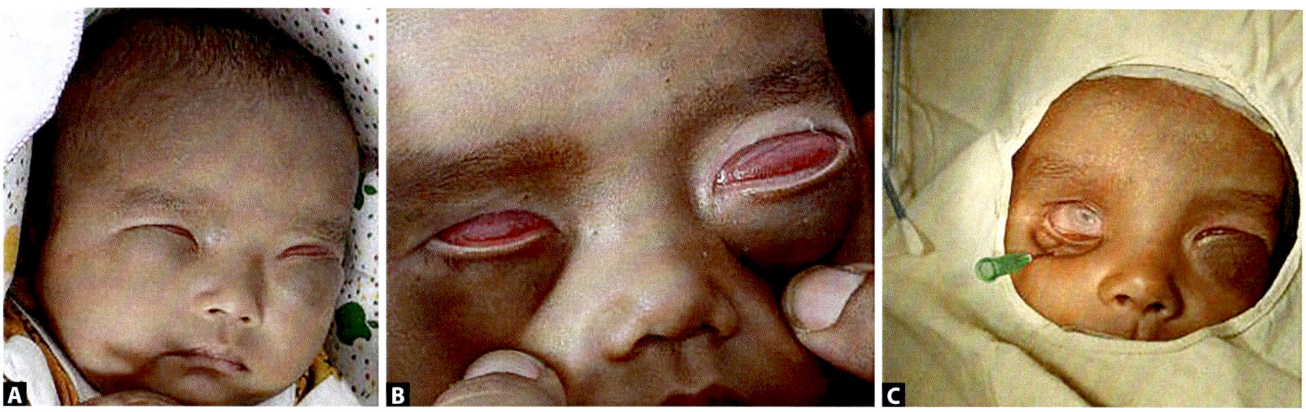

Figs. 24A to C: (A) Typical appearance of bilateral colobomatous cyst with upward displacement of the microphthalmic eye and protrusion of the lower eyelid secondary to a large inferior orbital cyst; (B) Overlying skin is pinchable but the eye is not visible; (C) After cyst aspiration, microphthalmic eye is visible.

and even blanches on pressure. It rapidly increases in size till 6 months of age followed by gradual involution by 2–3 years of age. It may be associated with Kasabach-Merritt syndrome (tumor causing thrombocytopenia and hemorrhage). Larger lesions may lead to amblyopia, astigmatism, corneal exposure, or optic neuropathy.

Diagnostic Evaluation

Computed tomography and MRI reveal an extraconal or intraconal orbital lobulated mass, well-circumscribed but can be ill-defined, enhancing mass **(Fig. 25B)**. Ultrasound demonstrates a poorly defined, hyperechoic mass, usually confined to the anterior part of the orbit. Doppler study may show abundant arterial and venous vascularization.

Treatment

For deep orbital lesions, systemic therapy with propranolol is the first line of treatment. The most common dose used is 2 mg/kg/day. Anteriorly located circumscribed capillary hemangioma often can be managed by complete excision. Other therapeutic options have been used, including intralesional **(Fig. 25C)** or systemic steroids, surgery, embolization, radiation, interferon therapy, and laser therapy. **Figure 25D** shows regression of tumor after local injection of Triamcinolone. Sometimes injection into orbital lesions carries the serious risk of retinal arterial embolization and blindness so a simultaneous dilated funduscopy during injection to detect emboli and immediate discontinuation of the infusion, if needed, can be done. Other complications include adrenal suppression, skin depigmentation, orbital fat necrosis, and localized calcification. Unresponsive lesions may benefit from interferon-α2a.

Lymphangioma

Overview

Lymphangioma is a benign vascular lesion that frequently affects the orbit.

Clinical Features

They present as painless unilateral proptosis **(Fig. 26A)** with a bluish hue after birth which may increase with an upper respiratory infection or on prone position. They may

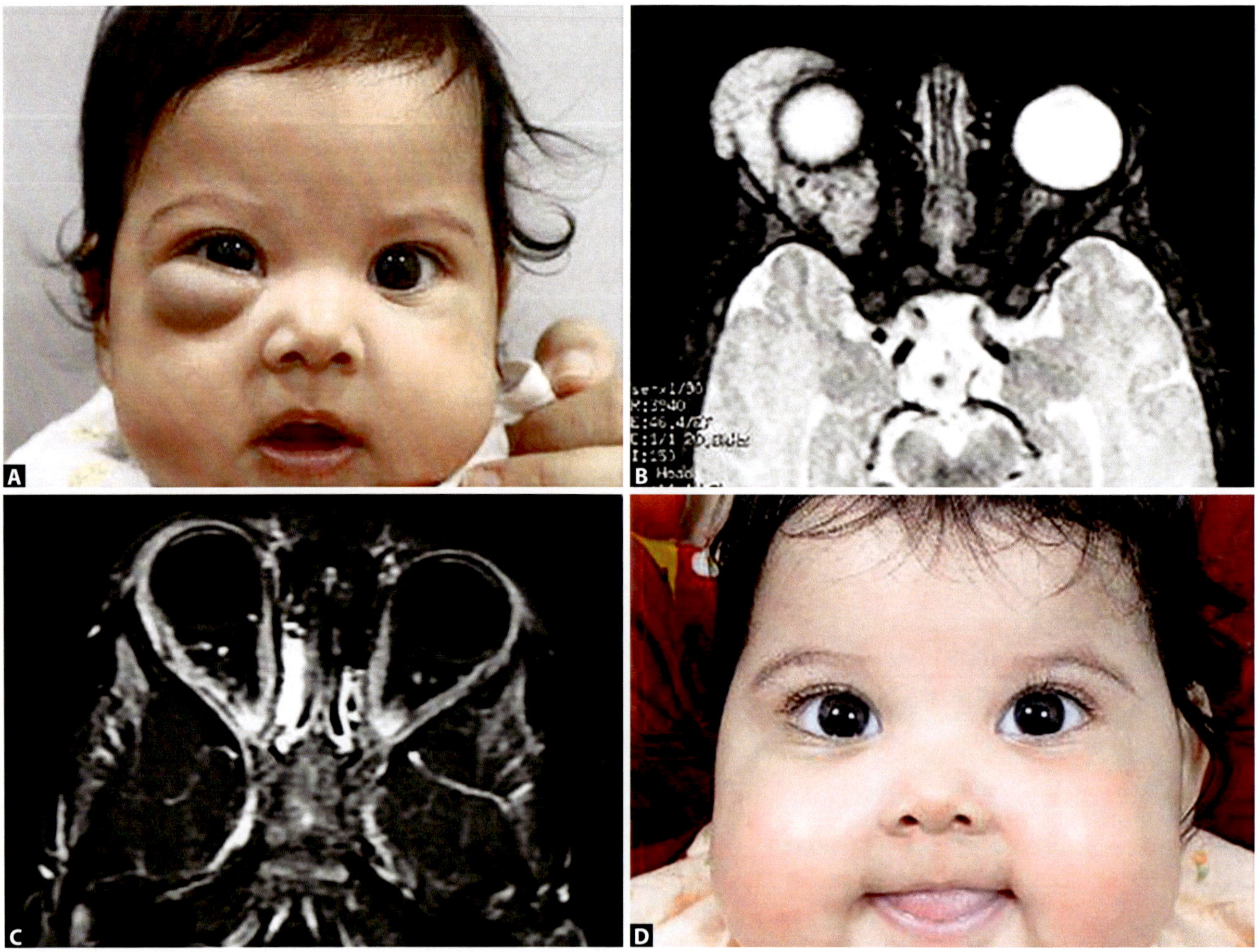

Figs. 25A to D: (A) Prominence of right lower eyelid secondary to orbital capillary hemangioma in a 6-month-old child; (B) Magnetic resonance imaging in T2-weighted image showing extensive hyperintense orbital mass involving orbital septum; (C) After intralesional injection triamcinolone (30 mg) slight residual retro-orbital component present; (D) Appearance at 1 year of age.

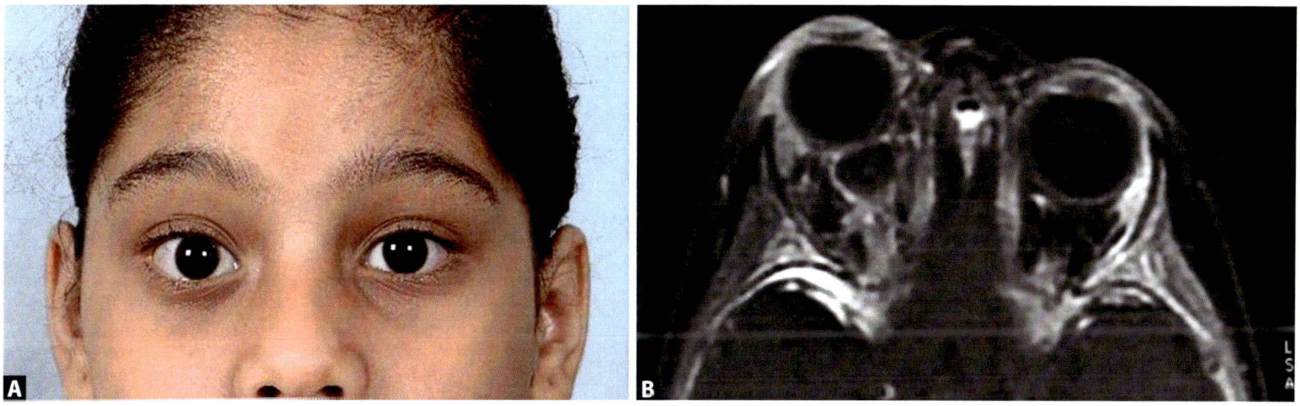

Figs. 26A and B: (A) Right eye orbital lymphangioma in a child presenting with unilateral proptosis; (B) MRI axial scan shows ill-defined mass with multiple cystic spaces intraconally.

have associated ptosis, strabismus, conjunctival or upper airway, and palate lesions. They become painful in case of internal bleeding forming hemorrhagic cysts which is called a "chocolate cyst".

Diagnostic Evaluation

It is type 1 arteriovenous (AV) malformation showing no evidence of venous or arterial flow. MRI and CT show suggestive features that can establish the diagnosis without resorting to an immediate biopsy. Gadolinium-enhanced MRI optimally delineates the cystic compartments with fluid levels **(Fig. 26B)**.

Management

Complete surgical resection is often not possible owing to poor definition of the lesion and excessive bleeding at the time of surgical manipulation. Various treatment modalities have been tried but they are only marginally effective. It includes surgical debulking, carbon dioxide laser, and sclerotherapy. It involves the use of a sclerosing agent that irritates the endothelial lining of the lymphangioma, which leads to inflammation, fibrosis, and involution. Sclerosing agents are hypertonic saline, ethyl alcohol, sodium tetradecyl sulfate, ethanolamine oleate, and OK-432. Nowadays, intralesional injection bleomycin at 6 mg/kg body weight is being used. Even systemic sildenafil and sirolimus have been used.

Juvenile Pilocytic Astrocytoma/Optic Nerve Glioma

Overview

In children, the most common cause of axial proptosis is optic nerve glioma. They are uncommon benign lesions accounting for 1.5–4% of all orbital tumors and 50–55% of all primary optic nerve tumors. They can be classified as anterior glioma (involve optic nerve only) or posterior glioma (involve chiasm and rarely can extend into the adjacent hypothalamus or third ventricle). The reported incidence of neurofibromatosis type 1 (NF1) among patients with optic gliomas varies from 10 to 70%, with an overall incidence of 29%.

Clinical Features

It generally affects children in the first decade of life. Children either come with progressive visual loss and axial proptosis **(Fig. 27A)**. All these children must be evaluated for NF1 features such as café-au-lait spots at back or chest, iris Lisch nodules, subcutaneous nodules, or neurofibroma. Sometimes these children can present with pulsatile proptosis secondary to the absence of the greater wing of the sphenoid bone. Posterior glioma presents with visual loss, strabismus, or nystagmus. In the early stages, fundus examination reveals an edematous optic disk and later the disk appears atrophic with a pale appearance.

Diagnostic Evaluation

Visual field analysis should be done if the chiasmal lesion is suspected. CT and MRI of the optic nerve typically show a fusiform swelling of the optic nerve **(Fig. 27B)**. For posterior gliomas, MRI is superior to CT. A characteristic kink in the midportion of the tumor is often present. Imaging studies reveal that enlargement of the optic canal can be demonstrated in up to 80% of patients with a glioma involving the optic nerves. Enlargement and J-shaped excavation of the sella turcica may be associated with chiasmal gliomas.

Treatment

Management is explained in **Flowchart 2**. It is generally believed that juvenile pilocytic astrocytomas (JPA) associated with NF1 is less aggressive and can show spontaneous regression. For gliomas initially confined to the optic nerve the mortality rate is 12%, typically from the intracranial extension. Chiasmal gliomas left untreated or that are partially excised show a mortality rate of 17% over a mean follow-up period of 10 years. In patients with chiasmal tumors plus hypothalamic or third ventricle involvement at the time of presentation, the mortality rate is 50% or more over 15 years.

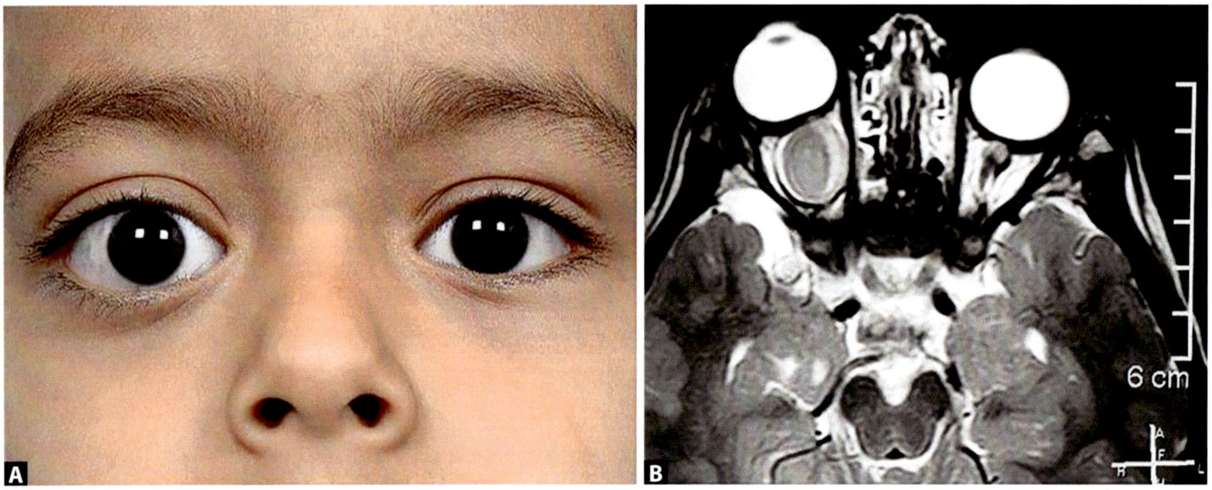

Figs. 27A and B: (A) Axial proptosis of right eye in a 4-year-old child; (B) MRI T2-weighted axial scan show a characteristic, well-defined, and ovoid mass affecting the optic nerve.

Flowchart 2: Management of optic nerve glioma.

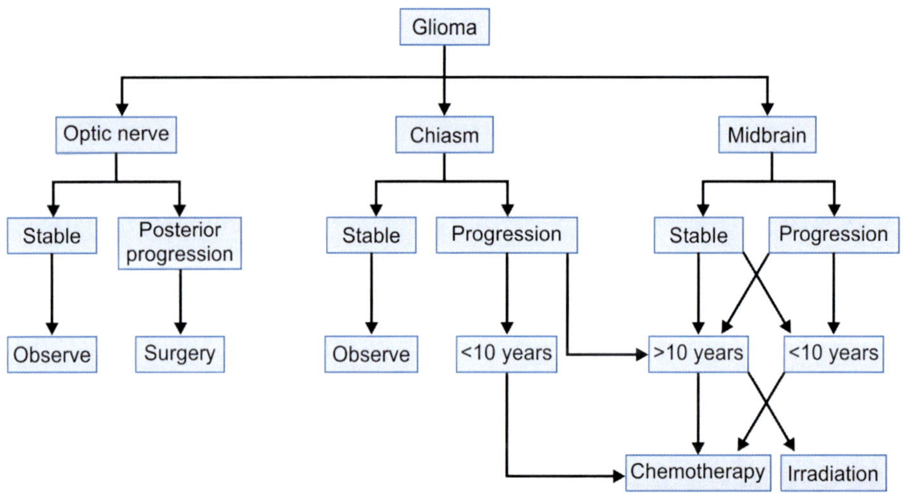

Rhabdomyosarcoma

Overview

The most common primary malignancy of the orbit in children is rhabdomyosarcoma. The tumor is derived from undifferentiated mesenchymal cells that have the potential to differentiate into striated muscle accounting for approximately 5% of all solid tumors in children. It is nonfamilial and is diagnosed typically at a mean of 7.5 years of age. Malignancy has occurred secondarily in patients after radiotherapy for RB and squamous cell carcinoma.

Clinical Features

Children present with rapidly progressive unilateral proptosis with a firm ill-defined mass may be associated with periocular inflammation **(Figs.28A and 29A)**. They are associated with motility restriction, hypogeous, diplopia, ptosis, eyelid erythema, chemosis, exposure keratopathy **(Fig. 29A)**, and masquerading as orbital cellulitis. The fundus examination may show choroidal folds or optic disk edema. Most commonly the lesion is found in the supranasal quadrant and sometimes may even occur from local spread from the adjacent sinus cavities, meninges, or other soft tissues of the head and neck.

Diagnostic Evaluation

A CT shows a moderately well-defined mass either extraconal **(Fig. 28B)** or intraconal (rare) of homogenous density with adjacent bony erosion **(Fig. 29B)**. It may displace the globe. Heterogenousity may be due to necrosis or intralesional hemorrhage associated with calcification. It enhances moderately with contrast. In MRI, mass is isointense relative to muscle or brain with T1-weighted sequences and hyperintense relative to muscle and brain with T2-weighted sequences. They show moderate contrast enhancement. Occasionally, invasion of the adjacent paranasal sinuses or intracranial contents may be seen reflecting the aggressive nature of the tumor.

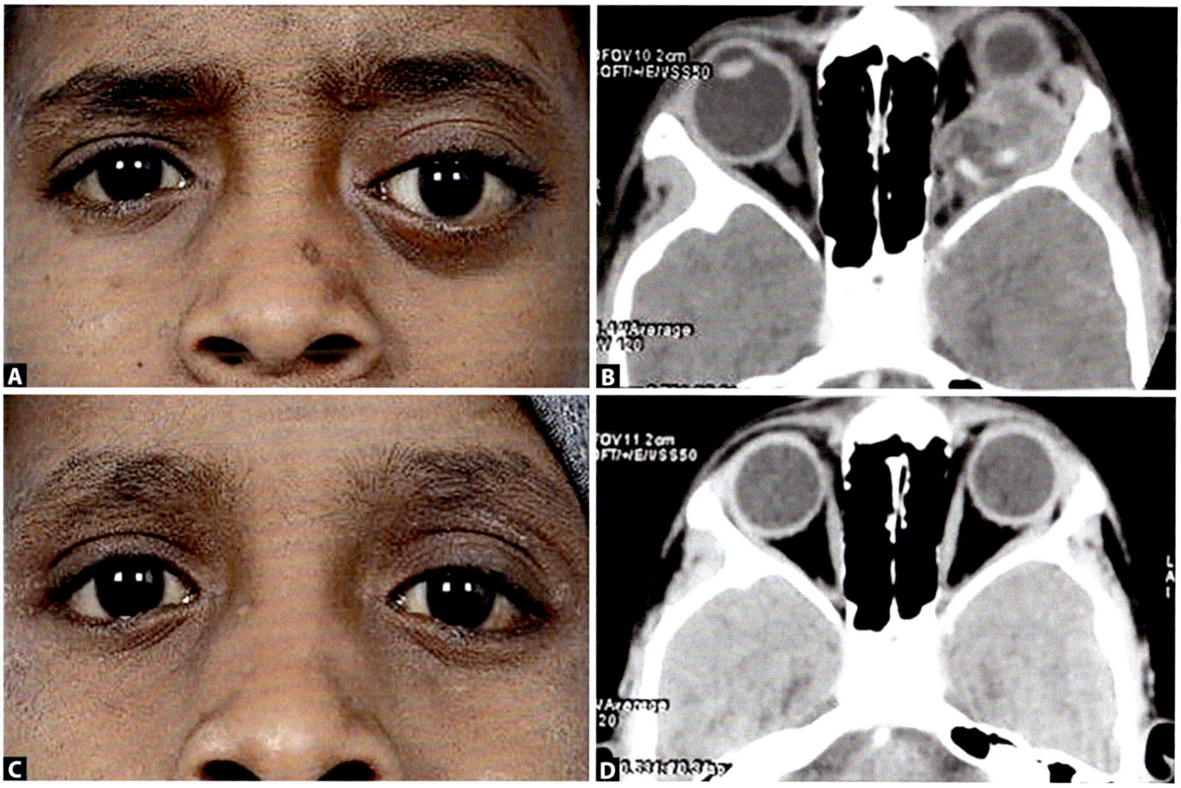

Figs. 28A to D: (A) A 8-year-old child presented with abaxial proptosis; (B) CT scan shows ill-defined extraconal heterogeneous mass; (C and D) After undergoing chemotherapy and surgical excision.

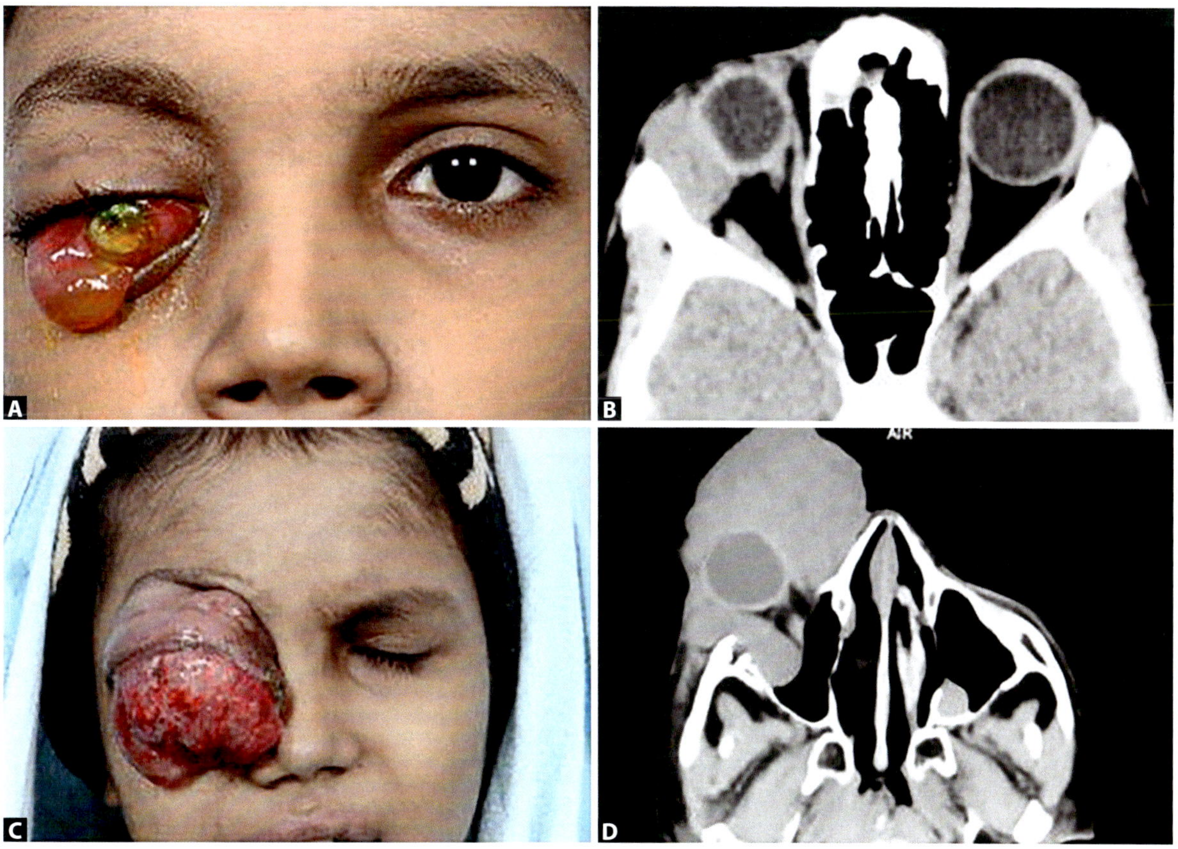

Figs. 29A to D: (A) An 8-year-old child showing abaxial proptosis, conjunctival chemosis, and exposure keratopathy; (B) CT scan shows well-defined extraconal mass associated with bony molding; (C) Child was lost to follow-up and returned with a fungating mass; (D) CT scan shows large ill-defined mass in the anterior, mid and posterior orbit, and indenting the globe.

Based on histopathology there are four variants: embryonal, alveolar, botryoid, and pleomorphic. Embryonal is the most common variant carrying a good prognosis while the alveolar type is the most malignant variant.

Treatment

Firstly, peripheral blood smear should be done to rule out chloroma and leukemia. Treatment depends upon the groups, as defined by the Intergroup Rhabdomyosarcoma Study Group **(Table 8)**. If left untreated then can lead to fungating growth **(Figs. 29C and D)** and systemic metastasis. **Figures 28C and D** show successful management after chemotherapy and surgical excision.

Langerhans Cell Histiocytosis

Overview

Langerhans cell histiocytosis is a rare group of disorders due to the clonal proliferation of histiocytes. It is a wide term encompassing histiocytosis X, Hand-Schüller-Christian disease, and Letterer–Siwe disease. It behaves aggressively in children.

Clinical Features

Children mostly present with unilateral proptosis, ptosis, or a decrease in vision **(Fig. 30A)**. Orbital involvement consists of fullness with irregular firm palpable lesion mainly in superotemporal quadrant and may be associated with bony

TABLE 8: Intergroup Rhabdomyosarcoma Study Group staging classification with treatment.

Group	Description	Management
I	Localized tumor	Neoadjuvant chemo(VA) + complete resection
II	Residual microscopic disease after surgery	Adjuvant chemo(VA) + RT
III	Tumors with gross residual disease after biopsy	Adjuvant chemo(VAC) + complete excision/exenteration + RT
IV	Distant metastases	Adjuvant chemo(VAC) + RT (local + distant)

(RT: radiotherapy; VA: vincristine, actinomycin; VAC: vincristine, actinomycin, cyclophosphamide)

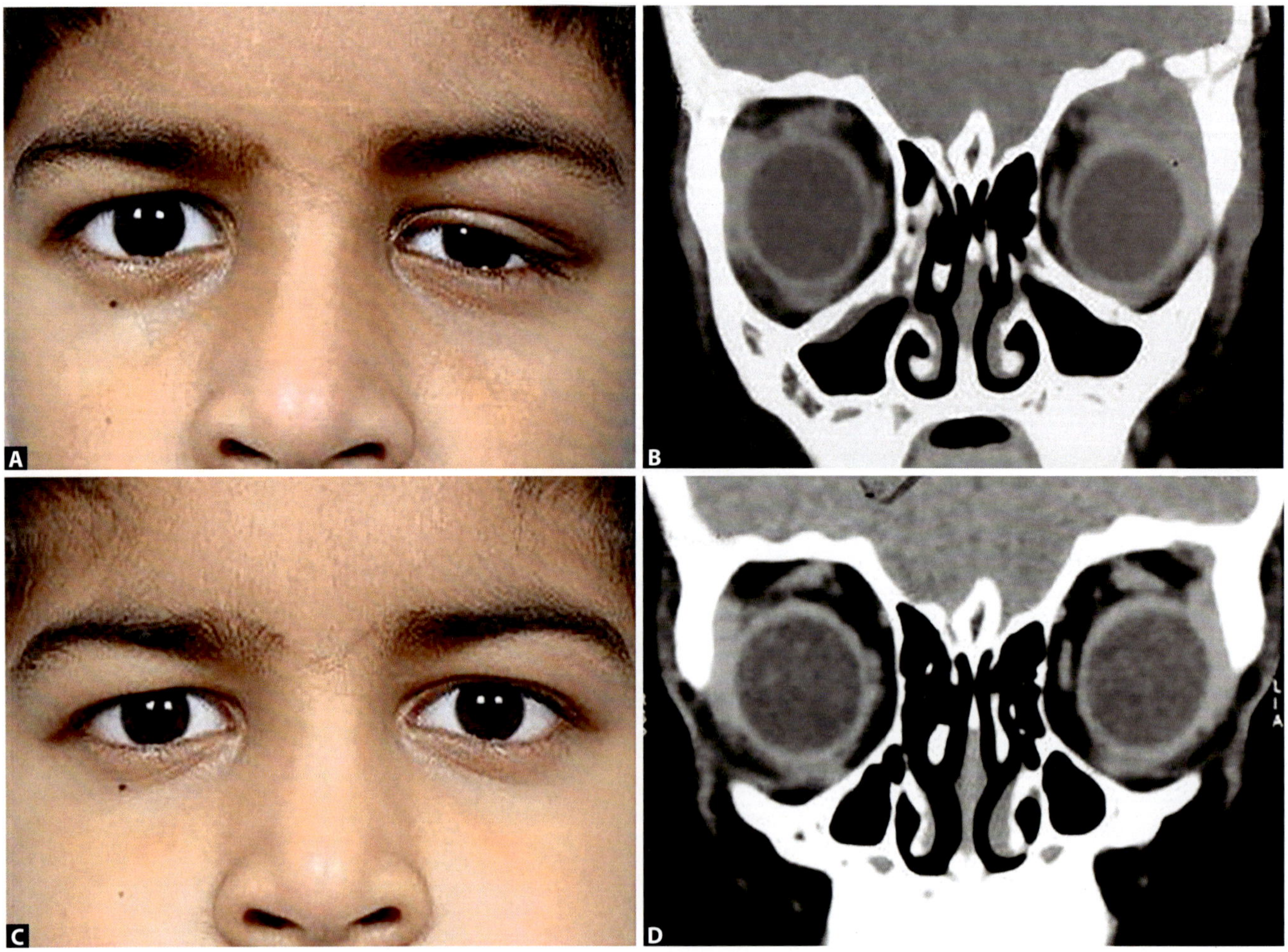

Figs. 30A to D: (A) An 8-year-old child with drooping of left eye upper eyelid; (B) CT scan coronal section shows ill-defined heterogeneous mass in superior quadrant eroding the bone to reach dura but dura is intact; (C) After undergoing multilevel incision biopsy and intralesional injection steroid, lid has come back to its normal position; (D) Bone remodeling seen.

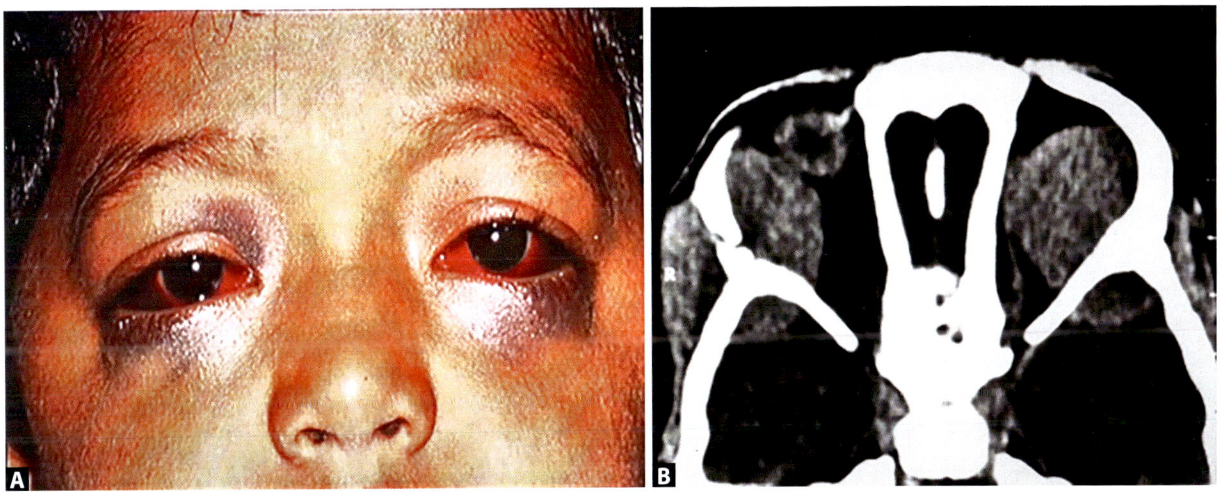

Figs. 31A and B: (A) Child with bilateral proptosis, raccoon eyes, and bitemporal fossa fullness; (B) CT scan axial section reveals ill-defined heterogeneous mass forming a triradiate lesion with bony erosion.

irregularity, if the bone is involved. Thus, orbital LCH can simulate the imaging appearance of rhabdomyosarcoma with bone invasion, although bone destruction in the former is typically more pronounced.

Diagnostic Evaluation

A CT scan shows a moderately differentiated lesion with bony erosion. Sometimes the erosion is too severe to lead to the intracranial extension **(Fig. 30B)**. Immunohistochemistry demonstrates a CD1a and S100 positive phenotype.

Treatment

If the lesion is well defined not involving vital structures then complete excision biopsy followed by close observation. If the lesion is ill defined and large enough to preclude excision biopsy then a multilayered incision biopsy with intraoperative frozen section diagnosis should be done. When the diagnosis is confirmed then intralesional injection triamcinolone can be given till the lesion resolves **(Fig. 30C)**. Spontaneous bone remodeling is also seen **(Fig. 30D)**.

Metastatic Neuroblastoma

Overview

Metastatic neuroblastoma is the second most frequent orbital malignancy of childhood after rhabdomyosarcoma. Neuroblastoma arises from embryonic neural crest tissue of the postganglionic sympathetic nervous system. The most common site for the primary tumor is in the abdomen.

Clinical Features

Most of them present before the age of 3 years. They present with rapidly developing unilateral or bilateral proptosis with periocular ecchymoses **(Fig. 31A)**. They may also present with opsoclonus, myoclonus, and metastases to the iris or choroids. CT scan shows both bony and soft tissue involvement with the intracranial extension **(Fig. 31B)**. Metastatic neuroblastoma often results in high levels of urine homovanillic acid and vanillylmandelic acid.

Treatment

Aggressive combination chemotherapy and total body irradiation are used, but the prognosis remains poor.

SUGGESTED READING

1. Ang M, Lee SY. Multifocal photodynamic therapy for diffuse choroidal hemangioma. Clin Ophthalmol. 2012;6:1467-9.
2. Cassoux N, Charlotte F, Sastre X, Orbach D, Lehoang P, Desjardins L. Conservative surgical treatment of medulloepithelioma of the ciliary body. Arch Ophthalmol. 2010;128(3):380-1.
3. Chanana B, Kumar V. Imaging findings in tuberous sclerosis with multiple retinal astrocytic hamartomas. J Pediatr Ophthalmol Strabismus. 2011;48(2):127-8.
4. Chawda SJ, Moseley IF. Computed tomography of orbital dermoids: a 20-year review. Clin Radiol. 1999;54:821-5.
5. Dahr SS, Cusick M, Rodriguez-Coleman H, Srivastava SK, Thompson DJ, Linehan WM, et al. Intravitreal anti-vascular endothelial growth factor therapy with pegaptanib for advanced von Hippel-Lindau disease of the retina. Retina. 2007;27(2):150-8.
6. Drolet BA, Esterly NB, Frieden IJ. Hemangiomas in children. N Engl J Med. 1999;341:173-81.
7. Dutton JJ, Byrne SF, Proia AD. Diagnostic Atlas of Orbital Diseases. Philadelphia: WB Saunders; 2000.
8. Egbert JE, Schwartz GS, Walsh AW. Diagnosis and treatment of an ophthalmic artery occlusion during an intralesional injection of corticosteroid into an eyelid capillary hemangioma. Am J Ophthalmol. 1996;121:638-42.
9. Elner VM, Mintz R, Demirci H, Hassan AS. Local Corticosteroid Treatment of Eyelid and Orbital Xanthogranuloma. Ophthalmic Plas Reconstr Surg. 2006;22(1):36-40.
10. Finger PT, Pro MJ, Schneider S, Kurli M, Shapira I, Hu K. Visual recovery after radiation therapy for bilateral subfoveal acute myelogenous leukemia (AML). Am J Ophthalmol. 2004;138:659-62.
11. Gambrelle J, Kivelä T, Grange JD. Sturge-Weber syndrome: decrease in intraocular pressure after transpupillary thermotherapy for diffuse choroidal haemangioma. Acta Ophthalmol. 2011;89(2):190-3.

12. Gandhi NG, Lin LK, O'Hara M. Sildenafil for pediatric orbital lymphangioma. JAMA Ophthalmol. 2013;131:1228-30.
13. Garcia-Arumi J, Sararols LH, Cavero L, Escalada F, Corcóstegui BF. Therapeutic options for capillary papillary hemangiomas. Ophthalmology. 2000;107:48-54.
14. Haik BG, Karcioglu ZA, Gordon RA, Pechous BP. Capillary hemangioma (infantile periocular hemangioma). Surv Ophthalmol. 1994;38:399-426.
15. Hidayat AA, Mafee MF, Laver NV, Noujaim S. Langerhans' cell histiocytosis and juvenile xanthogranuloma of the orbit. Clinicopathologic, CT, and MR imaging features. Radiol Clin North Am. 1998;36:1229-40.
16. Hill RH, Shiels WE, Foster JA. Percutaneous drainage and ablation as first line therapy for macrocystic and microcystic orbital lymphatic malformations. Ophthal Plast Reconstr Surg. 2012;28:119-25.
17. Honavar SG, Manjandavida FP. Tumors of the ocular surface: a review. Indian J Ophthalmol. 2015;63:187-203.
18. Horgan N, O'Keefe M, McLoone E, Lanigan B. Fundus fluorescein angiographic characterization of diffuse choroidal hemangiomas. J Pediatr Ophthalmol Strabismus. 2008;45(1):26-30.
19. Howard GM, Forrest AW. Incidence and location of melanocytomas. Arch Ophthalmol. 1967;77:61-6.
20. Jakobiec FA, Depot MJ, Kennerdell JS, Shults WT, Anderson RL, Alper ME, et al. Combined clinical and computed tomographic diagnosis of orbital glioma and meningioma. Ophthalmology. 1984;91:137-55.
21. Jeong J, Song Y-J, Seung-Il J, Kwon J-W. New surgical approach for limbal dermoids in children: simple excision, corneal tattooing, and sutureless limboconjunctival autograft. Cornea. 2015;34:720-23.
22. Kennedy R. Orbital dermoids. In: Hornblass A (Ed). Oculoplastic, orbital and reconstructive surgery. Baltimore: Williams & Wilkins; 1990. pp. 866-72.
23. Khurshid GS. Transvitreal endoresection of refractory retinal capillary hemangioblastoma after feeder vessel ligation. Ophthalmic Surg Lasers Imaging Retina. 2013;44(3):278-80.
24. Lang S, Böhringer D, Reinhard T. Surgical management of corneal limbal dermoids: retrospective study of different techniques and use of Mitomycin C. Eye. 2014;28:857-62.
25. Léauté-Labrèze C, Dumas de la Roque E, Hubiche T, Boralevi F, Thambo JB, Taïeb A. Propranolol for severe hemangiomas of infancy. N Engl J Med. 2008;358:2649-51.
26. Lee V, Ragge NK, Collin JR. Orbitotemporal neurofibromatosis. Clinical features and surgical management. Ophthalmology. 2004;111:382-8.
27. Lonngi M, Gold AS, Murray TG. Combined bevacizumab and triamcinolone acetonide injections for macular edema in a patient with astrocytic hamartomas and tuberous sclerosis. Ophthalmic Surg Lasers Imaging Retina. 2013;44(1):85-90.
28. Mahesh L, Krishnakumar S, Subramanian N, Babu K, Biswas J. Malignant teratoma of the orbit: a clinicopathological study of a case. Orbit. 2003;22:305-9.
29. Mennel S, Meyer CH, Eggarter F, Peter S. Autofluorescence and angiographic findings of retinal astrocytic hamartomas in tuberous sclerosis. Ophthalmologica. 2005;219:350-6.
30. Mullaney PB, Jacquemin C, Abboud E, Karcioglu ZA. Tuberous sclerosis in infancy. J Pediatr Ophthalmol Strabismus. 1997;34: 372-5.
31. Murthy R, Hanovaz SG, Naik M, Gopi S, Reddy VA. Ruthenium-106 plaque brachytherapy for the treatment of diffuse choroidal haemangioma in Sturge-Weber syndrome. Indian J Ophthalmol. 2005;53(4):274-5.
32. Murthy R, Honavar SG, Naik MN, Reddy VA. Retinoblastoma. In: Dutta LC (Ed). Modern Ophthalmology. New Delhi, India: Jaypee Brothers Medical Publishers (P) Ltd; 2004. pp. 849-59.
33. Nathan N, Thaller SR. Sturge-Weber syndrome and associated congenital vascular disorders: a review. J Craniofac Surg. 2006;17:724-8.
34. Parmar DN, Mireskandari K, McHugh D. Transpupillary thermotherapy for retinal capillary hemangioma in von Hippel-Lindau disease. Ophthalmic Surg Lasers. 2000;31:334-6.
35. Parsa CF, Hoyt CS, Lesser RL, Weinstein JM, Strother CM, Muci-Mendoza R, et al. Spontaneous regression of optic gliomas: thirteen cases documented by serial neuroimaging. Arch Ophthalmol. 2001;119:516-29.
36. Pirouzian A, Holz H, Merrill K, Sudesh R, Karlen K. Surgical management of pediatric limbal dermoids with sutureless amniotic membrane transplantation and augmentation. J Pediatr Ophthalmol Strabismus. 2011;49:114-9.
37. Polito E, Leccisotti A. Colobomatous ocular cyst excision with globe preservation. Ophthal Plast Reconstr Surg. 1995;11:288-92.
38. Raichura ND, Alam MS, Noronha VO, Mukherjee B. A prospective study of the role of intralesional bleomycin in orbital lymphangioma. J AAPOS. 2017;21:146-51.
39. Raynor M, Hodgkins P. Microphthalmos with cyst. Preservation of the eye by repeated aspiration. J Pediatr Ophthalmol Strabismus. 2001;38:245-6.
40. Rebuffini E, Zuccarino L, Grecchi E, Carinci F, Merulla VE. Picibanil (OK-432) in the treatment of head and neck lymphangiomas in children. Dent Res J. 2012;9(Suppl 2):S192-6.
41. Reddy SC, Jackson N, Menon BS. Ocular involvement in leukemia—a study of 288 cases. Ophthalmologica. 2003;217:441-5.
42. Rootman J, Hay E, Graeb D, Miller R. Orbital-adnexal lymphangiomas. A spectrum of hemodynamically isolated vascular hamartomas. Ophthalmology. 1986;93:1558-70.
43. Rosenthal G, Snir M, Biedner B. Corticosteroid resistant orbital hemangioma with proptosis treated with interferon alfa-2-a and partial tarsorrhaphy. J Pediatr Ophthalmol Strabismus. 1995;32:50-51.
44. Sangwan VS, Sridhar MS, Vemuganti GK. Treatment of complex choristoma by excision and amniotic membrane transplantation. Arch Ophthalmol. 2003;121(2):278-80.
45. Schmidt-Erfurth UM, Kusserow C, Barbazetto IA, Laqua H. Benefits and complications of photodynamic therapy of papillary capillary hemangiomas. Ophthalmology. 2002;109:1256-66.
46. Sharma T, Grewal J, Gupta S, Murray PI. Ophthalmic manifestations of acute leukaemias: the ophthalmologist's role. Eye. 2004;18:663-72.
47. Shields CL, Benevides R, Materin MA. Optical coherence tomography of retinal strocytic hamartoma in 15 cases. Ophthalmology. 2006;113(9):1553-7.
48. Shields CL, Fasiudden AF, Mashayekhi A, Shields JA. Conjunctival nevi: clinical features and natural course in 410 consecutive patients. Arch Ophthalmol. 2004;122:167-75.
49. Shields CL, Mashayekhi A, Ho T, Cater J, Shields JA. Solitary congenital hypertrophy of the retinal pigment epithelium: clinical features and frequency of enlargement in 330 patients. Ophthalmology. 2003;110:1968-76.
50. Shields CL, Pellegrini M, Ferenczy SR. Enhanced depth imaging optical coherence tomography (EDI-OCT) of intraocular tumors. From placid to seasick to rock and rolling topography. The 2013 Francesco Orzalesi Lecture. Retina. 2014;34:1495-512.

16

CHAPTER

Pediatric Community Ophthalmology

Vadrevu K Raju, Satya S Yalla, Srinivasa R Nambula, Leela V Raju

"Almost nothing need be said when you have eyes." "I shut my eyes and all the world drops dead; I lift my eyes and all is born again."

—Tarjei Vesaas, Sylvia Plath

INTRODUCTION

Community ophthalmology is delivery of eye care which involves preventive, curative, promotive, and rehabilitative activities, making it a holistic approach. With clinical ophthalmology at its core; it incorporates basic, clinical, and public-health sciences in its dimension. It highlights the realignment from individualized care to community-based eye care services. As ocular health is the end product of the interactions of the multifactorial determinants of disease that exist in the community, community or preventive ophthalmology has been attracting attention in the ophthalmological world.

Pediatric ophthalmology in particular is gaining importance in that its societal impact may surpass its impact on the individual. Considering the total number of disability-adjusted life years (DALYs) lost in those with adult blindness (number of years that a blind person lives after going blind), childhood blindness has a greater long-term impact, e.g., the difficulty in integrating the child socially and functionally, and the long-term burden on the caregiver and society.

For example, in India, childhood blindness results in 11.2 million blind-person-years resulting in longer DALYs loss as compared to 5.5 million blind-person-years of due to adult onset glaucoma.

CHILDHOOD BLINDNESS

Childhood blindness refers to a group of diseases and conditions occurring in childhood or early adolescence, which, if left untreated, result in blindness or severe visual impairment that are likely to be untreatable later in life. Childhood blindness and visual loss due to one of the most prevalent diseases, corneal disease, is important because of its significant impact on the child's development, education, future job opportunities, and quality of life.

World Health Organization Definition of Childhood Blindness and Visual Impairment

The World Health Organization (WHO) uses a definition of best corrected vision of <3/60 and a best corrected vision of <6/18 in the better eye in its definition of blindness. This definition ignores uncorrected refractive errors as an important cause of visual impairment in children. Because of this oversight, the WHO has changed its definitions to "presenting visual acuity" instead of "best corrected visual acuity". However, studies targeted towards refractive error have suggested that presenting visual acuity of <6/12 in the better eye may be a more appropriate criterion for defining visual impairment in children as ≥6/12 vision is essential for driving, some types of learning, and some sports.

Epidemiology of Childhood Blindness

Childhood blindness is a serious public health concern across the world and remains a significant problem due to cumulative loss of blind-person-years in young children. The magnitude of childhood blindness is relatively small when compared to extent of blindness in adults. The WHO has estimated that globally about 314 million people are visually impaired and among these there are 45 million children. About 19 million alone are children below the age of 15 years

Almost three quarters live in low-to-middle income countries where the prevalence is reported to be as high as 1.5 per 1,000 children in contrast to high-income countries where the prevalence is 0.3 per 1,000.

As per the available information from community-based studies, the prevalence of childhood blindness varied between 0.6 and 1.06/1,000 and prevalence of visual impairment varied between 2.05 and 13.6/1,000.

Causes of Childhood Blindness and Visual Impairment

The WHO system for classifying blindness and low vision in children uses two methods. The first method, a descriptive classification, refers to the anatomical site most affected. The following categories are used:

- Whole globe (e.g., anophthalmos and microphthalmos)
- Cornea (e.g., corneal scarring and keratoconus)
- Lens (e.g., cataract and aphakia)
- Uvea (e.g., aniridia)
- Retina (e.g., retinal dystrophies)
- Optic nerve (e.g., atrophy)
- Glaucoma
- Conditions where the eye appears normal (e.g., refractive errors, cortical blindness, and amblyopia).

The second method, an etiological classification, classifies blindness according to underlying cause. This method uses categories based on the time of onset of the condition:

- Hereditary (at conception), e.g., genetic diseases and chromosomal abnormalities.
- Intrauterine (during pregnancy), e.g., due to rubella or thalidomide teratogenicity.
- Perinatal (around birth), e.g., retinopathy of prematurity (ROP), birth injury, and neonatal conjunctivitis/ophthalmia neonatorum (ON).
- Childhood, e.g., vitamin A deficiency disorders, measles, and trauma
- Unknown/cannot be determined.

Childhood Blindness: Avoidable Causes

The term "avoidable" encompasses preventable and treatable causes with existing technology and resources. Conditions amenable to primary prevention (i.e., where the condition causing blindness could have been entirely prevented) include measles infection, vitamin A deficiency, ON, the use of harmful traditional eye medication remedies, and congenital rubella syndrome. Conditions that could have been treated early to prevent blindness (i.e., secondary prevention) include glaucoma and ROP. Causes of blindness where sight can be restored (i.e., tertiary prevention) include cataract and selected cases of corneal scarring.

In India, ocular trauma, infectious keratitis, corneal ulceration, and postinfectious keratitis and iridocorneal scars contribute significantly to pediatric ocular morbidity. Congenital corneal disorders are also an important cause of childhood blindness that usually result from hereditary dystrophies, congenital glaucoma, Peters' anomaly and other mesenchymal dysgenesis, birth trauma, and metabolic disorders.

Prevention and Control of Childhood Blindness

Educated and available primary healthcare providers along with personnel trained in comprehensive eye care are essential for the control of blindness in children. This applies particularly to developing countries, where a high proportion of blindness in children is due to preventable conditions described above.

The control of blindness in children, especially in India and similar developing countries, requires not only robust strategies but also a well-designed and functional integrated healthcare delivery system.

This integrated health system, for both screening and referral services, has to be tailored for both geographical accessibility and sociocultural acceptance.

Comprehensive Primary Eye Care

- Promotion of eye health, action in the community to prevent conditions which causes blindness, and recognition and treatment of common eye diseases by trained community-level health workers.
- Identification of children who need referral for special ophthalmological assessment and treatment, such as any blind child or a child with a white pupil or corneal ulcer.
- Different cadres of primary healthcare worker have different roles. Traditional birth attendants, for example, can prevent ON and examine the eyes of the newborn for structural abnormalities.

Secondary Level of Care

- An ophthalmologist who is able to carry out a complete examination and assessment, make a provisional diagnosis, manage corneal ulcers in children, and prescribe simple low-vision devices for children with less complex problems.
- School vision-testing programs to identify children with significant refractive errors should also be organized and supported.
- For effective referral, good communication needs to be established between staff working in the primary and tertiary levels.
- The management of conditions requiring surgical intervention is more complex in children than in adults, and requires a team of well-trained and well-equipped personnel.
- Effective communication with parents to ensure their involvement is also essential. An anesthetist may be required for young or uncooperative older children, and trained nurses, refractionists, and paramedics are all essential members of the team.

Care at Tertiary Centers

- Provide diagnostic and surgical services of high quality for the management of cataract, glaucoma, retinal disease, and corneal scarring.
- Ophthalmologists providing services for children at tertiary centers need a child-centered approach, and they

should also be trained in the required special pediatric diagnostic, medical, and surgical techniques.

- Standardized screening protocols for diagnosis and treatment of ROP, both in and out of nurseries, as well as the organization and provision of low-vision services.
- Tertiary centers should take responsibility for research; the training of trainers for primary- and secondary-level programs; and for supporting, supervising, motivating, and providing feedback to staff in secondary-level centers.

Global Initiatives

In 1999, the WHO along with the International Agency for the Prevention of Blindness (IAPB), established a joint venture called, "VISION 2020: The Right to Sight" which aims to eliminate avoidable blindness in the world by 2020 and targets the world's leading causes of avoidable visual impairment.

VISION 2020: The Right to Sight:

- *Targets for the control of childhood blindness*:
  - Eliminating corneal scarring due to vitamin A deficiency, measles, and ON.
  - Eliminate new cases of congenital rubella syndrome.
  - Making surgery for pediatric cataract accessible and available.
  - Setting up centers and increasing awareness to ensure that all babies at risk of ROP are examined at 6–7 weeks after birth and are provided appropriate treatment.
  - Ensure coverage of all schools by the School Eye Screening Programs and providing spectacles to all children with refractive errors.
  - Upgrading the available infrastructure to ensure that there is one refractionist/50,000 population, one trained person for low vision/5 million population, and one Pediatric Ophthalmology Unit/10 million population by 2020.
- *Human resources development*:
  - Ensure that prevention of childhood blindness is an explicit aim of all primary healthcare programs.
  - Ensure that all secondary-level eye clinics have facilities to provide appropriate glasses for children with significant refractive errors.
  - Provide training so that there will be one refractionist per 100,000/people by the year 2010.
  - Provide training so that there will be at least one worker to manage low vision/20 million people by 2010, and for every 5 million by 2020.
  - Ensure that one ophthalmologist is trained in the management of pediatric eye conditions for every 50 million people by 2010 and one per 10 million people by 2020.
- *Appropriate technology and infrastructure development*:
  - Ensure the development of low-cost, high-quality, low-vision devices, which should be widely available, even in low-income countries.
  - Establish a network of specialist "child eye care" tertiary centers.

Indian strategies and plans under VISION 2020: Right to Sight for control of childhood blindness:

- *Detection of eye disorders*: Like congenital blindness, refractive errors, squint, amblyopia, and corneal diseases
  - At the time of immunization
  - At school entry
  - Periodic checkup every 3 years for normal and every year for those with defects.
- *Preventable childhood blindness to be taken care of through cost-effective measures*:
  - Prevention of xerophthalmia is of utmost value in preventing childhood blindness.
  - Prevention and early treatment of trachoma by active intervention.
  - Refractive errors to be corrected at primary eye care centers.
  - Childhood glaucoma's to be treated promptly.
  - Harmful traditional/practices need to be avoided.
  - Prevention of ROP by proper screening and monitoring neonatal care in premature newborns.
- Curable childhood blindness due to cataract, ROP, corneal opacity, and other causes to be taken care of by the experts at secondary and tertiary level eye care.

Genetic Disorders

There is increasing prevalence of blindness due to whole globe diseases, e.g., anophthalmia, microphthalmia, and coloboma sequelae. There is also an increaswe in genetic (PAX2 & PAX6) diseases, use of alcohol and drugs, and environmental exposure to toxins like pesticides and fertilizers. However, some congenital defects may be the results of "genes + environment", an anomalous interaction between genes controlling retinoic acid signaling and maternal vitamin A deficiency.

Hereditary Disorders

Hereditary causes such as colobomas, anterior segment dysgenesis, corneal dystrophies, and systemic and ocular metabolic diseases contribute to the more serious forms of blindness in the newborn.

Intrauterine Causes

The greatest impact of community health has been the decreased incidence of rubella-related ocular morbidity through strict rubella vaccination coverage programs.

REFRACTIVE ERRORS AND FUNCTIONAL LOW VISION

The most common cause of visual impairment in children worldwide is uncorrected refractive errors. These children have been historically underrepresented in the data on childhood blindness. Over the past decade, a series of studies using a survey methodology, referred to as Refractive Error Study in Children (RESC), were performed in populations with different ethnic origins and cultural settings. These studies confirmed that the prevalence of uncorrected refractive errors is considerably high for children in low-and-middle-income countries. Worldwide, nearly 1% of all children in the age group 5–15 years are visually impaired from uncorrected or inadequately corrected refractive errors, with the highest burden reported in urban areas of Southeast Asia and in China. In India, it is estimated that 2–3% of school children in rural areas have refractive errors, the proportion being higher in urban areas.

Strategy for Control

It is essential that low-vision services be part of eye care services for children at all levels of service delivery. The most valuable method of identifying potentially treatable ocular abnormalities is vision screening and is best accomplished in the primary care setting in infants and school children. School and/or community vision screening programs substantially contribute towards prevention of vision loss and can be performed in various ways, including matching or verbal visual acuity charts or any of the many automated vision screeners studying showing high-positive predictive values. In developing countries, school nursing staff and teachers have been most commonly the ones performing vision screening of school children. In recent years; however, vision screening has also included preschool children. Current understanding of the natural history of refractive error and amblyopia is incomplete, thus limiting the prophylactic potential of early screening of preschool-age children. Improved access to optical services could reduce the burden of visual impairment and help accomplish the goals of Vision 2020 concerning refractive error and low vision.

CORNEAL BLINDNESS

The importance of corneal disease as a major cause of blindness in the world today remains second only to cataract, but its epidemiology is complicated and encompasses a wide variety of infectious and inflammatory eye diseases. The causes of corneal scarring in one large study were; vitamin A deficiency (19%), measles in 3%, ON in 1%, harmful traditional eye medicines in 1%, and trauma and keratitis in the remaining 3%. Xerophthalmia and ON were additional causes of corneal blindness in children. It is estimated that approximately half of all childhood blindness in India is preventable or treatable, to which vitamin A-associated corneal blindness is a significant contributor. Prevalence of corneal opacities of 0.08%, i.e., a total of three children <15 years were found to have corneal opacities due to ocular morbidity.

Many of the causes of corneal scarring in children would be prevented if the following essential elements of primary healthcare were in place:

- Immunization
- Maternal and child healthcare
- Health education
- Good nutrition
- Essential drugs
- Clean water supplies and good sanitation
- Control of endemic diseases
- Treatment of common conditions.

VITAMIN A DEFICIENCY AND MEASLES

Vitamin A deficiency is the single most frequent cause of blindness among preschool children in some developing countries. Recent studies show that vitamin A deficiency alone contributes to 19% of childhood blindness and severe visual impairment in India.

Xerophthalmia is a collective term for the ocular manifestations of vitamin A deficiency. It can affect any age group, but the most severe blinding complications affect children aged 6 months to 3 years.

Magnitude of Vitamin A Deficiency and Measles

During the 1980s, it was discovered that vitamin A deficiency was an important cause of child mortality and that high-dose vitamin A supplementation significantly reduced child deaths, even in communities with low levels of clinical xerophthalmia.

It has been estimated that 127 million preschool children under 5 years of age are vitamin A deficient, of whom 4.4 million have xerophthalmia.

The prevalence of vitamin A deficiency was found to be 23.4% even among school-aged children.

Ocular Manifestations of Vitamin A Deficiency

Vitamin A deficiency affects the retina, conjunctiva, and cornea, and the signs and symptoms tend to occur in a reliable sequence. The WHO classification of vitamin A deficiency is as follows:

- *XN*: Night blindness
- *X1A*: Conjunctival xerosis
- *XIB*: Bitot's spot
- *X2*: Corneal xerosis
- *X3A*: Corneal ulceration/keratomalacia involving one-third or less of the cornea
- *X3B*: Corneal ulceration/keratomalacia involving one-half or more of the cornea
- *XS*: Corneal scarring.

Strategy of Control

Linking vitamin A supplementation to routine immunization programs and distributing vitamin A supplements on immunization days is being adopted by many countries to increase coverage.

Measles immunization programs are reaching target coverage levels and the number of measles cases has dramatically reduced. There is anecdotal evidence that the success of the Expanded Program on Immunization (EPI) is also reducing corneal ulceration and scarring in children.

Our role as eye care professionals is to advocate for children when we see a child with corneal ulceration from vitamin A deficiency or following measles. We should not only treat the child, but also we should inform the relevant authorities so that they can improve their programs. Prevention can be best accomplished with dietary diversification, e.g., increasing vitamin A intake from available and accessible foods, nutritional education, social marketing, home or community garden programs, and measures to improve food security.

OPHTHALMIA NEONATORUM

Conjunctivitis is an inflammatory disease characterized by conjunctival erythema, a follicular and/or papillary reaction, edema, tearing, and discharge. ON, also called *neonatal conjunctivitis*, is an acute and mucopurulent infection occurring in the first 30 days of life and affects 1.6–12% of all newborns. The etiologies include chemical toxicity and bacterial or viral processes infections.

The prevalence of blindness or severe visual impairment due to ON is 0.8% in India.

Causes of ON include the following:

- Chemical
- *Bacterial*:
  - Sexually transmitted bacteria
    - *Chlamydia trachomatis*
    - *Neisseria gonorrhoeae*
  - Nonsexually transmitted bacteria
    - *Haemophilus* species
    - *Streptococcus pneumoniae*
    - *Staphylococcus aureus*
    - *Staphylococcus epidermidis*
    - *Streptococcus viridans*
    - *Escherichia coli*
    - *Pseudomonas aeruginosa*
    - Other
- *Viral*:
  - Adenovirus
  - Herpes simplex virus types 1 and 2.

Sexually Transmitted Bacteria

Gonorrheal Ophthalmia Neonatorum

Ophthalmia neonatorum remains a significant cause of childhood corneal blindness in developing countries, mainly from *Neisseria gonorrhoeae*. In the absence of adequate prophylaxis, 30–42% of infants born by vaginal delivery to infected mothers will develop gonococcal ON. Untreated or inappropriately treated gonococcal conjunctivitis can result in corneal perforation and vision loss within 24 hours. The mean duration of corneal perforation from untreated gonococcal conjunctivitis was 11 days.

Chlamydial Ophthalmia Neonatorum

Chlamydial ON is much more prevalent than gonococcal ON, and has historically been underdiagnosed, first, due to a lack of appropriate diagnostic techniques, and second, due to a lack of diagnostic techniques with appropriate sensitivity and specificity. An infant born vaginally to a mother with chlamydial cervicitis has a 50–75% chance of acquiring the bacteria in the nasopharynx, rectum, vagina, or conjunctiva. Of neonates with proven exposure to chlamydia, 30–50% will develop conjunctivitis. The prevalence of chlamydial infections is higher in the spring and summer months. The incubation period is typically 1 week after delivery; however, it varies from 5 to 14 days or earlier if membranes ruptured prematurely.

Nonsexually Transmitted Bacteria

Nonsexually transmitted bacteria account for 30–50% of cases of ON. Most commonly isolated microorganism is *Staphylococcus, commonly* cultured from the eyes of asymptomatic infants. Most cases of bacterial ON can be treated with topical antibiotics (aminoglycosides, polymyxin B sulfate–trimethoprim solution, macrolides, or fluoroquinolones). ON caused by *Pseudomonas* is rare but can present with eyelid edema, erythema, and purulent discharge causing corneal perforation, endophthalmitis, blindness, and possibly death. Presumptive diagnosis can be made from Gram stain results, and a definitive diagnosis is based on conjunctival culture results. Systemic antibiotics have poor penetration into the anterior chamber of the eye, and thus both systemic and topical aminoglycoside antibiotics, and occasionally subconjunctival injections, are required for effective treatment. These infants require isolation and assessment by an ophthalmologist.

Chemical Conjunctivitis

Chemical conjunctivitis accounts for most cases of ON, presenting as a mild, purulent conjunctivitis within the first 24 hours of life. It is most commonly associated with silver nitrate prophylaxis, or secondary to prophylaxis with other agents such as erythromycin or tetracycline. Chemical conjunctivitis is a self-limiting condition that does not require any diagnostic tests or treatment.

Prevention Strategy

- Primary prevention of the spread of sexually transmitted infections.

- Secondary screening of pregnant women for genital infection.
- Topical or systemic eye prophylaxis at birth.
- Tertiary prevention via early diagnosis and treatment of eye infections in neonates.

TRADITIONAL AYURVEDIC SYSTEM OF MEDICINE

The use of ayurvedic eye medicines (e.g., dried plant materials crushed into powder and dissolved in an aqueous medium; animal/human products such as breast milk, saliva, urine, etc.) is an important risk factor for ocular surface disease, specifically, corneal ulceration, in many developing countries. The use of ayurvedic eye medicines is a public health problem in many developing countries, including India, and an important risk factor for corneal blindness. The ayurvedic eye medicines are often contaminated and usually lead to delay in proper therapy. They also serve as a vehicle or culture media for spread and growth of pathogenic organisms. They may also cause corneal damage by their toxic effect.

Even as we educate the patients about these unproven, dangerous remedies, the original ayurvedic general health principles for health and longevity of life, cannot be ignored.

Prevention Strategy

Health education and awareness about primary eye care following trauma needs to be created in our community. Ayurvedic healers need to be educated and their cooperation must be sought in order to direct patients to appropriate healthcare facilities so that corneal blindness due to use of ayurvedic eye medicines may be prevented.

TRAUMA

Ocular trauma is one of the common causes of acquired unilateral blindness in pediatric age group. The consequences of childhood injury are harmful as it leads to permanent blindness and visual handicap. Ocular trauma in children accounts for 8–14% of the total injuries worldwide.

In the United States, eye trauma is the leading cause of noncongenital unilateral blindness in individuals younger than 20 years of age. The American Academy of Pediatrics (AAP) reported that 66% of all ocular injuries occur in individuals 16 years of age or younger, with the highest frequency occurring between 9 and 11 years of age.

Eye trauma constitutes 7% of all bodily injuries and 10–15% of all eye diseases.

Prevention Strategy

Childhood eye trauma includes a range of corneal surface abrasions to corneal and scleral perforations that are simply preventable by the supervision of the parents and baby caregivers.

Although most cases of eye injuries are preventable, current preventable strategies need more effective implementation. Today, preventive measures and protective eye wear have reached work places, and sport and leisure facilities; however, they are neither readily available for use, nor comfortable during related activities.

Hopefully, education about the hazards associated with specific activities, facilitating the availability of eye wear, accident prevention, and training for infant caregivers on how to prevent trauma in children, may prevent or decrease the mortality and morbidity of ocular injuries.

CONGENITAL AND DEVELOPMENTAL CATARACT

Introduction

Pediatric cataract is a leading cause of treatable childhood blindness. They are most often genetic and due to developmental anomalies of the lens fibers/and less commonly associated with metabolic disorders or ocular abnormalities. Cataracts in children require urgent diagnosis and treatment due to the unique sensitivity of the developing visual system and if left untreated may lead to amblyopia and irreversible loss of vision.

Epidemiology

Globally, it is estimated that 200,000 children are bilaterally blind from cataract. The overall incidence of clinically significant cataract (unilateral or bilateral) in childhood is unknown, but it has been estimated to be as high as 1 in 250 (0.4%).

Based on an etiological study of pediatric cataract in Western India, approximately 67% mothers of children with cataract had a history of maternal infections, especially toxoplasmosis, other agents, rubella, cytomegalovirus, and herpes simplex (TORCH) syndrome and 22% had taken medications for the same during pregnancy.

Management of Childhood Cataract

The management of cataract in young children has changed dramatically over the last 20 years. When intraocular lenses (IOLs) were first used in the late 1970s, they were thought not to be suitable for children. Over the last decade, smaller, high-power IOLs, suitable for children, have become available. Surgical techniques and equipment have also evolved. Many pediatric ophthalmologists now insert IOLs in children as young as 12 months of age. However, this technique requires considerable expertise and a vitrectomy machine, as the posterior capsule and anterior vitreous have to be removed in young children. Long-term follow-up is also crucial to manage visual axis opacities and to ensure the child is given optimal optical correction and low-vision devices, if required.

CHILDHOOD GLAUCOMA

Introduction

Glaucoma in children or even young adults cannot be looked upon in the same way as glaucoma in the adult. Diagnostic and treatment methods used primarily in adults may not be appropriate for the pediatric glaucoma. Children are not small adults so their disease must be assessed and treated accordingly. Diagnosis and treatment of pediatric glaucoma must take into consideration the age and developmental status of the child, other systemic signs, family history, the family psychosocial situation, and, in particular, the availability of follow-up and ongoing care. For those with internet access, a model for support and education for families can be found through the Pediatric Glaucoma and Cataract Family Association (*www.pgcfa.org*). Assistance for doctors treating children with glaucoma is available through Orbis Telemedicine, Cybersight at *www.cybersight.org*.

Epidemiology

Congenital glaucoma is responsible for 4–18% of childhood blindness worldwide. It is estimated that there are about 1.5–2 million children blind from glaucoma globally, of which two-thirds are in developing countries. In India, the disease accounts for 4.2–7% of all childhood blindness.

The incidence of congenital glaucoma is approximately 1 in 10,000 births in Western world.

The incidence of primary congenital glaucoma is increased when "founder effect" or a high rate of consanguinity are found in a population. The "founder effect" is a gene mutation observed in high frequency in a specific population due to the presence of that gene mutation in a single ancestor or small number of ancestors.

For glaucoma treatment, there is an inherent assumption that "success" is achieved in the patient who lives life with useful vision. More specifically, this might be called the treatment for the pediatric glaucoma. In children, life span may be many years past the initial diagnosis (life expectancy 37.2 years in Zambia and 83.2 years in Andorra); thus, the expected series of examinations and therapies through those years must address a number of issues and challenges that are not seen generally in an adult population.

Overview Basic Principles for Management of Glaucoma in Children

- The initial treatment may not be successful for the life span of the patient. A plan for the child must be formulated or at least appreciated by the first as well as subsequent doctors, so as to utilize all options in a logical and optimal sequence.
- Procedures done early should be planned not to interfere with, nor compromise the potential success of subsequent procedures.
- It must be recognized that each surgical intervention may have accompanying or potential future complications, many of which may not be apparent for months to years afterward (e.g., retinal detachments, macular edema, endophthalmitis, etc.). The extended life expectancy of the pediatric glaucoma patient will mean that these events, which might not be seen in adults, are more likely to appear over an extended time period. Short-term studies (<5–10 years), therefore, may not be as useful in planning longer or lifetime surgical options.
- A significant part of treating pediatric glaucoma is awareness of the need for timely diagnosis and appropriate treatment of strabismus, refractive amblyopia, and media opacities (cornea and lens). Even in successfully treated cases of pediatric glaucoma, these factors have a profound impact upon the degree of vision loss and therefore should not be overlooked.
- Other conditions and diseases associated with pediatric glaucoma must be considered during diagnosis and treatment (e.g., retinoblastoma, cataracts in rubella, corneal decompensation in aniridia, proptosis in neurofibromatosis, developmental delay in Lowe syndrome, etc.).
- Pediatric glaucoma is a family disease, which can affect other members directly by genetic transmission and indirectly by the demands of follow-up and care.

One principle that is in common with both childhood and adult glaucoma is the importance of early detection and appropriate intervention!

RETINOPATHY OF PREMATURITY

Retinopathy of prematurity is a potentially blinding eye disorder that primarily affects premature infants weighing 1,250 g or less that are born before 31 weeks of gestation. It is one of the most common causes of visual loss in childhood and can lead to lifelong vision impairment and blindness.

Retinopathy of prematurity has been rapidly increasing in many middle-income countries, with reports from Brazil, South Africa, India, and China. Recent Indian studies have shown that the incidence of ROP varies from 38 to 51.9% among low birthweight infants. With better neonatal care and increased survival of more preterm babies, it seems likely that ROP blindness will become another avoidable cause of blindness unless screening programs for premature babies are implemented in the neonatology units. In order to prevent the "spread of the ROP epidemic" being experienced by Latin America and Eastern Europe, programs for prevention and treatment need to be put in place, as is occurring in many cities in India and China.

A well-developed and implemented ROP screening program, with dedicated team, can significantly reduce the morbidity of ROP.

Blindness from ROP can be controlled through two broad approaches:

1. Reducing the incidence through excellent neonatal care
2. Detecting and treating infants who develop the severe stages of disease.

Population at Risk

- The WHO estimate that there are 15 million preterm births a year (born at <37 weeks).
- Infants born preterm contribute disproportionately to under 5 mortality rates (40% overall).
- Ministries of Health are highly likely to expand neonatal intensive care as a consequence this will lead to increased survival of preterm babies, so putting them at risk of ROP.
- The United Nations Children's Emergency Fund (UNICEF) is supporting the development of neonatal intensive care units in India.
- Those most at risk of ROP are those born at <32 weeks of gestational age; babies 32–37 weeks are at less risk.
- India has the largest number of preterm births of any country (WHO Born Too Soon, 2012).
- Only preterm babies cared for in neonatal intensive care units develop ROP.
- Factors which increase the risk of ROP include preterm birth, uncontrolled oxygen, sepsis, chronic lung disease, and poor nutrition.

Retinopathy of Prematurity the Disease

- Well-established classification system.
- *Natural history is known*: Signs develop 3–4 weeks after birth; progression is rapid, but in around 70% of infants the condition resolves without treatment (i.e., 5–10% of all babies screened). It is those who progress who need treatment.
- Clinical trials show that treatment of the disease once it reaches a critical stage is highly effective at preventing progression to blinding retinal detachment.

Strategies for Control

- *Prevent preterm birth*: This is a significant challenge as it is multifactorial.
- *Improve neonatal care*: Again, a challenge, but specific interventions such as reducing infection and controlled oxygen delivery in the incubator can reduce the risk.
- *Better oxygen monitoring requires*:
  - Systems for delivering oxygen in varying amounts (blenders).
  - Systems for measuring oxygen levels in the blood (probes and monitors).
  - Trained staff who understand the importance of controlling oxygen levels.
- *Detect infants with disease needing treatment*: This can be done in the following ways:
  - Neonatologist identifies infants to be examined according to gestational age, birth weight, etc.
- *Criteria*:
  - Ophthalmologists visit the neonatal unit on a fixed day and time each week to examine the infants using a portable retinal camera (widefield digital camera).
  - For each infant they have to decide (1) safe to discharge, or (2) see again next week, or (3) treatment needed.
  - *Advantages of retinal camera*: It can take images to track change over time; useful for educating staff and counseling parents. These cameras can be used in more than one unit.
  - The retinal camera can be used by a trained technician to captures the images. There are then two options:
    1. The technician is trained to interpret the images themselves and decide (1) safe to discharge, or (2) see again next week, or (3) needs to be seen by an ophthalmologist, or
    2. Images are uploaded onto the internet for remote reading by experts. *Challenge*: Report must be fed back to the screener within 48 hours in case treatment is needed—this requires 24/7 access to remote experts.

Challenge

Infants can develop the stages needing treatment after they have been discharged. They need to be examined too. Any system of detection has to be able to respond to this situation as well.

Treatment

- *Indications*: Infants who develop the constellation of clinical signs known as type 1 ROP.
- *Methods*: Laser retinal photocoagulation, under sedation or general anesthesia or intraocular injection of Bevacizumab (Avastin).
- *Timing*: Treatment is given within 72 hours as it can progress very rapidly to untreatable retinal detachment.
- Follow-up: Weekly to make sure getting better.

Long-term Follow-up

Infants with ROP have a massively increased risk of other pathology such as high degrees of myopia, strabismus, glaucoma, regressive late changes in the retina like blood vessel distortion with macular shift, retinal dragging, retinal folds and chorioretinal scarring, peripheral avascular areas, diffuse RPE lumping, and seldom retinal holes. They need regular follow-up so these problems can be detected and managed.

SUGGESTED READING

1. Acar U, Tok OY, Acar DE, Burcu A, Ornek F. A new ocular trauma score in pediatric penetrating eye injuries. Eye (Lond). 2011;25:370-4.
2. Aghadoost D. Ocular trauma: an overview. Arch Trauma Res. 2014;3(2):e21639.
3. Ajaiyeoba AI, Samaila E. Use of Bitot's spot in screening of vitamin A deficiency in Nigerian population. Afr J Biomed. 2001; 4:155-7.
4. Bhattacharjee H, Das K, Borah RR, Guha K, Gogate P, Purukayastha S, et al. Causes of childhood blindness in the northeastern states of India. Indian J Ophthalmol. 2008;56: 495-99.
5. Brophy M, Sinclair SA, Hostetler SG, Xiang H. Pediatric eye injury-related hospitalizations in the United States. Pediatrics. 2006;117(6):e1263-71.
6. Bućan K, Matas A, Lovrić JM, Batistić D, Borjan IP, Puljak L, et al. Epidemiology of ocular trauma in children requiring hospital admission: a 16-year retrospective cohort study. J Glob Health. 2017;7(1):010415.
7. Cao H, Li L, Zhang M, Li H. Epidemiology of Pediatric Ocular Trauma in the Chaoshan Region, China, 2001-2010. PLoS One. 2013;8(4):e60844.
8. Chander A, Chopra R, Batra N. Vitamin A deficiency: an eye sore. J Med Nutr Nutraceut. 2013;2:41-5.
9. Dandona L, Gilbert CE, Rahi JS, Rao GN. Planning to reduce childhood blindness in India. Indian J Ophthalmol. 1998;46: 117-22.
10. Dandona R, Dandona L, Srinivas M, Sahare P, Narsaiah S, Muñoz SR, et al. Refractive error in children in a rural population in India. Invest Ophthalmol Vis Sci. 2002;43(3):615-22.
11. Dandona R, Dandona L. Refractive error blindness. Bull World Health Organ. 2001;79:237-43.
12. Darville T. Chlamydia trachomatis infections in neonates and young children. Semin Pediatr Infect Dis. 2005;16(4):235-44.
13. Donham BP, Gibler WB. Images in emergency medicine. Gonococcal conjunctivitis. Ann Emerg Med. 2008;52(1):11.
14. Foster A, Volker K. Ophthalmia neonatorum in developing countries. New Engl J Med. 1995;332:600-1.
15. Foster A, Yorston D. Corneal ulceration in Tanzanian children: relationship between measles and vitamin A deficiency. Trans R Soc Trop Med Hyg. 1992;86:454-5.
16. Francois J. Congenital glaucoma and its inheritance. Ophthalmologica. 1972;181:61-73.
17. Genicek A, Genicekova A, Ferak V. Population genetical aspects of primary congenital glaucoma. Incidence, prevalence, Gene frequency, and age of onset. Hum Genet. 1982;61:193-7.
18. Gilbert CE, Foster A, Negrel AD, Thylefors B. Childhood blindness: a new form of recording causes of vision loss in children. Bull World Health Organ. 1993;71:485-9.
19. Gilbert CE, Foster A. Childhood blindness in the context of VISION 2020—The Right to Sight. Bull World Health Organ. 2001;79:227-32.
20. Gilbert CE. Causes of blindness and severe visual impairment in children in Chile. Dev Med Child Neurol. 1994;36:326-33.
21. Gupta N, Tandon R, Gupta SK, Sreenivas V, Vashist P. Burden of corneal blindness in India. Indian J Community Med. 2013; 38(4):198-206.
22. Heijl A, Leske MC. Cataract epidemiology. Ophthalmology. 2007;114:201.
23. Jaffar MS. Care of the infantile glaucoma patient. In: Reineck RD (Ed). Ophthalmol Annual. New York: Raven Press; 1988. pp. 15.
24. Kaid Johar SR, Savalia NK, Vasavada AR, GuptaIndian PD. Epidemiology based etiological study of pediatric cataract in western India. J Med Sci. 2004;58:115-21.
25. Kashima M, Kawakita T, Den S, Tomita M, Shimazaki J. Surgical management of corneal perforation secondary to gonococcal keratoconjunctivitis. Eye. 2009;23(2):339-44.
26. Khurana A, Khurana A. Comprehensive Ophthalmology. New Delhi: New Age International; 2007.
27. Livshitz I. Preventative strategies in the management of ROP: a review of literature. Open J Pediatr. 2015;5:121-7.
28. Matejcek A, Goldman RD. Treatment and prevention of ophthalmia neonatorum. Can Fam Physician. 2013;59(11):1187-90.
29. Murthy GV, Gupta SK, Ellwein LB, Munoz SR, Pokharel GP, Sanga L, et al. Refractive error in children in an urban population in New Delhi. Invest Ophthalmol Vis Sci. 2002;43:623-1.
30. Pradhan BK, Banerjee P. Community ophthalmology: dimensions. Community Ophthalmol. 2001;I:17-21.
31. Rahi JS, Sripathi S, Gilbert CE, Foster A. Childhood blindness in India: causes in 1318 blind school students in nine states. Eye. 1995;9(5):545-50.
32. Resnikoff S, Pascolini D, Mariotti SP, Pokharel GP. Global magnitude of visual impairment caused by uncorrected refractive errors in 2004. Bull World Health Organ. 2008;86(1):63-70.
33. Saxena R, Vashist P, Singh D, Tandon R. Preventing childhood blindness: Synergy between ophthalmology and community medicine. Indian J Community Med. 2015;40:149-51.
34. Singh V, West KP. Vitamin A deficiency and xerophthalmia among school aged children in south eastern Asia. Eur J Clin Nutr. 2004;58:1342-9.
35. Sommer A, West KP. Vitamin A deficiency: Health, Survival, and Vision. Oxford: Oxford University Press; 1996.
36. Thylefors B, Négrel AD, Pararajasegaram R, Dadzie KY. Global data on blindness. Bull World Health Organ. 1995;73:115-21.
37. Wadhwani M, Vashist P, Singh SS, Gupta V, Gupta N, Saxena R. Prevalence and causes of childhood blindness in India: a systematic review. Indian J Ophthalmol. 2020;68:311-5.
38. Whitcher JP, Srinivasan M, Upadhyay MP. Corneal blindness: a global perspective. Bull World Health Organ. 2001;79(3):214-21.
39. World Health Organization. Action plan for the prevention of avoidable blindness and visual impairment 2009-2013. Geneva: World Health Organization; 2010.
40. World Health Organization. Integration of vitamin A supplementation with immunization: policy and programme implications. Report of a meeting, 12-13 January 1998, UNICEF, New York. Geneva: World Health Organization; 1998.

17

CHAPTER

Pediatric Low Vision Care

Sarika Gopalakrishnan, TS Surendran

INTRODUCTION

Definition of Low Vision

A child with low vision is one who has impairment of visual functioning even after treatment and/or standard refractive correction, and has a visual acuity (VA) of <6/18 to light perception, or a visual field of <10° from the point of fixation in the better eye, but who uses, or is potentially able to use, vision for the planning and/or execution of a task for which vision is essential [World Health Organization (WHO), 1992] **(Table 1)**.

Impact of Low Vision

Functionally, low vision is described as irreversible visual loss and a reduced ability to perform many daily activities, such as recognizing people in the street, reading blackboards, writing at the same speed as peers, and playing with friends.

The purpose of "low vision clinic", is to enhance or maximize whatever vision (functional vision) is left with the patient, so that the daily tasks or best suited vocation can be carried out.

The major causes of blindness in children vary widely from region to region, being largely determined by socioeconomic development, and the availability of primary healthcare and low vision care services. The prevalence of blindness in children ranges from approximately 0.3/1,000 children in affluent regions to 1.5/1,000 in the poorest communities. Reliable population-based data on the causes of blindness in children are difficult to obtain in developing countries. There is an increasing awareness about the needs of students with low vision, particularly in developing countries where programs of integrated education are being developed. However, the appropriate low vision services are usually mandatory in order to improve their residual vision.

Functionally, low vision is described as irreversible visual loss and a reduced ability to perform many daily activities, such as recognizing people in the street, reading blackboards, writing at the same speed as peers, and playing with friends.

Causes of Low Vision

The major causes of visual impairment among children includes Stargardt disease, myopic degeneration, oculocutaneous albinism, retinitis pigmentosa, maculopathy, optic atrophy, corneal opacities, rod cone dystrophy, and other heredomacular degenerations. The list could be bigger but they can be broadly classified in terms of the impact on what the person with low vision sees.

These categories are depicted in **Figures 1 to 4**:

- Overall blurred vision
- Central field loss
- Peripheral field loss
- Multiple field loss.

TABLE 1: Categories of visual impairment.

Category	*Corrected VA—better eye*	*WHO definition*	*Working*	*Indian definition*
0	6/6–6/18	Normal	Normal	Normal
1	<6/18–6/60	Visual impairment	Low vision	Low vision
2	<6/60–3/60	Severe visual impairment	Low vision	Blind
3	<3/60–1/60	Blind	Low vision	Blind
4	<1/60–PL	Blind	Low vision	Blind
5	NPL	Blind	Total blindness	Total blindness

(NPL: no perception of light; PL: perception of light; VA: visual acuity; WHO: World Health Organization)

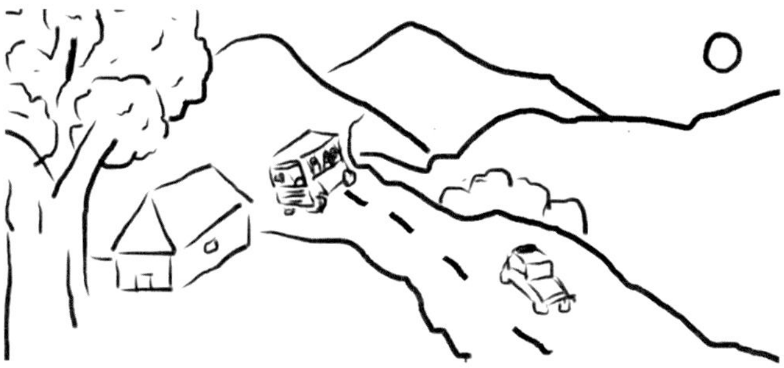

Fig. 1: Sample picture of a scenery seen by an individual with normal vision.

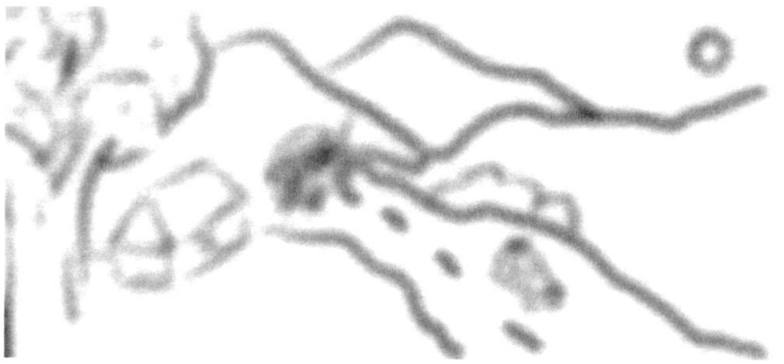

Fig. 2: Sample of scenery—as seen by a child with overall blurred vision.

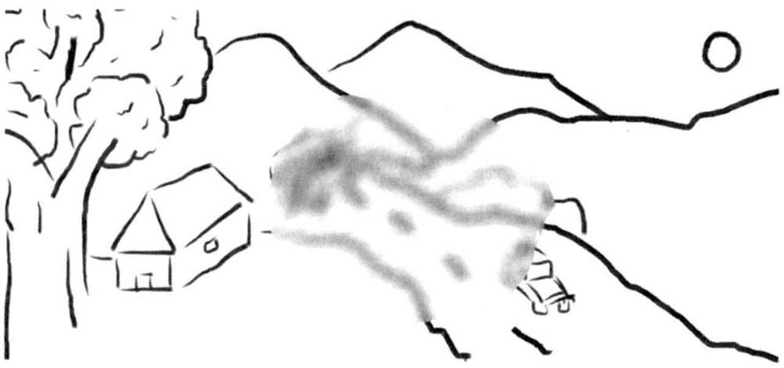

Fig. 3: Sample of scenery—as seen by a child with central field loss.

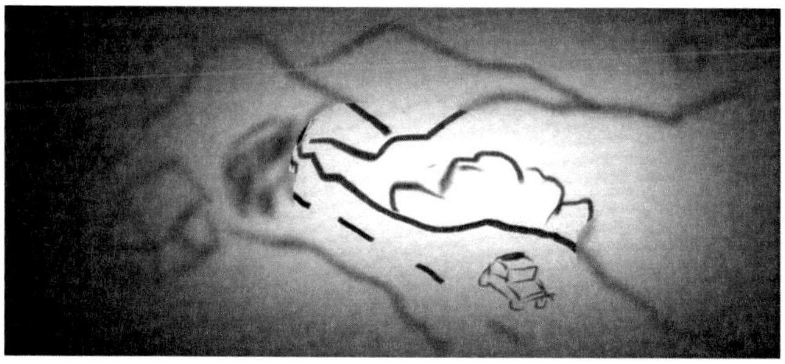

Fig. 4: Sample of scenery—as seen by a child with peripheral field loss.

LOW VISION ASSESSMENT

The first thing the clinician needs to understand is that the final management in the low vision clinic will have no impact on the ocular condition of the child. A child is referred to the low vision clinic after being diagnosed with a condition that cannot be improved further with treatment. The management aims to improve the way the existing vision is being used by the child.

Therefore, the low vision examination has two primary goals—(1) to identify and understand how well the child uses residual vision, i.e., functional vision assessment and (2) to explore conditions or modifications for maximizing or enhancing the existing visual performance.

Low Vision Examination

Steps in Examination of Child with Low Vision

- *Observation:* Observe how the child utilizes vision for moving or to locate an object or for communication from the time of entry into the clinic.
- *Interview (history taking):* Understand the difficulties the child has in utilizing vision for visual tasks and identify visual tasks that are important for the child to execute.
- *Assessment/functional vision:* Clinical assessment of visual functions—VA, contrast sensitivity, color vision, and visual fields.

External observation: The foremost step towards assessing a child with low vision begins even before the child enters the room. The clinician must carefully observe the mannerisms, visual habits, and body language of the child. The cues that an experienced practitioner can pick up from this initial assessment go a long way in successful counseling and management of the child. Details to observe before beginning the low vision evaluation are:

- *Level I: In the waiting room/waiting area*:
  How actively does the child use vision to gather input from the surrounding?
  - Does the child try to actively observe what is going on?
  - Does child make visual contact while interacting with family members/attender?
- *Level II*: *On entering the examination room*:
  How does the child navigate the environment?
  - With the help of the caregiver?
  - With the help of a cane?
  - Tries to use tactile input by trailing fingers along walls or furniture.
  - Is independent but visually (with or without additional head movement) scans the environment for obstacles.
  - Has poor navigation skills: Bumps into objects.
  - Walks independently, confidently without any aid.
- *Level III: Mannerisms/posture:*
  - Head down: May be due to glare or reduced inferior field of view
  - Squeezing eyes: Uncorrected refractive error/glare
  - Chin-up/chin-down posture
  - Head nodding
  - Eccentric viewing/fixation

- Eye-poking/rubbing
- Presence of nystagmus with/without compensatory head postures.

- *Level IV: Physical appearance:*
  - Shoddily dressed
  - Improperly buttoned
  - Poorly tied shoelaces
  - Untidy clothes
  - Unkempt appearance—matted hair
  - Spilt food stains on clothes
  - Frailty:
    - Any leg/arm weakness (favors a particular leg while walking or a particular hand for holding reading material)
    - Tremors
  - The last two are particularly important for deciding in the use of handheld devices.
  - Children diagnosed to have retinitis pigmentosa:
    - Obesity
    - Polydactyly
    - Clubbed fingers (syndactyly)
  - Albinism:
    - Sunburn
    - Nystagmus
    - Any unhealed lesions or deep abrasions on skin (may have poor platelet aggregation).
- *Level V: While interacting with the child*:
  - Does the child expect the caregiver/parents to be in close proximity? Is the child dependent on caregiver for the visual task?
  - Does the child interact directly with the examiner?
  - Mode of exploring surroundings—tactile/auditory/visual: Children with profound visual impairment may begin to depend on other senses to explore their surroundings, or continue to use vision—understanding their method for sensory input could help in suitable counseling on the mode of education
  - Voice modulation: Does the child talk with halts/in a monotone?
  - Does child make eye contact while talking or at least attempt to fixate eccentrically?
  - Child is enthusiastic about the outcome of the test/does not interact at all/is not interested in the test
  - Attempt to gauge the expectations of the child: High/reasonable/low.
- *Level VI: While interacting with the caregiver/parent:*
  - Is the caregiver/family aware about the ocular condition of the child
  - Are they over protective/deny care.

History taking:

- Child details:
  - Age.
  - Occupation/student.
  - Living situation and main caregiver (number of family members, care given, source of family income, etc., gives a general idea about the child's psychological outlook, need for independence and how much support will be available from the family).
  - General health (any medical condition, trauma, or surgery are important determinants of success of low vision management and also influence prognosis of the ocular condition)—in case of acquired conditions or worsening conditions, it would be a good practice to know when it was detected, specific milestones in disease history (worsening, surgeries, systemic/visual disability onset).
  - Relate ocular conditions to systemic syndromes, especially those that can be potentially life-threatening. For example, metabolic disorders, Wilms tumor in aniridia, and syndromes in children that can have impact on developmental milestones—for example: Bardet-Biedl syndrome in retinitis pigmentosa, etc.
  - Document family history of consanguinity or ocular disease to understand the mode of inheritance and the prognosis of the condition.
  - Other limitations such as physical handicap, hearing impairment, and mental retardation.
- Previous low vision care:
  - Has the child tried any device/devices before
  - Type of device
  - Details (magnification/color of tint)
  - For what purpose
  - How useful was it/success with device
  - Frequency of use
  - Duration of use.

  This gives an idea of what the child has tried before and how much success or failure has been faced on previous exposure to low vision care. Also, it would be a guideline to understand the child's demands and visual tasks.
- *Difficulty with visual tasks*: The most important thing to discern is about the difficulty with visual task and whether the problem is progressively worsening, stable, or if the vision is improving. Visual tasks are divided into three categories:
  1. Distance
  2. Intermediate
  3. Near

Distance visual tasks include tasks such as:

- Face recognition
- Seeing blackboard/reading (for students)
- Seeing PowerPoint displays
- Seeing signboards/bus numbers/shop names/street names
- Seeing curbs or steps
- General sightseeing/field of vision.

Near visual tasks may be broadly classified as:
- Reading textbooks/notebooks (school children)
- Reading office print/handwritten material at the office
- Reading newspapers/novels/magazines
- Reading bills/price tags/medicine labels
- Using mobile phone.

The examiner should take care to distinguish between difficulty in reading a text and difficulty in prolonged reading or reading in bright/dim light. Difficulty in writing should also be noted.

Intermediate visual tasks:
- Using computers.

Associated visual problems:

Various ocular conditions causing low vision can have problems such as:
- Photophobia
- Difficulty seeing in dim light
- Delayed dark adaptation
- Delayed light adaptation
- Glare—veiling.

Knowing the child's light sensitivity, one can help in modifying the daily environment of the child, providing modified optical devices such as filters or peaked caps to cope with bright light, etc.

Mobility Tasks

Differentiate between difficulty with navigating in familiar and unfamiliar environments to difficulty only with moving around in dim light or brightly lit surroundings.

Also question what compensating techniques the child uses such as:
- Having an assistant
- Help of the caregiver
- Use of walking stick/cane
- Does the child just sit at home due to mobility problems?

This question guides the practitioner in deciding the best mode of intervention for difficulty with mobility and determining the need for orientation and mobility training.

Activities of Daily Living

Activities of daily living (ADL) are those activities that are a part of daily life and are an absolute necessity:
- Personal grooming
- Personal hygiene/use of bathrooms
- Finding food on plate and eating
- Currency identification
- Inserting keys into doors
- Matching colors of clothes, etc.
- Managing stairs, if any.

Various techniques can be taught by rehabilitation therapists when optical devices do not help patients with low vision/visual impairment to perform ADL independently.

Parameters of Functional Vision Assessment

- Visual acuity
- Contrast sensitivity
- Color vision
- Visual field.

Ideal Visual Acuity Chart in Low Vision Clinic

- Standardized testing at different distances Logarithm of the Minimum Angle of Resolution (LogMAR)].

Recommendations for Visual Acuity Testing

- Chart lighting: 85–300 Cd/m^2
  - Use variable lighting to assess optimum lighting for best VA.
- Start at close working distance.
- Test better eye first, then worse eye and then binocularly. Document whether monocular (which eye) or binocular performance is better.
- Allow abnormal head postures and eccentric viewing.
- Do not point to letters or provide cues—allow to skip letters on a line (gives an idea of letters being skipped on a line due to scotoma).
- Allow time to scan and coax where required.
- Positively encourage further reading. Pointing to a letter, expecting a better performance on the test should be at the end and both visual acuities should be documented.
- Use of pinholes is not recommended when VA is assessed at <4 m *(<4 m cannot be considered optical infinity and therefore may not yield correct results for paraxial approximation. However, pinholes of larger aperture sizes are still used in some low vision clinics to detect uncorrected refractive error.)*. In the case of patients who have sufficient vision to respond at 4 m or larger distances may not always perceive an improvement, especially in cases of field loss (especially central) or impaired contrast sensitivity (due to luminance decrease with pinhole).

Large aperture pinholes are available for special use in the low vision clinic where indicated.

Note: The need for VA testing in the low vision clinic is to get an idea of functional vision or how the patient uses his vision in daily life and to also identify the smallest size of letters that can be read in ideal conditions such as a particular distance or given adequate time. This will assess the working distance best suited for the person in classroom or any vocational area.

Commonly used Visual Acuity Chart in the Low Vision Clinic

- Bailey-Lovie high contrast visual acuity chart **(Fig. 5)**
- Berkeley Rudimentary Vision Test kit (Bailey, 2012): Three pairs of cards (25 cm^2 area)
  - *First pair*: Single Tumbling E (STE)—100M, 65M, 40M, and 25M

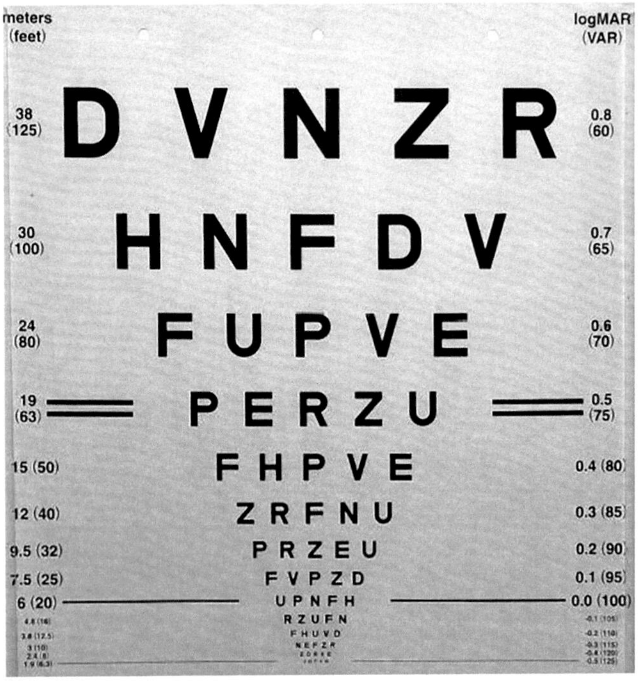

Fig. 5: High contrast Bailey-Lovie Chart.

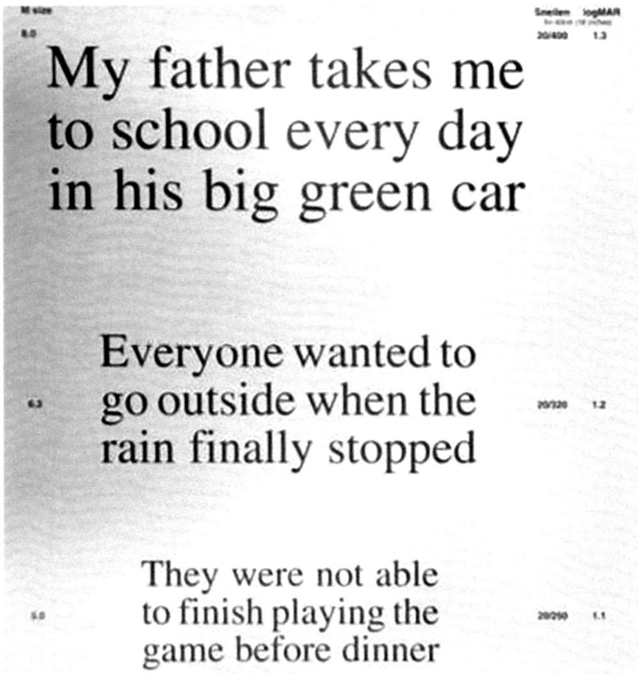
My father takes me
to school every day
in his big green car
Everyone wanted to
go outside when the
rain finally stopped
They were not able
to finish playing the
game before dinner

Fig. 6: MNREAD Chart.

- *Second pair*: Grating acuity: 200M, 125M, 80M, and 50M
- *Third pair*: White Field Projection and Black-White Discrimination.

Parameters to be documented when assessing VA in a child with low vision:

- Letter size
- Testing distance
- Qualitative components—missing letters, detects on pointing, speed of reading, etc.

Near Visual Acuity

Notations used in near visual acuity testing:

- N-notation (point notation)
  - Nonstandardized
  - Varies based on type of font
  - 1 point—1/72 of an inch (slug into which the text fits)
  - Actual size of lower case text: 1 (point—1/144 inch)
- M-notation
  - Sloan's M-notation can be converted based on the distance at which it is read
  - 1M subtends 5 minutes of an arc at 1 m
  - 8 points (N8) = 1M.

Snellen Equivalent

Near vision charts are calibrated for a certain working distance (usually 40 cm) and the corresponding Snellen acuity is given based on letter size.

Types of near vision cards:

- Single word
  - May be word, number, or symbol
  - Example: Lighthouse "game" or number cards
- Continuous text
  - Word reading
- Sets of unrelated words along a single line
- Example: Bailey-Lovie Word Reading chart
  - Continuous reading tests
- A complete sentence of about 10 words—usually simple and makes sense
- Example: MNREAD Card (Minnesota Near Vision Reading test) **(Fig. 6)**.

Recommendations for visual acuity testing—for near:

- Chart lighting: 85–300 Cd/m^2
  - Use variable lighting to assess optimum lighting for best VA
- Start at close working distance/allow patient to adjust for optimal comfort.
- Test better eye first, then worse eye and then binocularly. Document whether monocular (which eye) or binocular performance is better.
- Allow abnormal head postures and eccentric viewing.
- Allow changing orientation of text—vertical orientation is easier to read for patients with macular degeneration.
- Do not point to letters or provide cues—allow to skip letters on a line (gives an idea of letters being skipped on a line due to scotoma).
- Allow time to scan and coax where required.
- Positively encourage further reading. If you feel that by pointing to a missed letter/word the patient may perform better on the test, do it at the end and document both visual acuities.

Parameters to Document

- Letter size
- Working distance
- Illumination
    - *Reading speed*: Number of words read per minute (document for smallest text size that can be read)
    - *Critical print size*: Minimum print size for maximum reading speed. (Up to a certain acuity level, the patient may read fast and the reading speed may then drop off slowly. It is necessary to document this speed, as this is the speed the practitioner must aim to achieve with the use of the low vision device.)

Subjective Refraction

- Begin subjective refraction with the value obtained from objective refraction in trial frame.
- Use full aperture lenses.
- Use bracketing technique (just noticeable difference) to refine the endpoint.
- Just noticeable difference is the minimum power difference for which a patient will perceive a difference in quality of vision.
- For example: A person with 6/60 VA may not be sensitive to $\pm$ 0.25DS changes
- The minimum lens power for which a person with 6/60 will perceive a difference (just noticeable difference) can be calculated as follows:
    - *Just noticeable difference (in metric notation)*: Denominator of VA/30. (In this case: 60/30 = 2D). For this patient: The endpoint is arrived at by alternatively placing +1D and –1D in front of the eye and checking for improvement in vision.
    - For astigmatic error, stenopeic slit can be used for fine tuning.

Note: The endpoint of subjective refraction in children with low vision is not necessarily improvement in VA. Question the child if there is a perceived improvement in quality of vision such as contrast, identifying objects, face recognition, or contours in general.

Clinical Tips

- Always perform objective refraction using a retinoscope instead of an autorefractor, as the patient may not appreciate the target object.
- Provide a suitable fixation target for retinoscopy.
- Provide sufficient time for light adaptation before beginning subjective refraction.
- In case of people with high refractive errors or children already using habitual correction, refract over the glasses using clip-on trial frame clips (Halberg clips).
- Check if binocular acuity is better or worse than monocular VA. If monocular acuity is better or preferred, it may be beneficial to prescribe two sets of glasses:
    1. For mobility with preferred prescription for both eyes
    2. For specific purposes where use of distance vision is required with one of the eye occluded—use a frosted glass or neutral density filter.
- Preference for binocularity or monocularity may vary for distance and near. Check before prescribing occlusion for both.

Contrast Assessment

Fixed Contrast and Variable Acuity Tests

A Bailey-Lovie low contrast visual acuity chart can be used.

Screening for Impaired Contrast

In illiterate children, an alternative to assessing contrast sensitivity is to reduce the chart luminance to 10% of the original luminance level using a neutral density filter. This simulates a low luminance environment and thereby is an indicator of the subject's performance in low luminance conditions such as cloudy days or the evenings.

A difference in VA of more than two lines could be considered impaired or reduced contrast sensitivity.

Miscellaneous Assessment

Oculomotor Assessment

Check for extraocular motility as limitations would interfere with eye scanning to compensate for field loss

Saccades and Pursuits

Saccades: Ability to shift fixation or refixate from one object to another.

Test:

- Hold two fingers a few inches apart
- Ask patient to shift fixation from one finger to the other and back a few times
- Look for smooth eye movements and quick refixation.

Pursuit: Ability to track an object.

Test:

- Ask patient to look at a target such as a pencil, your finger, etc.
- Move a pencil or finger horizontally or vertically across
- Check for ability to follow without losing track.

Impaired saccades or pursuits could result in difficulty in using magnifiers comfortably for scanning text or tracking a line completely. Impairment could also indicate damage to higher order centers such as neural pathways or the cortex. This is most usually seen following cerebrovascular accidents (strokes), diffuse cerebral atrophy and causing hemianopias, altitudinal field defects, etc.

Low Vision Assessment for Preverbal Children

Goals for Low Vision Examination

- *Learning to communicate*:
  - An infant with low vision may not be able to make eye contact or imitate the mother smiles/coos.
  - A child with low vision who does not make eye contact could be affected in peer relationships, may be misunderstood by parents to be stubborn and face many problems in peer-groups, school as well as the home.

For the child with low vision in preverbal group, the usual area is home or play-school. As no formal learning is in place, the child is mostly involved in near activities of toys, or building blocks, or may be interested in riding a tricycle. It should be understood that these children have congenital reasons for low vision or trauma sequelae.

Attempts should be made to enhance activities best suited for the child's age or in which activities the child shows interest.

Aspects of vision that need to be evaluated have their application in:

- Communication
- Orientation and mobility
- ADL
- Sustained near vision tasks.

The examiner must explore what type of techniques will best help the child to carry out the above tasks:

- *Blind*: Use sensory substitution techniques for the tasks
- *Low vision techniques*: Needs optical enhancement/ magnification
- *Sighted techniques*: Can manage or needs environmental/ contrast enhancement.

It has been made amply clear that a child referred to low vision clinic has already undergone battery of tests to assess the child's vision and his/her visual performance regarding acuity—distance and near, field of vision, color vision, and light and dark adaptations, and contrast sensitivity has already been assessed. However, these can be repeated if the clinician deems it necessary. The following are the ways for examining VA in preverbal children:

- Lea's tests
  - Symbols: House, heart, apple, and circle
  - Numbers
  - Grating acuity tests/paddles
- HOTV chart
- Teller acuity cards
- Optokinetic nystagmus drum.

Refraction

- Perform manual retinoscopy with age-based cycloplegic drug.

Clinical Tip

- Perform dynamic retinoscopy to detect any accommodative insufficiency.
- Perform dynamic retinoscopy at working distance of the patient.

Contrast Sensitivity

- Lea's low contrast cards
- Lea's symbols at different contrast levels
- Patti Pics™
- Hiding Heidi

Color Vision

- Ishihara modified picture charts for children.

Visual Field

- Confrontation.

Functional Vision in Infants/Children with Learning Disability or Multiple Sensory Impairment

Visual Acuity

- Use small colored candy and look for ability to pickup.
- Small colored beads may also be used. In case of multisensory impairment, move beads on a string and look for visual attention and/or tracking.

Clinical Tip

- Tracking may not be smooth in children with multiple impairments, especially cerebral palsy.

Contrast

- Roll balls of different contrasts on the floor and look for ability to track/loss of interest
- Look for ability to pickup beads of different colors from different colored surfaces (gray beads on a white paper, black beads on white paper, red beads on yellow paper, and so on).

Color

- Use color pencils or building blocks and attempt matching.

Visual Field

- Confrontation with large interesting toys.

OPTICAL LOW VISION DEVICES

Magnifiers for Distance

The following types of telescopes prescribed in the low vision clinic:

- Monocular telescope **(Fig. 7)**:

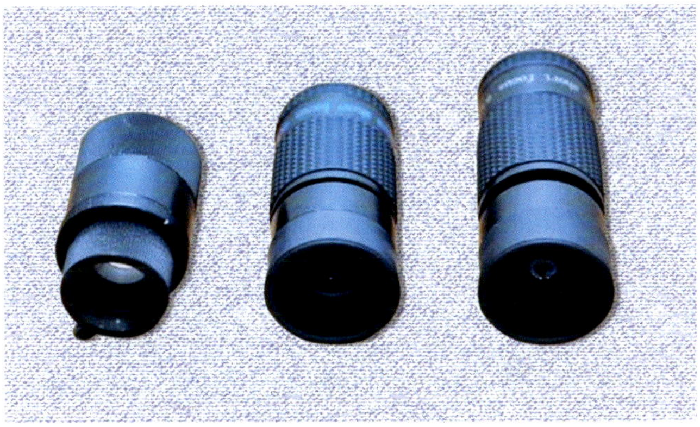

Fig. 7: Monocular telescope.

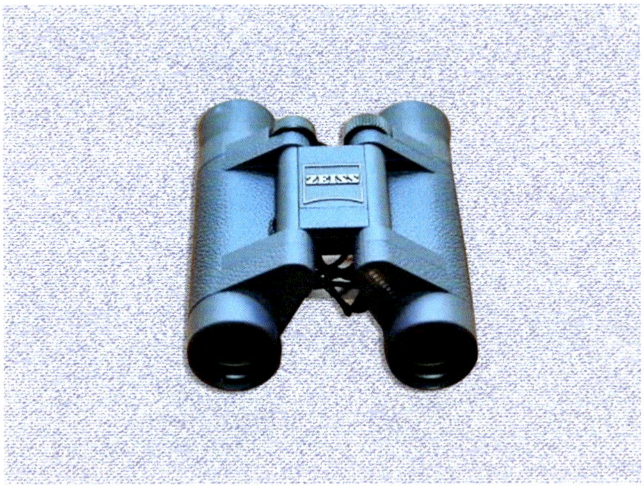

Fig. 8: Binocular telescope.

- These are used in front of a single eye
- Are portable
- Used for spotting tasks
- Can be used for copying from the blackboard in classrooms for students
- Can also be used for tourism and spotting
- Can be combined with a reading cap for near tasks
- Cannot be used for mobility

▪ Binocular telescope **(Fig. 8)**:
  - Similar to monocular telescopes except for larger field of view due to binocularity
  - Heavier than monocular telescopes
  - Less compact
  - Useful for spotting only
  - Cannot be used for long duration due to weight and bulk
  - Very useful for individuals who cannot tolerate occlusion due to nystagmus or reduced field loss

▪ Bioptic monocular telescope **(Fig. 9)**:
  - The individual can use the optics of the spectacle for general tasks and look through the telescope only when there is an object of interest.

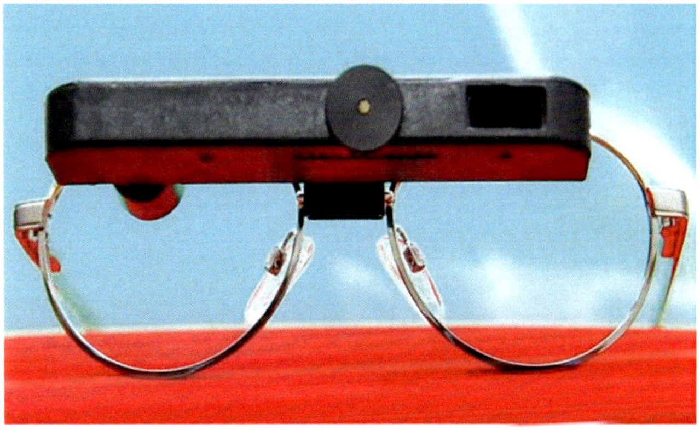

Fig. 9: Bioptic monocular telescope.

  - Especially prescribed for driving—following rigorous training program and special driving test in countries where it is approved.
  - Not approved in India.

Magnifiers for Near

▪ Spectacle magnifiers (+5D to +20.0D—higher plus can be prescribed subject to availability)
▪ Hand magnifiers (1.2X–14X)
▪ Stand magnifiers (4X–14X)
▪ Dome magnifiers (1.8X–2.2X)
▪ Bar magnifiers (1.5X–2.2X)
▪ Fresnel sheet magnifiers (up to 3X).

The above mentioned magnifications refer to the equivalent power of the system and not manufacture mentioned magnifications.

▪ Closed-circuit television (CCTV) systems

Spectacle Magnifiers (Relative Distance Magnification)

▪ Prescribing high near additions up to 5.0 D that can be incorporated in the spectacles.
▪ Prescribing separate reading glasses with addition higher than +5.00D.

If the spectacles are intended for binocular use, either decentration of the lenses or incorporation of base-in (BI) prism is necessary. This is because the interpupillary distance (IPD) will differ from that of near PD measured for 40 cm.

Clinical pearl: High powered lenses will have aberrations on moving away from the optical center of the lens. Therefore, decentration or incorporation of prisms is essential for best vision with the glasses. In case the patient has eccentric fixation or is not viewing the center of the lens, appropriate changes have to be made.

In decentration of higher near additions in spectacles, appropriate base-in prisms should be added.

TABLE 2: Power for magnifiers.

Power	*Base-in prism*
+6.0D	8 prisms for each lens
+8.0D	10 prisms for each lens
+10.0D	12 prisms for each lens

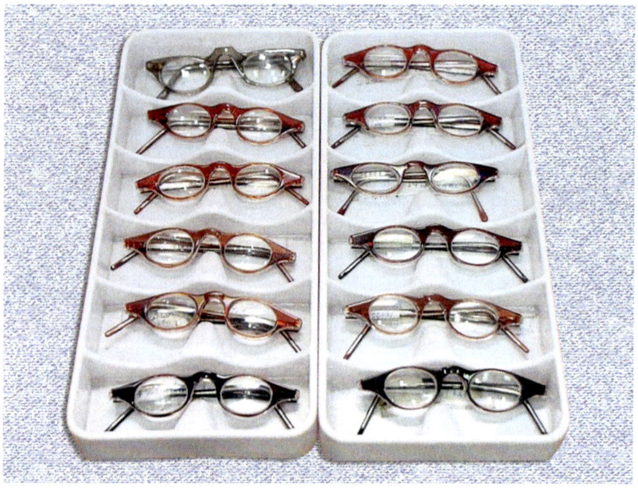

Fig. 10: Half-eyes.

Example:

1. Distance IPD 64 mm. Near Add 8D.

8 mm decentration = 8 Δ base-in for each eye's distance PD.

2. Distance IPD 68 mm. Near Add 10D. 10 mm decentration = 10 Δ base-in for each eye.

The higher the addition, more the meter angle of convergence and therefore, the requirement for more base-in prisms. If near PD is considered, the base-in prisms should be calculated for Near Adds over +3.0D only, i.e., for a 10D Near Add deduct 3D and calculate for 7D only.

A rule of thumb is to incorporate two prisms more than the power in each eye. For example: For +6.0D Near Add, 8 prism BI in each eye would equal 16 prism BI **(Table 2)**.

Half-eye frames can be used binocularly for reading powers of 6D–10D. Half-eye glasses give the wearer freedom to look over the frame for distance visual tasks **(Fig. 10)**.

Beyond +10.0D binocularity may not be possible in spite of equal or near-equal VA, primarily due to the close working distance.

Hand Magnifiers (Figs. 11 and 12)

A plus (convex) lens is held at a distance from the object such that the object is at the focal length of the lens. This makes the object appear closer and larger than the actual size of the object:

- The eye-to-lens distance and the lens-to-object distance can be varied making this a very flexible magnifier.
- The larger the eye-to-lens distance, the lesser the field of view and vice versa.

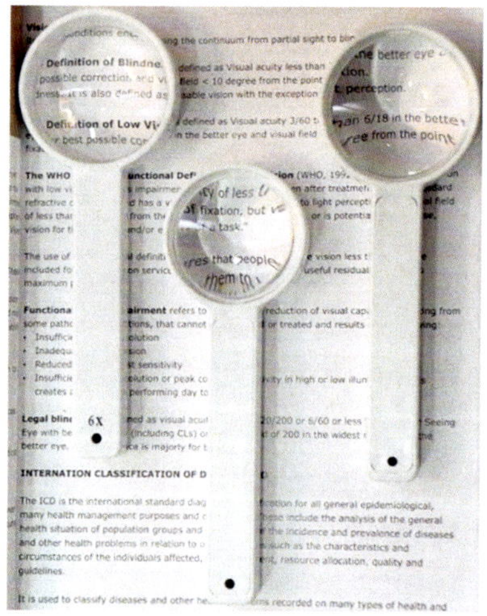

Fig. 11: Nonilluminated hand magnifier.

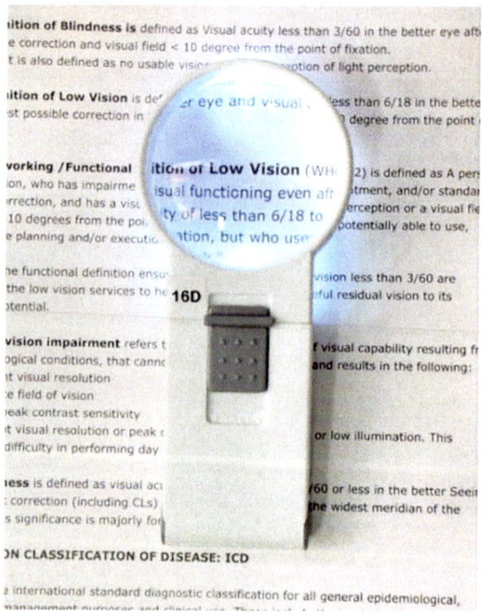

Fig. 12: Illuminated hand magnifier.

- The larger the lens-to-object distance, lesser the magnification.
- Can be prescribed in combination with a spectacle magnifier. The resulting magnification can be calculated using the formula for equivalent power:

$FE = F1 + F2 - dF1F2$ and the magnification = FE/4 where F1 and F2 are the powers of the plus lens and the hand held magnifier and d is the distance between the lens and the magnifier.

Pocket Magnifiers (Fig. 13)

- As the name indicates, they are constructed to be carried around in the pocket.
- These are hand-held magnifiers with slide-in mechanism into a case to protect the lens from scratching. The case itself functions as the handle of the "hand-held".
- They are intended for spot or quick reading.
- These are generally small aperture lenses:
  - 3.5X and 2.5X
  - 4.25X, 4X, and 3.75X

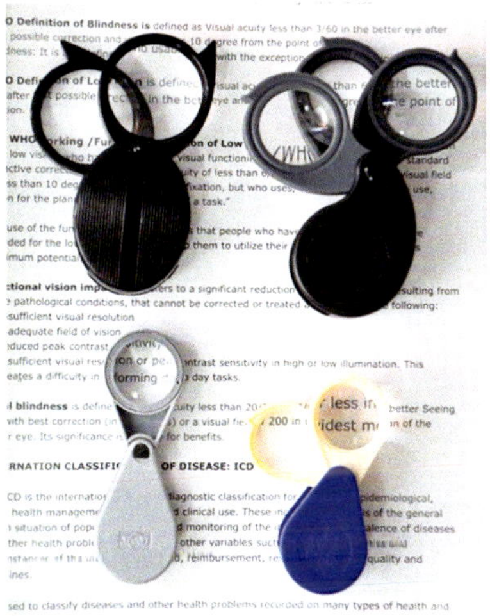

Fig. 13: Pocket magnifiers (clockwise).

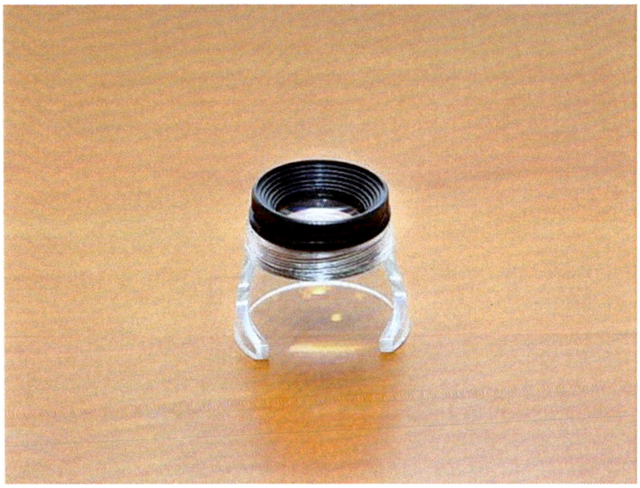

Fig. 14: 6X cutaway stand magnifier.

- 6X
- 4X and 10X.

Stand Magnifiers (Figs. 14 and 15)

- Option of choice for prolonged reading when higher levels of magnification are required.
- Magnifiers with internal illumination are available.
- Generally placed in contact with reading material. The height of the stand is the same as the focal length of the lens or lesser than the focal length of the lens.
- If the height of the stand is less than the focal length of the lens, the patient will have to accommodate or require Near Add to see clearly through the stand magnifiers.

Dome Magnifiers (Fig. 16)

- These are also called Visolett or bright field or paper weight magnifiers.
- These are magnifiers with a plano-convex construction and have better light gathering properties than other optical low vision devices. They are only possible with low magnification up to 4.0X.

Bar Magnifiers (Fig. 17)

- These are similar to dome magnifiers but are bar shaped and long (usually the width of a page). They use plus powered plano-cylindrical lenses to enlarge text vertically. Light gathering properties are similar to that of the dome magnifier.
- This is especially useful for people with subnormal near acuity or normal near acuity but requiring an increase in contrast for comfortable reading.
- They are also of use for people with constricted fields.

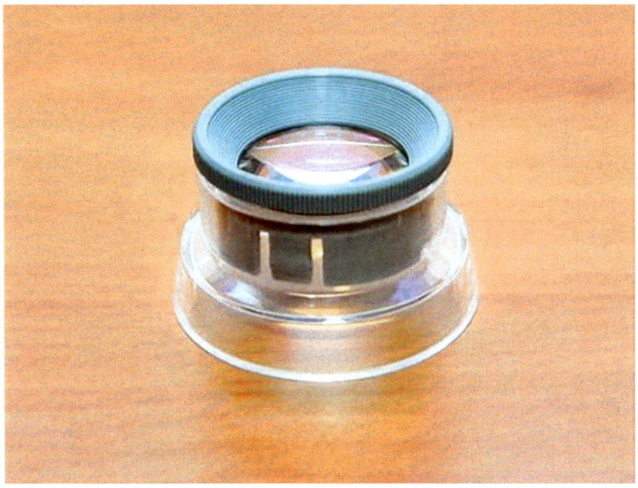

Fig. 15: 10X adjustable stand magnifier.

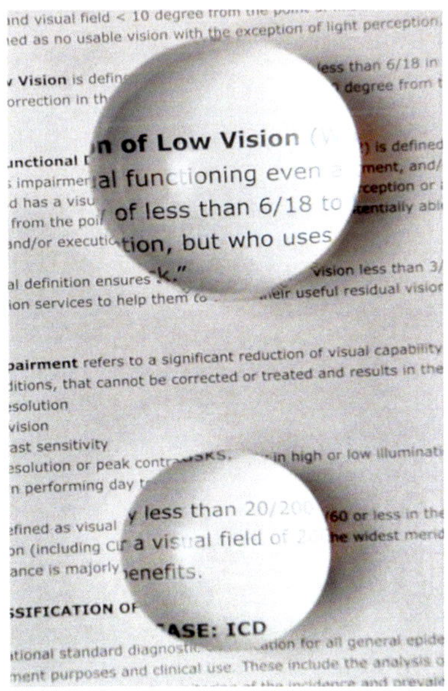

Fig. 16: Dome magnifier 4.0X (above) and 2.25X (below).

Fresnel Sheet Magnifiers (Fig. 18)

- These use Fresnel sheets to magnify the image (plastic sheet with concentric grooves cut into it). Higher magnification levels are not possible with this type of system as an increase in magnification would also increase distortions in the image formed by the Fresnel lens.

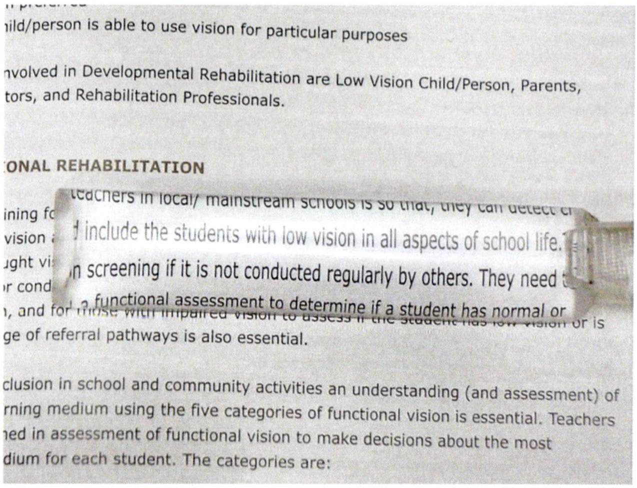

Fig. 17: Line or bar magnifier.

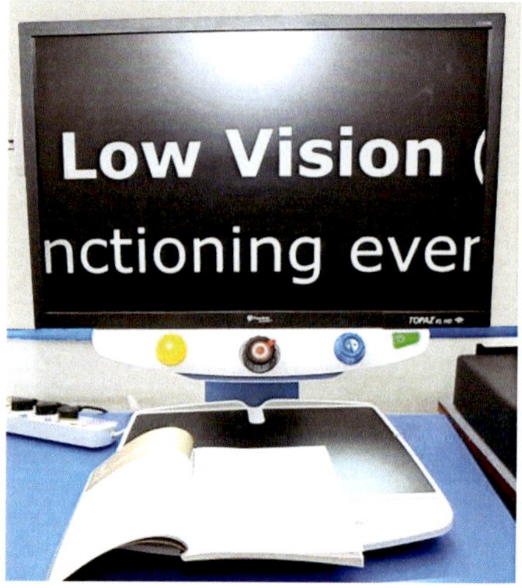

Fig. 19: Table top closed-circuit television (CCTV) (TOPAZ).

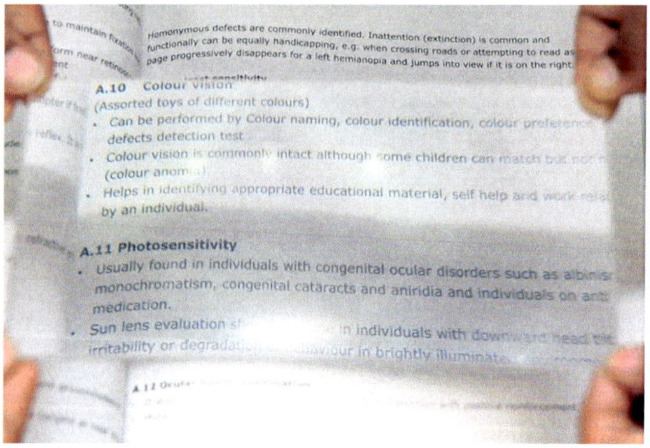

Fig. 18: Fresnel sheet magnifier.

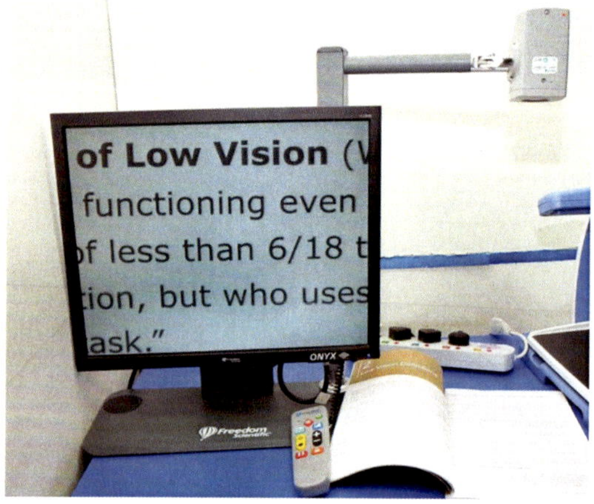

Fig. 20: Desktop closed-circuit television (CCTV) (ONYX CCTV).

- They are thin, lightweight, pocket-size or page size, and have good light gathering properties.

Closed-circuit Televisions

- In CCTVs, a camera projects the image onto a screen.
- As these system display images on an electronic screen, it is possible to alter the contrast and color and size of the text to suit the user's requirements.

Types of CCTVS:

- Table top CCTVs:
  - Consists of a monitor or screen placed on a table.
  - Attached camera has a viewing tray on which reading material is placed. The text is displayed on a screen, e.g., TOPAZ **(Fig. 19)**.
  - The camera can also be attached to a small stand that can be rotated and focuses for a range of distances (example: ONYX CCTV by Freedom Scientific). Instead of requiring an additional monitor, it can be connected to a personal computer (PC) **(Fig. 20)**.
- Mouse model:
  - The CCTV camera is hand held like a mouse and is attached to a television or PC screen.

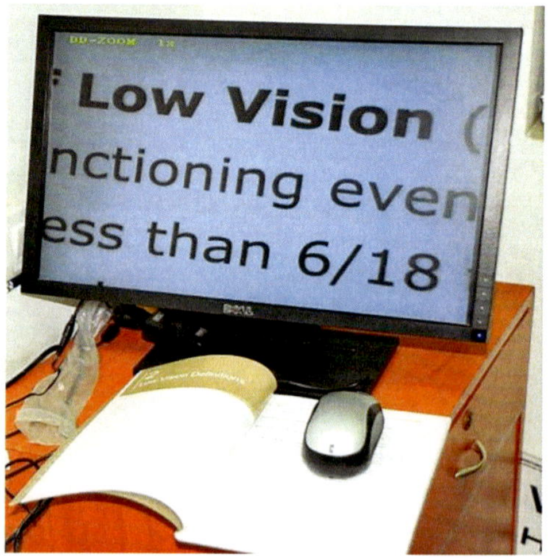

Fig. 21: Mouse model closed-circuit television (CCTV).

  - The text is placed under the mouse and displayed on the screen **(Fig. 21)**.
- Portable **(Figs. 22 to 24)**:
  - These are small video magnifiers with screen sizes that are between 2 and 5 inches.

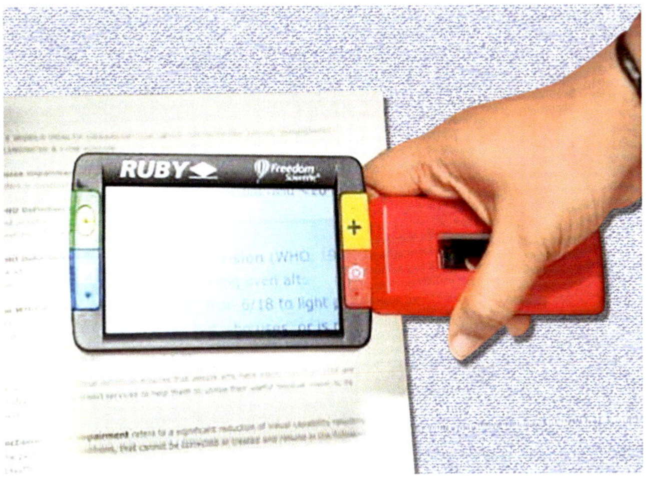

Fig. 22: Hand-held Ruby closed-circuit television (CCTV) (Freedom Scientific) being used for spotting.

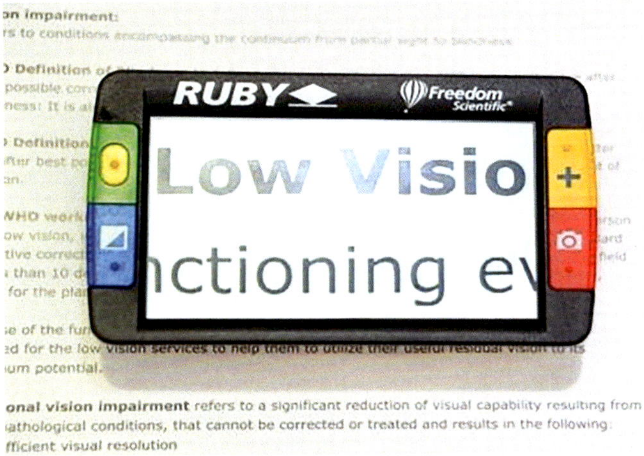

Fig. 23: Ruby closed-circuit television (CCTV) (Freedom Scientific) reading and continuous reading.

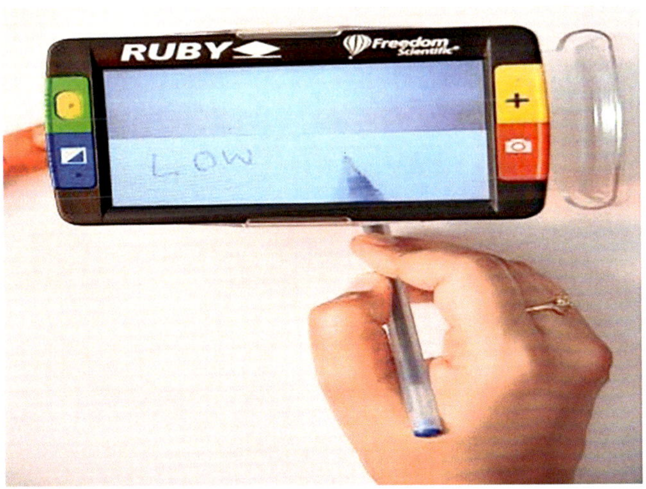

Fig. 24: Ruby closed-circuit television (CCTV) (Freedom Scientific) being used for writing tasks.

- The camera is inbuilt under the screen and the device can be moved directly over the material like a stand magnifier.

TABLE 3: Types of magnifier, magnification, magnification levels, and illumination.

Magnifier	Type of magnification	Magnification level	Illumination
Spectacle magnifier	Approach	1.5X–6X	External
Hand magnifier	Approach	1.5X–14X	Internal possible
Stand magnifier	Approach + angular	4X–14X	Internal possible
Dome magnifier	Approach + angular	2X-–4X	Light gathering
Bar magnifier	Approach	1X-–5X	Light gathering
Fresnel magnifier	Approach	1X-–3X	Light gathering + external possible
CCTV	Real image magnification	Up to 100X	Internal

(CCTV: closed-circuit television)

TABLE 4: Suitable tasks with specific type of magnifier.

Magnifier	Reading task	Spotting task	Writing task	Hands free
Spectacle magnifier	✓		✓	✓
Hand magnifier		✓		
Stand magnifier	✓		✓	
Dome magnifier	✓			
Bar magnifier	✓			
Fresnel magnifier	✓	✓	✓	
CCTV	✓	✓	✓	✓

✓ Indicates the usage.
(CCTV: closed-circuit television)

Table 3 discusses type of magnifier, type of magnification, available magnification levels, and type of illumination possible with the given magnifier.

Table 4 lists most suitable tasks with specific type of magnifier.

Prescribing Magnifying Devices

Prescribing for Distance Visual Tasks

Formula to calculate magnification:

Distance:
Magnification Required = Best corrected distance VA divided by required vision for distance.

For example, the best corrected distance VA of a 10-year-old boy is 6/36 and needed VA to view black board is 6/12. Required magnification is 36/12 = 3X

Near: Although there are several formulae to calculate the tentative magnification for near, the most acceptable formula which is in use now a days is the Equivalent viewing power [EVP]

The calculated magnification would be:

EVP	=	[BCVA/TVA] × [100/WD]
	=	[12/4] × [100/30]
	=	3 × 3.33 = 9.99D
	=	~10D → ~2.5X
EVP	=	[BCVA/TVA] × [100/WD]

Here BCVA is best corrected visual acuity, TVA is target visual acuity, and WD is working distance.

The options for prescription would be:

- A spectacle magnifier of +10.00D
- A stand magnifier of 2.5X magnification
- A hand magnifier of 2.5X magnification
- A near telescope of 2.5X magnification.

In this case, the option of choice would be a spectacle magnifier or a stand magnifier as they are apt for continuous reading such as for the newspaper/book.

Prescription of telescopes for near visual tasks requires a motivated patient who is very particular about working distance and is not worried about cosmesis or field of view.

Clinical Tip

The minimum field of view through the near magnifier should be 4–6 characters to ensure comfortable reading.

NONOPTICAL MANAGEMENT

A nonoptical device is a device that increases the ease of performance of a task just by increasing size, increasing contrast, reducing glare, or simply due to sensory substitution.

Nonoptical devices may be classified as follows:

- Relative size device
- Glare, contrast, and lighting control
- Postural devices
- Hand writing and written communication device
- Orientation and mobility techniques and devices
- Sensory substitution device
- Medical management and life skill device
- Assistive technology—computer and mobile modifications and computer and mobile software.

Relative Size Magnifying Device

These devices assist patients with low vision by mechanically increasing font size. For example, large print magazines, telephones with large numbers, large size playing cards, jumbo clocks, etc.

Glare Contrast and Lighting Control Device

- Filters
- Peaked cap for glare
- Use of table lamps to increase illuminance
- Typoscopes to improve contrast and cutoff specular reflection
- Hand held torch in dimly lit environments
- *Multiple pinhole spectacles*: Useful for multiple corneal opacities for glare reduction.

Tints and Filters

Types of Filters

- Contrast enhancing filters:
    - Yellow or yellow-orange filters
    - High absorption filters
    - Red/dark amber
    - Green
    - Gray.

Photochromatic Glasses

Prescribe with caution in children with delayed light adaptation or dark adaptation.

Sensory Substitution Devices

The visually impaired can make use of other senses such as touch (tactile), hearing (auditory), and smell (olfactory) to substitute for the lack of vision. Any device that makes use of these other senses and devices the visually impaired is called a sensory substitution device. For example: Braille (tactile), audio books, etc. Some people are trained to make a typical sound and determine their environment by the "echo" of that sound.

TECHNOLOGY IN LOW VISION MANAGEMENT

Advent of technology such as computers or CCTV systems has greatly enhanced learning for the visually handicapped children.

Using Computer

- *For mild near visual acuity* impairment (not accompanied by severe contrast sensitivity loss or severe field loss)—*basic computer modification is usually sufficient.*
    - Lower the screen resolution
    - Set the computer to extra-large fonts
    - Using high contrast desktop settings/themes
    - Change accessibility options to enlarge cursor size/icon size/scrollbar size/use high contrast settings
    - There are also modifications to customize the *font color, background, and font size* for every component of the Window such as the Menu bar.

- For moderate-to-severe near visual acuity impairment: Screen magnifier software
    - This software split the screen into a magnified window (whose size can be altered) and the regular window.
    - The "magnified window" can be set to suitable text size and color combination that is appropriate for the individual's acuity levels.
    - These software also have audio features to read text when required.
    - Individuals requiring up to 6X magnification (with the software) can generally function comfortably using this software. Beyond 6X, they tend to work easily with the audio function as the field of view is compromised beyond 6X.
- Severe visual acuity loss: Screen reader software
    - Screen reader software provides an audio output every time a key is pressed.
    - They have a wide variety of shortcut keys to enable easy use.
    - Job Access with Speech (JAWS) software by Freedom Scientific, Inc.) is the most commonly available software in India. It is also available with a voice having an Indian accent.

Reading Software and Devices

- Various software with optical character recognition (OCR) are available.
- These software use OCR technology to convert text on a scanned document to audio (example: Kurzweil and OpenBook).
- Standalone devices that use OCR technology are also available. These devices have a camera that captures an image of text and reads text aloud (example: SARA Stand-Alone Reading Appliance, Freedom Scientific, Inc., Intel Reader by Intel) **(Fig. 25)**.

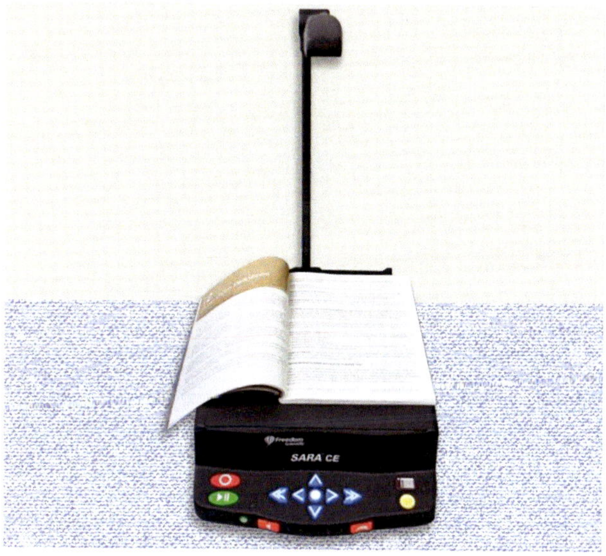

Fig. 25: SARA (Stand Alone Appliance, Freedom Scientific, Inc., Intel reader by Intel).

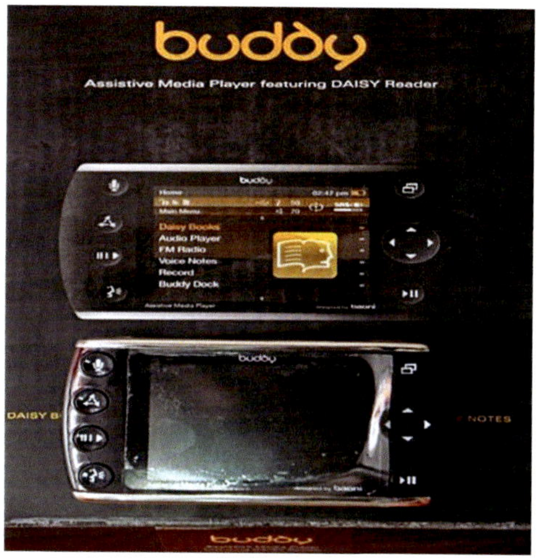

Fig. 26: BuddyPlayer.

Sensory Substitution Devices

Refreshable Braille Displays

These can be connected to a computer. The display then shows tactile dots on the screen that can be felt by the user. Some displays also have a Braille keyboard attachment that can be used to input text. Bluetooth displays are also available that can be connected to mobile phones.

Digital Book Reader Hardware/Software

Similar to music players, these devices convert electronic books into a digital accessible information system (DAISY) format. The books can be read in audio format and the user can toggle between chapters, pages, paragraphs or lines of text using buttons available on the player (Example: BookSense and BuddyPlayer) **(Fig. 26)**.

Digital talking books are audio/visual books that can be magnified and read, or listened to depending on the user's comfort.

GPS Devices

These devices use ultrasonic technology to detect objects/obstacles in the path of the user (example: Miniguide)

Barcode Readers

These devices help the individual identify items while shopping.

Mobile Phone Technology

Accessibility Settings

- *i-Phone*: Larger dynamic type setting can be activated, invert colors and grayscale features are available, and VoiceOver is a built in screen reader [Siri, Dictation, SpeakScreen, and Zoom are other available inbuilt apps].
- *Android*: Accessibility settings can be modified, Talkback is an in-built screen reader that will give an audio response to touch selection and gets activated with accessibility settings.

- *Other types of devices on mobile phones*:
  - Big screen clocks
  - Talking clocks
  - Talking calculators
  - *Global Positioning System (GPS) based*: Helps in navigation
  - Obstacle detectors
  - *Magnifying cameras*: Use mobile phone camera to convert smartphone to portable CCTV
  - *Picture search*: These compare a photo taken on a smartphone to images on the internet and help the user identify the object
  - *Organizer or reminder software*: These can be just audio based or can connect to Braille displays
  - *Money identifiers*: To identify currency
  - *Color ID*: To label colors.

Orientation and Mobility Devices

- Orientation is using the remaining senses to establish one's location in one's environment.
- Mobility is an art of moving from one place to another independently, safely, and gracefully.
- Mobility cane is the most commonly and widely used device in India. A cane with a "red-tip", indicates a visually handicapped device. Canes are available which can be carried in bag or pocket and assembled when needed **(Fig. 27)**.

Early Intervention Therapy in Children: What is it?

Early intervention is defined by Stephens and Tauber (2001) in two parts, early refers to the most critical period of a child's development between birth and 3 years of age. Intervention refers to program implementation designed to maintain or enhance the child's development in natural environments and as a member of a family.

Children with visual impairment face multiple problems:

- Lack of communication with parents and subsequent insecurity for both parents and children

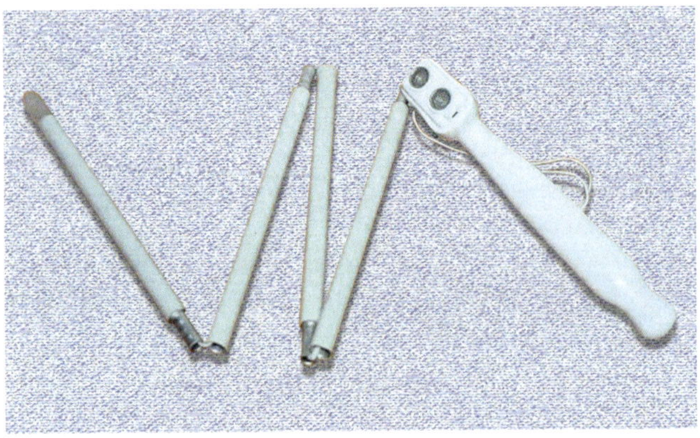

Fig. 27: Smart Cane.

- Inhibited learning experience due to lack of visual stimuli
- Delayed mobility, speech, and other milestones due to inability to see and learn. It is estimated that 80% of learning in children is through sight.

Early intervention services are aimed at infants/small children with some amount of residual vision. They attempt to enhance visual milestones using a standardized approach called "vision stimulation".

The aim of vision stimulation is to attempt to aid visual development in children and provide training in visual skills such as fixation, localization, scanning, searching, and tracking.

The early intervention therapist also works with the family to modify the child's environment to provide information that can be visually processed by the child. Further, the parents are taught various methods to interact with the child and aid further learning.

It is believed that provision of vision stimulation and early intervention therapy in infants with low vision can help in better utilization of vision when the child grows. However, early intervention is not a treatment aimed to improve the ocular condition.

Early intervention therapy is also of benefit for children with total blindness. The therapist works with the parent to teach them how to interact with the child and:

- Provide sensory cues for interaction such as touching and cuddling
- Provide sensory cues for environmental interaction
- Enhance other senses
- *Learn pre-cane skills*: Pre-cane skills can also be taught to children below the age of 5. This helps them to learn to navigate the environment at a young age and prepares them to use the cane easily in the future.

MANAGING FIELD LOSS

In general, people with field loss have difficulty staying on a line or reading continuously due to skipping or mixing lines. This can be managed by following compensating strategies:

- *Single finger guide*: Thumb of left hand is placed at beginning of sentence and moved for each sentence.
- *Double finger guide*: Thumb of left hand is placed at beginning of sentence while index finger of second hand is used to track the sentence. Left hand serves as guide to move back when the sentence is completed.
- *Ruler*: Ruler is placed under the sentence being read (as if to underline).
- *Typoscope*: Typoscope is used instead of ruler to track the line.

Central Field Loss

- Steady eye strategy
- Eccentric viewing training

- Subjectively:
  - Using Amsler grid
  - Using clock face
- Objectively:
  - Scanning laser ophthalmoscope
  - Microperimeter.

Managing Peripheral Field Loss (Table 5)

A visual field of >10° is sufficient for mobility in well-illuminated and noncluttered unfamiliar surroundings (Pelli DG, 1987).

A visual field of <10° requires the use of additional orientation and mobility techniques for mobility (Ferraro J and Jose RT, 1983).

Multidisciplinary Model of Management

Holistic management of the patient with low vision does not end with the low vision care practitioner. Rehabilitation is the road to comprehensive management of the patient.

The following is the basic skeleton of the multiple disciplines involved in management of the patient with low vision.

Whom to Refer and Where?

- *At the infant level*: Special educators and rehabilitation therapists are important to provide vision stimulation and vision training so that the child may learn to use residual vision and develop various visual skills to maximum use of functional vision.

TABLE 5: Management—a capsule.

Visual task	***Management options***	***Options for impaired contrast***
Distance		
Seeing blackboard	• Go closer to board (approach magnification)	• Use black board (avoid green board and white board)
	• Use telescope	• For white board, use black marker only
	• Use distance CCTV	• Avoid glare on board, use overhead light on board
Recognizing faces	• Use contrast cues	• Use voice/external mannerism as cue
	• Approach magnification	
Watching television	• Approach magnification	
	• Relative size magnification (large screen)	
	• Open field Galilean binoculars (SEETV)	
	• Bioptic (OR) spectacle-mounted monocular/binocular telescope	
Shop names/door numbers	• Approach magnification	
	• Monocular telescope	
	• Sighted guide assistance (SS)	
Traffic lights	• Bioptic telescope (if eligible to drive)	
	• Sighted guide assistance (SS)	
Crossing roads	• Telescope not recommended as it limits field of view	
	• Sighted guide assistance (SS)	
Driving	• Bioptic telescope (if vision with telescope eligible to drive)	
Seeing curbs or steps		• Use additional lighting
		• Contrast edge of steps
		• Use cane/sighted guide (SS)
Near		
Continuous reading	• Large print books reading	• Photocopy colored text to black and white
	• Near Add/spectacle magnifier	• Yellow overlay
	• Stand magnifier	• Illuminated magnifiers
	• CCTV	• CCTV
	• Screen reading software (SS)	• Use e-book readers where possible (flexible for glare control/color/ reversed contrast/magnification)
	• Reading stand	• Use additional lighting

Contd...

Contd...

Visual task	*Management options*	*Options for impaired contrast*
Cheque books/form filling/ writing	• Spectacle magnifier/Near Add	• Bold pen/marker
	• Bold tipped pen/marker	• Use additional lighting
	• Cutaway stand magnifier	• Portable CCTV
	• Large field hand magnifier	
	• Portable CCTV	
	• Reading/writing stand	
Price tags/bills/medicine labels/expiry date	• Spectacle magnifier/Near Add	• Use additional lighting
	• Hand held magnifier	• Portable CCTV
	• Portable CCTV	
Mobile phone	• Accessibility options/App	
	• Talks/mobile magnifier software	
Computer-based		
Reading text on screen	• Lower screen resolution	
Close working distance	• Increase font size	
	• Larger screen/monitor	
	• Screen magnifier software	
	• Adjustable laptop table for bringing laptop closer	Screen magnifier software (contrast settings)
Reading poor contrast		• Use black/white settings
Glare		• Screen magnifier software (contrast settings)
		• Window should be at right angles to screen
		• Avoid reflections on screen
		• Use glare reduction clip on screen/filter spectacles
Finding options on screen	Use keyboard shortcuts	
Using keyboard	Large print keyboard touch typing (SS)	High contrast keyboard
Mobility		
Staircases	• Sighted guide (SS)	Use contrast edges
	• Orientation and mobility techniques (SS)	Use additional lighting
Familiar places	• Sighted guide (SS)	Use contrast edges
	• Orientation and mobility techniques (SS)	Use additional lighting
Unfamiliar places	• Sighted guide (SS)	Use additional lighting
	• Orientation and mobility techniques (SS)	
Bumping into objects	• Sighted guide (SS)	Use contrast edges
	• Orientation and mobility techniques (SS)	Use additional lighting
Daily living tasks		
Matching clothes	• Organizing	Labels
	• Tactile labels (SS)	
Grooming	• Magnifying mirror	Use additional lighting
	• Sensory techniques	
Seeing food on table	Clock hour technique of food arrangement	• Contrast placemat/table color
		• Contrast plate/bowl color to food
		• Use additional lighting
Threading needle	• Thimble (needle threader)	
	• Chest resting/neck magnifier	

Contd...

Contd...

Visual task	***Management options***	***Options for impaired contrast***
Stitching/embroidery	Chest resting/neck magnifier	Use additional lighting
Currency identification	• Notex (SS) • Tactile cues (SS)	Use additional lighting
Finding objects in a group	Searching techniques	Use contrasting shelf liners/table/ countertop covers

Note: All of the above management options are just commonly available management options which have been mentioned as a guideline.
(CCTV: closed-circuit television; SS: sensory substitution)

- *At the school level*: It is the special educator and the rehabilitation therapist who play the major role. Once the device has been prescribed by the optometrist and various guidelines have been suggested, the special educator and rehabilitation therapist are necessary for implementation of the suggestions and for helping the child cope with their sighted peers.
  Modes of schooling available for children with low vision:
  - *Regular education*: Ordinary schooling with no specific modification except use of low vision devices if required.
  - *Integrated education*: Ordinary school with additional special educator who gives child special classes or attention when required. No changes are made in daily classroom and class teacher has no special training to handle special needs.
  - *Inclusive education*: Children of different types of disability in the same school or class. The class teacher is trained to handle children with special needs. Special concessions are made by the teacher to incorporate needs such as slow speed, use of special devices, and using sensory substitution when child cannot use visual means.
  - *Special education*: Special school where all children have some form of visual impairment and sensory substitution is the primary method of teaching.
- *At the adolescent level*: At this stage, the adolescent needs help from career counselors, special educators, and vocational trainers in order to decide the best vocation that will suit them for the future and acquire necessary skills for future career. This is the stage when the person is given special vocational training in areas where vision is not required, e.g., music, playing musical instrument, and counselors.
- *At the adult level*: The most important role would be played by:
  - *Rehabilitation therapist*: For training in use of devices
  - *Orientation and mobility therapist*: For independent mobility
  - *Social worker*: To help the individual and family cope with the onset of low vision

APPENDIX I: LETTER TO SCHOOL MANAGEMENT

Low Vision Care Clinic

Date:________

To Whomsoever It May Concern

This is to state that Master/Miss ________ who is studying STD in your school (Reference MRD No.: ________) was evaluated in the Low Vision Care Clinic. He was noted to have ________ ________________________ visual impairment in both the eyes due to retinal problem.

This vision will not be sufficient to view the black board comfortably. He needs to be seated closer to the black board (i.e., one meter distance) or in the front row (without rotation). Most of his learning will be through listening to the classes, so dictating as much as possible will help him in a large way.

Kindly allow him to copy notes from his friend's notebook in case he is not able to copy from the black board directly. In addition, he can be given compensatory time concession of minimum 30 minutes for all examinations (school level and for board exams) [Source: F.No.16-110/2003-DD. III, Government of India, Ministry of Social Justice and Empowerment, New Delhi, India].

Please extend your cooperation so that his ocular condition does not interfere with his academic performance. Thank you for your kind cooperation.

Yours sincerely,
(________) Optometrist
Low Vision Care Clinic

APPENDIX II: LETTER FOR DISABILITY CERTIFICATE

Low Vision Care Clinic

Date: ________

To Whomsoever It May Concern

This is to state that Mr/Ms ________ (Reference number: ________________) was evaluated in the low vision care clinic and was noted to have best corrected visual acuity of ________ in the right eye and ______________ in the left eye due to___.

He can be considered as_% visually handicapped [Source: No. 16-18/96-NI.I, Government of India, Ministry of Social Justice and Empowerment, New Delhi, India Category] and he is eligible for possible concessions and benefits according to this category.

Yours sincerely,
(________) Optometrist
Low Vision Care Clinic

APPENDIX III: REHABILITATION CENTER

Sample: Rehabilitation Wise Contacts

- Readers facility
- Blind school
- Early intervention center
- For children with learning difficulty
- Special school
- Integrated schools and special educators
- Inclusive school
- Braille training (preschool)
- Vocational training
- Disability certificate—State Resource Training Centre (SRTC)
- Computer software training
- Mobile software
- Job placement.

APPENDIX IV: SOURCES OF LOW VISION AND ASSISTIVE DEVICES

1. Karishma Enterprises
132, Market Tower B, Cuffe Parade, Mumbai 400005
India Phone: 022-22181853; Fax: 022-22153291
Email: ke@vsnl.com
Website: www.brailleworldindia.com
2. Barrier Break Technologies
101, Highway Commercial Complex
IB Patel Road, Goregoan (E), Mumbai-400063
India Phone: +91 (22) 26859730/26860485/6
Cell: +91 9920229081
E-mail: Vasu@barrierbreak.com Website: http://www.barrierbreak.com
3. Om Tao Scientific Apparatus 3-2-320/2, Chappal Bazar Kachiguda
Hyderabad-500027
Tel: 9885054759
Email: omtaosa@hotmail.com
4. JUTRON Vision
A-6, Nand Complex, Near Aims Oxygen Juna Padra Road
Baroda-390020
Phone: +91-99987-02020
Fax: 91-265-2321323
Email: mukul@jutronvision.com
5. ABISee, INC
141 Parker St, Suite 201, Maynard MA 01754, USA
Phone: 800-681-5909
Website: www.abisee.com
6. Telesensory
520 Almanor Avenue Sunnyvale, CA 94085, USA Website: www.telesensory.com Email: info@telesensory.com
7. Dolphin Computer Access Ltd. Technology House Blackpole Estate West Worcester, WR3 8TJ United Kingdom
Tel: +44 (0) 1905754577
UK Local Rate (from a BT landline): 08451305353
Fax: +44 (0) 1905754559
Email: info@dolphinuk.co.uk
8. Freedom Scientific 11800 31st Court North
St. Petersburg, FL 33716-1805, USA Phone: 1-727-803-8000 (worldwide)
Fax: 1-727-803-80
Web-site: www.freedomscientific.com

APPENDIX V: USEFUL WEB LINKS RELATED TO LOW VISION

1. For children with low vision—http://www.lowvisionkids.com
2. Visual perception and tracking skills—http://www.eyecanlearn.com/#Peripheral
3. Visual stimulation exercises—http://www.whiteboardroom.org.uk/LearningSystem/PortalHome/preDefault.asp?Resource=AEE03 C0E-AE07-497D-9FA7-989D8654B96F&ResourceID=7041
4. National Initiative for the Blind (NIB)-Centre for computer training—http://acharya.iitm.ac.in/projects/trgschools.php
5. International Council for Education of People with Visual Impairment (ICEVI)-Education for all children and youth with visual impairment—http://www.icevi.org/
Statewise contacts: http://www.udaan.org/parivaar/india.html
Countrywise contacts:
http://www.pediatriconcall.com/fordoctor/schools/view_schools.aspx?id=3&cat_id=Special%20Sch ools%20for%20mentally%20Handicapped%20&%20Spastic%20children
Ministry of social Justice: http://socialjustice.nic.in/policiesacts3.php
To know about concessions given for person with multiple disabilities: http://www.fourstepsindia.org/index.html
National Trust schemes: http://www.thenationaltrust.co.in/nt/index.php?option=com_ content&task=view&id=193&Itemid=26
6. Link to National trust for special children—http://thenationaltrust.in/NewWeb/snaplist.mht
7. Braille press and other provisions for persons with multiple disabilities—http://socialjustice.nic.in/brailpress.php

8. Job placement
   - www.enable-india.org—Enable India
   - http://www.eyeway.org/include/cl-jobs.php—Eyeway.org
   - http://www.disabilityindia.org/forum/viewtopics.cfm?Forum=13—Disabilityindia.org
   - http://www.ncpedp.org/employ/placements/viewopenings.php—NCPEDP
9. Information regarding available sources for all visually impaired (partially sighted, blind, etc)—http://www.sightlosssolutions.org/
10. ROPARD is The Association for Retinopathy of Prematurity and Related Diseases-awareness link for parents—http://www.ropard.org/information-for-parents?start=1
11. Blind resource center for visually impaired and Blind—http://www.nyise.org/speech/homepage.htm

SUGGESTED READING

1. Apfelbaum HL, Ross NC, Bowers AR, Peli E. Considering apical scotomas, confusion, and diplopia when prescribing prisms for homonymous hemianopia. Trans Vis Sci Technol. 2013;2(4):2.
2. Bailey IL, Jackson AJ, Minto H, Greer RB, Chu MA. The Berkeley rudimentary vision test. Optom Vis Sci. 2012;89(9):1257-64.
3. Brown B, Lovie-Kitchin JE. High and low contrast acuity and clinical contrast sensitivity tested in a normal population. Optom Vis Sci. 1989;66(7):467-73.
4. Colenbrander A. Assessment of functional vision and its rehabilitation. Acta ophthalmol. 2010;88(2):163-73.
5. Ferraro J, Jose RT. Training programs for individuals with restricted fields. In: RT Jose (Ed). Understanding Low Vision. New York: American Foundation for the Blind; 1983. pp. 363-76.
6. Gilbert C, Foster A. Childhood blindness in the context of VISION 2020: the right to sight. Bull World Health Organ. 2001;79(3):227-32.
7. Hassan SE, Hicks JC, Lei H, Turano KA. What is the minimum field of view required for efficient navigation? Vision Res. 2007;47:2115-23.
8. Hyvärinen L. (2000). How To Classify Paediatric Low Vision? [online] Available from: https://www.lea-est.fi/en/assessme/paediatric_low_vis.html. [Last accessed August, 2021].
9. Mufarriq S, Khan M, Khan MT, Khan MY, Saeed N. Causes of visual impairment in children with low vision. J Coll Physicians Surg Pak. 2011;21(2):88-92.
10. Onufryk M. Ophthalmic prismatic image relocating eye glasses for persons having retinitis pigmentosa and hemianopia and method for making same. USA Patent #5,323,190; 1994.
11. Pambakian A, Currie J, Kennard C. Rehabilitation strategies for patients with homonymous visual field defects. J Neuro-Ophthalmol. 2005;25(2):136-42.
12. Pelli DG. The visual requirements of mobility. In: Woo GC (Ed). Low Vision. New York: Springer; 1987. pp. 134-46.
13. Romayananda N, Wong SW, Elzeneiny IH, Chan GH. Prismatic scanning method for improving visual acuity in patients with low vision. Ophthalmology. 1982;89:937-45.
14. Sharma MK, Thapa H, Paudyal B, Adhikari RK, Dhakwa K. A profile of low vision among the blind school students in Lumbini Zone of Nepal. Nepal J Ophthalmol. 2010;2(2):127-31.
15. Smith HJ, Dickinson CM, Cacho I, Reeves BC, Harper RA. A randomized controlled trial to determine the effectiveness of prism spectacles for patients with age-related macular degeneration. Arch Ophthalmol. 2005;123:1042-50.
16. Stephens LC, Tauber SK. Occupational Therapy for Children, 4th edition. United States of America: Mosby Inc.; 2001.
17. Szlyk JP, Seiple W, Laderman DJ, Kelsch R, Ho K, McMahon T. Use of bioptic amorphic lenses to expand the visual field in patients with peripheral loss. Optom Vis Sci. 1998;75:518-24.
18. Verezen CA, Muelendijks CF, Hoyng CB, Klevering BJ. Long-term evaluation of eccentric viewing spectacles in patients with bilateral central scotomas. Optom Vis Sci. 2006;83(2):88-95.
19. VisionAware. (2021). Orientation and Mobility Skills. [online] Available from: http://www.visionaware.org/info/everyday-living/essential-skills/an-introduction-to- orientation-and-mobility-skills/123. [Last accessed August, 2021].

18

CHAPTER

Genetics and Pediatric Ocular Disorders

Srinivas Reddy, Vadrevu K Raju

INTRODUCTION

More than 60% of cases of blindness among infants and children are caused by inherited eye diseases which severely affect vision and almost 50% of children with strabismus have a family history of the disease. Till date, about 4,000 disorders are caused by genetic aberrations in humans and one-third of all cases of inherited genetic diseases have ocular abnormalities. Till date, about 350 ocular disorders have recognizable genetic abnormality. Worldwide, 1 in 1,000 people are affected with genetic eye disease!

During the last two decades, there has been an exponential increase in knowledge and understanding of ocular genetic disorders and syndromes. The number of human eye diseases that have a genetic component continues to increase. Since treatment of many congenital defects and degenerations may not be possible, but for others, early recognition of signs and symptoms may not only prevent morbidity, but can also be life-saving. More than half of these diseases are associated with an identifiable genes. The cause of these ocular manifestations may range from mutation of a single gene to mutations of several genes. Phenotypic presentations may vary based on variable expressivity, and vision can range from within normal limits to complete blindness. Many of these disorders present congenitally, while others develop later in life.

Therefore, knowledge of clinical and molecular features of ocular genetics and inherited eye disorders is important for appropriate diagnosis and patient management, and as our understanding of the pathogenesis of these diseases will increase, more customized therapy including gene therapy can be anticipated. This chapter is important as all genetic disorders are inherited, most of them presenting in childhood, some may manifest later, but the ophthalmologist must be aware of the consequences. Detailed description of each and every disorder is not possible here, but some important and common disorders are briefly described.

GJ Mendel (1822-1884), known as Father of Genetics, first described the basic characteristics of genetics with his laws of segregation, law of independent assortment, and law of dominance. He described the pairing of genes and that only one gene is transmitted from each parent. Certain genes may be dominant and its representation is strong, while others may be recessive and altogether skip its representation. Autosomal dominant diseases affect all generations and both genders; while the recessive may not show in offspring. If only males are affected within a family, the presentation is "X" linked, which means mother is the carrier. In cases where clear cut inheritance pattern is not observed, de novo mutations have occurred.

BASICS OF GENETICS

Genes define who and what we are! They carry the blueprint of our traits and ironically also of diseases.

Walther Flemming, in 1889, first recognized the easily stainable material in cell nuclei and termed it "chromatin," but it was WB Sutton in 1902 who suggested that the Mendel's factors of inheritance are transmitted by this chromatin, and by 1952, it was confirmed that this genetic chromatin consisted primarily of deoxyribonucleic acid (DNA). Later chromatin, scientifically was labeled as "chromosome." By chemical analysis, each chromosome consists mostly of DNA, but small quantities of ribonucleic acid (RNA) and two classes of proteins are also found, which are subclassified as histones and non-histones. Most of DNA in a cell is present in chromosomes and a small percentage in cell mitochondria, where it orchestrates oxidative metabolism.

Chromosomes

Normally DNA is densely packed along with proteins called histones into a highly coiled structure called chromatin or chromosome. The chromosomal structure is visible only at the time of cell division when the chromatin undergoes condensation into chromosomes. Every nucleated cell in the human body except sperm and ovum has 23 pairs of chromosomes. The first 22 pairs, numbered 1 to 22, are called as autosomes. The remaining pair is the sex chromosomes: XY in males and XX in females. Each chromosome has two arms; the shorter arm is called "p," and the long arm is called "q." Both the arms join at a central constriction called "centromere." The terminal part of a chromosome is the telomere. Each chromosome is further subdivided into regions based on banding patterns that appear after staining with various chemical agents. Numbering of subsections on each arm starts from the centromere and proceeds toward the telomere. Uracil substitutes for thymine in RNA. DNA is transcribed into messenger RNA (m-RNA) which is then translated into protein.

In the nucleus of each cell, DNA exists as a double-stranded helix, in which the order of bases on one strand is complimentary to that on the other. During cell division, the two DNA strands separate, and each acts as a template for the synthesis of a new strand. The genetic code is therefore, maintained during cell division and each cell contains an existing and a newly synthesized strand of DNA. If the helix of DNA is unwound, linearly it would be 2 m long **(Figs. 1A and B)**.

Genes

A gene is the basic physical and functional unit of heredity. In humans, genes vary in size from a few hundred bases to >2 million bases. The Human Genome Project estimated that humans have between 20,000 and 25,000 genes in every cell of our body. Every person has two copies of each gene, one inherited from each parent, one on each pair of 22 autosomal chromosomes. An *allele* is an alternate form of a gene found at the same locus on homologous chromosome. Males have only one X chromosome and therefore, only one set of alleles for all genes on X, while females have paired alleles on their sex chromosomes. Each set of instructions along the DNA strand is a gene, and so genes are expressed as to form proteins. The final result of a genetic expression is known as genotype. A DNA molecule or "strand" consists of a backbone of deoxyribose sugar units linked by phosphate groups. The purine bases, adenine (A), guanine (G), cytosine (C), and thymine (T), are attached to the deoxyribose base and their sequence along the strand constitutes the genetic code (genes).

Each gene has a promoter which is responsible for turning on the gene. The sequences that code for protein are called *exons* and noncoding sequences segments between exons are called *introns*. Exons make up for only 3% of human DNA, while the remaining 97% are introns. The exon region of a

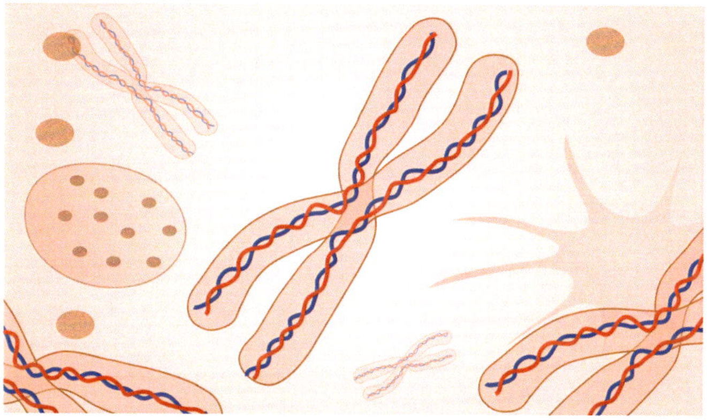

A

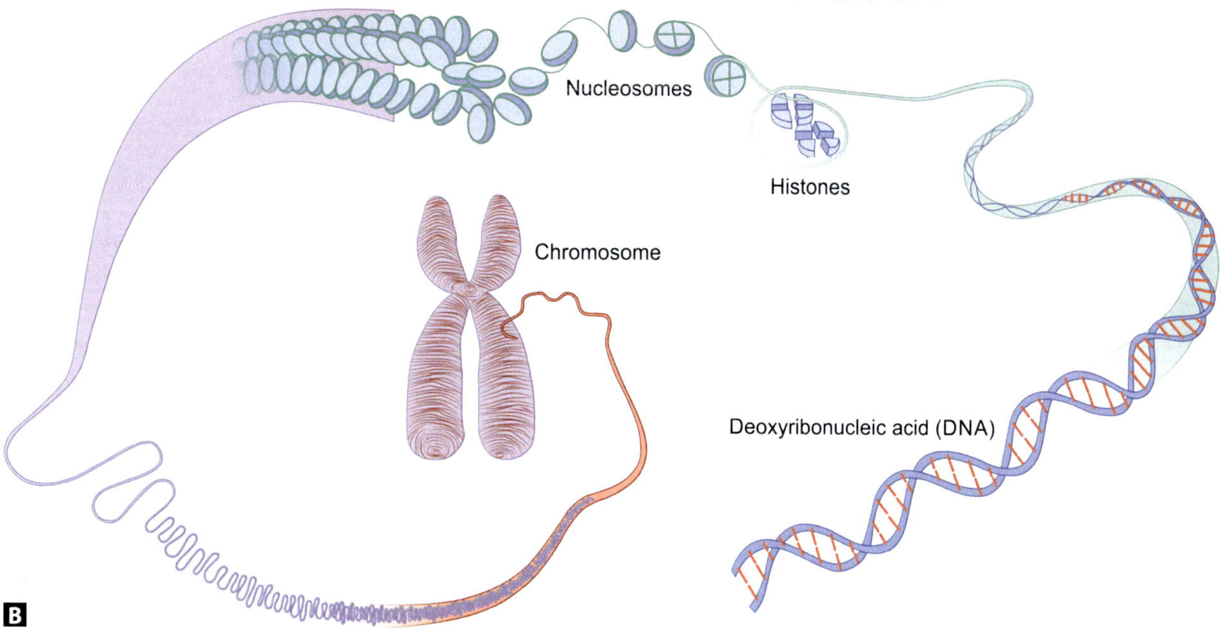

B

Figs. 1A and B: (A) Chromosome structure: Double helix; (B) Chromosome unwound.
Source: (A) istockphoto.com2; (B) genome.gov

gene acts as a set of instructions for the order of amino acids from which the protein is made. Within each exon, triplets of nucleotide bases form codons that correspond with specific amino acids.

Mutation

Any structural derangement in a gene is termed as mutation. Mutations can be:

- *Hereditary*: In this the mutations are inherited from either of parent with all the cells of the index patient having the concerned mutation. Since the parent's egg or the sperm (germ cells) might have had the same mutation, it is also known as germline mutation. The index case has the chances of passing the mutation to offspring.
- *Somatic*: The concerned mutation occurs in later part of its life and the concerned DNA changes are seen in the somatic cells. There are no chances of somatic mutation, further to subsequent generations.
- *De novo or sporadic mutations* can be hereditary or somatic. In some cases, the mutations occur only in the germ cells of the parent which gets passed on to offspring. In another scenario, the mutation occurs just after fertilization. In both the conditions, the affected person has the mutation afflicting all his cells and has the chances of passing it on to offspring. A person with a de novo mutation has the chance of passing the mutation to his offspring, none of his parents would have been affected as the mutation is "de novo."

EPIGENETICS

Epigenetics is the study of heritable changes in the gene expression without any change in the DNA sequence. This includes DNA methylation, histone modification, chromatin remodeling, and the use of noncoding RNAs. Abnormal DNA methylation and abnormal miRNA expression are the two most important epigenetic mechanisms that can be applied to human ophthalmic disease. The methylation of DNA at the gene promoter modifies DNA accessibility to transcription factors or helps recruit silencing-associated proteins. This abnormal methylation results in gene silencing and hence, gene expression alterations. Noncoding RNAs include nuclear, nucleolar, ribosomal as well as regulatory RNAs: Micro RNAs, long noncoding RNAs, and small-interfering RNA. These noncoding RNAs mediate post-transcriptional downregulation of gene expression. Knowledge of these epigenetic regulatory mechanisms helps in understanding the interactions between gene expression changes and environmental exposures and thereby, understanding the pathophysiology processes of ophthalmic disease such as age-related macular degeneration (AMD), cataract, pterygium, retinoblastoma (RB), and uveal melanoma. Epigenetic-targeted therapy may be the future treatment of ocular cancers, such as RB or uveal melanoma, and benefit from the development of an epigenetic map. Recently, clinical trials of epigenetic therapeutics in ophthalmic disease are focused on small RNA-based therapeutics for the retina, particularly for AMD. In the future, specific therapeutics to epigenetic alterations will be a more effective treatment modality to provide hope to prevent irreversible vision loss.

INHERITANCE PATTERNS

The inheritance patterns can be broadly classified as Mendelian disorders and non-Mendelian patterns of inheritance.

Mendelian Disorders

Mendelian disorders are caused by mutations in single genes and follow the principles of inheritance initially described by Gregor Mendel.

Autosomal Dominant

Autosomal dominance is a pattern of inheritance characteristic of some genetic traits or diseases. "Autosomal" means that the gene in question is located on one of the autosomal chromosomes or *autosomes,* numbered 1 to 22. "Dominant" means that a single copy of the disease-associated mutation is enough to cause the disease. The affected persons have 50% chances of passing it on to future generations. Each generation gets affected. Both males and females transmit the disease and are equally affected. In some pedigrees with an autosomal dominant disease, some individuals who carry the defective gene do not have the affected phenotype. However, these individuals can still transmit the disease gene to offspring and have affected children. This phenomenon is called reduced penetrance and is disease-gene-specific. The gene responsible for retinoblastoma 1 (*RB1*) is only 90% penetrant, which means that 10% of the individuals who inherit a mutant copy of the gene do not develop the tumor.

Autosomal Recessive

Diseases or traits that occur only when both copies of a gene are mutated are inherited as recessive pattern. Heterozygous carriers of mutant genes are usually clinically normal. When mutations in both copies of the gene are identical, the individual is homozygous. If the mutation on each allele is different, the individual is a compound heterozygote. Autosomal recessive disorders are more common in consanguineous marriages and constricted gene pools.

In a family with recessive disease, both parents are unaffected carriers, each having one wild-type gene (allele) and one mutant gene (allele). Each parent has a 50% chance of transmitting the defective allele to a child. Since a child must receive a defective allele from both parents to be affected, each child has a 25% chance of being affected, while 50% of the offspring will be carriers of the disease. If the parents are related, they may be carriers of the same rare mutations and there is a greater chance that a recessive disease can be transmitted to offspring. Males and females have an equal chance of transmitting and inheriting the disease alleles.

X-linked Recessive

The mutations on the X chromosome leads to distinctive patterns of inheritance because males have only one X chromosome. Most of the gene mutations on X chromosome are inherited in X- linked recessive pattern. In an X-linked recessive disorder, males who have the mutation on their single X chromosome manifest the phenotype, while females act as carriers but do not manifest the disease as their second X chromosome has a normal copy of the gene. For offspring of female carriers, the risk of a son being affected is 50% and for daughters, there is a 50% chance of being a carrier, with each conception. There is no male-to-male transmission as an affected male transmits his Y chromosome to son. In a pedigree, there is a predominant affliction of males.

In females, one of the X chromosomes is inactivated in every cell, a process called lyonization. In normal individuals, this is a random process which results, on an average, half of the cells of any organ using one X and half using the other X. A female might be affected with an X-linked recessive disorder either due to skewed X inactivation, if she has a mutation in both copies of the X chromosome gene, or if she has Turner syndrome (XO). If the gene mutation frequency is high in a population (e.g., red-green color deficiency), it is possible that affected males could mate with female carriers resulting in daughters who inherit the mutation from each parent thus becoming affected compound heterozygotes or homozygotes. Ocular albinism, juvenile retinoschisis, some forms of congenital stationary night blindness, and Lowe syndrome are other examples of X-linked recessive disorders.

Non-Mendelian Patterns of Inheritance

Mitochondrial Inheritance

Mitochondria have their own DNA which is distinct from nuclear DNA. All mitochondria are inherited from the mother. All children born to affected females have the mutated mitochondrial DNA (mtDNA). Severity of disease in each child depends upon the proportion of abnormal mitochondria in affected tissues. Affected males do not transmit the disease to their children. Examples include Kearns-Sayre syndrome, mitochondrial encephalopathy with lactic acidosis and seizure-like episodes (MELAS), and Leber hereditary optic neuropathy (LHON). Females and males are usually affected equally. The one exception is LHON for which there is preferential affectation of males.

Genetic Disorders Caused by Expansion of Repeat Nucleotides

Repeat nucleotide sequences occur in some human genes. Within a limit, these repeated nucleotide sequences do not disease phenotype. An excess number of repeats may disrupt the gene function leading to disease. The number of repeat sequences increases in subsequent generations resulting in earlier and more severe manifestations. Myotonic dystrophy and fragile X syndrome are examples.

Digenic and Triallelic Inheritance

When involvement of two different genes is required to manifest a phenotype, the pattern is digenic. Digenic retinitis pigmentosa (RP) is caused by a co-existing mutation involving ROM1 and peripherin/RDS (PRPH) genes. In Bardet-Biedl syndrome, triallelic disease has been observed: For example, co-existing mutations in two copies of one gene and one mutation in a second gene. Polygenic disease involves more than two genes.

Chromosomal Aberrations

Sometimes whole chromosomes, or chromosomes pieces, may be deleted or duplicated. Most chromosomal aberrations are lethal, as deletions or duplications almost always involve more than one gene. Patients usually have multisystem involvement, often including developmental delay. A karyotype examines chromosomes microscopically for deletions/duplications.

Deletion/duplication results in a contiguous gene syndrome. WAGR syndrome (Wilms tumor, aniridia, genital abnormalities, retardation) is due to deletion at 11p13 involves several genes including PAX 6 and WT1. Deletion of a portion of 13q causes dysmorphic facial features and RB. Contiguous gene syndromes should be suspected when patients present with features not usually seen together with a single gene disorder.

Translocation refers to transfer of genetic material from one chromosome to another. Reciprocal translocation involves an exchange of segments between two chromosomes. In balanced translocations, there is no net loss of genetic material and the individual is usually normal unless the break causes a disruption of a single gene. Offspring may have an unbalanced translocation with either excess or deficient chromosomal material leading to a phenotype, usually with more than one organ system involved. Karyotype is essential for diagnosis as translocation.

Mosaicism

After fertilization of the egg, the zygote begins to divide. Mutation or chromosomal aberration that develops in one cell thereafter will affect all progeny of that particular cell type. The patient will then have a separate population of cells throughout the body or localized to a region if the mutation occurs late in development. This is mosaicism. Mosaicism can affect somatic cells (somatic mosaicism) or sperm or unfertilized eggs (germline mosaicism). Mosaicism is not heritable unless germ cells are affected. Down syndrome may be caused by mosaic trisomy 21.

Loss of Heterozygosity

Retinoblastoma was the first disease to be described as secondary to a "two hit process" known as loss of heterozygosity. The first mutation usually occurs in the germ cells such that it is present in every cell in the body. RB develops only when a "second hit" occurs in a somatic cell, thus causing that cell to contain a mutation in both copies of the gene.

GENETICS OF SELECT OCULAR DISORDERS

Corneal Genetics

A brief account of corneal dystrophies are described as primary, inherited, bilateral affections of the cornea that occur unaccompanied by systemic disease. Affected corneas show no new vessels or inflammation, though secondary inflammation may occur. Age of onset, symptomatology, mode of progression, and inheritance vary with individual dystrophy.

Most of the corneal dystrophies present by the second decade, though the phenotypic expression may vary.

The clinical features remain true within a given pedigree.

Dystrophies of the Epithelium and Bowman's Layer of the Stroma

- Dystrophic recurrent erosion
- Meesmann epithelial dystrophy (may be completely asymptomatic)
- Ring-shaped dystrophy (Reis–Bücklers)
- Anterior membrane dystrophy (Grayson and Wilbrandt)
- Honey comb dystrophy (Thiel and Behnke)
- Inherited band-shaped keratopathy
- Anterior crocodile shagreen (Vogt).

Stroma

- Granular dystrophy (Groenouw I)
- Macular dystrophy (Groenouw II)
- Lattice dystrophy (Biber-Haab-Dimmer)
- Central crystalline dystrophy (Schnyder)
- Marginal crystalline dystrophy (Bietti)
- Central cloudy dystrophy (François)
- Deep parenchymatous dystrophy (Pillet)
- Speckled dystrophy (François and Neetens)
- Congenital stromal dystrophies
- Progressive dystrophy (Waardenburg and Jonkers).

Pre-Descemet Dystrophies

- Cornea farinata
- Deep filiform dystrophy
- Other forms.

Endothelium and Descemet Membrane

- Cornea guttata
- Late hereditary endothelial dystrophy (Fuchs')
- Congenital hereditary endothelial dystrophy (Maumenee)
- Posterior polymorphous dystrophy
- Annular endothelial dystrophy (François–Evens)
- Ectatic dystrophies
- Keratoconus.

Practical Considerations

Dystrophic Recurrent Erosions

Epithelial erosions are not uncommon in certain inherited corneal dystrophies. Such attacks are typical of the anterior membrane dystrophies and of macular and lattice dystrophies, less often in granular dystrophies, and have been described in unaffected family members of the families with inherited stromal dystrophies.

Cogan described an epithelial microcystic dystrophy with no inheritance of the disorder. Bilaterality, symmetry, and avascularity suggest that the changes may be dystrophic.

Meesmann Dystrophy

Meesmann dystrophy may be completely asymptomatic.

Reis–Bücklers Dystrophy

Reis–Bücklers dystrophy is a corneal disorder involving abnormality in Bowman layer of stroma. Symptoms may present at about the age of 5 years, with prolonged and painful attacks of recurrent erosions. A diffuse scarring at the level of Bowman layer can occur.

Anterior Membrane Dystrophy

Anterior membrane dystrophy may be a variant of Reis-Bücklers disorder.

Inherited Band-shaped Keratopathy

Band-shaped keratopathy occurs as a secondary manifestation in certain inherited disorders such as Norrie disease. Anterior crocodile Shagreen (Vogt): The cornea shows flat, gray, polygonal opacities at the level of Bowman membrane. A dominant inheritance has been described. A small proportion of patients develop band-shaped keratopathy. Anterior crocodile shagreen has been observed in association with megalocornea which is inherited as an X-linked recessive. Central anterior shagreen may have a variable effect on vision according to the density of the change.

Stromal Dystrophy: (Groenouw 1)

This presents with the appearance of discrete, discoid, or nodular white opacities in the anterior stromal layers of the axial cornea just deep to or at the level of Bowman layer. The number of opacities increase with time and they spread both peripherally and centrally. The deepest layers usually remain clear **(Fig. 2)**. The condition is inherited as autosomal dominant, though sporadic cases are described.

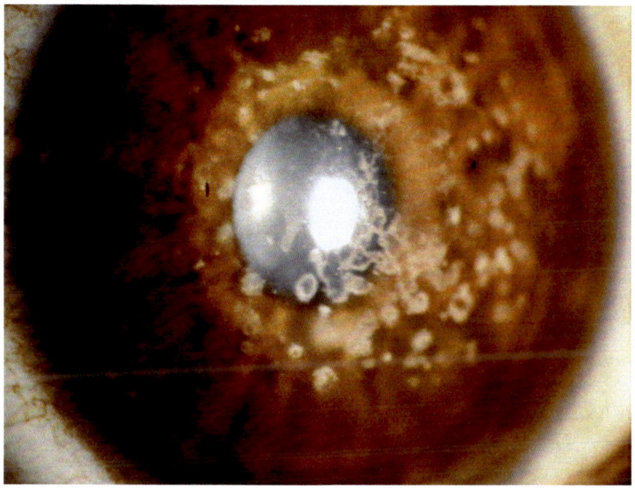

Fig. 2: Stromal dysytrophy (Groenouw 1).

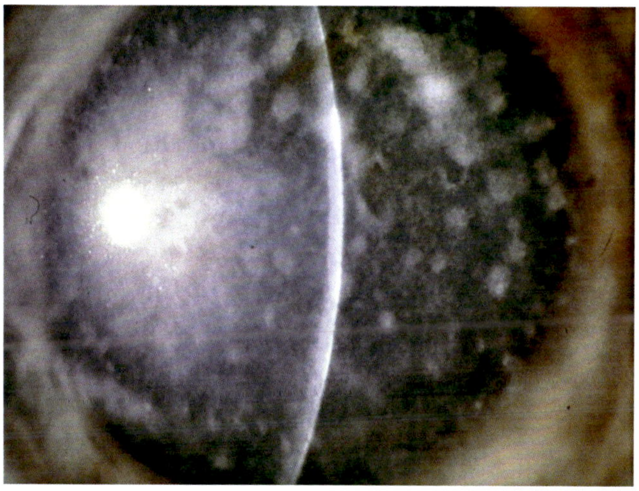

Fig. 3: Macular dystrophy (Groenouw 2).

Macular Dystrophy (Groenouw 2)

The onset is first seen between 5 and 9 years of age, when diffuse clouding is seen in superficial portions of the central cornea. The clouding increases in density and extent during the second decade and finally involves the whole thickness of the stroma, extending out to the limbus **(Fig. 3)**.

Corneal sensation is reduced. Attacks of irritation and photophobia may occur, and patients are essentially blind (or have very poor vision) by the age of 30–40 years. Inheritance is autosomal recessive. Ultrastructural studies suggest that there is a primary defect in the metabolism of the keratocytes, leading to mucopolysaccharide storage leading to improper glycosaminoglycan accumulation.

Lattice Dystrophy (Biber-Haab-Dimmer)

Lattice dystrophy has been observed as early as at the age of 2 years, though commonly presents at around 10 years. Symptoms of recurrent erosion or visual disturbance may lead to diagnosis. The changes begin in the anterior and middle of axial stroma, where double-contoured, relucent, branching filaments are found. They form an irregular lattice work resembling the arrangement of the corneal nerve net **(Fig. 4)**. Between the filaments, fine dots, flakes, and star-shaped opacities are seen in some, but not all families. Progressive clouding of the central stroma occurs. Corneal sensation may be lost over the central opacity, but retained in the periphery. As a rule, both corneas are affected, but both unilateral cases and those with sectoral involvement of the cornea have been described. A prominent and even presenting feature of lattice dystrophy is the occurrence of recurrent erosion. It is interesting to note that recurrent erosions have been reported in family members unaffected by the dystrophy. Secondary vascularization of the cornea may follow inflammatory episodes. Vision is affected early and shows progressive deterioration; by the age of 40 years, the patient may be unable to work. The condition is inherited as an autosomal dominant. Electron microscopy and immunofluorescent studies confirmed the material as amyloid. It is of interest that an inherited form of systemic amyloidosis, giving rise to skin changes and polyneuropathy is reported in association with corneal changes of lattice dystrophy.

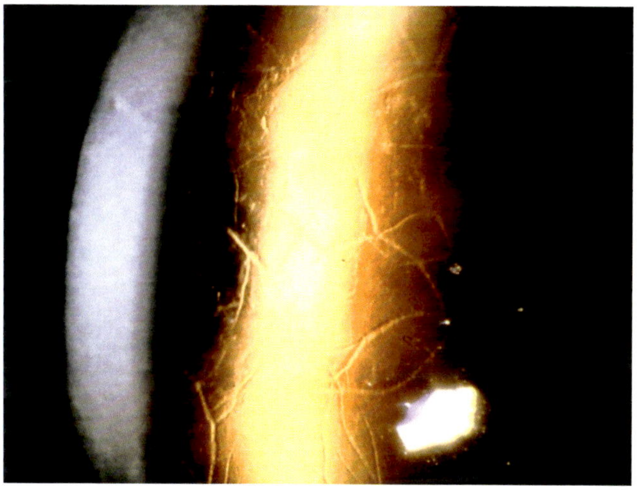

Fig. 4: Lattice dystrophy.

Central Crystalline Dystrophy (Schnyder)

This dystrophy is reported occurring as early as at 18 months. There may be little or no progression throughout life. It occurs bilaterally as asymmetrical crystalline deposits in the anterior third of the corneal stroma including Bowman layer. Vision is usually good, but corneal transplantation may be necessary in a small number of patients. Following the histochemical identification of the crystals as cholesterol, there has been great interest in the serum cholesterol level in this disorder. There are no conclusive studies suggest correlation.

Deep Parenchymatous Dystrophy

The central opacities affect the posterior, middle, and to a lesser extent, the anterior stroma. The corneal changes have only a slight effect on vision. Corneal sensitivity is normal, and patients do not often complain of discomfort.

Speckled Dystrophy (François and Neetens)

This is a benign, nonprogressive dystrophy of the corneal stroma. It is characterized by the presence of small, semi-opaque, flattened opacities scattered sparsely throughout the full thickness of the stroma, except in Bowman layer. It involves peripheral as well as central stroma.

Congenital stromal dystrophies (recessive and dominant forms), progressive dystrophy (Waardenburg and Jonkers), and pre-Descemet dystrophies have been described and are rare.

Dystrophies of the Endothelium and Descemet Membrane

Cornea Guttata

Cornea guttata is characterized by the formation of numerous fine wart-like excrescences on Descemet membrane that appear centrally and spread peripherally with age. On specular reflection, the warts are seen as dark guttate spots **(Fig. 5)**. Although the endothelium is morphologically abnormal, there are no clinical signs of disturbed endothelial function in terms of corneal edema. The incidence and severity of cornea guttata increases with age. The sex inheritance is equal. An inheritance pattern is not always demonstrable, but it may occur as an autosomal dominant and also been described in siblings who are the offspring of unaffected parents.

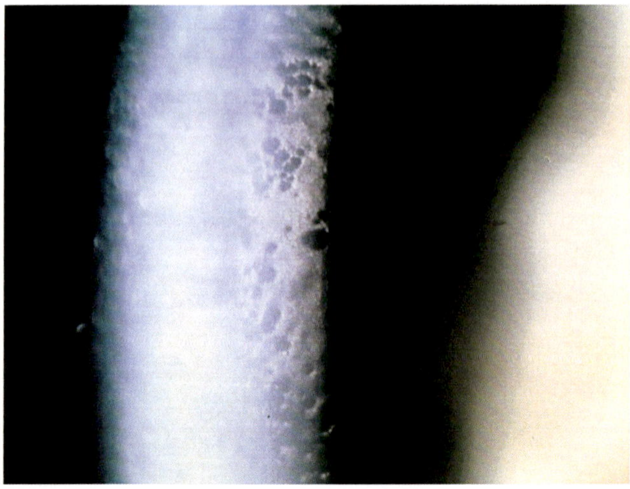

Fig. 5: Corneal guttata.

Fuchs' Dystrophy

The term Fuchs' dystrophy may be properly applied to a dystrophy of the endothelium resulting in corneal edema manifesting after the fourth decade. Cornea guttata may be the precursor of Fuchs' dystrophy **(Figs. 6A and B)**. The edema results from a decreased pumping and barrier function of the endothelium. This is expressed as stromal edema first and epithelial edema later. Fuchs' dystrophy tends to be progressive disorder over a variable period of time. In the early stages of epithelial edema, visual symptoms are worst on waking. In advanced cases, rupture of epithelial bullae accounts for repeated attacks of pain. Burning sensation may be moderately reduced at a later stage. The sex incidence is roughly three females to one male.

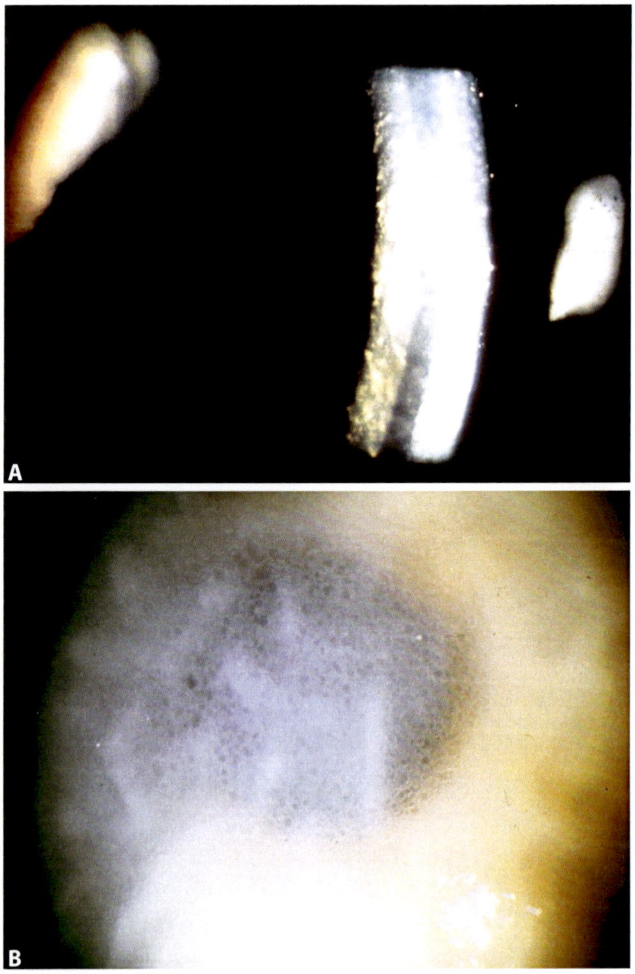

Figs. 6A and B: (A) Corneal dystrophy in Fuchs' dystrophy; (B) Fuchs' endothelial dystrophy.

Congenital Hereditary Endothelial Dystrophy (Maumenee)

A number of pedigrees have been reported of families exhibiting a dominantly or recessively inherited dystrophy of the corneal endothelium, and expressing itself as corneal edema present at birth. Affected corneas show diffuse milky or ground-glass opacification of the stroma. Vision varies according to the degree of corneal clouding. The condition differs from juvenile Fuchs' dystrophy, in that no guttate changes are seen in Descemet membrane. Large bullae are not seen despite the massive stromal edema that occurs. This is thought to be due to the unusually tight adhesion between epithelium and the underlying Bowman layer. Corneal sensation is normal, and vascularization is rare. Histopathologically, the findings vary from a paucity to generalized absence of endothelial cells and an overall increase in the thickness in Descemet membrane. In contrast to Fuchs' dystrophy, wart-like excrescences are not found. The stroma is thickened, and the lamellae are separated by numerous fluid clefts. The keratocytes show degenerative changes.

Posterior Polymorphous Dystrophy

Posterior polymorphous dystrophy is a bilateral, congenital disorder of Descemet membrane and endothelium. It is dominantly inherited. Descemet membrane exhibits a variable number of round, elliptical or irregular lesions that may be vesicular in appearance, bulge forward into stroma, or otherwise form ridge-like projections into the anterior chamber. A degree of posterior stromal opacity may also be present.

The condition is generally benign and nonprogressive, with little effect on vision. The severity of the disorder may vary within the same pedigree. Corneal edema following cataract surgery may occur.

Summary: Treatment of Corneal Dystrophies

Exceptional advances have occurred during the last three decades in eye banking, procurement, preservation, and corneal transplantation surgery. Full thickness corneal transplantation, Descemet stripping endothelial keratoplasty (DSEK), Descemet membrane endothelial keratoplasty (DMEK), and potential artificial corneas are being performed as outpatient surgery, because of our understanding of basic sciences and improvements in technology and instrumentation. With early diagnosis, coupled with accessibility and affordability, corneal blindness can be prevented or cured. This is of utmost importance, especially in children, as 80% of learning is through vision.

GENETICS OF CONGENITAL CATARACT

It is possible to identify a genetic mutation in up to 90% of cases of bilateral cataract with current genetic testing **(Figs. 7A and B)**. The main lens proteins associated with congenital cataract include crystallins, membrane proteins, cytoskeletal structural proteins, and transcription factors. Some of these genes are also involved in the development of other ocular structures; hence, in approximately 15% of cases, mutations can lead to associated eye abnormalities.

Crystallins

Crystallins, α, β, and γ-crystallins, are the main structural refractive protein of the human lens; thus mutations in this family of genes result in congenital cataract. In addition, α-crystallins act as molecular chaperones, where they assist in the folding or unfolding of other damaged or denatured proteins such as β and γ-crystallins, and can inhibit apoptosis. Approximately 50% of nonsyndromic hereditary cataract are due to mutations in genes coding for crystallin proteins. More than 100 mutations, mostly missense, encoding 12 different human α, β, and γ crystallin genes have been identified.

Cytoskeletal Structural Proteins

Beaded filament structural proteins (BFSPs) are a type of intermediate filament protein that are expressed in various cells of the body, such as epithelial, glial, and muscle cells. *BFSP1* and *BFSP2* are genes encoding Filensin and Phakinin, respectively, which are proteins expressed exclusively in the lens. They are intimately associated with crystallins, where they form part of a highly organized cytoskeleton and are also thought to have an important role in lens development and differentiation. Mutations in the *BFSP2* gene is known to cause cataract which is inherited as autosomal recessive fashion. Heterogeneous carriers of this mutation may also be predisposed to develop age-related cataract and myopia.

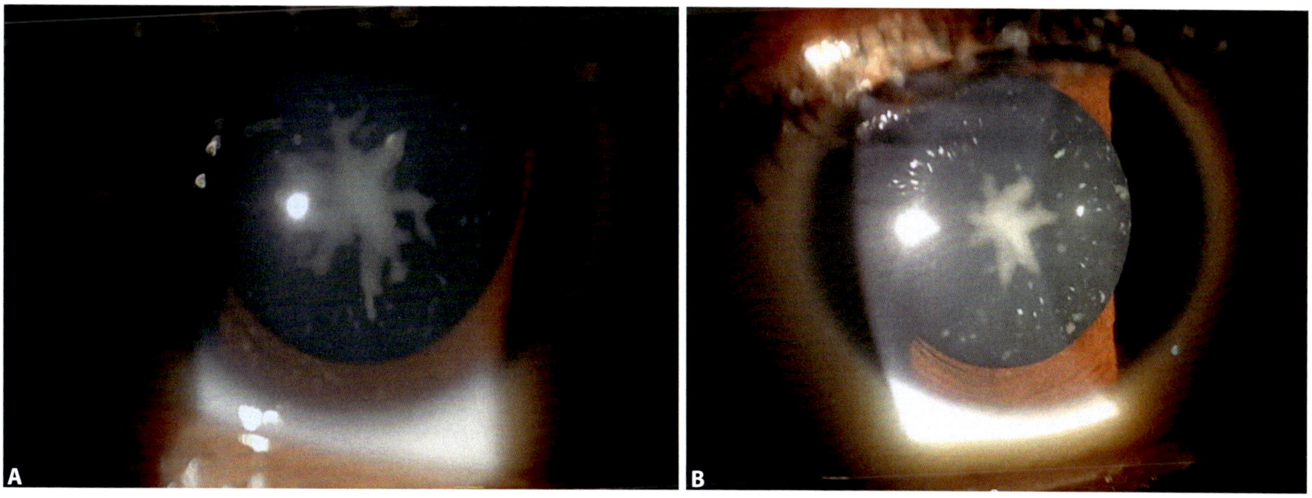

Figs. 7A and B: Bilateral congenital cataract in a child. (A) Right eye and (B) Left eye.

Membrane Proteins

Connexins

As the lens is an avascular structure, membrane proteins have an important role in maintenance and metabolic homeostasis. Genetic mutations in over 10 membrane protein genes lead to inappropriate transport of ions, solutes, and water between cells in the human lens. Gap junction channels are made up of two connexons composed of six subunits called connexins. Connexins have an important role in lens microcirculation, particularly in the supply of metabolites and nutrients toward the center of the lens, and outward flow of unwanted ions and by-products to the periphery. Mutations in *GJA3* and *GJA8* genes that encode connexins have also been implicated in the formation of cataract. These mutations are mostly missense mutations and are most commonly associated with zonular and nuclear pulverulent cataracts with varying progression.

Major Intrinsic Protein

Mutations in genes encoding major intrinsic proteins (MIPs) account for 5% of all inherited cataract. Aquaporin-0 is the most expressed membrane protein in the human lens and variants are inherited in an autosomal dominant pattern producing a variety of cataract phenotypes. Lens intrinsic membrane protein-2 (LIM2) is the gene responsible for a membrane protein with four transmembrane domains called MP19, which contribute to lens transparent. Three LIM2 missense mutations have been described that cause autosomal recessive cataract mostly cortical in nature.

Other proteins working at the membrane include EPHA2 and DNMBP. EPHA2 mutations are most often associated with autosomal dominant posterior polar cataract. DNMBP encodes a protein that regulates the configurations of cell junctions through binding to tight junction protein. Biallelic loss-of-function variants have been shown to result in autosomal recessive cataract with other ocular features, including pupil abnormalities, strabismus, and nystagmus.

Transcription Factors

Heat shock transcription factor 4 (HSF4) protects lens proteins from cell stressors and has a regulatory role in the differentiation of lens fiber cells. Mutations in HSF4 most often produce lamellar cataract, which can be present at birth or develop in early childhood, and can be inherited in a dominant or recessive mode.

MAF encodes a transcription factor containing the basic-leucine zipper (bZIP) domain which has a critical role in eye development. Mutations in bZIP domain are associated with congenital cataract and ocular defects such as iris coloboma, glaucoma, microcornea, microphthalmia, myopia, nystagmus, and Peters anomaly.

FOXE3 is one of a family of genes encoding transcription factors with a "forkhead" DNA binding domain and has a role in lens embryology. 24 unique mutations have been shown to affect various ocular structures, including cornea, iris, lens, and retina.

Pituitary homeobox 3 (PITX3) proteins are transcription factors that have been shown to play an important role in controlling lens epithelial cell maintenance and lens fiber cell differentiation. Mutations in *PITX3* genes most often cause posterior polar cataract with or without anterior segment dysgenesis (ASD), that can result in other ocular defects such as corneal opacity, microphthalmia, microcornea, nystagmus, and glaucoma.

GENETICS OF GLAUCOMA

Genetic factors contribute to the development of most types of glaucoma. Early-onset glaucoma before the age of 35 years exhibits autosomal dominant or autosomal recessive inheritance. The inheritance of adult-onset glaucoma is complex due to the influence of multiple genetic and/or environmental risk factors. Current genetic and genomic methodologies have identified genes responsible for early-onset glaucoma as well as genetic risk factors contributing to adult-onset glaucoma.

CONGENITAL GLAUCOMA

Currently two genes are known to cause congenital glaucoma, CYP1B1 coding for cytochrome P450 1B1 and LTBP2 (latent transforming growth factor-β binding protein 2). Mutations in both genes cause autosomal recessive congenital glaucoma.

Developmental Glaucoma

Axenfeld–Rieger syndrome, aniridia, and glaucoma associated with ASD are caused by mutations in PITX2, PAX6, and FOXC1, respectively. These genes code for transcription factors active in ocular development. Mutations in these genes cause dominantly inherited disease.

Juvenile Open-angle Glaucoma

Approximately 20% of patients with open-angle glaucoma before the age of 35 years have mutations in *MYOC* coding for myocilin. The first-degree relatives of *MYOC* mutation carriers have a 50% chance of inheriting the mutation (dominant inheritance) and should undergo genetic testing and regular eye examinations. Patients with *MYOC* mutations may benefit from therapeutic approaches that relieve endoplasmic reticulum stress such as phenyl butyrate. Because several MYOC mutations cause adult-onset disease, genetic screening for MYOC mutations should also be considered for patients who develop the disease after the age of 35 years and have a family history of glaucoma.

Familial Normal-tension Glaucoma

A duplication of the TBK1 gene causes a rare form of familial normal-tension glaucoma (NTG). *TBK1* interacts with optineurin, a protein encoded by optineurin gene (OPTN) that can also cause NTG. Patients with NTG who have family members can be screened for TBK1 and OPTN gene mutation. Because both genetic products are involved in tumor necrosis factor-α signaling, it is possible that these patients could benefit from tumor necrosis factor-α inhibitors.

Adult-onset Primary Open-angle Glaucoma

Recent advances in genomic technologies have made it possible to study the genetic etiologies of common forms of adult-onset glaucoma. Many genome-wide association studies for primary open-angle glaucoma (POAG) have been completed, that identified DNA sequence variants in the CAV1/CAV2 gene region associated with POAG. *CDKN2BAS* and *TMCO1* genes mutations have been found in patients with POAG. Research suggests that TMCO1 is associated with elevated intraocular pressure (IOP), whereas *CDKN2BAS* may primarily affect the optic nerve's susceptibility to degeneration.

Primary Angle-closure Glaucoma

Studies have identified mutations in *PLEKHA7* and *COL11A1* genes and an intergenic region between *PCMTD1* and *ST18* on chromosome 8q in patients with primary angle-closure glaucoma (PACG). However, it is not clearly understood how these genes may contribute to primary angle-closure glaucoma, although potential mechanisms include the regulation of cellular permeability, scleral rigidity, and ocular growth have been hypothesized.

Exfoliation Syndrome and Glaucoma

Genome-wide association studies identified *LOXL1* as a major genetic risk factor for exfoliation syndrome, in populations worldwide. The frequency of *LOXL1* risk alleles is high in both affected and unaffected individuals which suggest that other factors, which could be genetic or environmental, may also contribute to the disease.

RETINITIS PIGMENTOSA

Retinitis pigmentosa is a heterogeneous group of diseases characterized by progressive rod-cone dysfunction. Patients initially present with nyctalopia from rod photoreceptor loss, progress to tunnel vision, and ultimately experience central vision loss. RP is also the most common form of inherited retinal degeneration, affecting one in 3,000 people. The described inheritance patterns of RP include autosomal dominant (30–40%), autosomal recessive (50–60%), X-linked recessive (5–20%), and mitochondrial. As RP is a genetically heterogeneous set of disorders, the specific mutation involved in any given case of RP dictates the inheritance pattern and strongly influences the prognosis. More than 100 gene loci that cause RP have been mapped or identified.

Autosomal Dominant Retinitis Pigmentosa

Mutations in >25 genes have been identified that cause autosomal dominant retinitis pigmentosa (ADRP). Patients with ADRP usually present late in life. The disease is less severe and it progresses slowly. The macula usually remains spared for a long period **(Figs. 8A to D)**.

Molecular Genetics of Autosomal Dominant Retinitis Pigmentosa

RHO Gene

Mutations in the *RHO* gene are the most common cause of ADRP, accounting for 20–30% of all cases. This gene encodes for making rhodopsin protein, which is predominantly present in rods. The cytogenetic location of *RHO* gene is 3q22.1.

PRPF3 Gene

The removal of introns from nuclear pre-mRNAs occurs on spliceosomes, which are made up of four small nuclear ribonucleoproteins (snRNPs). This gene participates in pre-mRNA slicing and mutations lead to abnormality of this function. The cytogenetic location of *PRPF3* gene is 1q21.2.

RP1 Gene

The *RP1* gene encodes a doublecortin domain, which binds microtubules and regulates microtubule polymerization. This microtubules-associated protein is needed for correct stacking of the outer segment disk mutation in this gene. The cytogenetic location of *RP1* gene is 8q11.23–q12.1.

Autosomal Recessive Retinitis Pigmentosa

Autosomal recessive retinitis pigmentosa (AR-RP) accounts for about 50–60% of all cases of RP. Clinically, it shows all the classic features of RP, such as attenuated retinal blood vessels, intraretinal pigmentation, and waxy pallor of the optic disk.

Molecular Genetics of Autosomal Recessive Retinitis Pigmentosa

Phosphodiesterase 6

The phosphodiesterase (PDE) complex has one α, one β, and two γ subunits. The complex encodes a protein that plays an important role in rod phototransduction and maintenance of the intracellular cyclic guanosine monophosphate (cGMP) level. *PDE6G* might be associated with early-onset RP.

RP25 or EYS (Eyes Shut Homolog)

This gene accounts for 10–20% of AR-RP in Spanish populations. The cytogenetic location of this gene is 6q12.

TULP1 (Tubby-like Protein 1) Gene

The protein encoded by the *TULP1* gene is thought to play a role in the physiology of photoreceptors. The cytogenetic location of this gene is 6p21.31.

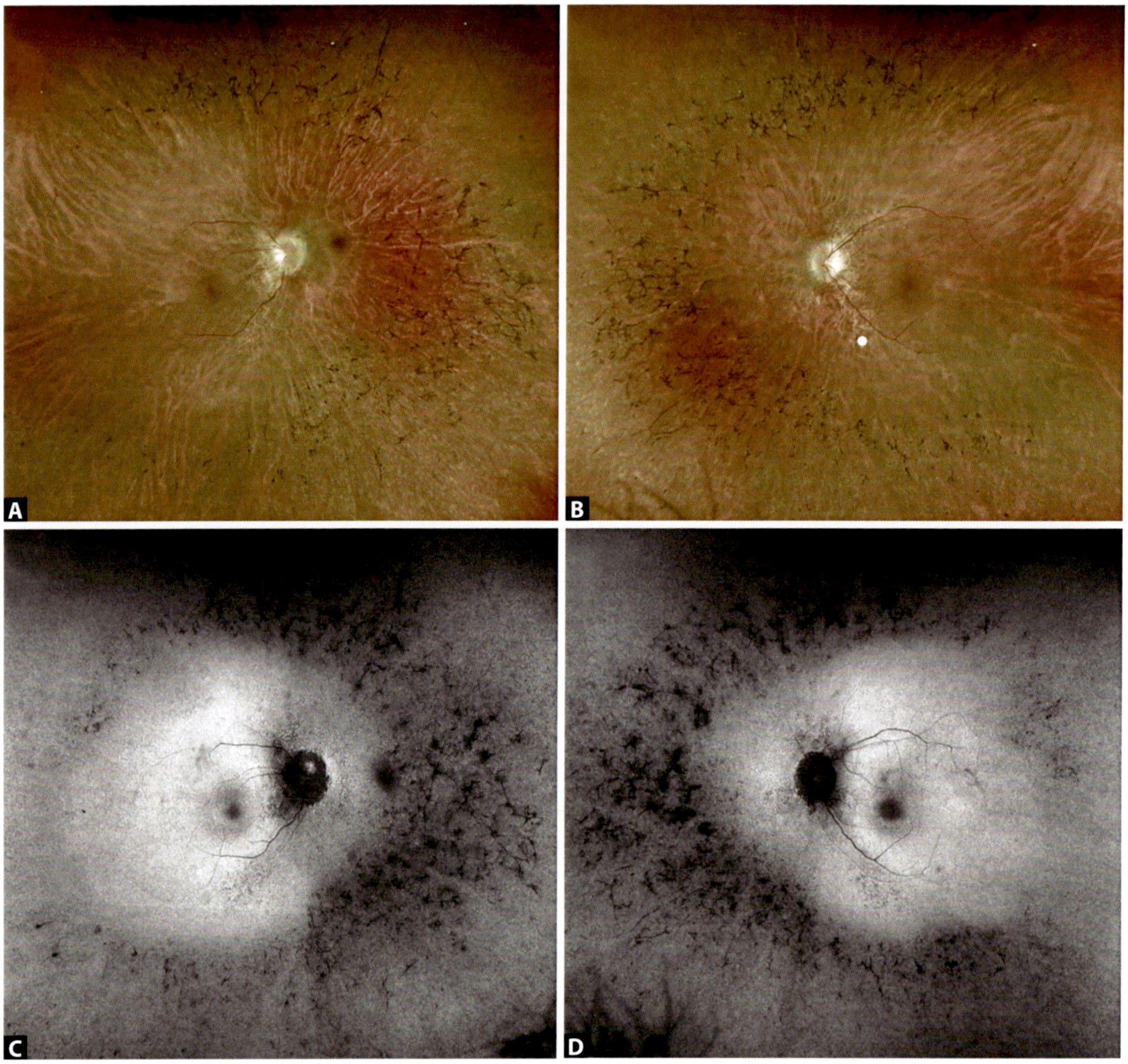

Figs. 8A to D: (A and B) A case of autosomal dominant (AD) retinitis pigmentosa (RP) showing all the classic features, but sparing the macula; (C and D) Fundus autofluorescence imaging of the same patient showing ring-shaped hyper autofluorescence around the macula.

CERKL (Ceramide Kinase-like) Gene

This gene encodes a protein with ceramide kinase-like domains; the protein may be a negative regulator of apoptosis in photoreceptor cells. The cytogenetic location of this gene is 2q31.3.[35]

RPE65 Gene

This gene is expressed in the retinal pigment epithelium (RPE) and is vital for converting all- *trans*-retinyl esters into 11-*cis*-retinal, an important step in the regeneration of visual pigment. The *RPE* gene mutations are responsible for around 2% of AR-RP and 16% of Leber congenital amaurosis. The cytogenetic location of this gene is 1p31.3.

X-linked Retinitis Pigmentosa

X-linked retinitis pigmentosa (XLRP) is considered to be one of the most severe forms of RP. It accounts for about 5–20% of all RP cases. It primarily affects males. Patients usually present with night blindness in the first decade of life, with reduction in the visual fields in the second decade, and severe visual loss usually less than about 20/200 by the fourth decade. Fundi show all the characteristic features of RP: Bone spicule-like pigmentary deposits in the retina, attenuation of retinal arterioles, waxy pallor of the optic disk, and grossly reduced or absent amplitude on electroretinogram (ERG) **(Fig. 9A and B)**.

The fundus examination of the female carriers may show only peripheral RPE changes, including pigmentary deposits. ERG may show a reduced amplitude to white light or delayed cone-wave implicit times. The carrier may also show a characteristic tapetal reflex—a golden, metallic luster in the perimacular area. About 50% of female carriers may have these abnormalities such as tapetal reflex, pigmentary alteration, and ERG changes.

Molecular Genetics

The most frequent single cause of X-linked RP is a mutation in the RP guanosine triphosphatase (GTPase) regulator

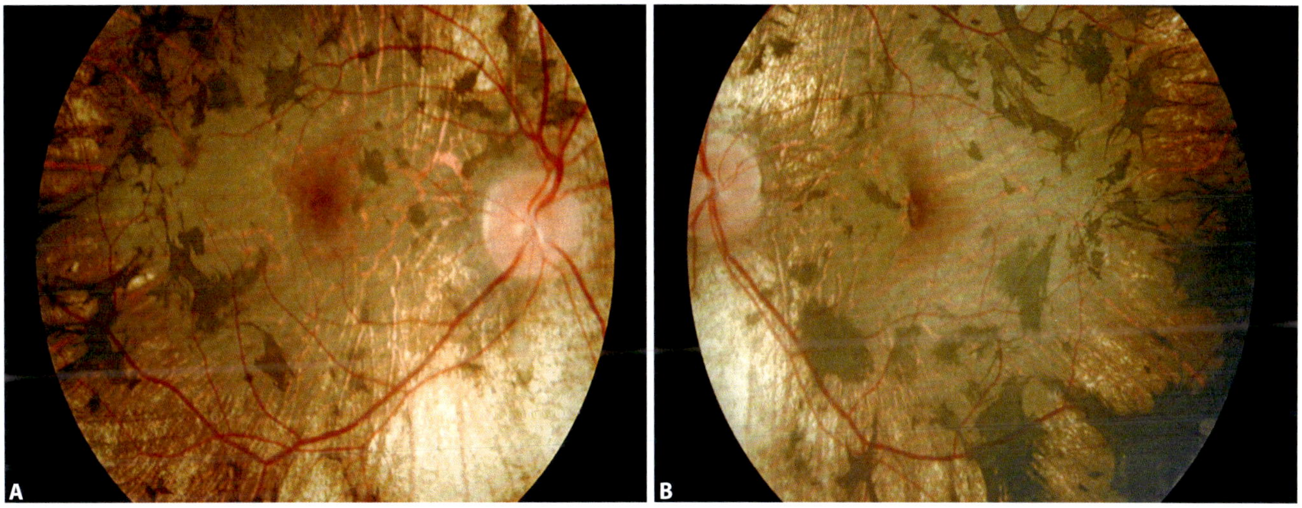

Figs. 9A and B: A case of X-linked retinitis pigmentosa showing extensive pigmentary changes. (A) Right eye and (B) Left eye.

gene (*RPGR*). The other gene involved in the mutation is *RP2*. About, 35–55% of mutations in RPGR gene different versions of RPGR protein, one of which contains an ORF15 exon. This is expressed predominantly in the photoreceptors and plays an important role by regulating the function of RPE cilia. A few mutations in the *ORF15* exon result in cone-rod dystrophy, cone dystrophy, and atrophic macular degeneration.[35] Some affected individuals with the *RPGR* mutation have chronic respiratory and sinus infections, recurrent otitis media, and hearing loss. These effects could be due to disruption of the function of cilia. Mutation results in an abnormally short and malfunctioning protein. The cytogenetic location of the gene is Xp11.4 (short arm of the X chromosome at position 11.4).

The *RP2* gene encodes a protein, which may be involved in transporting proteins within photoreceptor cells. More than 70 mutations have been identified in subjects with XLRP. The mutations result in a short version of the RP2 protein. The cytogenetic location of this gene is Xp11.3 (short arm of the X chromosome at position 11.3).

X-LINKED RETINOSCHISIS

X-linked retinoschisis, or X-linked juvenile retinoschisis (XLRS) is a rare congenital disease of the retina caused by mutations in the *RS1* gene, which encodes retinoschisin, a protein involved in intercellular adhesion and likely retinal cellular organization. X-linked retinoschisis has also been referred to as juvenile retinoschisis, congenital retinoschisis, juvenile macular degeneration/dystrophy, degenerative retinoschisis, and vitreous veils of the retina. X-linked juvenile retinoschisis occurs exclusively in males and is characterized by visual loss that begins in early childhood. The patients are usually school-age and are experiencing visual disturbances, especially in reading. The prevalence is estimated to be 1 in 15,000–30,000 men. XLRS has complete penetrance but variable expressivity. Carrier females generally remain asymptomatic.

General Features

Visual acuity depends on the amount and location of schisis. On presentation, most affected males have a visual acuity of 20/60 to 20/120. It deteriorates slowly over the next few decades and may later progress to legal blindness (<20/200) by the fifth or sixth decade. The characteristic finding is foveal schisis seen as stellate or fine radial striae in a sort of spoke-like pattern radiating from the fovea **(Figs. 10A to D)** due to small cystoid spaces. Unlike cystoid macular edema, these spaces do not show leakage on fluorescein angiogram. The schitic areas are seen as dome-shaped elevation of a thin layer of retina and are more easily identified with red-free light. The peripheral retina may show RPE alteration. The splitting occurs predominantly within the inner retinal layers (neural retina). The inner retina of the retinoschisis can develop large oval holes. Peripheral retinoschisis is present in about half of patients, and is visible as large holes, which may be so large as to extend from the arcade to the equator. Peripheral vision may be normal in the unaffected areas. Absolute scotomas may be present in areas of peripheral retinoschisis, which are often inferotemporal. Color vision is often normal. In the inner retina, the retinal blood vessels are freely floating which is called a vitreous veils. Rarely, these vessels rupture and patients present with vitreous hemorrhage. Retinal detachment may occur in 5–20% of cases. Patients who develop vitreous hemorrhage or rhegmatogenous retinal detachment may benefit from vitreoretinal surgery. Patients above 50 years old commonly have pigmentary changes and retinal pigment epithelium atrophy in the macula.

Fundus autofluorescence (FAF) shows modification of normal foveal autofluorescence with a radial pattern **(Fig. 10D)**. Over time, FAF can document progression in terms of RPE changes.

Optical coherence tomography (OCT) shows schisis in the superficial neural retina and thinning of the retina.

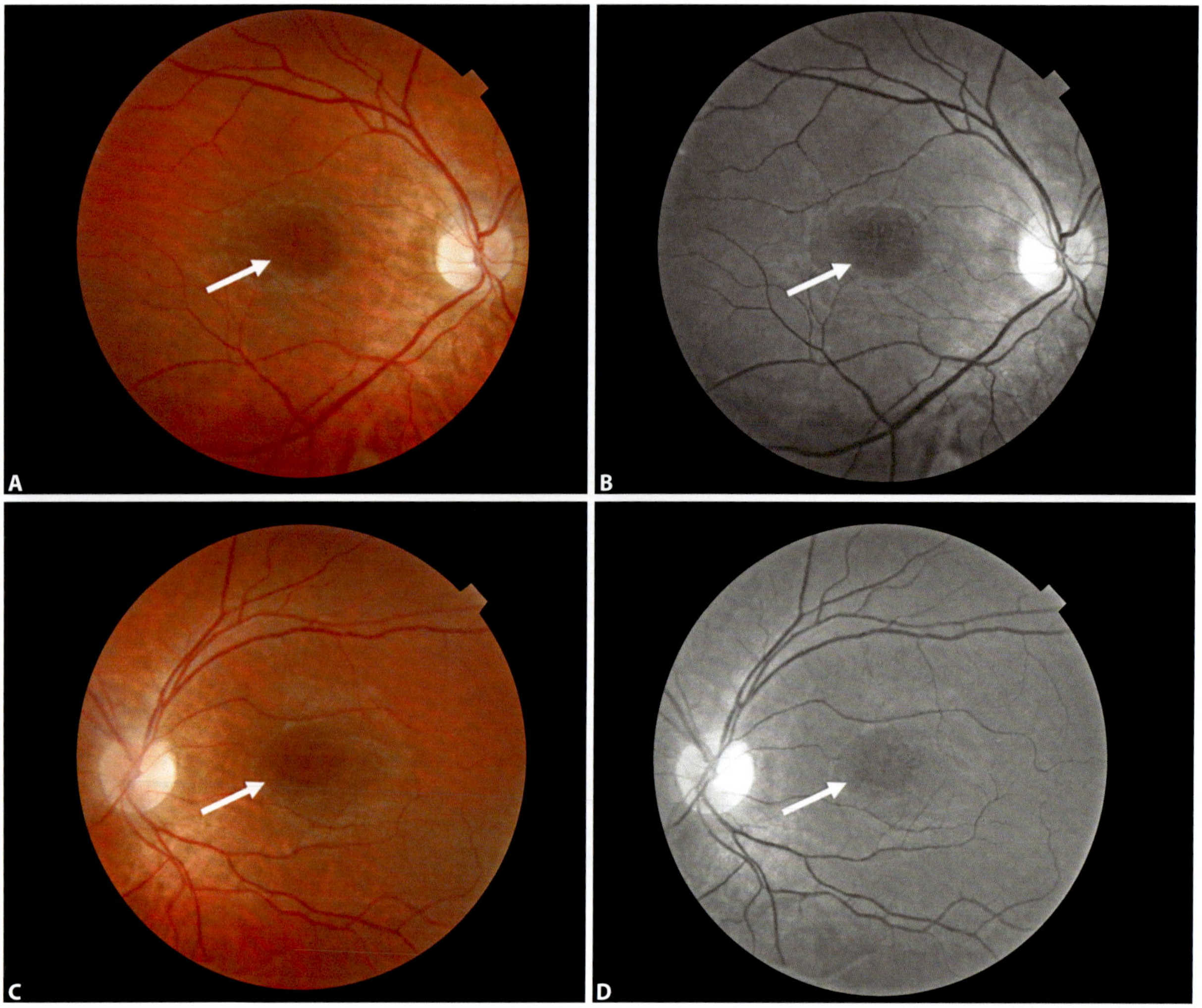

Figs. 10A to D: Color fundus and red free photographs of a patient with X-linked juvenile retinoschisis. (A and B) Right eye and (C and D) Left eye. The central macula shows cystic changes around the fovea, in a spoke-like pattern indicated by arrows.

OCT shows small cystic-like spaces perifoveal and large cystic-like spaces within the fovea. With increasing age, these cystic spaces may not be evident because of flattening of the cysts.

Electroretinography (ERG) shows a negative waveform. The a-wave is preserved, but the amplitude of the b-wave is reduced; the alteration of the ratio of these waves (a-wave amplitude exceeding the b-wave amplitude) is an important diagnostic feature. Multifocal ERG also demonstrates reduced amplitude, along with longer implicit time in the central macular area.

Molecular Genetics

The gene responsible for XLRS is *RS1*, which encodes a protein called retinoschisin; the gene encodes a 224-amino acid protein called *retinoschisin*, which is secreted by photoreceptors. This protein is important for cell adhesion among all neuronal cells, including Müller cells. *RS1* gene mutations cause a complete loss of functional retinoschisin protein, so the maintenance and organization of cells in the retina are disrupted. As a result, the retina splits.

About 220 mutations of the *RS1* gene have been reported. Most mutations involve single amino acid change in the retinoschisin protein.

STARGARDT DISEASE

General Features

Stargardt disease (STGD) is the most common childhood recessively inherited macular dystrophy. The condition has a genetic basis due to mutations in the *ABCA4* gene, and results from the accumulation of visual cycle kinetics-derived by-products in the RPE with secondary photoreceptor dysfunction and death. STGD accounts for about 7% of all retinal degenerations, grossly affecting 1 per 10,000 individuals. The disease usually manifests itself in early childhood or adolescence, but later onset has also been reported. As with all autosomal conditions, males and females are equally affected.

Stargardt patients may be asymptomatic but most commonly present with bilateral central visual loss, photophobia, color vision abnormalities, central scotomas, and slow dark adaptation. Vision deterioration is rapidly progressive and its age of onset highly variable, but it most often occurs between childhood and adolescence. At presentation visual acuity may range between 20/20 and 20/400, with prior visual acuity being frequently normal, and very few patients further deteriorate their vision to counting finger or hand motion level. The visual prognosis is highly dependent on age of disease onset, with patients presenting with significantly compromised vision at an earlier age, have poorer outcomes. An autosomal recessive pattern of inheritance is most common. Color vision using Hardy-Rand-Rittler or Ishihara color plates usually shows a mild red-green dyschromatopsia in patients with STGD. Moreover, when these patients are submitted to a Farnsworth-Munsell Hue Test, a tritan defect (or short wavelength) may also be noted.

Stargardt disease affects the macula with variable centrifugal expansion. Fundus examination is frequently normal early on the course of disease. Later on, typical fundus manifestations arise, including pigment mottling, frank macular atrophy, a bull's eye maculopathy or beaten-bronze appearance, and with or without fundus flecks. Fundus flecks are *pisciform*, round or dot-like yellow-white lesions typically found in Stargardt patients. Flecks are indeed accumulation of lipofuscin in the RPE but may also represent areas of regional depigmentation and atrophy. Fleck distribution may change over time, does not correlate well with the visual loss, form individual or confluent patterns, and have a central distribution, with variable mid-periphery involvement. However, STGD presents with highly variable phenotypes, influenced by a combination of several factors.

Visual field testing in Stargardt patients is often normal in early disease stages. Over time, relative central scotomas develop, further progressing to absolute central scotomas. Usually Stargardt patients have preserved peripheral visual fields. However, in severe cases, with widespread retinal atrophy, visual constriction can occur. Another particularly important finding is the change in preferred retinal locus of fixation.

Fluorescein angiography reveals a "dark-choroid" sign in up to 62% of patients due to lack of early choroidal hyperfluorescence, which is blocked by high-grade lipofuscin accumulation in the RPE. Fundus flecks are seen as small irregular hyperfluorescent lesions.

Autofluorescence imaging provides a fast noninvasive way to study the health and viability of the RPE. Abnormally increased autofluorescence represents excessive lipofuscin accumulation in the RPE. Inversely, decreased areas of autofluorescence relate to low-level RPE metabolic activity which normally underlies local atrophy with secondary photoreceptor loss.

Electroretinogram in Stargardt patients reveals that they typically maintain normal or subnormal full-field electroretinographic scotopic (rods) and photopic (cones) responses. However, patients with more widespread disease can present with notably abnormal scotopic and photopic responses on full-field ERG.

Optical coherence tomography shows early detection of lipofuscin accumulation in the RPE and photoreceptor layer disorganization.

Molecular Genetics

Mutation in *ABCA4* gene, which encodes an ATP-binding cassette (ABC) transporter protein, expressed in the outer segment (OS) of rods. ABCA4 protein transports potentially toxic substances out of photoreceptor cells. These substances are formed after phototransduction. Buildup of the toxic substance lipofuscin in the RPE and photoreceptor cells causes cell death. The cytogenetic location of this gene is 1p22.1.

The genetics is extremely heterogeneous and may be responsible for wide variations in clinical presentations. Mild reduction in ABCA4 activity results in about 95% of cases of STGD; moderate loss of activity results in cone-rod dystrophy (about 30–50% of cases); and complete loss results in RP with complete loss of rod and cone function (about 8% of cases of AR-RP). Other mutations, accounting for the remaining 5% of STGD cases, are in the dominant genes *STGD4* and *ELOVL4* and *PRPH2*. The ELOVL4 protein plays a role in making very long-chain fatty acids. Mutations in the *ELOVL4* gene lead to the formation of ELOVL4 protein clumps in the cells, interfering with their activity and eventually leading to cell death. The cytogenetic location of *ELOVL4 is* 6q14.1.

BEST VITELLIFORM DYSTROPHY

Best vitelliform macular dystrophy (VMD) is one of the most common macular dystrophies, affecting 1 in 10,000 individuals.

Clinical Features

The clinical presentation varies, depending on the stage of the disease at which the patient presents, usually one of these five stages:

1. Previtelliform
2. Vitelliform
3. Pseudohypopyon fundus
4. Vitelliruptive
5. Atrophic

The vitelliform stage is characterized by an egg yolk-like appearance in the central macula, due to deposition of yellowish material in the subretinal space. As the material breaks down, there is clear fluid in the upper part and yellowish material in the lower part, giving a picture of pseudohypopyon. As the condition progress, the yellow material breaks down and resembles a scrambled egg, and eventually appears as an atrophic scar. Surprisingly, vision remains good until the last stage of geographic atrophic appearance. A choroidal neovascular membrane develops in about 20% of cases and may account for decreased visual acuity.

Fundus autofluorescence shows the yellowish material (photoreceptor outer segment and lipofuscin-like material) intense hyper fluorescence, but the pattern may change as the lesion passes through various stages. OCT shows neurosensory detachment at the macula; rarely, choroidal neovascular membrane and scarring are also visible. The material involved is shed photoreceptor outer segments. ERG is normal, but electrooculography (EOG) is always abnormal, with an Arden ratio of about 1.0 or <1.5. This is an important marker in those with a normal fundus or poorly defined lesion. Some *BEST1* mutation carriers (previtelliform stage) do show an abnormal EOG, but the fundus may be normal or just show some RPE alterations.

Molecular Genetics

Mutations in the *BEST1* gene cause Best VMD. The *BEST1* gene encodes for a multifunctional protein called bestrophin-1. Bestrophin-1, a chloride channel protein, is located on the basolateral membrane of the RPE. Abnormal function results in accumulation of lipofuscin in the RPE and subretinal space. Prolonged neurosensory retinal detachment and overloading of the RPE with lipofuscin eventually result in photoreceptor and RPE dysfunction. About 200 mutations have been described in *BEST1*, with a broad range of phenotypes. The phenotypes most often associated with *BEST1* mutations are Best VMD and adult-onset foveomacular vitelliform dystrophy, confined to the macular area. The cytogenetic location of this gene is 11q12.3.

Subtypes

Adult-onset Foveomacular Vitelliform Dystrophy

This disorder resembles VMD, but its onset is at a higher age (30–60 years) and patients have normal EOG. The gene involved is *PRPH-2/RDS*. This gene makes a protein called peripherin 2, found in the photoreceptors. Mutation in *PRPH2* usually causes adult-onset foveomacular vitelliform dystrophy. The cytogenetic location is 6p21.1

Autosomal Recessive Bestrophinopathy

Autosomal recessive bestrophinopathy is a rare ocular genetic disease. It was defined by Burgess in 2008. It results from bi-allelic mutations in gene BEST1, and is characterized by multifocal vitelliform dystrophy with subretinal fluid. An association with hyperopia and angle closure has been described.

Autosomal Dominant Vitreoretino Choroidopathy

These patients show a characteristic hyperpigmented band from equator to ora serrata (almost 360°), along with peripapillary atrophy. The patients are usually hyperopic.

ACHROMATOPSIA

Achromatopsia is a rare, bilateral inherited retinal degeneration affecting all three types of cone photoreceptor cells that result in reduced visual acuity, photophobia, hemeralopia, and severe loss of color discrimination. Achromatopsia is estimated to affect approximately 1 in 30,000 individuals worldwide. The disease can be complete with total lack of cone function, also known as rod monochromacy, or incomplete with reduced cone function. Achromatopsia is also distinguished from more common forms of color blindness by the fact that all three types of cones are defective.

Clinical Features

Visual acuity ranges from 20/200 or worse in complete achromatopsia to 20/80 in incomplete achromatopsia. Color vision testing is severely or completely diminished and pupillary examination in children can demonstrate a paradoxical pupil, where the pupil initially constricts on dimming of light. Fundus examination can appear normal early in the course and later patients can develop retinal pigment epithelial mottling and atrophy.

Electroretinography is the gold standard for the diagnosis of achromatopsia. Cone function is severely or completely diminished while rod function is normal.

Optical coherence tomography shows a hyporeflective "optical gap," which can be found at the fovea although not specific corresponds to foveal loss of photoreceptor outer segments.

Molecular Genetics

Achromatopsia is inherited in autosomal recessive fashion and it affects all three types of retinal cones. The most common mutations affect genes that code for or regulate cone cyclic nucleotide-gated (CNG) cation channel subunits, including CNGB3 in 50% of cases and CNGA3 in 25% of cases. The CNG channels are located on photoreceptor outer segment cell membranes and are involved in signal transduction. These mutations result in a significant decline in cone function. Other implicated genes include GNAT2, PDE6C, PDE6H, and ATF6.

OCULOCUTANEOUS ALBINISM

Albinism refers to a group of hereditary disorders that involve an abnormality of melanin synthesis or distribution. Clinically, albinism presents as a pigmentation abnormality of the skin, the hair, and/or the eyes. Albinism can be divided into two broad categories: Oculocutaneous albinism and ocular albinism. Oculocutaneous albinism involves both the skin and the eyes, whereas ocular albinism mainly affects the eyes with minimal to no skin involvement.

Clinical Features

The primary morbidity of both oculocutaneous albinism and ocular albinism is eye related. Signs and symptoms include photophobia, refractive errors, strabismus, pendular nystagmus, iris transillumination defects, foveal hypoplasia, and abnormal decussation of the optic nerve fibers. The visual acuity in patients with albinism is variable and ranges from 20/40 to 20/400. Fundus examination reveals hypopigmented fundus revealing underlying large choroidal blood vessels. OCT can demonstrate an absence of the foveal pit. These ocular manifestations are almost always present in both forms of albinism; however, the degree of their presentation can vary depending on the type of albinism and the racial background of the patient. The inheritance pattern of albinism is also quite variable. Oculocutaneous albinism is mostly an autosomal recessive disorder, whereas ocular albinism is transmitted as a sex-linked or autosomal recessive disease.

Oculocutaneous albinism is divided into approximately 10 different types. Two of the more common forms are type I (tyrosinase negative) and type II (tyrosinase positive) oculocutaneous albinism. Patients with type I disease have no skin or ocular pigmentation, whereas those with type II disease can develop some pigmentation as they grow older.

Another important form of oculocutaneous albinism is type IB, which was previously called yellow mutant oculocutaneous albinism. Patients with type IB are similar to those with type I but can exhibit some pigmentation of their skin, hair, and ocular structures.

Two additional rare types of oculocutaneous albinism with important systemic findings and an increased risk of mortality are *Hermansky-Pudlak syndrome and Chédiak-Higashi syndrome*. *Hermansky-Pudlak syndrome* features include easy bruising and severe bleeding due to a defect in platelet adhesion. *Chédiak-Higashi syndrome* features include severe infection due to neutropenia or bleeding due to thrombocytopenia. Ocular albinism type I is an X-linked disorder associated with the *OA1* gene. Type I is the most common form of ocular albinism. Female carriers can show minor signs, whereas males with ocular albinism can show a constellation of any of the above-mentioned findings.

Molecular Genetics: Ocular Albinism

Ocular albinism is caused by mutations in the G protein-coupled receptor 143 (*GPR143*) gene, also known as *OA1*. More than 60 *GPR143* mutations have been identified. Most of the mutations in the *GPR143* gene alter the size or shape of the GPR143 protein. This protein controls the growth of melanosomes, a cellular structure that produces and stores melanin pigment. Without functional GPR143 protein, melanosomes can grow abnormally large (macromelanosomes). It is not clearly understood how these large melanosomes are related to vision loss and other eye abnormalities. The cytogenetic location is Xp22.2, the short arm of the X chromosome at position 22.2.

Oculocutaneous Albinism

The enzyme tyrosinase is produced by the *TYR* gene, and this enzyme (located in the melanocytes) is needed for the synthesis of melanin. Tyrosinase converts a protein building block, the amino acid tyrosine, to another compound called dopaquinone, and a series of other reactions converts dopaquinone to melanin. The cytogenetic location is 11q14.3, the long arm of chromosome 11 at position 14.3. The mutations in *TYR* gene that are responsible for the types of OCA are type 1: *TYR* gene and type 2: *OCA2* gene.

LEBER CONGENITAL AMAUROSIS

Leber congenital amaurosis (LCA) is a part of the spectrum of early-onset retinal dystrophy (EORD). It usually presents in the first few years of life, most often before the age of 1 year. The prevalence is about 1:30,000 to 1:80,000.

General Features

Leber congenital amaurosis is also known as congenital RP. The patients have wandering nystagmus, with reduced vision from birth. The best corrected visual acuity (BCVA) ranges from no light perception (in nearly one-third of cases) to no better than 20/400, often with a hyperopic refraction (≥5.0 D). Patients have absent pupillary reflex and some of them have keratoconus. Oculodigital reflex (eye rubbing or poking) is a common association.

The retina appears normal initially. However, a variety of abnormalities may develop either in isolation or combination later. These changes include chorioretinal degeneration and atrophy centered around the fovea, "bone-spicule" like pigmentation, subretinal flecks, "marbled" fundus, pigmented nummular lesions at the level of the RPE, optic disk abnormalities, and "Coats like" reaction.

Electroretinogram shows nonrecordable/extinguished or severely reduced scotopic and photopic responses. Normal ERG responses rule out a diagnosis of LCA.

Autofluorescence imaging shows variable of autofluorescence in LCA, which varies by subtype. For example, autofluorescence is normal in GUCY2D mutation but absent in RPE65 mutations.

Molecular Genetics

Leber congenital amaurosis is a group of hereditary (usually autosomal recessive) retinal diseases. 17 phenotypes (LCA1 to LCA17) with 25 genotypes have been identified that account for 70–80% of cases, with more genes are yet to be identified. These genes are known to be important in several retinal developmental and physiologic pathways. Genes with known mutations are GUCY2D, RPE65, SPATA7, AIPL1, LCA5, RPGRIP1, CRX, CRB1, NMNAT1, CEP290, IMPDH1, RD3, RDH12, LRAT, TULP1, KCNJ13, GDF6, CABP4, CNGA3, ALMS1, IQCB1, and MYO7A. The other genes causing LCA are unknown. CEP290 (15%), GUCY2D (12%), and CRB1 (10%) and RPE65 (8%) are the most frequently mutated LCA genes.

The pathophysiology of LCA is related to the inability of the eye to undergo phototransduction due to a disruption of the visual cycle. The visual cycle is a series of enzymatic reactions between the RPE and the neurosensory retina to metabolize dietary vitamin A into 11-*cis* retinal to generate photopigment. Without 11-*cis* retinal, the "phototransduction cascade" cannot be initialized; thus, visual neuronal signals are not propagated to the visual cortex. A dysfunctional mutation of any of the genes encoding for proteins that catalyze any of the series of enzymatic reactions to generate 11-*cis* retinal can block the visual cycle and lead to symptoms of LCA.

CHOROIDEREMIA

Choroideremia is an X-linked chorioretinal dystrophy characterized by the diffuse, progressive degeneration of the RPE, photoreceptors, and choriocapillaris. Its prevalence is about 1 in 50,000–100,000 people. Men are predominantly affected due to its X-linked etiology, but women can be asymptomatic carriers or rarely can be affected by the dystrophy as well. Northern Finland has the highest reported prevalence.

General Features

On fundus examination, the earliest manifestation is widespread pigment clumping at the level of the RPE in the mid-periphery in the mid-periphery; these spread centripetally. Subsequently, patients develop well-defined regions of atrophy with visible underlying sclera and large choroidal vessels, most commonly in the equatorial region just outside the vascular arcades. In the involved areas, scalloped areas of diffuse chorioretinal atrophy are present. Underlying larger choroidal and overlying retinal blood vessels are preserved. Unlike in RP, patients with choroideremia do not show intraretinal pigmentation; the central visual acuity is preserved until the fifth decade of life, and retinal blood vessels are not attenuated. The macular area remains intact until late in the disease course, with good visual acuity. In addition, choroideremia exhibits no optic atrophy, unlike the waxy pallor of optic disks seen in RP. Carrier patients can have mild RPE changes, and in severe cases, patchy RPE degeneration and areas of atrophy. This phenotypic variability in carriers is due to lyonization in which one copy of the X chromosome is randomly silenced early in embryogenesis. Other associated ocular findings are posterior subcapsular cataract, macular edema, and choroidal neovascularization.

Fluorescein angiogram shows diffuse loss of choriocapillaris throughout the fundus, except for the macular area. *Visual field* reveals ring scotoma at the midperiphery to start with; the scotomas later progress to complete loss of the peripheral field.

Fundus autofluorescence typically shows loss of fluorescence in areas of chorioretinal atrophy and an intact RPE/choriocapillaris patch in the macular area.

Optical coherence tomography images showing histopathological changes seen in choroideremia. The affected retina shows areas of RPE and choriocapillaris atrophy and corresponding thinning of outer retinal layers. In some cases, outer retinal tubulations may be seen, denoting end-stage photoreceptor degeneration.

Molecular Genetics

Choroideremia is caused by a mutation in the *CHM* gene, which encodes for a geranyl transferase Rab escort protein-1 (REP-1 protein). Rab proteins are involved in intracellular trafficking; as an escort protein, REP-1 attaches to Rab proteins in the cells and directs them to the membranes of various cell organelles. Mutations in the REP-1 protein affect intracellular trafficking, so the cells die prematurely. More than 140 mutations in the *CHM* gene have been found to cause choroideremia. Most mutations result in protein truncation by replacement of an arginine residue with a stop codon. The cytogenetic location is Xq21.2, the long arm of the X chromosome at position 21.2.

GYRATE ATROPHY

Gyrate atrophy of the choroid and the retina is a rare autosomal recessive retinal dystrophy characterized by progressive chorioretinal degeneration, early cataract formation, and myopia. It is caused by a deficiency in the enzyme ornithine aminotransferase (OAT), which results in a 10- to 20-fold increase in plasma ornithine concentrations. The highest rate is in Finland with one case per 50,000 individuals. There is no predilection for gender.

Clinical Features

Patients initially present with myopia and nyctalopia that begins in late childhood. As the disease progresses in the second decade of life, patients report progressive loss of peripheral vision. Visually significant posterior subcapsular cataracts develop early in virtually all patients, by the second decade of life. Vision loss secondary to cystoid macular edema is common. Fundus examination early in the disease course shows bilateral patchy, sharply demarcated circular areas of chorioretinal atrophy with hyperpigmented margins in the mid to far periphery. Typically, during the second decade of life, the peripheral atrophic lesions coalesce and spread toward the posterior pole, forming a confluent lesion with a scalloped border at the junction of healthy and diseased retinal pigment epithelium. The remaining healthy RPE in uninvolved areas is hyperpigmented, distinguishing this disease from choroideremia. The macula and thus central vision is spared until late in the disease course, often preserved into the fourth or fifth decade of life. However, later in the course of the disease chorioretinal atrophy involves the macular area also.

Molecular Genetics

Gyrate atrophy occurs due to various mutations in the OAT gene, which is found on chromosome 10q26. Inheritance is autosomal recessive. More than 50 variants of the genetic mutations have been identified, with missense mutations occurring most frequently. These mutations lead to truncation of the enzyme OAT, causing protein degradation. A subset of patients carry a genetic variant that is favorably responsive to supplementation with co-factor pyridoxine (vitamin B6), which has been shown to partially restore the function of the OAT enzyme.

The underlying biochemical defect of gyrate atrophy is in OAT, a vitamin B6-dependent mitochondrial matrix enzyme. OAT catalyzes the conversion of L-ornithine, a nonproteinaceous amino acid, to proline and glutamic acid, serving in the exchange of molecules between the urea and Krebs cycle. OAT plays a critical role in cellular detoxification by disposing of ornithine derived from dietary arginine. Deficiency of OAT, thereby leads to ornithine accumulation, with levels 10- to 20-fold above normal. The mechanism by which a deficiency of OAT and the consequent accumulation of ornithine leads to the chorioretinal degeneration is not fully understood. Possibilities include a direct toxic effect of the accumulated ornithine or one of its metabolites. The RPE is the site of the initial insult due to its reliance on OAT activity for metabolic functions. RPE injury then leads to a breakdown of the outer blood retinal barrier causing photoreceptor cell exposure to toxic agents from choroidal circulation.

■ LEBER HEREDITARY OPTIC NEUROPATHY

Leber hereditary optic neuropathy is the most common inherited mitochondrial disorder and typically affects young males. It typically begins as a unilateral progressive optic neuropathy with sequential involvement of the fellow eye months to years later.

Individuals eventually diagnosed with LHON may initially be asymptomatic, or experience mild blurring of the central visual field of one eye. Males are more likely to be affected than females, with some reported ratios as high as 9:1. Age of onset is typically between 10 and 30 years, though onset in the seventh or eighth decade has been reported. Symptoms may progress from mild unilateral visual loss to severe bilateral visual loss, usually worse than 20/200. Visual field testing typically shows a worsening central or centrocecal scotoma. Color testing reveals decreased red-green discrimination Examination may initially reveal normal or pseudoedematous optic nerves, with optic nerve pallor and atrophy appearing subsequently. Individuals may harbor concurrent disease including cardiac conduction abnormalities, dystonia, and multiple sclerosis-like illness, is referred to as "LHON Plus" disease.

Genetics of Leber Hereditary Optic Neuropathy

Leber hereditary optic neuropathy is classically associated with mitochondrial base pair mutations G11778A (guanine to adenine at position 11778), T14484C (tyrosine to cytosine), and G3460A. These mutations primarily affect respiratory chain complex I genes, mitochondrial genes ND1, ND4, and ND6 among others.

The G11778A is the most common, reported to account for 70% of cases in Northern European populations, and 90% in Asian populations. It is associated with more severe disease, with less chance of significant visual recovery. The T14484C mutation is associated with the best overall prognosis, with some visual recovery in 37–58% of cases. This typically occurs after reaching a visual "nadir." French Canadians with LHON commonly exhibit this mutation variant. The G3460A mutation usually portends a more intermediate course and has the worst prognosis.

Many mitochondrial diseases display heteroplasmy. Each cell contains numerous mitochondria, and in 10–15% of patients with LHON mutations, only a certain percentage of these mitochondria may have mutant DNA. Those with a "mutation load" less than threshold (60–75%) may not exhibit a disease phenotype and may never lose vision. It has been postulated that due to the heteroplasmy seen in this disorder, the right and left eye may have different amounts of affected mtDNA. It is unknown why males are preferentially affected. Theories include the presence of a "susceptibility locus" on the Y chromosome.

Mitochondrial mutations cause defects in several nicotinamide adenine dinucleotide hydrogen (NADH)-ubiquinone oxidoreductase chains. This is thought to impair glutamate transport and increase reactive-oxygen species production. This leads to retinal ganglion cell through apoptosis, though it is unclear why these cells are particularly vulnerable. Atrophy and demyelination are subsequently noted in the optic nerves, chiasm, and tracts.

In acute LHON, macular changes precede peripapillary retinal nerve fiber layer swelling. The thickening of these layers is acute and is then followed by thinning chronically. It has been suggested that this is process is due to a state of pseudohypoxia, followed by a compensatory response. Optical coherence tomography angiography (OCTA) performed in LHON patients demonstrates vascular dilation and tortuosity, which may be seen clinically.

The introduction of exogenous DNA into the mitochondrial genome with mitochondrial targeting of viral vectors is promising therapy and is shown to improve vision in patients effected by the 11778A mutation. However, such gene therapy trials are at preliminary stages and need further studies.

GENETIC TESTING

Recognizing genetic eye disorders affords patients and doctors the opportunity for very accurate diagnosis and prognosis, genetic counseling about the risk of recurrence in future children, and potentially gene replacement or causative-gene directed treatment. It is important for pediatric ophthalmologists to recognize which ocular disorders in children are possibly genetic in order to institute the appropriate workup or refer to a specialist for further evaluation. The ophthalmologist should strive to make the most detailed and specific clinical diagnosis possible to aid in the proper ordering and interpretation of the test. The indications for genetic testing can be divided into five broad categories: treatment, diagnosis, prognosis, counseling, and research.

Karyotyping is mainly useful to detect structural and numerical abnormalities of chromosomes. It is most useful when the patient has multiple congenital anomalies, suggesting involvement of multiple genes, or when a parent has had multiple miscarriages. Disorders that result from copy number variations may not be detected by karyotype. For such disorders, microarray or fluorescence in situ hybridization (FISH) technology may then be useful. FISH uses fluorescent probes that bind to specific chromosome loci. Microarray technique screens the entire genome for copy number variations. Microarray cannot detect single gene mutation.

Single gene testing is useful for diseases such as X-linked retinoschisis (*RS1* gene), choroideremia (*CHM* gene), STGD (*ABCA4* gene), and vitelliform macular dystrophy (*PRPH2* or *BEST1* genes).

Multigene testing, also called *panel testing,* is needed for a condition like RP, in which 100 or more causative genes are known.

Whole exome sequencing (WES) allows multiple strands of DNA to be sequenced simultaneously. The exome is the coding region of DNA. It makes up about 2% of an individual's entire genome and is thought to contain the majority of disease-causing mutations.

Whole genome sequencing (WGS) studies or sequences the entire genome, and therefore reveals the impact of variation within the exome/coding region and the noncoding region of the genome. WGS provides the option to "sequence once, study often." Currently, we can analyze the area of the genome we understand, but if the whole genome has been captured, we can revisit other areas as we learn more without the need to obtain additional samples from the patient.

GENE THERAPY

Gene therapy is a mechanism to deliver a functional gene to a cell or to inactivate an abnormal gene. In vivo gene therapy involves the delivery of genetic material directly to living organisms, while ex vivo gene therapy delivers the genetic material to cultured cells, which are then transplanted into the host. In vivo gene therapy employs a *viral vector* to insert genetic material into host cells. Having a thorough understanding of the pathogenesis of the disease is imperative in gene replacement therapy. Any disease in which gene replacement will not change the outcome should be excluded.

The goal of gene therapy is to achieve stable expression of the inserted genetic material in the host cell while avoiding complications from inflammation or deleterious off-site effects. Ophthalmic disorders are especially attractive targets for "in vivo" gene therapy, because local therapy can easily be delivered to the eye and inflammatory responses may be limited because the eye is an immune-privileged organ. Recently, there has been greater focus on gene therapy to treat ocular disease in vivo largely due to the successful treatment of *RPE65*-associated Leber congenital amaurosis.

Gene therapy can also be used to selectively target and destroy dividing cells. RB is the most common malignant ocular tumor in children and results from a mutation in "tumor suppressor" gene. In RB, an adenoviral vector was used to deliver the herpes simplex thymidine kinase gene into rapidly dividing tumor cells. The only complication was inflammation. Though adenovirus vectors have been successfully used, lentiviral vectors are also used, specifically inactivated human immunodeficiency virus.

Inserting Genetic Material into Living Cells

Current methods to deliver genetic material in vivo can be categorized as viral and nonviral methods. Viruses, by nature, infect cells and insert their genetic material into the host cell's nucleus. After removing pathogenic viral genes, viral vectors can be used to insert a desirable gene [or complementary DNA (cDNA)] into the host. Viral vectors either integrate their genetic material directly into the host's genome (lentivirus and retrovirus) or insert their genetic material as stable extrachromosomal episomes (adenovirus, herpesvirus, and adeno-associated virus). Nonviral methods of gene delivery rely on chemical or physical methods to insert naked DNA into a cell's nucleus. These methods include electroporation, iontophoresis, liposomes, and nanoparticles, such as cell-penetrating peptides. Nonviral methods have the benefits of production scalability, lower immunogenicity, and the ability to deliver large genes. However, they are less efficient than viral vectors at targeting cells in vivo.

Ocular Diseases Targeted for Gene Therapy

Currently, inherited retinal diseases and other retinal diseases targeted for gene therapy rely on gene augmentation. A normal copy of a gene is inserted by a recombinant virus to reestablish normal cell function. This transgene exists in extrachromosomal DNA as an episome, and there is no direct replacement of the abnormal gene. This strategy will work for loss-of-function mutations, but not for dominant gain-of-function alleles.

In 2017, US Food and Drug Administration (FDA) approved first in vivo gene therapy for a genetic disease approved was voretigene neparvovec luxturna for *RPE65*-associated retinal dystrophy. Patients with pathogenic variants in both alleles of *RPE65* typically present clinically with autosomal recessive LCA or RP. Vision loss is progressive and variable and may be severe in early childhood. The *RPE65* gene is expressed in RPE and is one of the critical enzymes in the visual cycle, necessary for converting all-trans-retinol to 11-cis-retinal required for proper photoreceptor health and function. Human *RPE65* cDNA is delivered using an AAV2 vector injected into the subretinal space after pars plana vitrectomy. The treated patients had significant improvements in navigation in dim light, full-field light sensitivity threshold, and visual field.

Success of gene therapy for LCA and FDA approval led to many gene therapy trials, that are currently on-going for various inherited diseases such as choroideremia, achromatopsia, X-linked RP, X-linked retinoschisis, STGD, Usher syndrome, and also for other diseases such as AMD.

Future Directions of Gene Therapy

As our understanding of the pathogenesis of genetic diseases increase, targets and methods for genetic therapy will further develop. Success has been shown in several disorders such as LCA, juvenile retinoschisis, and LHON, using animal models. Human phase-1 clinical trials are already under way. Further research is needed to create ideal vectors with increased specificity for target cells and to minimize side effects.

Current gene therapy strategies involve gene augmentation, which works by supplying a functional gene product. This strategy, however, is ineffective for disorders involving gain-of-function variants. Inhibition of the gene product would be necessary. One strategy would be delivery of RNAi or microRNAs, which act to silence expression of genes. Both viral and nonviral delivery approaches can be used.

Gene Editing

Gene editing technology using the CRISPR/CAS9 system would also be well-suited to correcting dominant gain-of-function mutations. A CRISPR/CAS9-based approach would involve editing out the pathogenic variant in a targeted fashion. A viral vector could possibly deliver a guide RNA and the CAS9 nuclease. However, low efficiency and off-target effects would need to be overcome before CRISPR/CAS9 can be used in vivo.

SUGGESTED READING

1. Alkozi HA, Franco R, Pintor JJ. Epigenetics in the eye: an overview of the most relevant ocular diseases. Front Genet. 2017;8:144.
2. Alward WL, Kwon YH, Khanna CL, Johnson AT, Hayreh SS, Zimmerman MB, et al. Variations in the myocilin gene in patients with open-angle glaucoma. Arch Ophthalmol M. 2002;120(9):1189-97.
3. Bell SJ, Oluonye N, Harding P, Moosajee M. Congenital cataract: a guide to genetic and clinical management. Therap Adv Rare Dis. 2020.
4. Berson EL. Retinitis pigmentosa and allied diseases. In: Albert D, Miller J, Azar D, Blodi B, (eds). Albert and Jakobiec's Principles and Practice of Ophthalmology, 3rd edition. Philadelphia, PA: Elsevier; 2008.
5. Berthoud, VM, Ngezahayo, A. Focus on lens connexins. BMC Cell Biol. 2017;18(Suppl 1):6.
6. Chacon-Camacho OF, Zenteno JC. Review and update on the molecular basis of Leber congenital amaurosis. World J Clin Cases. 2015;3(2):112-24.
7. Cideciyan AV, Aleman TS, Swider M, Schwartz SB, Steinberg JD, Brucker AJ, et al. Mutations in ABCA4 result in accumulation of lipofuscin before slowing of the retinoid cycle: a reappraisal of the human disease sequence. Hum Mol Genet 2004;13(5):525-34.
8. Daiger SP, Bowne SJ, Sullivan LS. Genes and mutations causing autosomal dominant retinitis pigmentosa. Cold Spring Harb Perspect Med. 2014;5(10):a017.
9. Dijkstal JM, Cooley SS, Holleschau AM, King RA, Summers CG. Change in visual acuity in albinism in the early school years. J Pediatr Ophthalmol Strabismus. 2012;49(2):81-6; quiz 87.
10. Fingert JH, Robin AL, Stone JL, Roos BR, Davis LK, Scheetz TE, et al. Copy number variations on chromosome 12q14 in patients with normal tension glaucoma. Hum Mol Genet M. 2011;20(12):2482-94.
11. Fujinami K, Zernant J, Chana RK, Wright GA, Tsunoda K, Ozawa Y, et al. Clinical and molecular characteristics of childhood-onset Stargardt disease. Ophthalmology. 2015;122(2):326-34.
12. George NDL, Yates JRW, Moore AT. Clinical features in affected males with X-linked retinoschisis. Arch Ophthalmol. 1996;114(3):274-80.
13. Issa PC, Maclaren RE. Non-viral retinal gene therapy: a review. Clin Exp Ophthalmol. 2012;40(1):39-47.
14. Jain N, Jia Y, Gao SS, Zhang X, Weleber RG, Huang D, et al. Optical coherence tomography angiography in choroideremia: correlating choriocapillaris loss with overlying degeneration. JAMA Ophthalmology. 2016;134(6):697-702.
15. Kaiser-Kupfer M, Kuwabara , Uga S, Takki K, Valle D. Cataracts in gyrate atrophy: clinical and morphologic studies. Invest Ophthal Vis Sci. 1983;24(4):432-6.
16. Khan KN, Islam F, Moore AT, Michaelides M. Clinical and genetic features of choroideremia in childhood. Ophthalmology. 2016;123(10):2158-65.
17. Kumaran N, Moore AT, Weleber RG, Michaelides M. Leber congenital amaurosis/early-onset severe retinal dystrophy: clinical features, molecular genetics and therapeutic interventions. Br J Ophthalmol. 2017;101(9):1147-54.
18. Lam BL, Feuer WJ, Abukhalil F, Porciatti V, Hauswirth WW, Guy J. Leber hereditary optic neuropathy gene therapy clinical trial recruitment: year 1. Arch Ophthalmol. 2010;128(9):1129-35.
19. Li W, Liu J, Galvin JA. Epigenetics and common ophthalmic diseases. Yale J Biol Med. 2016;89(4):597-600.
20. Lim SH, Tran-Viet KN, Yanovitch TL, Freedman SF, Klemm T, Call W, et al. CYP1B1, MYOC, and LTBP2 mutations in primary congenital glaucoma patients in the United States. Am J Ophthalmol. 2013;155(3):508-17.
21. Lyraki R, Megaw R, Hurd T. Disease mechanisms of X-linked retinitis pigmentosa due to RP2 and RPGR mutations. Biochem Soc Trans. 2016;44(5):1235-44.
22. Molday RS, Kellner U, Weber BHF. X-linked juvenile retinoschisis: clinical diagnosis, genetic analysis, and molecular mechanisms. Prog Retin Eye Res. 2012;31(3):195-212.

23. Newman NJ. Treatment of Leber hereditary optic neuropathy. Brain. 2011;134(Pt 9):2447-50.
24. Ohden KL, Tang PH, Lilley CC, Lee MS. Atypical Leber hereditary optic neuropathy: 18 year interval between eyes. J Neuro-ophthalmol. 2016;36(3):304.
25. Pasquale LR, Loomis SJ, Kang JH, Yaspan BL, Abdrabou W, Budenz DL, et al. CDKN2B-AS1 genotype-glaucoma feature correlations in primary open angle glaucoma patients from the United States. Am J Ophthalmol M. 2013;155(2):342-53.
26. Pasquay C, Wang LF, Lorenz B, Preising MN. Bestrophin I - phenotypes and functional aspects in bestrophinopathies. Ophthalmic Genet. 2015;36(3):193-212.
27. Patel, A, Hayward, JD, Tailor, V, Nyanhete R, Ahlfors H, Gabriel C, et al. The oculome panel test: next-generation sequencing to diagnose a diverse range of genetic developmental eye disorders. Ophthalmology. 2019;126(6):888-907.
28. Preising M, Ayuso C. Rab escort protein 1 (REP1) in intracellular traffic: a functional and pathophysiological overview. Ophthalmic Genet. 2004;25(2):101-10.
29. Reis LM, Tyler RC, Volkmann Kloss BA, Schilter KF, Levin AV, Lowry RB, et al. PITX2 and FOXC1 spectrum of mutations in ocular syndromes. Eur J Hum Genet M. 2012;20(12):1224-33.
30. Roh M, Zhang Y, Murakami Y, Thanos A, Lee SC, Vavvas DG, et al. Etanercept, a widely used inhibitor of tumor necrosis factor-α (TNF-α), prevents retinal ganglion cell loss in a rat model of glaucoma. PLoS One M. 2012;7(7):e4.
31. Russell S, Bennett J, Wellman JA, Chung DC, Yu ZF, Tillman A, et al. Efficacy and safety of voretigene neparvovec (AAV2-hRPE65v2) in patients with RPE65-mediated inherited retinal dystrophy: a randomised, controlled, open-label, phase 3 trial. Lancet. 2017;390(10097):849-60.
32. Sadagopan KA, Capasso J, Levin AV. Genetics for the ophthalmologist. Oman J Ophthalmol. 2012;5(3):144-9.
33. Sergouniotis PI, Davison AE, Lenassi E, Devery SR, Moore AT, Webster AR. Retinal structure, function, and molecular pathologic features in gyrate atrophy. Ophthalmology. 2012;119(3):596-605.
34. Shaffer L, Tommerup N. ISCN. In: Shaffer LG, Tommerup N (Eds). An International System for Human Cytogenetic Nomenclature. Basel, Switzerland: Karger Publications; 2005. pp. 9-35.
35. Shen BW, Hennig M, Hohenester E, Jansonius JN, Schirmer T. Crystal structure of human recombinant ornithine aminotransferase. J Mol Biol. 1998;277(1):81-102.
36. Shiels, A, Hejtmancik, JF. Molecular genetics of cataract. Prog Mol Biol Transl Sci. 2015;134:203-18.
37. Spritz RA. Molecular genetics of oculocutaneous albinism. Hum Mol Genet. 1994;3 Spec No:1469-75.
38. Tanna P, Strauss RW, Fujinami K, Michaelides M. Stargardt disease: clinical features, molecular genetics, animal models and therapeutic options. Br J Ophthalmol. 2017;101(1):25-30.
39. Thomas CE, Ehrhardt A, Kay MA. Progress and problems with the use of viral vectors for gene therapy. Nat Rev Genet. 2003;4(5):346-58.
40. Thorleifsson G, Magnusson KP, Sulem P, Walters GB, Gudbjartsson DF, Stefansson H, et al. Common sequence variants in the LOXL1 gene confer susceptibility to exfoliation glaucoma. Science M. 2007;317(5843):1397-400.
41. Tsang SH, Vaclavik V, Bird AC, Robson AG, Holder GE. Novel phenotypic and genotypic findings in X-linked retinoschisis. Arch Ophthalmol. 2007;125(2):259-67.
42. Tsybovsky Y, Molday RS, Palczewski K. The ATP-binding cassette transporter ABCA4: structural and functional properties and role in retinal disease. Adv Exp Med Biol 2010;703:105-25.
43. Valle D, Simell O. In: The Metabolic and Molecular Bases of Inherited Disease. Scriver C, Beaudet A, Sly W, Valle D, (Eds). New York: McGraw-Hill; 1995. p. 114.
44. Wygnanski-Jaffe T, Levin AV. Introductory genetics for the ophthalmologist. American Academy of Ophthalmology, Focal Points. Clin Module Ophthalmol. 2005;23:1-11.

SECTION 2

Strabismus

19

CHAPTER

Evaluation of Sensory Status and Adaptations in Strabismus

Rohit Saxena, Karthikeyan Mahalingam

INTRODUCTION

Evaluation of binocular sensory status in strabismus involves the determination of visual functions other than visual acuity. The sensory examination reveals the fusional status of the patient and any adaptations that may have evolved in response to strabismus or blurred image. The relevant tests comprise of three categories: stereo acuity tests, diplopia tests, and fovea-to-fovea tests.

Binocular single vision is the virtue we have where two separate images from the two eyes are fused together in the brain to form one image. This is *sensory* fusion. The term fusion is also used to describe *fusional vergence* where eye movements serve to align the two eyes so that a single image can occur. This is *motor fusion.* Sufficiently dissimilar objects presented to the eyes, may not be fusible. Retinal rivalry may result in such a situation where superimposed but non-fusible portions of images are seen in alternation. Confusion is another sensory phenomenon which may occur in such situations.

Whatever is imaged on the fovea is experienced by the person as straight ahead or in *Herring's principal visual direction.* A fundamental of binocular single image of best acuity is that both foveas carry the subjective straight - ahead position (Herring's law of *identical visual direction.)* Corresponding points are a pair of retinal elements, one from each eye, that have the same subjective visual direction. Thus, objects in the binocular field of vision will be seen single because they stimulate the corresponding points on retina.

In 1838, Wheatstone discovered the adequate stimulus for *stereopsis* and demonstrated it with his stereoscope. Stereopsis is a unique sensation, elaborated under conditions of simultaneous binocular vision. It is based on the differences in the horizontal positions of visual counters, nearer or further away than the fixation point. This geometric disparity in position of binocularly observed contours, expressed as an angle, is the feature for stereopsis. In actuality, for a retinal element in one eye, a range of elements exists around the exactly corresponding point in the other eye, any of which can fuse with the corresponding point in the first eye. But these points have to be within an area where the non-corresponding points are fusible. This is called *Panum's fusional* area.

Under optimal conditions the foveal stereoscopic threshold is 10 sec arc., corresponding at arms length to a depth difference of 0.2 mm. 'Seconds of arc' is the quantification of stereoacuity. A circle has 360 degrees; each degree is divided into 60 minutes and each minute into 60 seconds. Normal stereoacuity is around 40 sec of arc.

There is another area related to vision. A *Horopter* is an imaginary line in space where objects located can be fused to obtain a single image. If a circle is drawn in space, points on that circle having zero disparity, fall on corresponding retinal elements and will be fused to provide single vision. This circle is known as Vieth-Müller circle. Fusion for singleness of vision and stereopsis are different neurophysiologic processes. One can have fusion without stereopsis and vice-versa.

The main sensory disorders arising in strabismic patients are diplopia, suppression, amblyopia, confusion, rivalry, loss of stereopsis, and adaptations like anomalous retinal correspondence and mono-fixation syndrome.

SENSORY ASSESSMENT IN STRABISMUS

Sensory assessment is done to check the presence of binocularity and the nature of the correspondence between the two eyes. We elicit the presence/grade of stereopsis, presence/type of diplopia, presence of suppression, and presence/type of anomalous retinal correspondence (ARC). The motor assessment gives the measures needed for planning the strabismus surgery, while sensory assessment helps to determine the prognosis. Sensory assessment can reveal if the binocular fusion with a functional improvement is possible or only cosmetic alignment can be achieved after the surgery. They are broadly divided into binocularity tests and stereoacuity tests.

Binocularity Tests

Bagolini Striated Glass Test

It consists of lenses with linear striations, oriented obliquely at 45° and 135°. It is the least dissociating test, so has the advantage of free binocular viewing. After wearing the glasses, the patient is asked to see a source of light **(Figs. 1A to C)**.

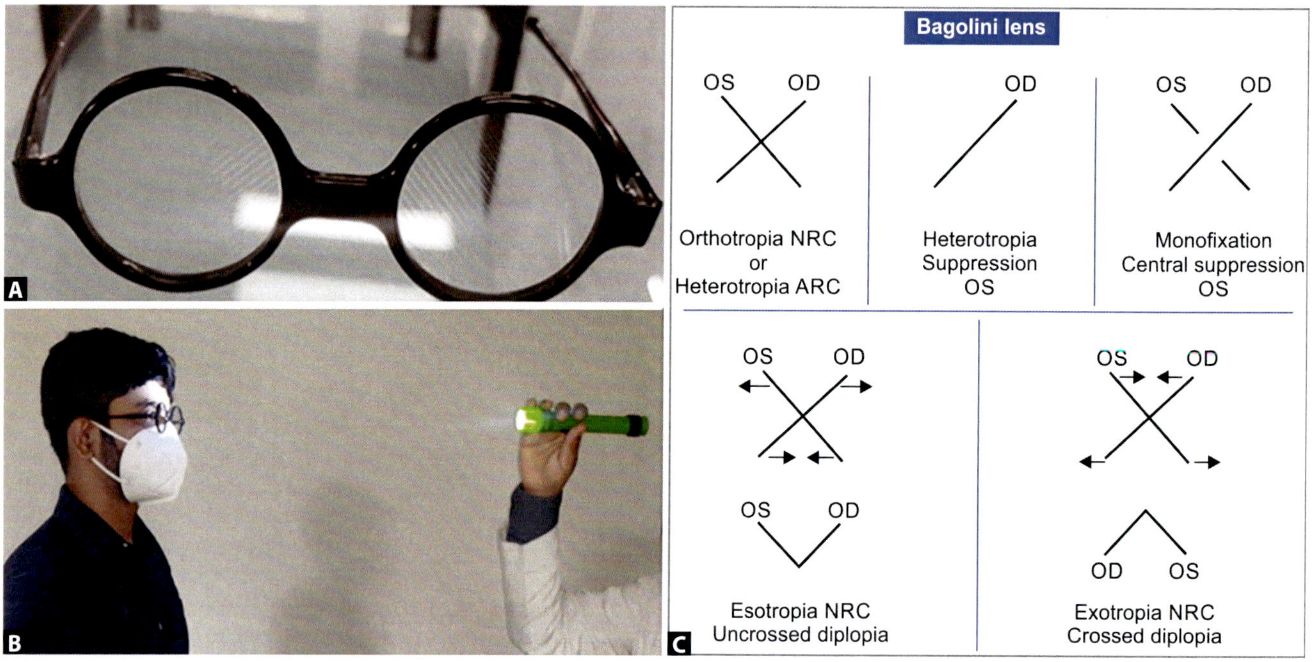

Figs. 1A to C: (A) Bagolini glasses; (B) Bagolini test being performed; (C) Various responses seen in the test.

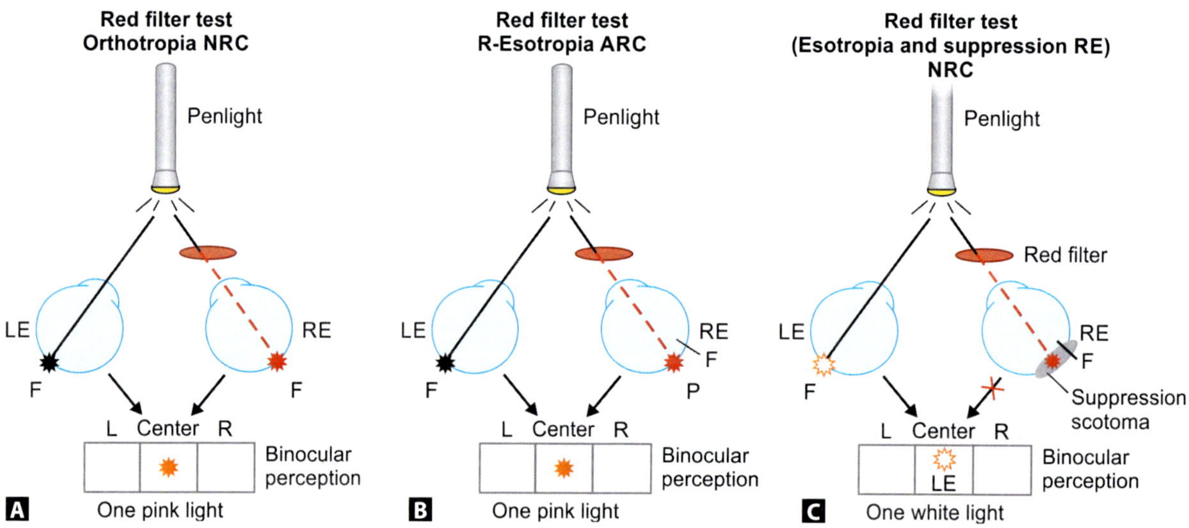

Figs. 2A to C: (A) Red filter test being performed in a straight eye with normal retinal correspondence (NRC); (B) Strabismic eye (right eye esotropia) with anomalous retinal correspondence (ARC); (C) Strabismic eye (right eye esotropia) with suppression scotoma and NRC.

- *Symmetrical cross response that is two lines cross each other at center*: Seen in aligned eyes with normal retinal correspondence (NRC) and also in strabismic (manifest) eyes with ARC (harmonious).
- *Asymmetrical cross response (two lines cut at a point other than the center)*: Seen in incomitant strabismus with NRC.
- *Cross response with central gap*: Seen in monofixation syndrome.
- *Single line seen*: Indicates suppression of one eye.

Red Filter Test

This is a simple test where a red glass is placed in one eye and the patient is asked to look at a light source (or an accommodative target).

Single light is seen:

- Patients having aligned eyes with NRC will see one pinkish-red light **(Fig. 2A)**.
- Patients having strabismus with ARC will see a single pinkish-red light **(Fig. 2B)**. The partial neutralization of deviation with prism will result in diplopia.
- Strabismus patients with suppression will see either white light or red light depending upon the fixing eye **(Fig. 2C)**.
- Patients with alternate fixation will see alternating red and white light. But only one light at a time.

Double light seen: Uncrossed diplopia (two lights: White and red seen with the red light on the same side of the red filter) is seen in esotropia with NRC. Crossed diplopia (red light seen on the opposite side of the red filter) is seen in exotropia with NRC. In both these conditions, the diplopia disappears and both images will be superimposed after neutralizing with prism.

Worth Four Dot Test

Red-green color dissociation is used in the Worth four dot test. The patient wears a red-green glass with red glass over the right eye. There are two green lights horizontally, one red light over the top and white light over the bottom. The lightbox is placed at 6 m so separated by 1.25°. For the near test, the light is at 1/3 m, so dots are separated by 6°. In cases of central scotoma larger than the mentioned size, the patient cannot see the dots and then patients can be moved accordingly.

- *Four dots response*: Seen in aligned eyes with NRC **(Fig. 3)** and also in strabismic (manifest) eyes with ARC (harmonious)
- *Five dots response*: Seen in eyes having manifest strabismus with NRC
  - *Uncrossed pattern (red on the right side):* Seen in esotropia
  - *Crossed pattern:* Seen in exotropia
  - *Vertically displaced sets:* Seen in vertical strabismus
- *Three dots response*: Seen in right eye suppression
- *Two dots response*: Seen in left eye suppression

Synoptophore

It has a special set of slides to check the three levels of binocular vision **(Figs. 4A to D)**:

1. *Simultaneous perception slides*: Detects the basic level of binocularity. There two dissimilar slides but overlapping the same retinal areas (e.g., the lion and the cage) **(Fig. 4B)**.
2. *Fusion slides*: It is more physiological than simultaneous perception slides. The two slides have a similar main image with dissimilar parts in the periphery acting as a control. Example: First slide—a tree with person in right, second slide—a tree with person in left **(Fig. 4C)**.
3. *Stereopsis slides*: There are two similar slides, but they do not stimulate corresponding retinal points due to horizontal disparity. But they fall in the Panum's fusional area, so they fuse to give the perception of depth or third dimension. This is the highest grade of binocular vision **(Fig. 4D)**.

After Imaging Test

It is the most dissociating test. The true fovea (or eccentric fixation point) of both eyes are stimulated separately with

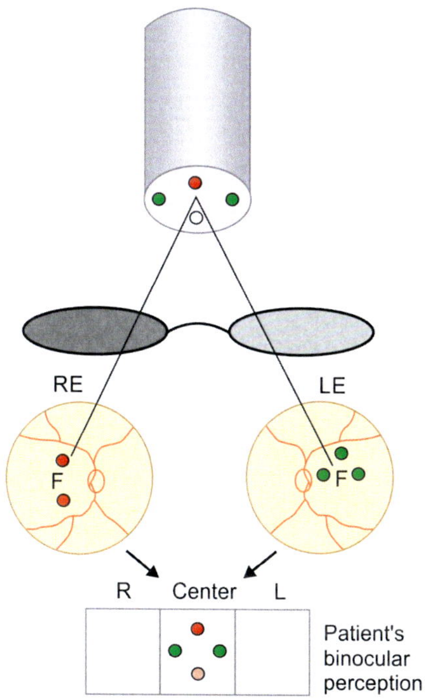

Fig. 3: Worth four dot test in a patient with straight eye and normal retinal correspondence (NRC).

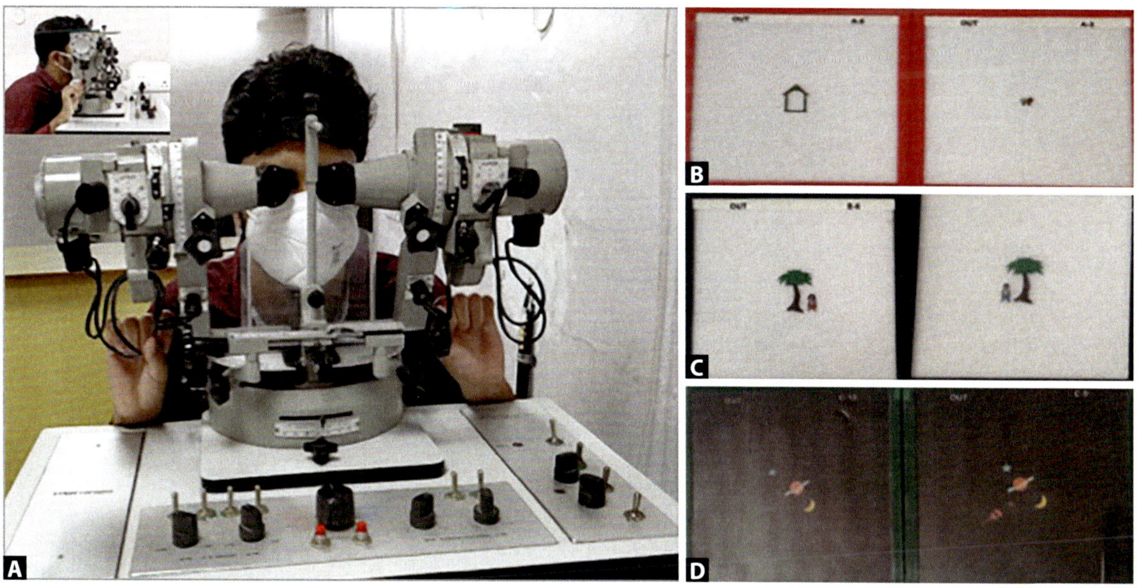

Figs. 4A to D: (A) Synoptophore; (B) Simultaneous perception slides; (C) Fusion slides; (D) Stereopsis slides.

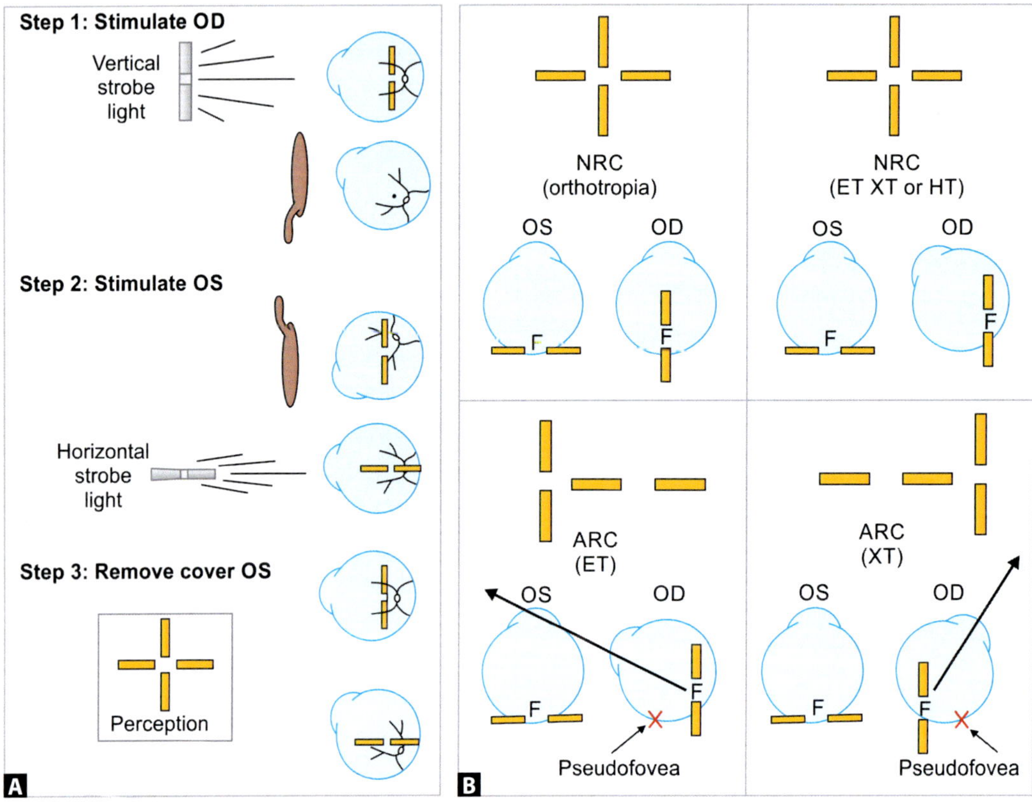

Figs. 5A and B: (A) After imaging test being performed; (B) Various responses seen in after imaging test.

flashes of light after occluding the other eye. One eye is stimulated with the vertical strobe of light and another eye is stimulated with the horizontal strobe of light **(Figs. 5A and B)**.

- *Symmetrical crossing response*: Seen in all patients with NRC (also in eccentric fixation) where both the true foveae are stimulated irrespective of where the eyes are aligned or deviated.
- *Asymmetrical crossing response*: Seen in ARC, the centers of horizontal and vertical lines are separated. The distance of separation depends on the angle of anomaly (AA).
- *Single line seen*: Indicates suppression of one eye.

Stereoacuity Tests

Depth perception has certain cues which can be observed monocularly or binocularly. Monocularly perceivable cues include the apparent size of objects already known, interposition of a near object on more distant one, linear perspective (e.g., converging railway tracks), loss of contrast, effects of light and shade, and gradients of texture. All these cues can be incorporated in pictures and therefore interfere in true stereopsis evaluation. Hence, tests for stereopsis are staged according to age and cognitive abilities in tests where minimal monocular cues are available. For testing stereoacuity, we dissociate the two eyes and each eye gets a slightly different view of the same object which then fuses to form a single three-dimensional image. The following principles are used for dissociation in stereoacuity testing:

- *Anaglyph*: Dissociation of both eyes is provided by colored glasses. Conjugate colors (red/green) are used to form a stereo-paired object. It is viewed through red (over one eye) and green (over another eye) glasses to perceive a three-dimensional scene. For example: The Netherlands Organisation Test (TNO).
- *Haploscopic principle*: Angled mirrors placed in front of each eye projected through a hollow tube are used for dissociation. The right eye sees the right temporal field while the left eye sees the left temporal field. For example: Synoptophore.
- *Panographic principle*: It is a real depth stereogram. The objects are placed at different depths. No special glasses or tubes are needed for dissociation. For example: Frisby Davis Distance Stereotest.
- *Vectographic principle*: Special polarizing method is used to print the polarizing targets and is viewed through the glasses with a Polaroid filter to get the three-dimensional view. For example: Titmus fly test and Randot stereopsis test.

Near Stereoacuity Tests

- *The Netherlands Organisation Test*:
  - Red-green glasses are used and the seven plates are serially viewed at a 40 cm distance **(Figs. 6A and B)**.
  - The first three plates are for gross stereopsis (up to 1,980 seconds of arc).
  - Plate IV is to test suppression, plates V to VII for qualitative estimation (15–480 seconds of arc).
  - Only plate V can be used for quick screening.

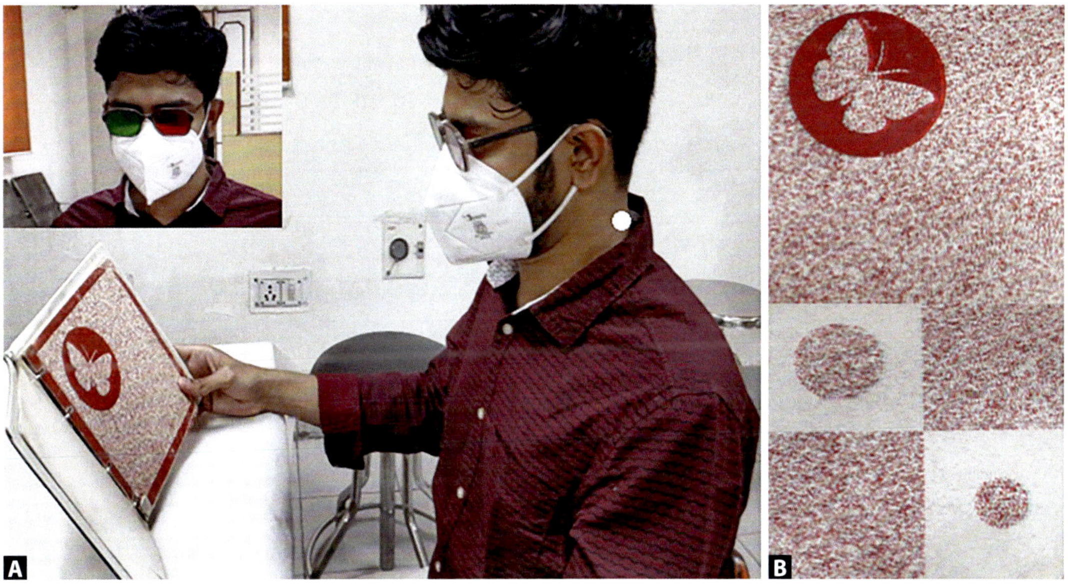

Figs. 6A and B: (A) The Netherlands Organisation Test (TNO) being performed with subject wearing red-green glasses; (B) TNO plates.

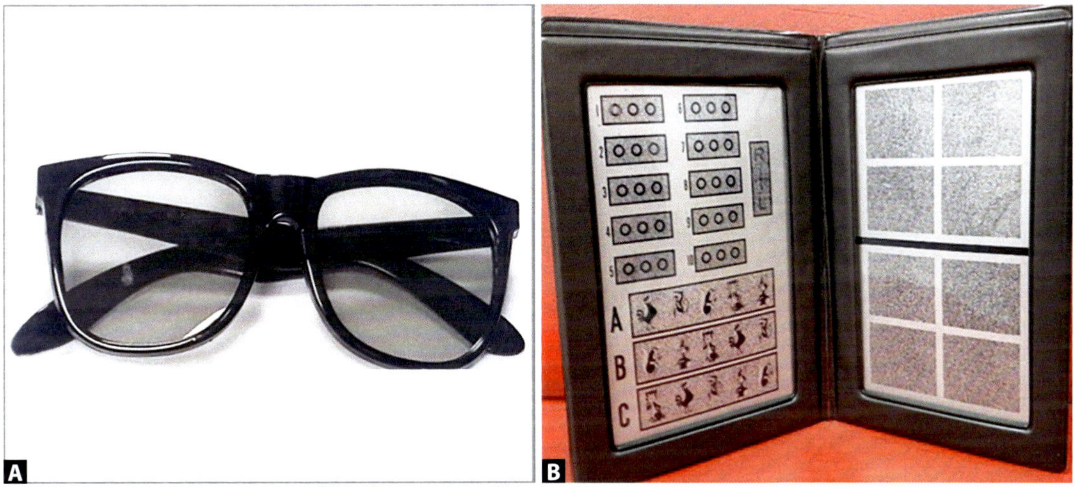

Figs. 7A and B: (A) Polarized glasses; (B) Random dot stereogram images.

   - Used as a screening tool for stereopsis in age group >3 years.
   - *Limitation*: It cannot be used in color blind individuals.
- *Titmus fly test*:
   - Based on vectographic principle, uses a Stereo fly card and polarized glasses.
   - *Grade of stereopsis*: Fly—3,500 seconds of arc, Graded circle test—800 to 40 seconds of arc, and Animal test for children—400, 200, and 100 seconds of arc.
   - Allows effective screening of gross stereopsis and fine depth perception in age group >3 years.
   - *Limitation*: Specific disparate images look different from the rest, so they can be pointed without having stereopsis, i.e., using monocular clues.
- *Stereo butterfly test*:
   - Has hidden configuration of butterfly within the random dots. Rest all similar to Titmus fly test.
   - *Grade of stereopsis*: Upper wings 2,000 seconds of arc, lower wings 1,150 seconds of arc, and abdomen 700 seconds of arc.
- *Random-dot stereogram*:
   - Based on the vectographic principle it consists of random-dot stereogram rather than contour patterns **(Figs. 7A and B)**.
   - *Advantage*: Offers no monocular clues and thus guessing can be avoided.
   - *Grade of stereopsis*: 400 to 20 seconds of arc.
- *Lang test*:
   - There is a panographic presentation of a random dot pattern **(Figs. 8A and B)**.
   - A separate image is provided to each eye through cylindrical lenses imprinted on the surface lamination of the test card.
   - *Advantages*: No glasses are needed, relatively cheap and convenient

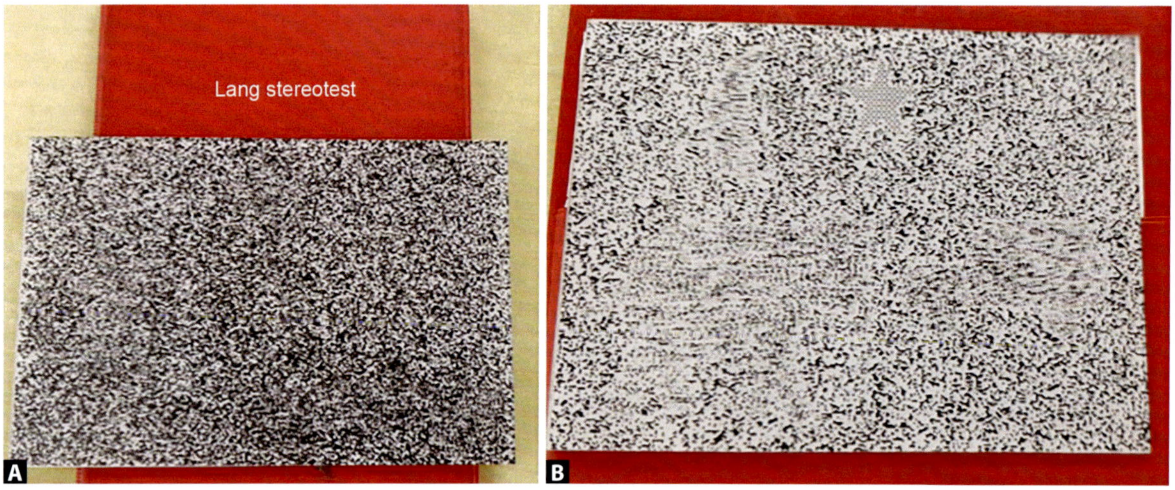

Figs. 8A and B: Lang stereotest.

- *Grade of stereopsis*: Moon-200 seconds of arc, Truck-400 seconds of arc, and Elephant-600 seconds of arc.
- *Lang two-pencil test*:
  - To detect gross stereopsis (3,000–5,000 seconds of arc)
  - Examiner holds one pencil, moves it quickly and the patient is asked to touch the examiner's pencil tip with their pencil tip.
  - *Advantages*: Easily performed, no special instruments are needed.
  - Has 100% sensitivity and negative predictive value.
- *Stereopsis slides placed in synoptophore carrier*:
  - The patient is instructed to view the stereopsis slides are placed in the slide carrier.
  - Two sets of slides are available:
    - *Paratrooper and plane:* The patient is asked whether the paratrooper is in front of the plane or not
    - *Four stars:* One star appears in front when viewed binocularly
  - *Grade of stereopsis:* 720 to 90 seconds of arc

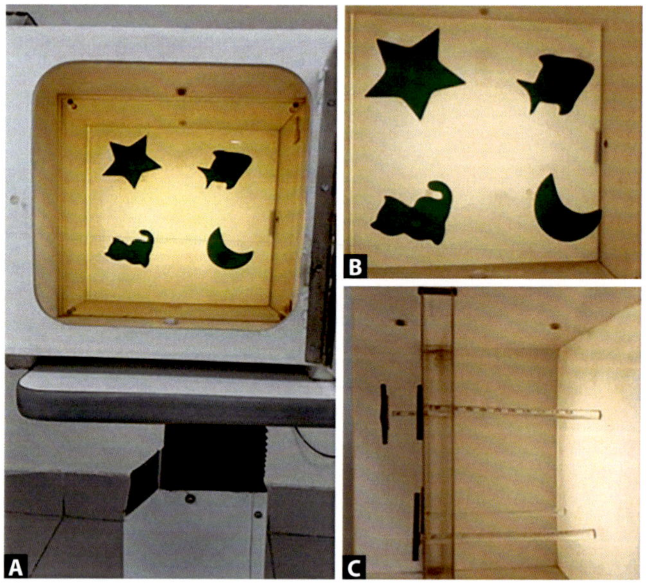

Figs. 9A to C: (A and B) Frisby Davis Distance Stereotest; (C) Side on view showing that one geometric shape is placed ahead of others.

Distance Stereoacuity Tests

- *Frisby Davis Distance Stereotest (FD2 test)*:
  - Based on the panographic principle, the real depth stereogram. It is similar to the Frisby Stereotest for near **(Figs. 9A to C)**.
  - There are either four geometric shapes or four animals (that are translucent), mounted in a transparent frame pointing towards the observer, giving the appearance that the shapes are free-floating.
  - One of the shapes is kept ahead of others and the patient is asked to identify the shape that is ahead.
  - Used in children older than 3 years of age.
  - *Advantages*: No need for polarizing/red-green glasses. It cannot be memorized.
  - *Grade of stereopsis*: 5–50 seconds of arc at 6 m.
- *Distance Randot Stereotest*:
  - It is based on a vectographic random-dot stereogram.
  - Consists of polarized glasses and a Distance Randot Stereotest card.
  - *Grade of stereopsis*: 400 to 60 seconds of arc.
  - *Advantage*: Offers no monocular clues and thus guessing can be avoided.
- *Mentor B-VAT II SG video acuity tester*:
  - Video system with monitor B-VAT II using Random Dot E (BVRDE) and Contour circles (BVC).
  - *Grade of stereopsis:* 240-15 seconds of arc.
- *AO vectographic project-O-chart slide*:
  - Uses phoropter with polarizing lenses
  - *Grade of stereopsis:* 480 to 30 seconds of arc

SENSORY ADAPTATIONS IN STRABISMUS

Sensory adaptations are the neurodevelopmental modifications occurring as a result of changes in binocular

Flowchart 1: Sensory adaptations in strabismus.

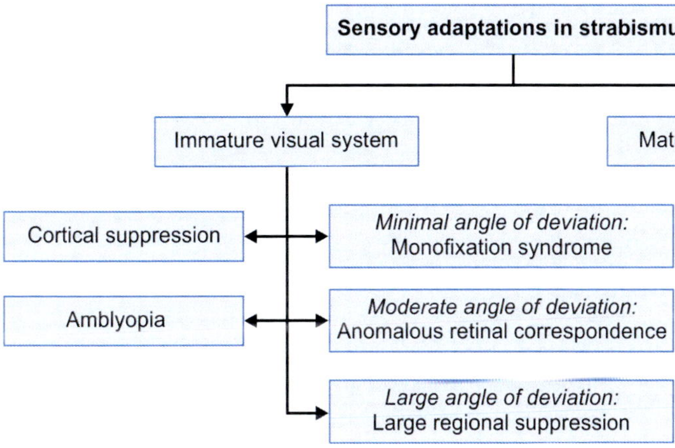

architecture and loss of binocular cells due to a disruption in binocular neural connection caused by strabismus/blurred retinal images. The type of sensory adaptations depends on the time of onset of sensory insult, its severity, and the type of binocular disruption. Based on the time of onset of sensory insult, sensory adaptations are broadly divided into two sections **(Flowchart 1)**:

- Adaptations in the mature visual system
- Adaptations in the immature visual system

Adaptations in the Mature Visual System

Diplopia and confusion can occur if strabismus develops after the development of bifoveal fusion, i.e., when the visual system is mature. The neurophysiological development of the visual system continues till 7–8 years and after that, there is minimal visual-neurological plasticity. There are some exceptions where visual plasticity has been reported in adulthood.

Diplopia

Double vision usually develops in patients over 7 or 8 years with acquired strabismus. Transient diplopia (2–4 weeks) can be seen in younger children with acquired strabismus before cortical suppression develops. Two different objects fall in the fovea of both eyes and the fovea of the deviated eye is suppressed. Thus patient will see the object falling on the fovea of the fixating eye and a diplopic image of the same object falling in the perifoveal retina of the deviated eye. The image from the fixating eye will be clear and the diplopic image from the deviated eye will appear blurred (as it comes from the peripheral retina).

If the diplopic image is on the same side of the deviated eye, the condition is called uncrossed diplopia and if it is on the opposite side, the condition is called crossed diplopia **(Figs. 10A and B)**. Uncrossed diplopia is seen in esotropia as the image falls on the nasal retina of deviated eye and is projected temporally **(Fig. 10B)**. Crossed diplopia is seen as exotropia as the image falls on the temporal retina of deviated eye and is projected nasally.

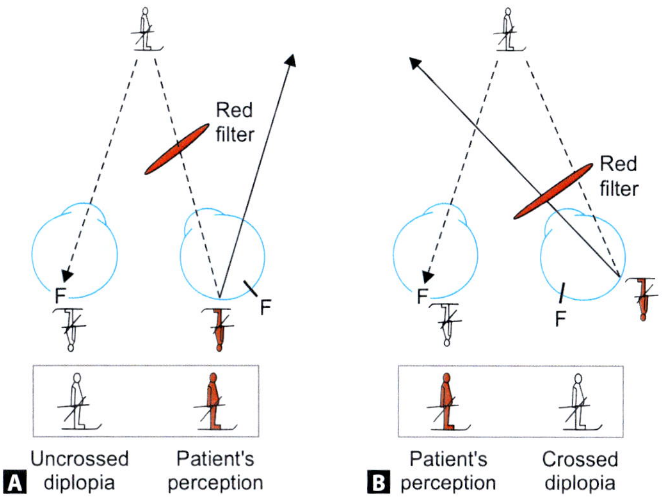

Figs. 10A and B: (A) Esotropia with uncrossed diplopia; (B) Exotropia with crossed diplopia.

Anisometropia causes differences in image size between two eyes (aniseikonia) and can also lead to diplopia. Usually an aniseikonia up to 7% is tolerated and >10% causes diplopia.

Confusion

Confusion also occurs in acquired strabismus developing after a period of visual-neurological plasticity. Here also two different objects fall on the fovea of fixating and the deviating eye. But under rare circumstances instead of suppressing the foveal image of the deviated eye (as in diplopia), images from both the fovea superimposes. For example, if the fovea of fixating eye sees a dog and the fovea of deviated eye sees a cat, the patient will finally see an image of the dog superimposed over the cat. This simultaneous perception of images from the fixing fovea and deviating fovea is called confusion.

Confusion is very rare because in most cases there is cortical suppression of image from the deviated eye leading to diplopia. It has been reported in a glaucoma patient with acquired strabismus and tunnel vision in the deviated eye. Probably the absence of peripheral retinal stimulation by diplopic image in the deviated eye could not cause the foveal suppression and thus leading to confusion instead of diplopia.

Adaptations in the Immature Visual System

It is seen if the sensory insult occurs in the first few years of life, usually before 6 years of age. The basic mechanism seen in almost all the sensory adaptations of the strabismus is cortical suppression. Other adaptations are amblyopia, monofixation syndrome, ARC, large retinal suppressions.

Cortical Suppression

In patients with strabismus, dissimilar images fall on corresponding retinal areas of both eyes. These images cannot be fused, if there is a greater dissimilarity between them. The visually immature individuals adapt by inhibiting the cortical activity from the deviated eye. It is termed cortical suppression and it usually involves the central portion of the visual field. An area of suppression scotoma is formed as the image is not perceived in the area of cortical suppression. In cases of suppression, pattern visual evoked potential (VEP) shows the reduced amplitude of the first positive peak (P1 wave). Suppression is likely to occur at or before the primary visual cortex development, as the P1 wave reflects early visual processing at the level of the striate cortex. So for suppression to develop a constant, large-angle deviation during early childhood is necessary. Cortical suppression results in poor binocular vision and stereopsis. If suppression occurs only in binocular conditions, it is called facultative suppression, i.e., if the dominant eye is occluded, there is no suppression scotoma/reduced visual acuity in the suppressed eye. But constant suppression of one eye can cause obligatory suppression (the suppression scotoma/reduced visual acuity persists even after occluding the dominant eye) leading to amblyopia.

Amblyopia

Amblyopia is defined as the reduction of best-corrected visual acuity of one or both eyes caused by form vision deprivation and/or abnormal binocular interaction that cannot be attributed exclusively to a structural abnormality of the eye. Clinically diagnosed as a reduction in visual acuity by two or more lines compared to fellow eye (uniocular conditions) or compared to normal visual acuity (binocular conditions). It can occur due to strabismus, visual axis obstruction, uncorrected refractive errors, or a combination of the above.

Strabismic amblyopia occurs in patients having constant tropia (usually large angle) who show strong fixation preference to one eye (dominant eye) and constant cortical suppression of another eye (deviated eye). The neuronal connection to the deviated eye is degraded due to constant cortical suppression. Moderate-to-severe amblyopia can occur in these cases.

Amblyopia does not occur if the patient shows alternate fixation and suppression. Amblyopia occurs in approximately half of patients with infantile esotropia (constant tropia). It is very uncommon in intermittent exotropia (alternate fixation and suppression) and incomitant strabismus such as Brown syndrome or Duane syndrome due to maintenance of central fusion by compensatory head posture.

Monofixation Syndrome

Monofixation syndrome is a sensory adaptation when a small central suppression scotoma in the deviated eye, allows for peripheral fusion. It is also termed peripheral fusion syndrome. Prerequisites: Small-angle strabismus [<10 prism diopters (PD)] or unilateral mild-to-moderate image blur and the sensory insult must be at a younger age or infancy. It is classified as strabismic monofixation (due to small-angle strabismus occurring usually after strabismus surgery) or blurred image monofixation (due to anisometropia, partial ptosis, partial cataract, etc.). Common causes of monofixation syndrome include hypermetropic anisometropic amblyopia or corrected strabismus.

In the central retina, small interocular differences in image clarity/position are recognized as it has small receptive fields and high spatial resolution potential. But in peripheral retinal, small interocular image differences are not recognized as it has large receptive fields and relatively low spatial resolution potential. In monofixation syndrome, there is suppression in central 4–5° and there is peripheral fusion where small interocular image differences are not recognized. Patients with a greater angle of strabismus (>10 PD) or severe image blur would not have monofixation syndrome as the peripheral fusion is also affected.

They often have large underlying phoria in addition to small tropia because of motor fusion, so-termed as a phoria-tropia syndrome. They have stereoacuity in the range of 3,000 to 70 seconds of arc. In Bagolini striated lens test **(Fig. 11A)**, patients see a cross with a gap in the center of the line corresponding to the deviated eye is seen. The gap represents the central scotoma of the deviated eye. It is a facultative scotoma, as the suppression scotoma of deviated eye vanishes after occluding the dominant fixing eye. Worth four dot test: Patient can fuse for near Worth four dot test (as it subtends 6° or 12 PD) but not distance Worth four dot test, as it subtends 1.25° or 2.5 PD falling within suppression scotoma **(Figs. 11B and C)**. Patients with monofixation syndrome can have mild amblyopia.

Anomalous Retinal Correspondence

In normal conditions, the fovea of one eye has a binocular relationship with the fovea of another eye, functionally linked together at the occipital cortex. This is called normal retinal correspondence (NRC). In cases of moderate infantile strabismus, the brain allows the fovea of fixing eye to have a binocular relationship with the extrafoveal point of the deviated eye and thus the foveal image (fixing eye) and the extrafoveal image (deviated eye) superimposes at the occipital cortex. This is called anomalous retinal

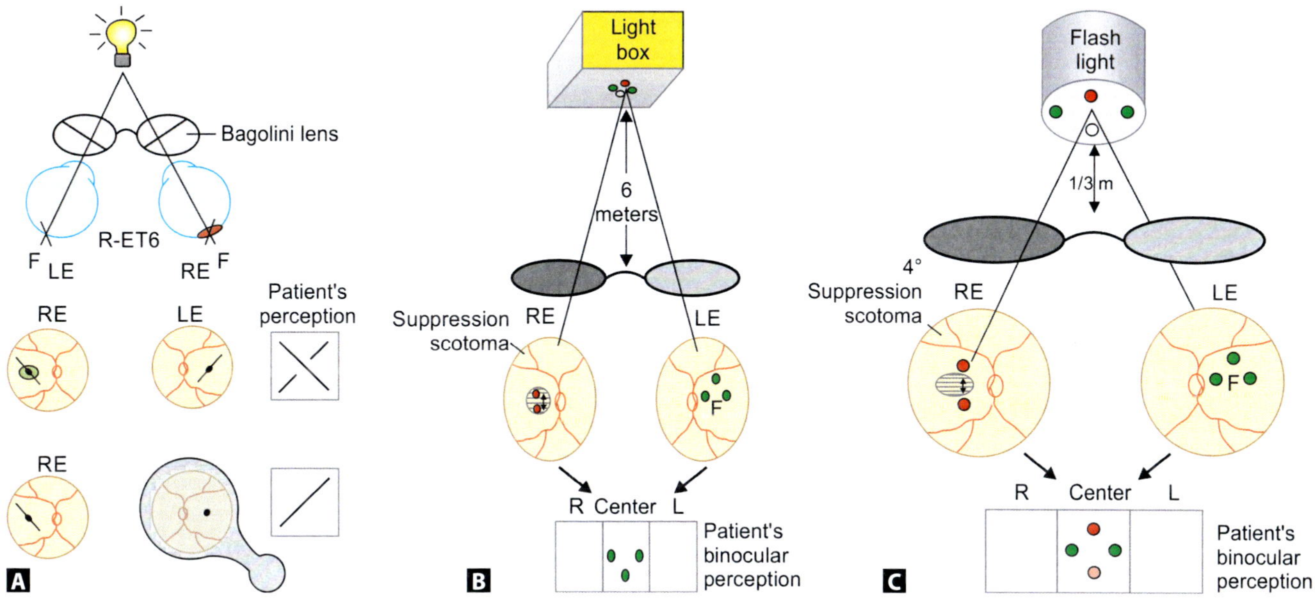

Figs. 11A to C: (A) Bagolini test; (B) Distance and (C) near Worth four dot tests in monofixation syndrome.

correspondence (ARC). The deviation must be around 15–30 PD, i.e., too large to allow for monofixation. Thus ARC is a binocular functional adaptation to strabismus at the cortical level to avoid diplopia. A new fovea called pseudofovea is established that corresponds to the true fovea of fixing/dominant eye.

Requirements for anomalous retinal correspondence

- Early-onset strabismus (during immature visual system)
- Constant angle of deviation, very rarely in intermittent deviation
- Moderate angle deviation (15–30 PD)
- Good vision or mild amblyopia
- Esotropia, but can occur rarely in exotropia.

If the fixing eye is occluded, the true fovea of the previously deviated eye takes fixation from the pseudofovea. Thus ARC and pseudofovea exist only in the binocular conditions.

In patients with ARC, if strabismus surgery or prisms corrects the angle of deviation either partially or fully, still the pseudofovea (of the previously deviated eye) will correspond with the true fovea of the other eye. Thus the patient will have diplopia even if the image falls on the true fovea (of the previously deviated eye) and it is called paradoxical diplopia **(Fig. 12A)**. This paradoxical diplopia usually vanishes after few weeks after the strabismus surgery.

Anomalous retinal correspondence should not be confused with eccentric fixation. Eccentric fixation presents in both binocular and monocular viewing conditions, while ARC presents only in binocular viewing conditions. There is no true fusion in ARC; it provides a crude binocular vision with superimposition of the retinal images. So they do not have fusional vergence amplitude or stereoacuity.

Harmonious and unharmonious anomalous retinal correspondence: The AA is the offset of pseudofovea from the true fovea. Objective angle (OA) of deviation can be measured using prism bar cover test, cover-uncover test in synoptophore, etc. Subjective angle (SA) of deviation can be measured by after-image test, synoptophore, Worth four dot test, Bagolini striated glass test, etc.

If the position of pseudofovea completely compensates for the angle of deviation (OA), then it is called the harmonious ARC. In other words, the AA is equal to the OA of deviation and there is no SA of deviation (AA = OA, SA = 0). In some cases, where there is SA deviation, the position of pseudofovea does not correspond with the angle of deviation(OA). This condition is called an unharmonious ARC. Here, AA = OA – SA. In NRC, there is no psuedofoveal offset, i.e., AA = 0 and the OA of deviation is the same as the SA of deviation (OA = SA). The differentiation of harmonious and unharmonious ARC is not of much clinical importance **(Fig. 12B)**.

Large Regional Suppression

Large suppression scotoma develops in patients with large-angled strabismus (or severe unilateral retinal image blur) to eliminate the disparity of images from both eyes **(Fig. 13)**. It is usually seen in infantile esotropia with a large angle of deviation, where there is no binocularity, peripheral fusion, or ARC. Large regional suppression can also occur intermittently. For example, patients with intermittent exotropia switch from a state of binocular fusion to monocular vision and suppression. Intermittent regional suppression can also be seen in congenital incomitant strabismus (Duane syndrome and congenital superior oblique palsy) where the eyes can be aligned with a compensatory face turn.

Horror Fusionis

Once established, the normal sensory and motor fusion is usually permanent. Loss of binocular fusion can occur when

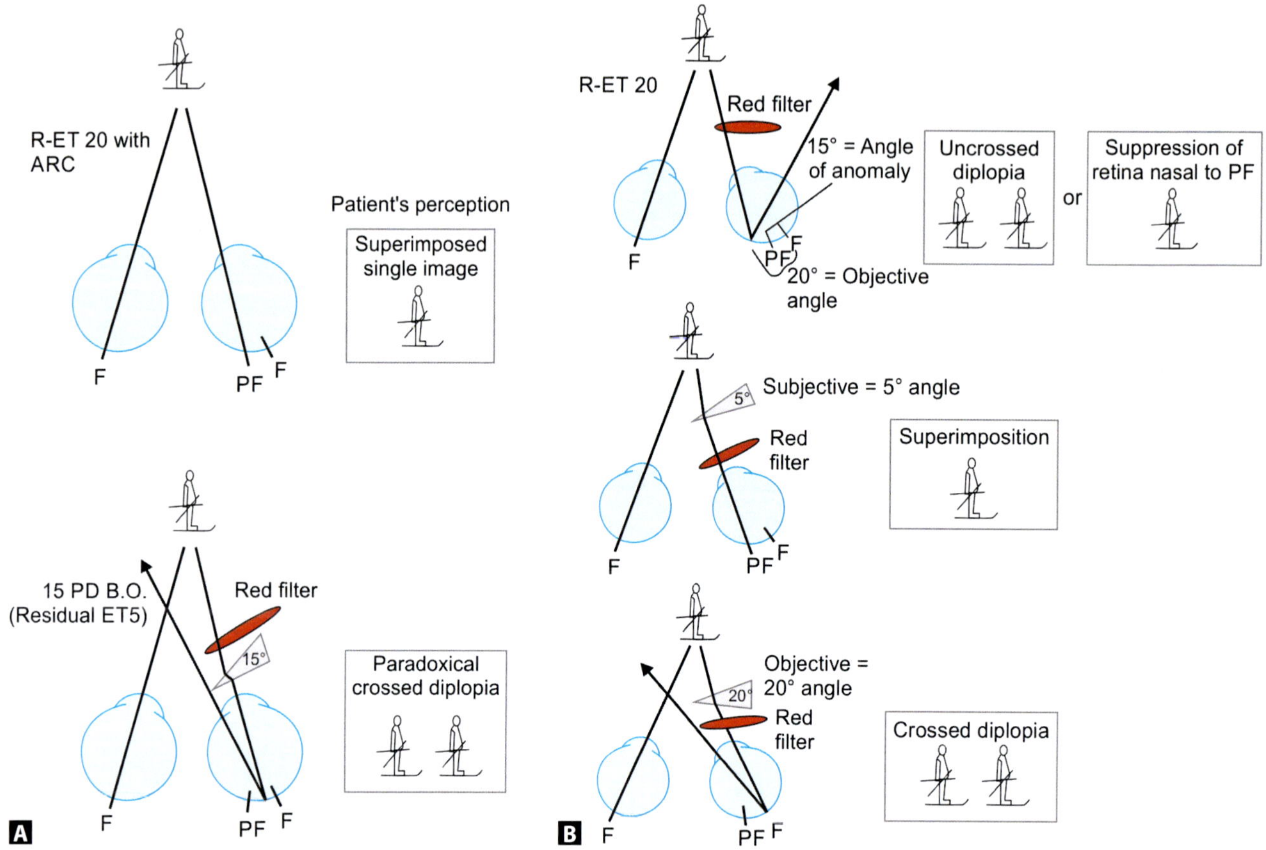

Figs. 12A and B: (A) Paradoxical diplopia in a patient with anomalous retinal correspondence (ARC); (B) Unharmonious ARC in a patient with esotropia.

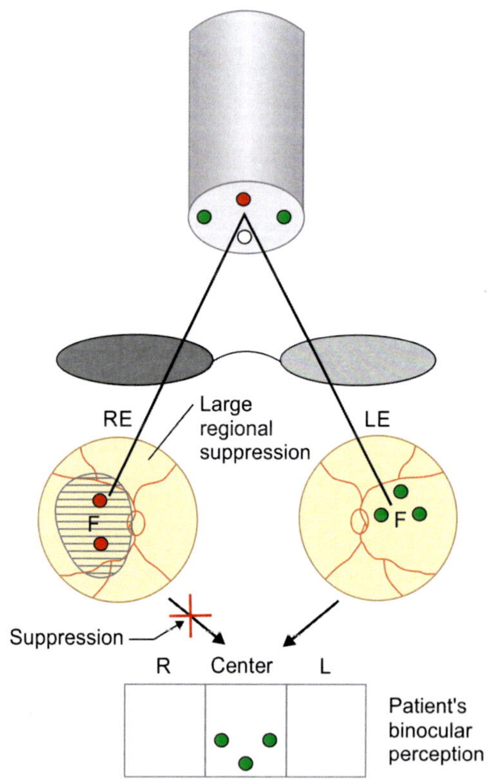

Fig. 13: Worth four dot test in a patient having large regional suppression in right eye.

there is long-term occlusion of one eye (usually dominant eye). If this loss of binocularity occurs in a period where the patient cannot suppress (late childhood or adulthood), horror fusions can develop. Horror fusionis is the acquired disruption of central fusion, where the patients can neither fuse nor suppress the image causing intractable diplopia. It can occur in cases with unilateral acquired cataracts in older children. It can also be seen in cases of adults with previous strabismus/amblyopia developing cataracts in the dominant eye. It can also occur after antisuppression therapy, where the nondominant eye is forced to fix after placing a dense red filter in the dominant eye of patients with strabismus.

SUGGESTED READING

1. Hoyt CS, Taylor D. Pediatric Ophthalmology and Strabismus, 4th edition. St. Louis: Elsevier Saunders; 2013.
2. Rosenbaum AL, Santiago AP. Clinical Strabismus Management: Principles and Surgical Techniques. Philadelphia: David Hunter; 1999.
3. Sharma P. Strabismus Simplified, 2nd edition. New Delhi: CBS Publishers and Distributors; 2016.
4. Von Noorden GK. Binocular Vision and Ocular Motility: Theory and Management of Strabismus, 6th edition. St. Louis: Mosby; 2002.
5. Wright KW, Strube YNJ. Pediatric Ophthalmology and Strabismus, 3rd edition. New York: Oxford University Press; 2012.

20 CHAPTER

Ocular Motility and Evaluation of Strabismus

Miho Sato

INTRODUCTION

In the clinical examination of eye position, attention must be paid to the position of the head and eyelids. Head position many times gives a clue to strabismus, as is usually positioned to minimize the deviation. For example, with left lateral rectus palsy, gaze will be to the right and head turned to left. In superior oblique palsy, the head is tilted away from the side of palsy to use gaze directions away from the field of action of the paretic muscle, and chin slightly depressed to avoid extreme downgaze to avoid diplopia. These maneuvers are compensatory to find binocular single vision. Similarly, the eyelids may give a false impression of esotropia, as in case of telecanthus or epicanthus-inversus.

The position of eyes, in cases of no head or eyelid anomaly, can also be misleading. A large angle kappa can give a false appearance of tropia. Angle kappa is the angle between the visual axis and the optical axis. Optical or anatomical axis is a line passing through center of cornea and intersecting retina slightly nasal to the fovea. The visual axis is a line passing through the center of cornea and intersecting at the fovea. Therefore, when a person fixates on an object, the eyes would appear to be slightly deviated outward, and a penlight reflection on the cornea would be nasal to the center of cornea and will give an impression of exotropia. This presentation is normal and is called positive angle kappa. In large negative angle kappa, the light reflection would be temporal to the center of cornea, and will give an impression of esotropia. Donders found that the average angle kappa is 4-5° in emmetropic eyes, 7.5° in hyperopic eyes, and 2° in myopic eyes. A large angle kappa could result from temporal drag of fovea in retinopathy of prematurity.

Clinically, deviation of eyes can be evaluated by objective methods (corneal reflection methods, cover tests, and haploscopic methods) or by subjective methods (red-glass, Lancaster-green, or Hess screen tests). Objective methods do not require any psychophysical judgment or decision by the patient and are especially helpful in children and uncooperative patients. Subjective tests are more accurate but are tedious and require full cooperation by the patient.

UNDERSTANDING OCULAR MOTILITY

The extra-ocular muscles are unique in number of ways. They are the fastest acting muscles in the body. They are the only muscles to have two different types of muscle fibers. Each muscle fiber is extensively innervated. The neuromuscular tone is so balanced that the eyes can be held still in any direction for any length of time.

Abnormality in ocular motility severely affects functioning of a person.

Fixation and Gaze Holding

In an awake person, the eyes are never still ! Fixation is interrupted by three distinctive 'miniature' movements; a) micro-saccades b)micro- drifts, and c) micro-tremors. These are physiological movements, and some researchers relate them to 'scanning' movements on a particular point object.

Laws of Motility

1. **Fick's Law**: This states that the eye rotates around a fixed point that lies 13.5 mm posterior to the corneal apex and 1.5 mm nasal to the geometric center of the eye.
   All movements of the eyeball around this hypothetical center are around three axis perpendicular to each other. These axis, as described by Fick in 1854, are called X,Y and Z axis.
   X-axis in horizontal, around which the eye rotates vertically.
   Y-axis is parallel to the visual axis, and eye rotates torsionally.
   Z-axis is vertical, around which eye rotates horizontally.
2. **Herring's law**: This law states that 'equal' amount of innervation flows to the 'yoke' muscles, so that movement of both eyes in that direction is conjugate and equal.
3. **Sherrington's law**: This states that when one muscle is contracting, an equal amount of decreased innervation goes to the opposite (antagonist) muscle, so that it is equally relaxed (reciprocal innervation).
4. **Donder's rule**: This rule states that visual axes of the two eyes for a particular gaze, will always move synchronously in the same way to take up that position.

Symptoms of Oculomotor Disorder

Whenever the synchronicity of ocular motility is disturbed, a number of visual difficulties appear, such as diplopia, visual confusion, blurred vision, ocular asthenopia, and vestibular symptoms of vertigo, oscillopia, or tilting.

1. **Diplopia**: Misalignment of eyes causes the image of an object to fall on non-corresponding points of the two retina, usually fovea of one eye and an extra-foveal point of other eye, resulting in a sensory phenomena of diplopia. Diplopia due to ocular misalignment is sudden and very disturbing as in cases of paralysis of any muscle and does not appear in gradual long-standing misalignment.
   Diplopia due to strabismus is always a "binocular" phenomena and disappears with either eye closed. "Monocular" diplopia, with blurring of vision, occurs due to intraocular disease, most commonly cataract. Monocular diplopia or polyopia can sometimes occur with cerebral disorders. It is present with either eye closed but the vision is clear. The cause is unknown.
2. **Visual confusion**: Visual confusion occurs when the two foveas have different direction in space and are viewing two "dissimilar" objects. The images cannot be fused and the patient experiences two images superimposed.
3. **Blurring of vision**: In some cases of strabismus, the patient experiences "blurring of vision", instead of visual confusion. This is because the disparate points on retina are so close together that person senses only blurring.
4. **Vestibular symptoms**: Vertigo and tilting of space are often the chief complaints of torsional strabismus. Careful exclusion of oblique muscle paresis should be done in these cases.

MOTOR EVALUATION OF STRABISMUS

Objective Tests

Hirschberg and Krimsky Tests

While the examiner is holding a penlight about 30 cm in front, the patient is asked to look at the penlight. The reflections from cornea are observed while the patient is fixating at the flashlight. When the eyes are aligned properly, the reflection from the corneas is seen in the center or slightly nasal from the center of the pupil and symmetrical in position. This method is called the Hirschberg test. It should be remembered that it is not a reflex, but corneal *reflection* as the first purkinjee image from the front surface of cornea. This test may not give precise measurement of angle of strabismus because the angle kappa may affect the evaluation, but this method is useful in young children or patients with very poor vision. When the reflection does not locate in the center of the cornea, the angle of strabismus is estimated by the distance from the center. The distance of the reflection from the center of the pupil is converted to the angle of deviation. One millimeter (mm) shift of corneal reflection from the center, amounts to 7.5° or 15 prism diopter (PD) of deviation. In practice, measuring this deviation on the cornea is done by the location of the reflection from the center of pupil (assuming the center of cornea and pupils coincide). Taking the normal size of pupil to be 4 mm, a reflection on the edge of pupil, that is, at 2 mm, a deviation of 15° or 30 PD is recorded. The Hirschberg test has inherent fallacies regarding the position of pupil, size of pupil, near reflex problems, etc., and thus is practiced in infants and small children and in persons who cannot fixate due to very poor vision.

Krimsky test is a method to evaluate the angle of strabismus by using a prism placed in front of the fixing eye. When the prism is placed in front of the fixing eye, the fixing eye may move toward the apex of the prism and the nonfixing eye may move toward the same direction in accordance with Hering's law. By reading the amount of the prism by which the corneal reflection of the nonfixing eye comes to the center of the cornea is used as the amount of strabismus. This method is used only on patients with young children or on poor vision patients same as Hirschberg test.

Both Hirschberg test and Krimsky test are defined by the corneal reflection, therefore, when the patient has large angle Kappa, the evaluation is faulty. Pseudoesotropia with epicanthus inversus and telecanthus has already been stated. When the macula locates temporally after retinopathy of prematurity (ectopia macula), a large positive angle kappa may cause pseudoexotropia or may conceal true esotropia **(Figs. 1A to C)**. In all these cases, determination of true or pseudostrabismus is difficult with these corneal reflection tests and one needs to perform a cover test.

Cover Test

Cover test should be performed to determine manifest misalignment of visual axis.

Procedure: A cover is placed briefly before the eye that appears to fixate while the patient looks at a target. The test should be done at distance and near fixation to establish any differences between the two conditions. One may use the palm of the hand or some form of occluder or paddle can be used as an occlusion instrument. If the patient has a heterotropia and the nonfixating eye is covered, the seeing eye will not move. If the fixating eye is covered, the opposite eye will make a movement from the heterotropic position to normal position and the covered eye may move toward the same direction with the heterotropic eye under the cover. When the patient has exotropia, the heterotropic eye moves toward the nose, and when the patient is esotropia, the heterotropic eye moves toward the temple **(Figs. 2A to G)**.

Cover-Uncover Test

When no manifest strabismus is present (no movement of the fellow eye when either eye is covered), a cover-uncover test will determine whether the patient has a latent deviation or phoria **(Figs. 3A to F)**.

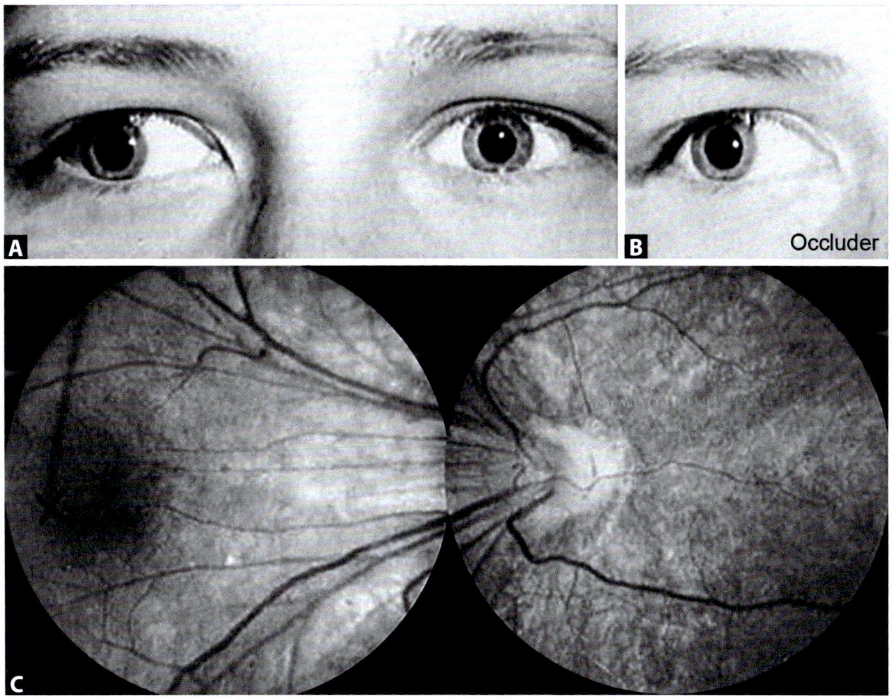

Figs. 1A to C: Pseudostrabismus caused by ectopic macula. (A) The patient appears to have a large right exotropia (XT). The Hirschberg test showed an XT of 20–25°; (B) No shift of OD occurs when OS is covered; (C) Fundus photographs reveal an ectopic macula. The tip of the fixation target (X) indicates the position of the fovea, which is displaced several disk diameters temporally. The retinal blood vessels are pulled over temporal ward. This patient had been born prematurely and for several weeks was kept in an incubator with high oxygen concentration.

Source: von Noorden GK. Atlas of Strabismus, 4th edition. St Louis: Mosby–Year Book; 1983. pp. 35.

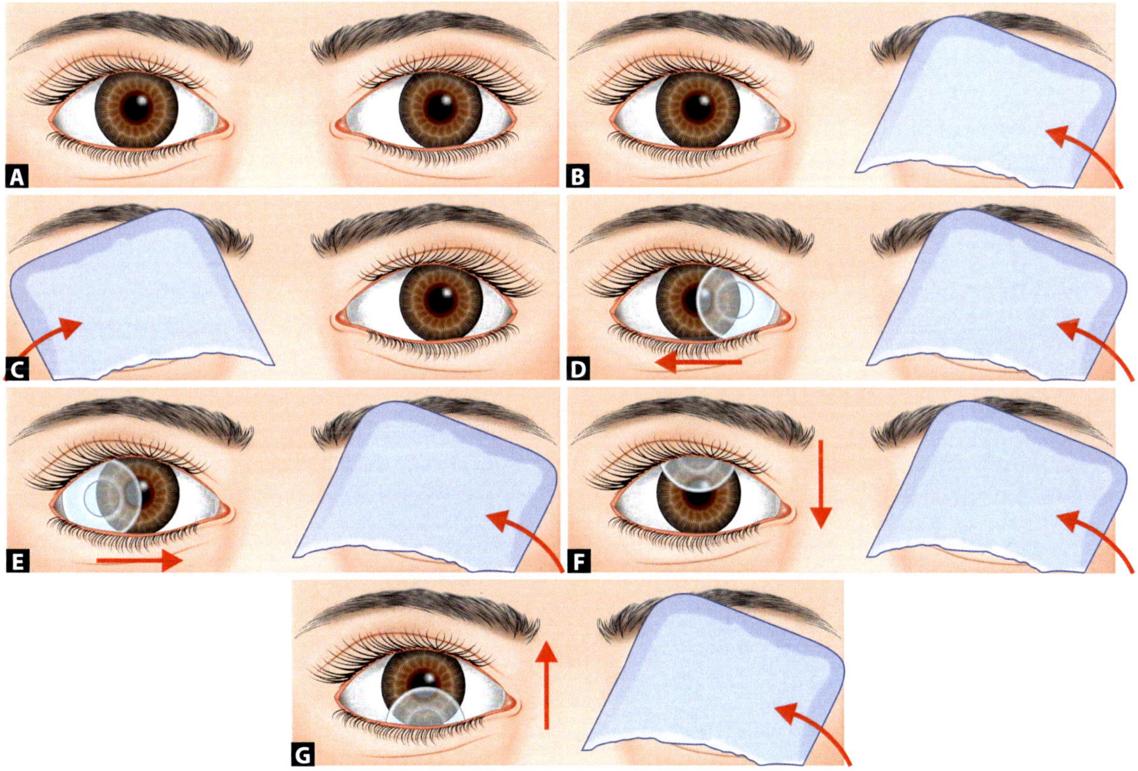

Figs. 2A to G: The cover test. (A) Position of patient's eyes before the test; (B) Cover placed over OS from the left does not elicit a fixation movement of OD—no deviation of OD is present; (C) Cover placed over OD from the right does not elicit a fixation movement of OS—no deviation of OS is present; (D) OD moves outward to fixate when OS is covered—esotropia; (E) OD moves inward to fixate when OS is covered—exotropia; (F) OD moves downward when OS is covered—right hypertropia; (G) OD moves upward when OS is covered—right hypotropia.

Source: von Noorden GK. Atlas of Strabismus, 4th edition. St Louis: Mosby–Year Book; 1983. pp. 39.

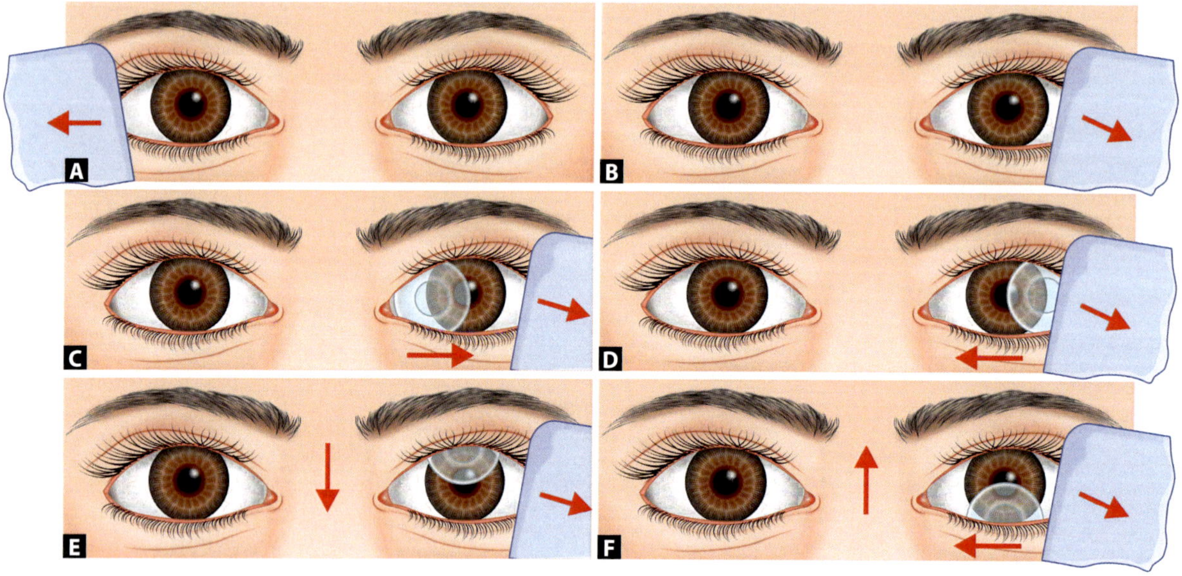

Figs. 3A to F: The cover-uncover test. (A) Cover has been removed from OD, and no movement of OD can be detected—no latent deviation of OD; (B) Cover has been removed from OS, and no movement of OS can be detected—no latent deviation of OS. If conditions A and B are present, the patient has no phorias that can be detected with this test; (C) When uncovered, OS moves outward to fixate—esophoria; (D) When uncovered, OS moves inward to fixate—exophoria; (E) When uncovered, OS moves down to fixate—left hyperphoria; (F) When uncovered, OS moves up to fixate—left hypophoria. The cover-uncover test must be performed on both eyes.

Source: von Noorden GK. Atlas of Strabismus, 4th edition. St Louis: Mosby–Year Book; 1983. pp. 43.

Cover-uncover test is same with cover test as a maneuver, but the examiner should pay attention to the eye while the occluder is removed.

The possible results of the cover and cover-uncover tests may be summarized as follows:

- *On covering the seemingly fixating eye*:
  - *No movement of the other eye*: There was binocular fixation before applying the cover.
  - *Movement of redress of the other eye*: A manifest deviation was present before applying the cover.
- *On uncovering the eye:*
  - See the movement of the uncovered eye. No movement shows no phoria.
  - If the eye takes a redressal movement from outward to inwards, it is exophoria; if movement from inwards to outward, it is esophoria.
  - If comitant strabismus is present, the cover-uncover test will also reveal the dominance of eye.
- *Alternate cover test:* The cover is moved alternately over each eye in turn. This elicits the summation of tropia plus phoria, i.e., total strabismus. The importance of this fact is that if surgery is decided, the total strabismus is taken into account.
- *Prism and cover test*: Prism and cover test should be performed both at near and distance with the accommodative fixation target not with a penlight. The reason for using accommodative fixation objects rather than a simple penlight is to control accommodation during measurement of the deviation at near and distance fixation. To perform this test, a cover is placed alternately in front of each eye while the patient maintains fixation. The prisms used in testing can be loose prisms or stacked in prism-bar or ladders, consisting of a row of prisms of increasing power. When using prism bars, two bars are necessary: one to measure the horizontal deviation and one to measure the vertical deviation. One also may use the horizontal bars with loose prisms held vertically **(Figs. 4A to C)**.

After cover-uncover test, the approximate power of prism is placed in front of the deviating eye.

Prisms should be placed as base-out for esotropia, base-in for exotropia, and when the patient shows right hyper tropia, a base-down prism should be placed in front of the right eye. When the patient shows both horizontal and vertical deviation, horizontal and vertical prisms can be placed on the same eye. But when the patient shows large deviation that exceeds the maximum available prism, another prism should not be added on the same eye, but it should be separately placed over both eyes. According to Thompson and Guyton, the effect produced by adding a 5 prism over a 40 prism is not 45 but 59. This error can be minimized by holding one prism before each eye.

Combinations of horizontal and vertical deviations are frequent. In such patients, it is best to first neutralize the horizontal deviation with prisms and then to add prisms to stop the vertical deviation. At that point, it may be necessary to further correct the horizontal deviation. The amount of prism strength required to offset all movements of redress is a measure of the deviation. Cyclodeviations cannot be

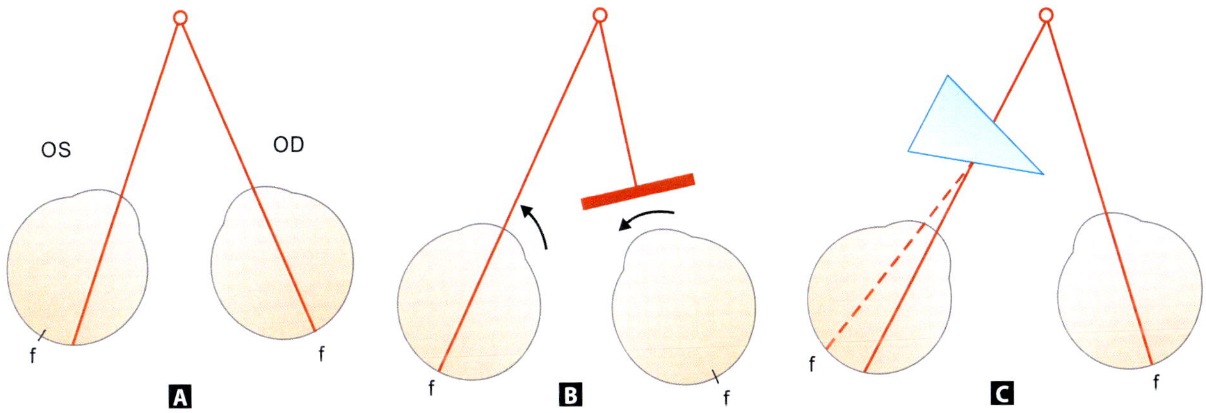

Figs. 4A to C: Optical principles of prism and cover test. (A) Image of object fixated by OD is projected on the nasal half of the retina of OS; (B) When OD is covered, OS moves outward to take over fixation. Under the cover, OD performs an inward movement of equal amplitude, following Hering's law of equal innervation; (C) When a prism of sufficient power offsets the nasal displacement of the image; OS will no longer change its position when OD is covered.

Source: von Noorden GK. Atlas of Strabismus, 4th edition. St Louis: Mosby–Year Book; 1983; pp. 51

measured in this fashion, and must be determined either subjectively or with the major amblyoscope.

Maximal dissociation of the eyes must be achieved to make the correct diagnosis, especially in patients with heterophoria. Such patients have a strong compensatory innervation that keeps their eyes aligned and it is not immediately suspended when one eye is covered. *It is necessary to dissociate the eyes for some time to bring out the full amount of the deviation.* The test must not be performed hurriedly, and the cover should be placed alternately over each eye a few times. Most importantly, the patient should never be permitted to regain fusion while the cover is being transferred. In patients with an exodeviation, one eye may have to be occluded for 30–45 minutes. The difference in measurements before and after occlusion may be significant.

Another way to ensure full dissociation and obtain the full amount of the deviation is to add prism power not only until redress is stopped but also until a reversal of the direction of movement is noted. In so doing, one frequently finds that the endpoint is higher than originally thought. This technique is recommended for routine use.

The prism and alternate cover test **(Figs. 5A to F)** should be performed for distance and near fixation with the patient first wearing refractive correction and then with the correction removed. Comparison of these four figures allows one to draw conclusions about the part played by accommodation in the patient's deviation. The deviation measured in distance fixation while the patient is wearing full correction excludes accommodation. The fusion factor must be excluded as far as possible by a properly performed prism and cover test. If correction of the refractive error is inadequate, accommodation is uncontrolled and one then obtains the *dynamic deviation* or dynamic angle of squint. Likewise, in the case of insufficient dissociation of the eyes, persistent strong compensatory fusional innervation during the prism and cover test will cause dynamic factors to override and obscure the static deviation.

Another useful modification of the prism cover test is to repeat it while the patient is fixating at 33 cm distance and looking through +3.00D lenses, clipped over the distance correction or, in the case of emmetropia, placed in the trial frame. With the accommodative demand for near fixation thus eliminated, the deviation at near should now approximately equal that at distance. It is recommended that the prism and cover test also should be performed with either eye fixating. To do this, one eye is made to fixate while the other is alternately covered and uncovered and a prism is placed before the covered eye to stop movement of that eye. The process is then repeated with the other eye fixating. Differences in the amount of prism power required for each eye indicated the presence of a *primary and secondary deviation* or an *incomitance.*

Prism and Cover Test in Diagnostic Positions of Gaze

The prism and cover test is useful in determining incomitance in otherwise comitant deviations, confirming by measurement the degree of a paresis, and establishing what muscle or muscles are involved in a paralytic condition. To this end, the deviation should be measured in the *nine diagnostic positions of gaze.* The first is the primary position; next come the secondary positions of right, left, up, and down; and last the tertiary positions of up and right, up and left, down and right, and down and left. To determine whether a deviation is paretic or paralytic, the relative position of the eyes in diagnostic positions should be measured with either eye fixating, as has been described for the primary position. In practical performance of the prism and cover test in diagnostic positions of gaze, varying procedures are followed. Accommodative fixation targets should be used as fixation

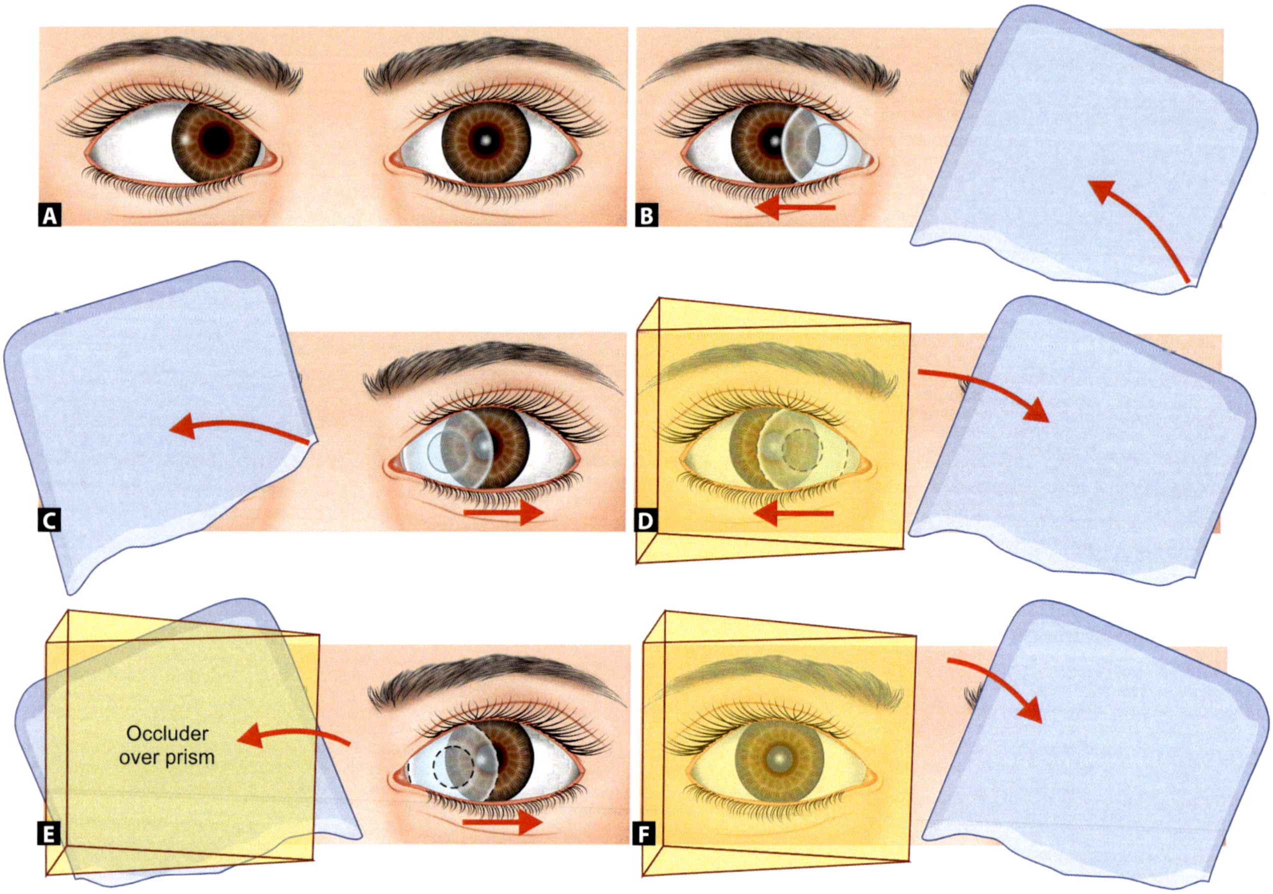

Figs. 5A to F: The prism and alternate cover test. (A) Right esotropia; (B) When OS is covered, OD moves outward to take over fixation; (C) When the cover is transferred to OD, OS moves out to take over fixation; (D) A prism, base-out, is held before OD; the cover is transferred to OS. There is still outward movement of OD when taking over fixation, although the amplitude of this movement is decreased by the effect of the prism (compare with B); (E) The cover is again transferred, and a prism of greater power is held before OD; (F) Transfer of cover to OS does not elicit fixation movement of OD. The deviation is offset by the prism, and the power of this prism equals the deviation.

Source: von Noorden GK. Atlas of Strabismus, 4th edition. St Louis: Mosby–Year Book; 1983. pp. 49.

objects to minimize variability of the deviation resulting from variations in accommodation. Such a target may be handed to the patient to hold and the hand placed successively in the desired positions, leaving the examiner's hands free to perform the test.

DUCTION/VERSION

Determination of the deviation amount in the nine diagnostic positions of gaze by means of the prism and cover test or by one of the subjective tests establishes certain important points in the diagnosis. These points must be amplified by a study of the extent to which the eyes, singly or together, perform movements in various directions of gaze. When examining *ductions,* cover one eye and have the patient follow a penlight or other fixation target, bringing the eye to the farthest possible position in the directions right, left, up, down, up and right, up and left, down and right, and down and left. The examiner observes whether movement lags or is excessive in any direction.

In maximal adduction, an imaginary vertical line through the lower lacrimal punctum should coincide with a boundary line between the inner third and the outer two-thirds of the cornea **(Fig. 6A)**. If more of the cornea is hidden, the adduction is excessive **(Fig. 6B)**. If more of the cornea is visible on maximal adduction and if some of the sclera remains visible, adduction is defective **(Fig. 6C)**. If abduction is normal, the corneal limbus should touch the outer canthus **(Fig. 6D)**. If the limbus passes that point and some of the cornea is hidden, the abduction is excessive **(Fig. 6E)**. If some of the sclera remains visible, abduction is defective **(Fig. 6F)**.

The Kestenbaum limbus test **(Fig. 7)** for measuring of muscle actions is particularly useful for paretic muscles. The test is performed by holding a transparent millimeter ruler horizontally in front of the cornea. In measuring abduction, the location of the nasal limbus point is noted on the ruler in primary position and in maximum abduction. The difference immediately gives the degree of abduction in millimeters. Adduction is measured similarly by determining the positions of the temporal limbus. To measure elevation and depression, hold the ruler vertically. The examiner should test each eye with his or her own homonymous eye. Normal values established by Kestenbaum are 10 mm for adduction, abduction, and depression, and 5–7 mm for elevation.

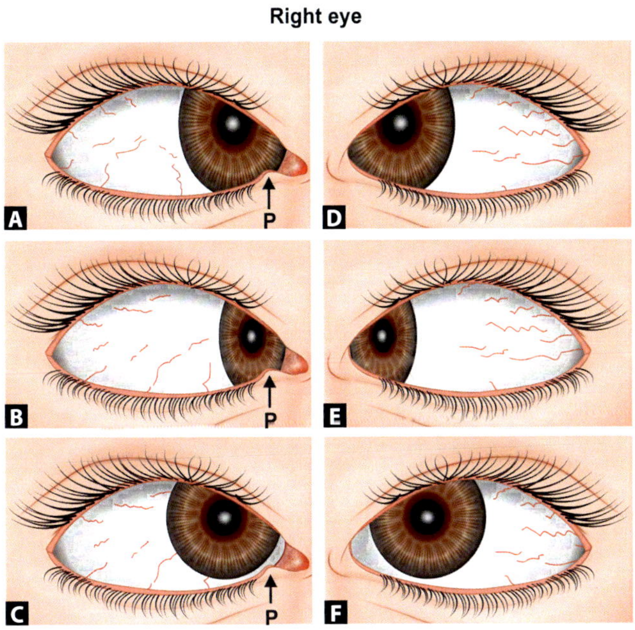

Figs. 6A to F: The ductions of the eyes. (A) Normal adduction; (B) Excessive adduction; (C) Defective adduction; (D) Normal abduction; (E) Excessive abduction; and (F) Defective abduction; lacrimal punctum. While the versions are being tested, the fellow eye is kept open and, as a rule, fixates. The left eye is not shown in this figure.

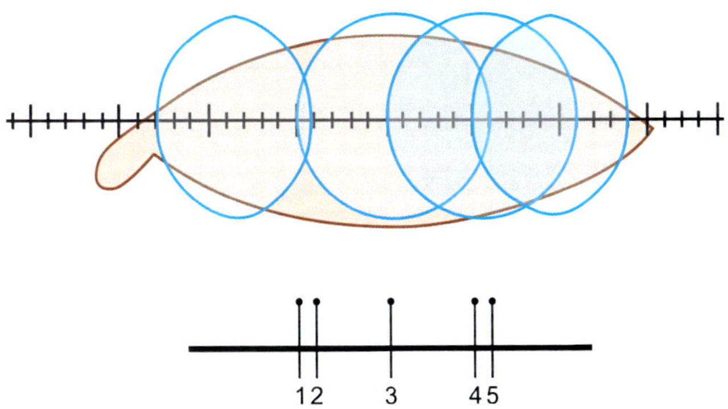

Fig. 7: The limbus test of Kestenbaum.

Source: Kestenbaum A. Clinical Methods of Neuro Ophthalmologic Examination, 2nd edition. New York: Grune & Stratton;1961. pp. 237.

Versions

Synchronous simultaneous movements of the two eyes in the same direction are called *versions*. To study the *versions*, one places a penlight in the midline before the patient's eyes and moves it in the various directions, keeping the penlight at such a distance that one can always observe the corneal reflections in both eyes. While doing so, carefully watch for excessive or defective movements in any direction. Remove the patient's glasses to observe the movement of the eyes in peripheral positions of gaze.

When studying the versions, one often finds the adducted eye to be elevated. The phenomenon may be unilateral or bilateral. This elevation in adduction is called *upshoot in adduction*. It is often overlooked but important to note that *overaction of the inferior oblique muscle* is but one of several causes for this phenomenon. Depression of the adducted eye, also called *downshoot in adduction,* is seen with overaction of the superior oblique muscles, paralysis of the contralateral inferior rectus muscle, atopic muscle pulleys, and may also occur with Duane retraction syndrome.

Vergence

Synchronous simultaneous movements of the two eyes in opposite directions are called *vergences*. Versions are fast and vergences are slow eye movements. There is an upper limit in vergences.

The limit determines the *amplitude of motor fusion,* which is usually greatest for convergence movements and smallest for vertical vergence movements. In normal subjects, the amplitudes vary considerably from individual to individual. They vary with the state of alertness, that is, whether the subject is tired or rested or under the influence of a toxic agent. They depend on the type of visual activity prior to the measurement, the procedure by which the amplitudes are measured, and to a large extent on the state of the individual's neuromuscular apparatus. Horizontal and vertical fusional amplitudes are determined by prisms or with some haploscopic device.

While measuring vergence, the patient is seated comfortably and asked to fixate the appropriate object. A rotary prism is then placed in front of one eye and moved to produce the desired fusional movement. The prism may be hand-held, or it may be part of a phorometer or phoropter. The prism strength is increased slowly and stepwise, and the patient is asked to report when the fixation object appears double. When the patient reports diplopia, at which point the two images are rather suddenly quite far apart, the required amount of prism power is noted. It represents the limit of the patient's fusional amplitude in the direction tested, the so-called breakpoint. The prism power is then reduced, again slowly and stepwise, and the point at which the patient regains, single vision is noted. This is the so-called *recovery point.*

Because convergence after effect reduces the amount of divergence, the following order in testing fusional amplitudes is recommended—prisms base-out (convergence), prisms base-up (deorsumvergence), prisms base-in (divergence), and prisms base-down (sursumvergence).

Vergences should always be tested both in distance and near fixation. Frequently they are tested at one fixation distance only (e.g., in distance fixation), especially when the divergence amplitudes are determined with a major amblyoscope.

Near Point of Convergence

The near point of convergence (NPC) is determined by placing a fixation object at 30–40 cm in the midplane of the patient's head; the patient is then asked to maintain fixation on the object. The object is then moved toward the eyes until one of the eyes loses fixation and turns out. The distance at which this occurs is the NPC. It is measured by a Prince ruler or similar device. This NPC lies approximately in the plane of the centers of rotation of the eyes. The NPC should be at 8–10 cm. A distance closer than 5 cm is excessive. An NPC farther away than 10 cm is defective or remote.

Measurement with a Major Amblyoscope

When vergences are measured with a major amblyoscope, the point of departure is the heterophoric position, that is, the arms are set at the patient's angle of deviation. From this position, various vergence movements are induced by moving the arms (for the horizontal vergences) or the targets (for vertical and cyclovergences). This procedure determines total vergence amplitudes, but no information is gained about the fusional reserve beyond the straight position of the eyes. This test can be done also in heterophoric patients by starting with the arms of the major amblyoscope at zero. These measurements correspond to those obtained with the rotary prism. Ordinarily, the major amblyoscope is adjusted for optical infinity. Placing minus lenses of appropriate strength in front of each eye and setting the arms at 18 D adapt the instrument for near fixation, and vergences can also be measured for near visual distance. Targets that incorporate fusible material must be used to measure vergence amplitudes when a major amblyoscope is used. Using targets that contain larger or smaller amounts of fusible material allow the effect of the amount of fusible material on the amplitudes to be determined.

Measurement of Dissociated Vertical Deviation

Dissociated vertical deviation (DVD) is characterized by the spontaneous drifting of either eye upward when the patient is fatigued or daydreaming or when fusion is artificially interrupted by covering one eye **(Figs. 8A and B)**. When the elevated eye is covered, it may perform pendular and vertical movements. When the cover is removed, the elevated eye will move slowly downward and settle in the primary position.

In patients with DVD, the alternate cover test reveals that each eye turns upward under cover in contrast to the situation in vertical heterophoria. After removal of the cover, the eye makes a slow downward movement to reach the midline, at times even going below it, accompanied by incycloduction **(Fig. 8A)**. The translucent occluder of Spielmann is especially useful in the diagnosis of this condition and in demonstrating it to the patient's parents **(Fig. 8B)**. A precise measurement of the vertical excursions of each eye during DVD is nearly impossible because of the variable nature of this condition.

An accurate quantitative assessment of DVD may be obtained, provided visual acuity in each eye is sufficient to visualize the fixation target, using a modification of the prism and cover test. As the patient focuses on the fixation target at 6 m distance, the occluder is quickly shifted to the fixating eye, allowing the previously dissociated and elevated eye to take up fixation. The cover is then returned to the nonfixating eye. As the alternate cover test is continued, increasing amounts of base-down prisms are held under the occluder in front of the nonfixating eye until the downward fixation movement of that eye is neutralized. The procedure is then repeated with the fellow eye fixating.

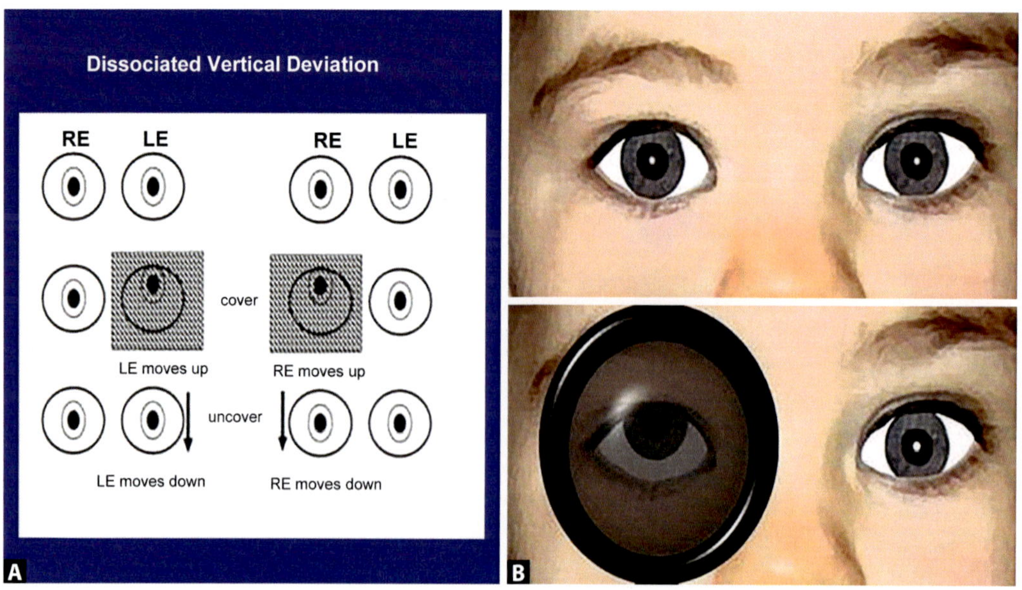

Figs. 8A and B: (A) Bilateral DVD with updrift of either eye under cover and slow return to primary position on removal of the cover; (B) Right eye manifesting DVD under cover with a translucent occluder of Spielmann.

Source: Spielmann A. A translucent occluder for study of eye position under unilateral or bilateral cover test. Am Orthoptics J. 1986;36:65.

First, in DVD the covered eye becomes elevated in abduction, primary position, and adduction. Conversely, with overaction of the inferior oblique muscles, each eye becomes elevated primarily in adduction and never in abduction unless there is coexisting contracture of the ipsilateral superior rectus muscle. Unlike DVD, overaction of the inferior obliques is commonly associated with a V-pattern esotropia. The reason for elevation in adduction in a DVD is that the adducted eye becomes occluded by the nasal bridge and fusion is suspended. In children under the age of 2–3 years, the nasal bridge has not yet fully developed and the upshoot in adduction is rarely seen.

Second, DVD is found also in patients in whom there is no noticeable overaction of the inferior oblique muscles and actually occurs frequently in those with underacting inferior oblique and overacting superior oblique muscles.

RESTRICTION OF EYE MOVEMENTS

When, there exists limitation in eye movement, paralytic strabismus and restrictive strabismus should be differentiated. Forced duction, active force generation, and saccadic velocity tests are used to evaluate them.

Measurement of Paralytic Strabismus

Although evaluation of ductions and versions is enough to identify gross defects of ocular motility, a quantitative study of the angle of deviation in diagnostic positions of gaze with either eye fixating will reveal more subtle forms of paralysis. These measurements are obtained using objective (prism and cover test) or subjective (diplopia fields) methods. Such tests, with the patient fixating first with one eye and then the other, are of fundamental diagnostic importance, since a difference between a *primary deviation* (nonparetic eye fixating) and a *secondary deviation* (paretic eye fixating) clearly distinguishes paralytic from nonparalytic strabismus; *the secondary deviation is always greater than the primary deviation.* According to Hering's law of equal innervation, the innervation flowing to the yoke muscles of both eyes is always determined by the fixating eye.

FORCED DUCTION TEST

Forced duction test **(Figs. 9A to C)** can be performed in the office setting, after applying drops of 4% lidocaine hydrochloride (Xylocaine). The eye is then moved with two-toothed forceps applied to the conjunctiva near the limbus *in the direction opposite that in which mechanical restriction is suspected.* For instance, to distinguish between lateral rectus paralysis and mechanical restriction involving the medial aspect of the globe, we apply the forceps at the 6- and 12-o'clock positions and move the eye passively into abduction. If no resistance is encountered, the motility defect is clearly caused by paralysis of the lateral rectus muscle. If resistance is encountered, mechanical restrictions do exist medially and contracture of the medial rectus muscle, conjunctiva, or Tenon's capsule, or myositis of the medial rectus muscle must be considered.

ACTIVE FORCE GENERATION TEST

The active force generated by a contracting muscle can be estimated by stabilizing the eye with forceps while the patient tries to move the eye against this. Mechanical determination of muscle force can be useful in assessing the function

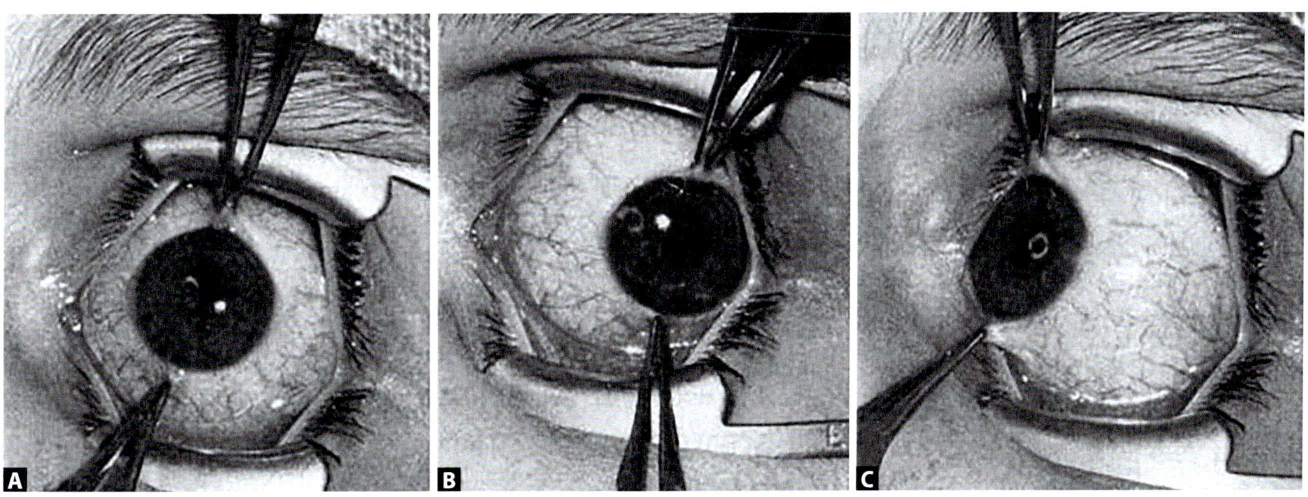

Figs. 9A to C: The forced duction test—(A) Conjunctiva and episcleral are grasped near the limbus with two fixation forceps; (B) The eye is moved temporally; (C) Nasally to test for mechanical restriction of ocular motility. Note that the eye must not be depressed into the orbit during the test to avoid false positives.

Source: von Noorden GK. Atlas of Strabismus, 4th edition. St Louis: Mosby–Year Book; 1983.

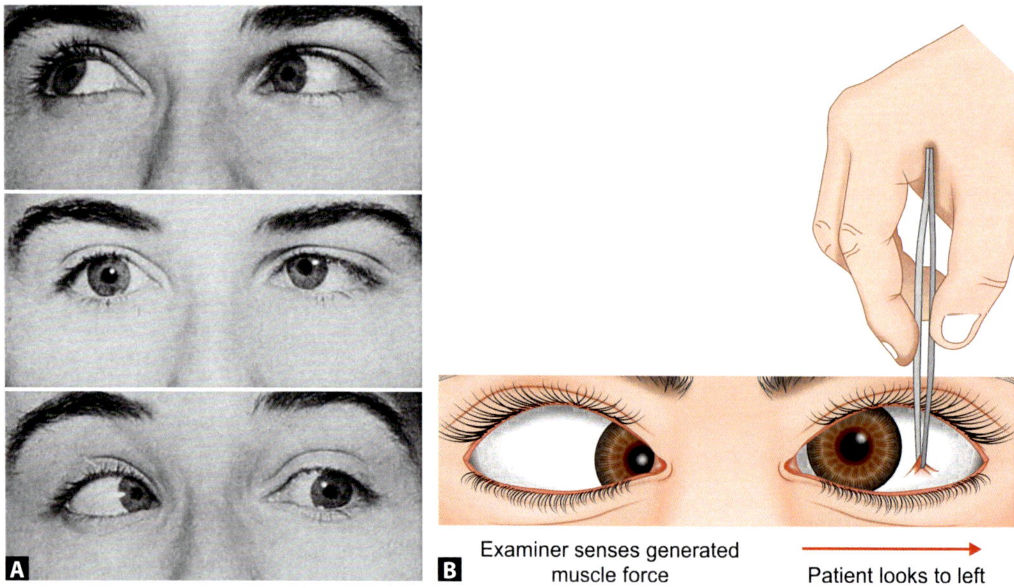

Figs. 10A and B: Estimation of force generation test. (A) Patient with a left lateral rectus paresis shows movement of the left eye from adduction toward primary position on levoversion and slightly beyond. This movement may be active (residual lateral rectus innervation) or passive (medial rectus relaxation). In the first instance, maximal recession of the medial rectus and resection of the paretic lateral rectus may be indicated. In the second situation, a muscle transposition procedure may be considered; (B) The examiner senses a tug on the forceps as the paretic eye moves from adduction toward primary position. The tug is a sign of residual innervation of the lateral rectus muscle and incomplete paralysis. Absence of the tug is a sign of complete paralysis.

Source: von Noorden GK. Atlas of Strabismus, 4th edition. St Louis: Mosby–Year Book; 1983.

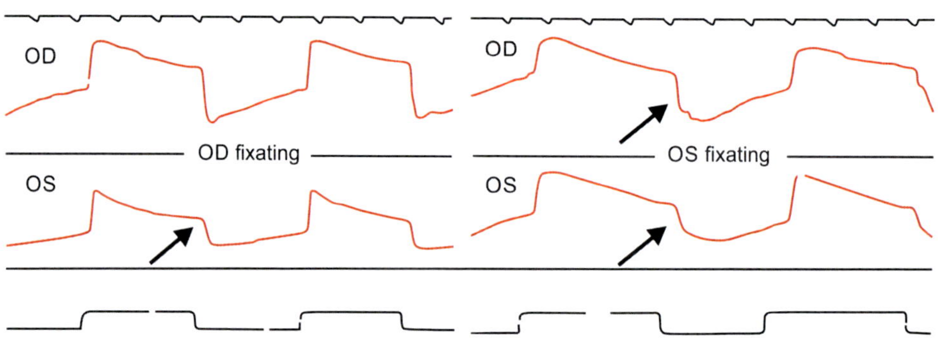

Fig. 11: Electro-oculographic registration of eye movements in a patient with left cranial nerve VI paresis. Positive deflection, gaze to right. Negative deflection, gaze to left. *Arrows* denote decreased saccadic velocity upon gaze into the paretic field of gaze.

Source: Mackensen G. Okulographie. In: Hamburger FA, Hollwich F (Eds). Augenmuskella hmungen, vol 46. Stuttgart: Ferdinand Enke Verlag; 1966.

of apparently paretic muscles with contracture of their antagonists **(Figs. 10A and B)**.

Eye Movement Velocity

A study of saccadic velocity may be used also in conjunction with other diagnostic methods, such as the forced duction test or determination of generated muscle force, to assess the function of a paralyzed muscle. If paralysis exists, the velocity of eye movement into the field of action of the paralyzed muscle will be markedly decreased **(Fig. 11)**, the normal rapid saccade being replaced by a slow and drifting eye movement. If the motility defect is caused by a mechanical obstacle, the saccadic velocity of an eye movement into the field of apparent paresis will be normal.

SUBJECTIVE TESTS

Diplopia Tests (Red-Glass Test and Others)

In the diplopia type of test, one determines the subjective localization of a single object imaged on the fovea of the fixating eye and an extrafoveal retinal area in the other eye. In esotropia, where the image of the fixation point in the deviated eye falls on a retinal area nasal to the fovea, there should be *uncrossed diplopia*. In exotropia, where the image of the fixation point in the deviated eye falls on a retinal area temporal to the fovea, there should be *crossed diplopia*. If retinal correspondence is normal, double images not only should be properly oriented but also should have a distance equal to the angle of squint. The distance of the double images is then a measure of the deviation; but even with spontaneous diplopia it is difficult if not impossible for the patient to state whether the images are crossed or uncrossed. The two visual fields must be differentiated and for this purpose a red glass is placed in front of one eye (hence, *red-glass test*), usually in front of right eye, as a convention. The patient fixates a small point light source and states whether the red light is to the right or to the left and above or below the white light. If the white fixation light is in the center of a *Maddox cross*, the patient must state the numbers at which the red light is seen. If the patient is seated at the correct distance, these numbers indicate the amount of deviation. The Maddox cross test is now seldom used. More accurate are achieved by using Red-Green Maddox rods and distance fixating white target.

Maddox cross is seldom used now-a-days. A simpler test using 'Red-Glass' or the 'Maddox Rod' is commonly used for subjective evaluation of deviation.

The Red-Glass test is done by placing a red-glass in front of one eye, creating a red and white image of fixating white point light. Horizontal and vertical prisms are then placed in front of other eye, until the patient reports that the two point lights are superimposed. The deviation is then read off from the prisms used.

Maddox-Rod Test

This is similar to the Red Glass test. But does not need the Maddox cross and also the red streak is more precise in measuring the amount of deviation. As we know, the Maddox rod consists of high power cylinders, stacked parallel to each other, which convert a point light into a streak, perpendicular to the placement of rods. A green color Maddox can be placed in the other (left) eye, which further facilitates the positioning of streaks. Prisms can then be placed to bring the streaks in alignment and the deviation measured. The test is more valuable to detect and measure phorias.

In esotropia/esophoria, the red streak in right eye will be on the right side of the point light (homonymous or uncrossed diplopia while on the other side in exotropia/phoria (heteronymous or crossed diplopia). In hyperphoria, it will be below and above the point light in hypophorias.

Haploscopic Tests

Haploscopic tests differ from diplopia tests in their mode of stimulation. Two test objects rather than one are presented to the patient, who is required to place them in such a fashion that they appear superimposed **(Fig. 12)**. Again, assuming that correspondence is normal, the two objects are placed to stimulate the foveae of the two eyes. The common methods of identifying the images are by color, red-green lights and red-green colors (Lancaster test, Hess screen) or by mirrors (Lee's screen, major amblyoscope).

The *Lancaster red-green test* **(Figs. 13A and B)** uses a window shade type of screen that can be rolled up when not in use. The screen is ruled into squares of 7 cm so that at a distance of 2 m each square subtends approximately 2°. The patient is equipped with red-green reversible goggles. Two projectors are used, a green projector, handled by the patient, and a red projector, handled by the examiner. The image formed by the projector is linear. The red filter may be placed in front of either eye to investigate differences

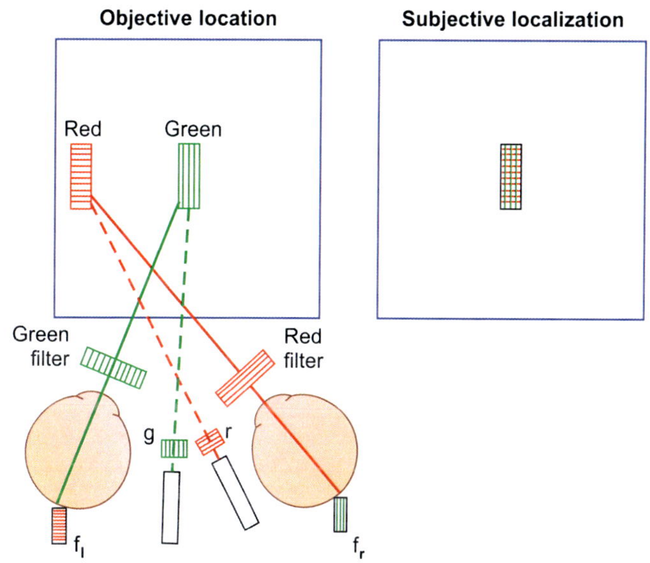

Fig. 12: Principle of haploscopic tests.

Source: Burian HM. Normal and anomalous correspondence. In: Allen JH (Ed). Strabismus Ophthalmic Symposium, II. St Louis: Mosby–Year Book: 1958. pp. 184.

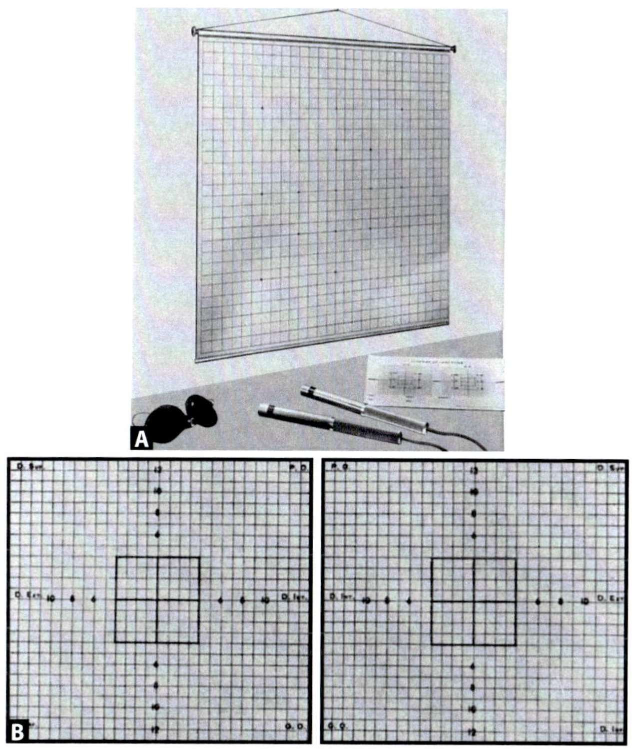

Figs. 13A and B: Lancaster red-green test. (A) Equipment for the test; (B) Charts to record results.

(*Courtesy*: Luneau and Couffignon, Chartres, France.)

caused by changes in fixation. Instead of inverting the glasses, the examiner can exchange projectors with the patient. The examiner projects the line from his or her projector onto the screen at any desired place, the patient's head is held steady, and the patient is asked to place the streak from his or her projector so that it appears to the patient to coincide exactly with the other streak. If one assumes that correspondence is normal, the two streaks will be separated objectively on the screen by an amount corresponding to the deviation of the visual axes. The positions of the streak shown by the patient are entered into a small chart on which the screen is reproduced.

The Hess screen test **(Figs. 14A and B)** is based on the haploscopic principle. This test is useful in particular for diagnosing possible paretic or paralytic conditions in patients with normal correspondence. To perform this test, a black cloth 3 ft wide by 3½ ft long, marked out by a series of red lines subtending between them an angle of 5°, is used. At the zero point of this coordinate system and at each of the points of intersection of the 15° and 30° lines with one another and with corresponding vertical and horizontal lines, there is a red dot. These dots form an inner square of 8 dots and an outer square of 16 dots. An indicator is provided consisting of three short green cords knotted to form the letter Y. The end of the vertical green cord is fastened to a movable black rod 50 cm long. The ends of the other two cords are kept taut by black threads that pass through loops to small weights at corresponding upper corners of the screen. This arrangement enables the patient to move the indicator freely and smoothly over the whole surface of the screen in all directions. The patient wears red-green goggles and is seated 50 cm from the screen, preferably with his or her head fixed in a headrest. The patient now sees the red dots with one eye and the green cords with the other and is instructed to place the knot joining the three green cords over each of the red dots in turn. The examiner marks the positions indicated by the patient on the small card with a reduced copy of the screen. The points found by the patient are connected by straight lines and permit the examiner to determine which, if any, muscles react abnormally. To change fixation, the red-green goggles are reversed with the red filter now in front of the left eye.

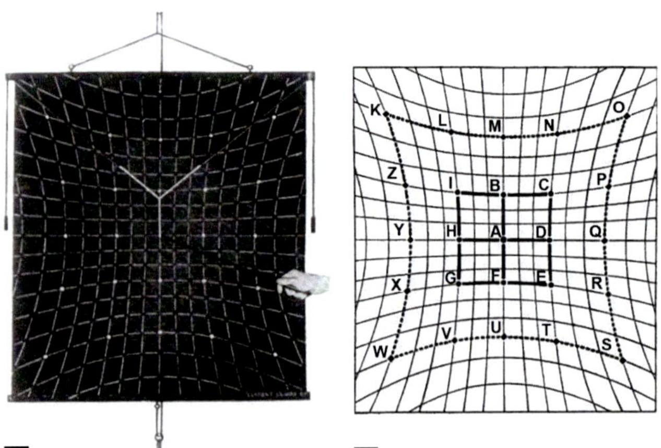

A **B**

Figs. 14A and B: The Hess screen test. (A) The screen; (B) Chart for recording the results.

Source: Lyle TK, Wybar KC. Lyle and Jackson's Practical Orthoptics in the Treatment of Squint [and the Anomalies of Binocular Vision], 5th edition. Springfield, IL: Charles C Thomas; 1967.

MEASUREMENT OF CYCLODEVIATIONS

Qualitative Diagnosis Based on Position of Double Images

The measurement of cyclodeviations in clinical practice relies largely on subjective tests. In patients who have spontaneous diplopia or who can be made to appreciate diplopia by interrupting fusion with alternate covering of the eyes, cyclodeviations can be grossly estimated by holding a ruler horizontally with the straight edge in front of their eyes and slightly below the midline. If one of the cyclovertical rotators is involved, there will be vertical diplopia. By alternately covering the eyes, the examiner then ascertains to which eye the higher or lower image belongs and asks whether the two rulers seen by the patient appear closer on the right or on the left. To avoid any misunderstanding, one should draw a horizontal line and then let the patient add the obliquely seen line.

For quantitative determination of cyclotropia the Lancaster red-green test may be used. *The tilt of the retinal image is opposite the tilt of the horizontal line, as seen by the observer.* **Figures 15A to C**.

Maddox Double Rod Test

For quantitative determination of a cyclodeviation, red and white Maddox rods are placed in a trial frame, the red before the right eye and the white before the left eye **(Fig. 16)**.

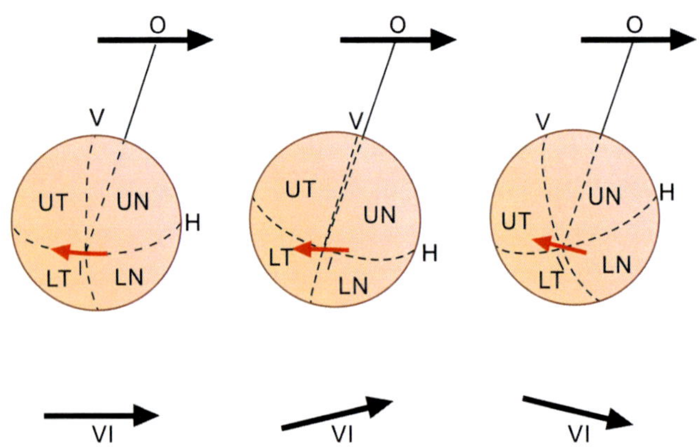

A **B** **C**

Figs. 15A to C: Subjective appearance and retinal image of a horizontal line seen by the left eye. (A) In the absence of a cyclodeviation; (B) with incyclotropia; (C) with excyclotropia.

(V and H: the vertical and horizontal meridians of the retina; UT: upper temporal; UN: upper nasal; LT: lower temporal; and LN: lower nasal, the upper and lower temporal and nasal quadrants of the retina; VI: the resulting visual impression)

The direction of the glass rods is aligned with the 90° marks of the trial frame. A small scratch on the metal frame of the Maddox rods facilitates this alignment. The patient looks through the Maddox rods and is shown a penlight, the images of which appear as horizontal streaks. A vertical prism may be added to separate the images for easier identification. If one of the lines (say, the red one) appears slanted toward the nose **(Fig. 16A)**, excyclotropia of the right eye is present. The red Maddox rod is then turned by the ophthalmologist (or by the patient) until the red line is seen parallel with the white line **(Figs. 16A and B)**. In the presence of bilateral cyclotropia, for instance, excyclotropia of the right and left cyc in bilateral traumatic superior oblique paralysis, both the red and white lines will be seen slanted toward the nose. The settings are repeated two or three times. With good observers, the measurements are extremely accurate. To test the cyclodeviation outside the primary position, shift the penlight to the right, left, above, and below, and repeat the test. To avoid this artifact and the influence of peripheral visual clues, that red Maddox rods will be placed before both eyes and that the test will be performed in a dark room. To distinguish which eye is cyclodeviated one Maddox rod is then slightly rotated back and forth in the trial frame and the patient is asked whether it is the horizontal or tilted luminous line that is "rocking."

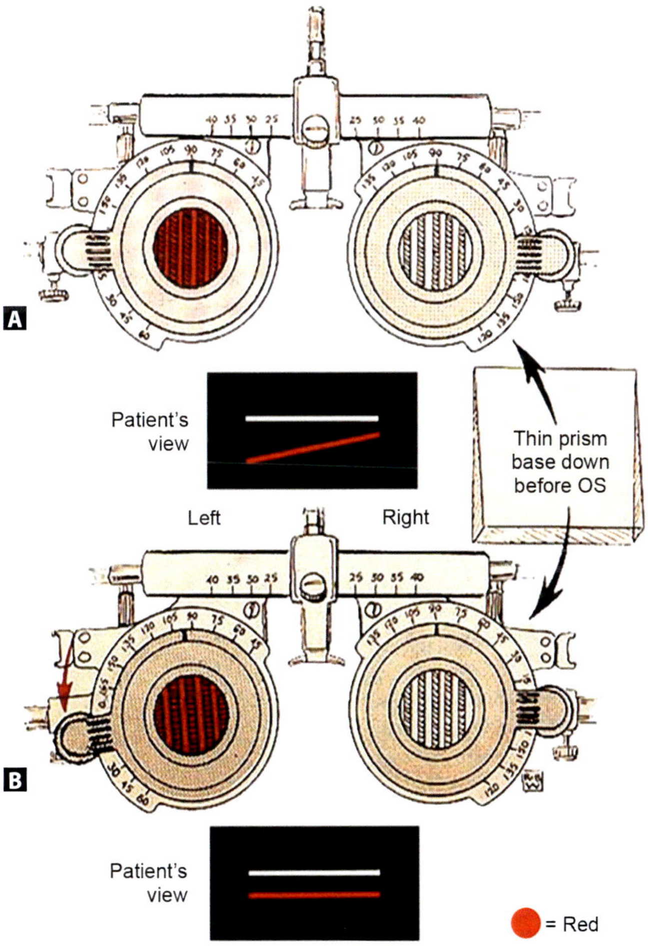

Figs. 16A and B: The Maddox double-rod test.
Source: von Noorden GK. Atlas of Strabismus, 4th edition. St Louis: Mosby–Year Book; 1983. pp. 57.

Bagolini Striated Glasses

To test for cyclotropia under casual viewing conditions, we replace the Maddox rods with the striated glasses of Bagolini. Like Maddox rods, these glasses produce an image of a streak of light, perpendicular to the axis of the striations when viewing a punctate light source, without, however, obstructing surrounding fusible visual details. The glasses are placed in the trial frame with the axes of striation pointing toward the 90 mark. If the patient is unable to fuse the two vertical lines, the glasses are turned until fusion occurs and the amount and direction of the cyclotropia are read off the trial frames as during the Maddox double rod test.

Measurement of Cyclotropia with Major Amblyoscope

To test for cyclotropia, the targets positioned in the arms of this instrument are rotated around an axis until there is no more movement of redress of the eye that takes up fixation. The amount of cyclodeviation, expressed in degrees, can be read off the instrument.

Ophthalmoscopy and Fundus Photography

Indirect ophthalmoscopy and fundus photography are useful auxiliary methods to diagnose cyclotropia. Normally, the average location of the fovea in relation to the optic nerve head is 0.3 disk diameter below a horizontal line extending

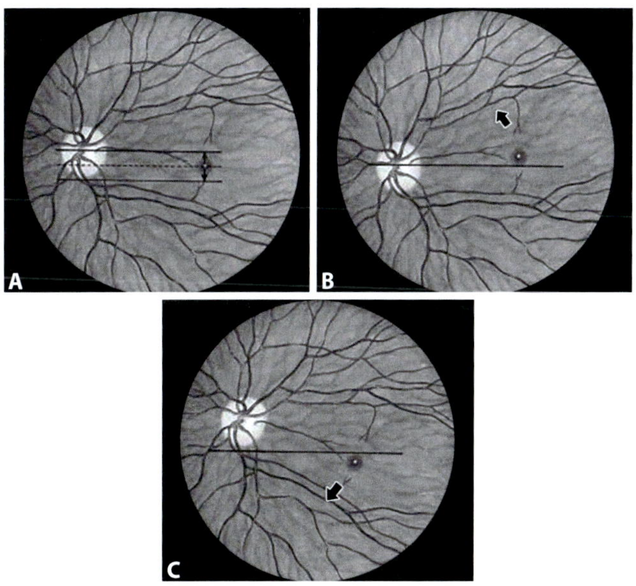

Figs. 17A to C: (A) Average foveal position (dashed line) and range of normal (solid line); (B) Fundus in patient with incyclotropia; (C) Fundus in excyclotropia.
Source: Bixenmann WW, von Noorden GK. Apparent foveal displacement in normal subjects and in cyclotropia. Ophthalmologica. 1982;89:58.

through the geometric center of the optic disk. From this position, an imaginary horizontal line will cross the optic nerve head just below the halfway point between its geometric center and lower pole. Incyclotropia is present when the fovea appears above a line extending horizontally from the center of the optic nerve head, and excyclotropia is present when the fovea is below a line extending horizontally from just below the lower pole of the optic disc **(Figs. 17A to C)**.

THE "NEW CYCLO TEST"

The New Cyclo Test, introduced by Awaya and coworkers, is similar in principle to the Awaya test for aniseikonia and based on haploscopic image separation with red-green spectacles. A red half-moon is viewed through the green glass and a green half-moon through the red glass. In a series of printed figures, the green halfmoon is tilted in a stepwise fashion. The patient selects the figure in which the two half-moons appear to be aligned and the amount of cyclodeviation in degrees is then read off this figure.

SUGGESTED READING

1. Bahil AT, Brokenbrough A, Troost BT. Variability and development of normative data for saccadic eye movements. Invest Ophthalmol Vis Sci. 1981;21:116-25.
2. Derespines PA, Naidu E. Calibration of Hirschberg test photographs under test conditions. Ophthalmology. 1989;96: 944-9.
3. Guyton DL. Exaggerated traction test for oblique muscles. Ophthalmology. 1982;88:1035.
4. Jampel RS. The fundamental principle of action of oblique ocular muscles. Am J Ophthalmol. 1980;69:623.
5. Podos S, Yanoof M. Textbook of Ophthalmology: Strabismus and Pediatric Ophthalmology. United States: Mosby & co.; 1995.
6. Spiegel P, Wright K. The Requisits: Pediatric ophthalmology & Strabismus. United States: Mosby & co.; 1999.
7. Wright K. Pediatric Ophthalmology and Strabismus. United States: Mosby & co.; 1995.

21

CHAPTER

Childhood Esotropia

Nils Mungan

INTRODUCTION

Esotropia is a convergent misalignment of the eyes. About 2% of all children will develop esotropia. It is the most frequent type of strabismus encountered in non-Hispanic Caucasian children in the United States, accounting for 71% of cases, although exotropia is more common among other ethnic groups, especially Asian children.

Traditionally, childhood esotropia has been classified as congenital or acquired, comitant (that is, approximately equal in all directions of gaze) or incomitant, and by etiology. Likewise, congenital esotropia, more accurately labeled as "infantile esotropia (IET)," has typically been the first entity addressed in textbooks. However, accommodative esotropia (AET) is actually far more common than IET. Therefore, it is more clinically relevant to begin by classifying childhood esotropia as accommodative or nonaccommodative, and then subclassify it by comitancy and etiology **(Box 1)**.

BOX 1: Major types of childhood esotropia.

- *Accommodative esotropia*:
  - Fully accommodative ("refractive")
  - Partially (or deteriorated) accommodative
  - High AC/A (accommodative convergence to accommodation) ratio ("nonrefractive")
- *Nonaccommodative esotropia*:
  - Comitant (in horizontal gaze):
    - Infantile esotropia ("congenital esotropia")
    - Esotropia associated with neurodevelopmental conditions
    - Sensory esotropia
    - Consecutive esotropia
    - Acquired nonaccommodative comitant esotropia (ANAET or AACE)
    - Other types (rare): Nystagmus blockage syndrome, convergence spasm, and cyclic esotropia
  - Incomitant (uncommon):
    - Paretic:
      - Duane syndrome
      - Mobius syndrome (rare)
      - Sixth nerve palsy (rare)
      - Childhood myasthenia gravis (rare)
    - Restrictive:
      - Medial orbital fracture
      - Congenital fibrosis of the extraocular muscles (rare)

(AACE: acute acquired comitant esotropia)

PSEUDOESOTROPIA

It is important to recognize that up to 50% of children referred for esotropia to pediatric ophthalmologists do not actually have esotropia. Prominent epicanthal folds and a wide, flat nasal bridge can give the false impression of esotropia by obscuring the nasal sclera. This is known as pseudoesotropia. Because of its association with prominent epicanthal folds, it is more common among children of East Asian descent **(Fig. 1)**.

Parents will often present photographs of the child purporting to show an esodeviation, but on closer inspection, the child's head is often noted to be turned slightly to one side, causing the adducted eye to appear crossed. It is important, however, to recognize that even children with pseudoesotropia can later develop true esotropia, as may any other child. Therefore, if there are risk factors for esotropia present, such as high hyperopia or family history, it is prudent to continue following children with pseudoesotropia. In addition, several studies have shown an incidence of true esotropia as high as 12% following apparent pseudoesotropia, which is much higher than the prevalence of strabismus in the general population, which ranges between 2 and 3%.

ACCOMMODATIVE ESOTROPIA

Accommodative esotropia is the most common form of esotropia, comprising over 50% of all cases of childhood esotropia in most studies. It affects up to 2% of the population in the USA. Mohney found that it is up to 10 times more frequent than IET **(Table 1)**. AET results from the interaction between accommodation and accommodative convergence in the presence of insufficient fusional divergence amplitude. AET may be divided into "refractive" or "nonrefractive" types, or divided into "fully accommodative" or "partially accommodative" forms.

Purely refractive AET, also known as just "refractive" AET, is associated with a large amount of hyperopia leading to a correspondingly large accommodative effort to maintain clear vision. On the other hand, high AC/A (accommodative

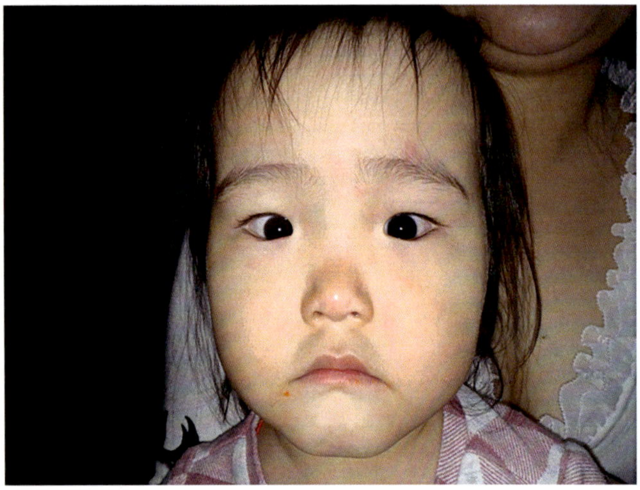

Fig. 1: Pseudoesotropia.
The broad flat nasal bridge and epicanthal folds give a false impression of esotropia in this child, but the corneal light reflex is centered in each pupil.
(*Courtesy*: Miguel Paciuc-Beja, MD; Denver, Colorado, USA)

TABLE 1: Observed forms of esotropia among 221 consecutive patients.

Esotropia type	No.	%
Accommodative:	117	52.9
• Pure	69	
• Partial	48	
Central nervous system defects:	38	17.2
• Congenital	32	
• Acquired	6	
Acquired nonaccommodative	23	10.4
Sensory	15	6.8
Congenital	12	5.4
Paralytic	7	3.2
Unknown age at onset (nonaccommodative)	9	4.1

Source: Adapted from Mohney BG. Common forms of childhood esotropia. Ophthalmology. 2001;108:805-9. Reprinted by permission of Elsevier.

convergence to accommodation) ratio AET, also known as "nonrefractive" AET, is associated with an excessive convergence response at near to a normal amount of accommodative effort. However, as a high AC/A ratio can be associated with any type of refractive state including myopia, astigmatism, emmetropia, or hyperopia, the current author prefers not to refer to this entity as "nonrefractive" AET to avoid giving the false impression that a significant refractive error is always absent. More information on high AC/A ratio esotropia is provided in the separate section next.

"Fully" (also known as "pure") AET responds completely to spectacle correction, whereas "partially" AET has a nonaccommodative component that does not respond to optical correction by spectacles. The term "deteriorated" implies that a previously fully AET later became partial. The distinction between "partial" since presentation and "deteriorated" does not meaningfully impact management.

Fully AET is the most common form of AET, representing about 59% of cases, while partially AET represents 41% of cases. About 15% of all patients with AET have a high AC/A ratio, which can be associated with a distance esotropia and can also be fully or partially accommodative. Therefore, high AC/A ratio AET is actually a subset of both prior categories.

All forms of AET usually begin as an acquired, intermittent esodeviation that gradually becomes constant over time. In some cases, the onset of a constant esotropia is more acute, rarely with diplopia. Occasionally, the esotropia is also noted following illness or trauma, but it is likely that these events precipitated the manifestation of a preexisting latent esophoria, rather than causing it. The average age of onset is 2.5 years, with an average range of 1.5–4 years, although it can occur as early as 2 months of age or as late as 10 years.

All cases of AET with a normal AC/A ratio, whether fully or partially accommodative, are associated with hyperopia, usually of at least +2.00 diopters, and averaging +4.00–+4.75 diopters. Patients with a high AC/A ratio are also usually hyperopic, averaging +2.25 diopters, but may also have any other refractive state.

Risk factors for all types of AET include a positive family history of AET, prior history of surgically repaired IET and anisometropia. Approximately, 75% of patients have a close relative with AET. Several studies indicate that IET is a risk factor for later developing AET. One study reported that up to 60% of children with surgically corrected IET later develop AET within 4 years. These children also tended to develop AET at lower thresholds of hyperopia than other children. The risk of developing AET after IET doubled in the presence of increasing hyperopia, a duration of constant misalignment in infancy of >3 months, or absence of any demonstrable stereopsis. The authors postulated that preexisting sensory abnormalities interfere with maintenance of motor fusion and may thereby allow AET to develop at a lower threshold of hyperopia. A similar mechanism may explain the higher incidence of AET in patients with neurodevelopmental defects. Patients with anisometropia also can develop AET at lower levels of hyperopia compared to other patients.

Fully Accommodative Esotropia

Fully AET is not only the most common type of AET, but the most common form of all strabismus. It begins as an acquired, intermittent esotropia of moderate angle that becomes constant over time. It is always associated with significant hyperopia, and the esodeviation is adequately reduced by spectacle wear alone. If the AC/A ratio is also normal, which it is 85% of the time, then this type is also called "refractive" AET.

Clinical Evaluation

The typical presenting history of all forms of AET has been covered above. The clinical evaluation consists of a full ophthalmology examination, paying special attention to visual acuity, alignment, and refraction. Amblyopia is present on first evaluation in 59–61% of patients. Versions and ductions should be carefully assessed and will be normal in this type of esotropia. The esodeviation is usually relatively small on alternate cover testing, 20–40 prism diopters (PD) (10–20°), variable over time, comitant, and equal within 10 PD at near compared to distance fixation. Cycloplegic refraction reveals hyperopia averaging +4.75 diopters, with a range from +3.00 to +10.00 diopters. Patients with high levels of hyperopia (mean +6.50), however, may have straight eyes with bilateral amblyopia rather than esotropia. On the other hand, children with a history of neurodevelopmental issues, prematurity, corrected IET, subnormal sensory fusion, or anisometropia may develop esotropia at considerably lower levels of hyperopia (+1.00–+2.00).

Management

Spectacles: The mainstay of treating AET is spectacles to correct the hyperopia **(Figs. 2A and B)**. This should be accomplished as soon as possible because a delay of even a few months can cause permanent damage to the child's binocularity. Children who experienced 4 or more months of constant esotropia before receiving spectacle correction were 33 times more likely to have no stereopsis compared to children who received spectacles sooner, and 4.6 times more likely to have subnormal stereopsis. The duration of constant esotropia is more important than the age at onset of the AET and the age at alignment in determining the ultimate sensory outcome. There is also evidence that a delay in wearing spectacles increases the chance of decompensation to a non-AET requiring surgery. Therefore, any patient referred for possible AET should be seen and treated promptly, regardless of age.

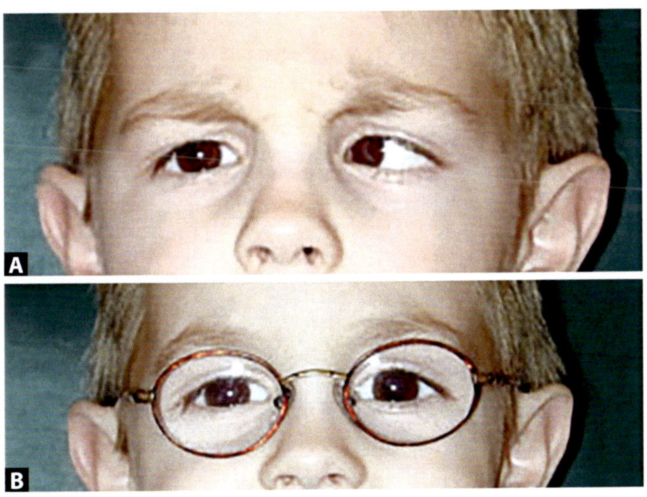

Fig. 2A and B: Fully accommodative esotropia. Spectacles consisting of the full cycloplegic refraction have completely corrected this child's esotropia.

(*Courtesy*: Brown S, Arbor A, Michigan, USA; under open license from https://commons.wikimedia.org/wiki/File:Esotropia-uncorrected.jpg and https://commons.wikimedia.org/wiki/File:Esotropia-corrected.jpg).

The minimum threshold to prescribe glasses for hyperopia is lower when esotropia is present: +2.00 diopters if the child is <age 2, but +1.50 if over age 2, and any amount if anisometropia >1.00 diopter is present.

Traditional teaching dictates that the first spectacle prescription in esotropic patients should consist of the full cycloplegic refraction. Some authors have shown that an undercorrection of as little as 1.00 diopter <the full cycloplegic refraction can lead to a continued manifest esotropia in 40% of patients. However, other clinicians contend that many children will not relax their accommodation fully and therefore have blurry vision in their full prescription glasses, leading to poor compliance with spectacle wear. Poor compliance has been shown to lead to poor motor and sensory outcomes. If the esodeviation is small and the hyperopia large, it may be reasonable to undercorrect the hyperopia by 1–2 diopters and follow the patient closely to ensure that decompensation does not occur. After all, a weaker pair of glasses that the patient actually wears is always better than a stronger pair of glasses that is left at home. Park et al. found that visual acuity, stereoacuity and motor fusion did not deteriorate in the vast majority of children while wearing undercorrected spectacles over 2 years of follow-up. In the few such patients who did worsen on follow-up, only a few did not improve by returning to the full cycloplegic prescription. Therefore, judicious undercorrection of high hyperopes with small esodeviations seems reasonable if accompanied by close follow-up.

The parents should be counseled that the glasses should be worn at all times, as children will continue to have esotropia when they are not wearing the glasses, and will have trouble relaxing their accommodation if they are worn only intermittently, which will cause blurry vision and will decrease compliance. It is helpful to use language that parents can understand, such as explaining that "the glasses do the focusing esotropia, but only control the esotropia while the glasses are actually being worn". In fact, the esotropia without glasses often becomes worse after the glasses are initiated, because the child becomes accustomed to the clear vision obtained with correction. It is also important to explain to the parents that the glasses do not cure the glasses off, a greater accommodative effort may occur to recover this clear vision. This is best explained beforehand; otherwise many parents will feel that the glasses have made their child's esotropia worse or made their child become "dependent" on glasses.

If a child will not comply with glasses despite the parents' best efforts, the cycloplegic refraction should be repeated to ensure its accuracy. The new glasses should be inspected while on the patient's face to ensure that the size and fit are correct, as a poor fit will lead to poor compliance. Reducing the strength of the hyperopic prescription in appropriate situations may improve compliance. If compliance is still poor, temporary use of cycloplegic drops at home may be used for 1–2 weeks to give the child an "optical incentive" to wear the glasses.

Anticholinesterase ("miotic") drops: Anticholinesterase eye drops such as phospholine iodide (PI), also known as echothiophate iodide, and diisopropyl fluorophosphate (DFP) can sometimes be effective as an alternative to glasses for AET, especially when a high AC/A ratio is present. By prolonging the action of acetylcholine on the ciliary body, these agents can reduce the "accommodative effort" required to achieve a given level of accommodation, thereby also reducing the accommodative convergence. However, the drops are only 42% as effective as spectacles. There are also numerous adverse effects, the most common ocular being iris cysts in 20–40%. The concurrent use of phenylephrine drops may prevent iris cysts. The drops can also cause angle closure, cataract and retinal detachment in adults, although these effects have never been reported in children. Systemic effects include brow ache, headache, abdominal cramps, and nausea, but most significantly, prolonged paralysis after the use of depolarizing muscle relaxants such as succinylcholine during general anesthesia. Finally, neither PI nor DFP is currently available in the USA. Miotic drops are seldom used today, although they may have a small role in patients who are noncompliant with glasses or otherwise unable to wear glasses.

Refractive Surgery

Some authors have investigated the possibility of performing photorefractive keratectomy (PRK) or laser-assisted in situ keratomileusis (LASIK) in patients who are noncompliant with spectacles, usually older patients with cognitive and behavioral impairments. In most cases, alignment within 10 PD was achieved, and many had improvement in uncorrected visual acuity and stereopsis. However, follow-up was short in many cases. Challenges included the fact that many refractive errors are not stable until adulthood, and that the amount of hyperopia needing to be corrected exceeded current capabilities of LASIK. In addition, general anesthesia is often required, reducing the accuracy and safety of the procedure. Loss of fusion has been reported after LASIK in patients with AET, even in a 22-year-old patient. Use of refractive surgery in AET patients remains investigational.

Follow-up/Course

After prescribing spectacles, the child should be seen back in 4–8 weeks as it takes this amount of time for the full relaxation of accommodation and reduction of esotropia to become apparent. Testing the patient with the prescription in trial frames in the office does not give a true picture of the full effectiveness of the glasses. The goal is to achieve alignment within 8 PD of orthotropia, as this allows at least peripheral fusion and gross stereopsis to occur. If the child is well aligned in glasses and without amblyopia, further follow-up can occur every 6 months. If the child is not well aligned in glasses at both distance and near, then partially AET is present (see separate section below). If the child is well aligned at distance but not at near, then a high AC/A ratio is likely present (see next).

Amblyopia: If amblyopia is present, it may improve with glasses alone, by a process originally called "refractive adaptation" by British authors, but later called "optical treatment" by American researchers. Of 146 children with strabismic or combined mechanism amblyopia, 25% resolved with spectacles alone. Amblyopia improved even if the strabismus did not improve in glasses, and the improvement in amblyopia was independent of either the degree of the refractive error or esotropia. The maximum improvement was seen in 50% of patients by 9 weeks, and 90% of patients by 18 weeks. Therefore, in patients with amblyopia, the current author follows patients for several weeks to months after prescribing glasses and only prescribes patching or atropine, if the visual acuity does not continue improving. This may increase the chance of compliance with the glasses by not initiating two treatments at the same time (i.e., glasses and occlusion), and may also facilitate compliance with later patching if needed, by improving the visual acuity of the unpatched eye beforehand.

It has been shown that unilaterally withholding optical correction from the sound eye does not significantly improve the effect of atropine.

If surgery for the esotropia is needed, the traditional recommendation is to first wait until all amblyopia treatment is completed, although differences of opinion exist (see management of partially AET for further information).

Deterioration: Cycloplegic refraction should be repeated every 6–12 months depending on the patient's age, and also whenever the visual acuity or esotropia is found to worsen on follow-up. Even if the initial alignment in spectacles is good, the esotropia may deteriorate over time into a partially AET. Deterioration has been reported to occur in 10–40% of cases. It usually occurs by age 5 and rarely after age 7. The risk of deterioration might be higher if there was a delay in initiating spectacle wear, very early onset of the esotropia (before age 2), a high AC/A ratio, larger esodeviation, smaller hyperopia, or presence of amblyopia. However, the data are conflicting on many of these claims. Deterioration may be caused by gradual contracture of the medial rectus muscles or surrounding tissues.

Weaning: One of the most common questions asked by parents is whether their child will always need to wear glasses.

Lambert et al., found that 60% of children with 5.00 diopters or less of hyperopia could be gradually weaned out of glasses starting at the age of visual maturity, that is, at a mean of 8 years old. The spectacles were reduced no more frequently than every 6 months by 0.50 diopter steps, as warranted by a change in the refraction. The odds of successful weaning increased if baseline hyperopia was 3.00 diopters or less, if no increase in hyperopia by >1.00 diopter had occurred since baseline, and if patients had had strabismus surgery. Weaning is less likely to be successful if there is a history of premature birth, high hyperopia, a high AC/A ratio, or anisometropia. In contrast to the study by Lambert, however, a population-based study by Mohney found that the rate of spectacle discontinuation was only 8% at 5 years, 20% at 10 years, and 37% at 20 years after diagnosis. It is clear that many patients will continue to require optical correction to control their esotropia during adulthood.

Long-term Sensory Outcomes

Although binocular vision matures by age 18 months, it is still susceptible to damage until at least 4 years of age. Timely prescription of the full cycloplegic refraction is thought by many to prevent adverse binocular sensory outcomes. Although crude stereopsis is possible with 8 PD of esotropia, Lee found that high quality stereopsis was only possible with 4 PD or less of residual esotropia in glasses. While 59–61% of patients may have amblyopia at presentation, only 15–23% had amblyopia after 4.5–5 years of follow-up. About 70–89% had gross stereopsis but only 24–25% had high grade stereopsis on long-term follow-up. High-grade stereopsis was more likely to be present if patients were treated before the esotropia became constant, and if they did not require bifocals or surgery.

Partially Accommodative Esotropia

Partially AET is defined by the persistence of 10 or more PD of esotropia at both distance and near after the patient has been wearing his full cycloplegic refraction for at least 4–6 weeks. The risk factors for having or developing a nonaccommodative component to the esotropia were discussed above (section on "deterioration" in fully AET).

Clinical Evaluation

Any time that a possibly nonaccommodative component is present, the clinician should first recheck the cycloplegic refraction to ensure that the entire amount of hyperopia is in fact being corrected with glasses. The risk of amblyopia is higher in partially AET than fully accommodative cases. Otherwise the evaluation is as described above for fully AET.

Management

Partially AET requires surgical correction. Most commonly, a bilateral medial rectus recession is performed, but in the case of irreversible decreased visual acuity, a unilateral recess-resect procedure on the worse-seeing eye may be preferred. Surgery should not be delayed, as even 4 months of untreated residual esotropia may permanently harm binocular vision. Approximately one-third of all patients with AET ultimately require surgery. Patients and parents should be counseled that glasses will still be required after surgery. The goal of surgery is not to eliminate glasses, but to align the eyes while the glasses are worn. The one exception to this is that surgery can also be considered in older teen-age or adult patients with fully AET and minimal hyperopia who wish to discontinue glasses.

There are differences of opinion as to the timing of surgery around amblyopia, and what the target angle of deviation for surgery consists of.

It is usually advisable to wait until amblyopia therapy is complete before doing surgery. Preoperative amblyopia treatment may improve, or, rarely, worsen the esotropia and therefore change the surgical plan. Surgery on patients with moderate-to-severe amblyopia has a lower success rate, both by motor and sensory criteria. Amblyopia treatment may interfere with the reestablishment of fusion after surgery. Also, the risk of consecutive (postoperative) exotropia has been reported to be higher in the presence of amblyopia. Amblyopia is easier to detect in a preverbal child by fixation preference testing before the eyes are aligned. Finally, parents may be less motivated to treat amblyopia after surgery, when an external abnormality to the eye is no longer visible to them. On the other hand, in some cases, amblyopia treatment itself may be facilitated by aligning the eyes beforehand.

The largest area of controversy concerns the dosage of surgery that should be performed, which in turn depends on what preoperative deviation is "targeted" for surgical alignment. There are essentially four measured esodeviations—the distance versus the near deviation, and whether measured with or without spectacle correction. The standard approach has been to operate for the distance deviation with correction, which is the smallest deviation. However, this results in a high undercorrection rate of 25%. To compensate for this unacceptably high rate of undercorrection, many surgeons simply add an additional 0.5–1.0 mm of recession to their surgical nomogram or target the near angle with correction instead. Wright developed an "augmented" surgical formula which targeted the mean of the near deviation with correction and the near deviation without correction. This increased the success rate to 93%, however, it also increased the overcorrection rate to 7%. All of the patients with consecutive exotropia had a high AC/A ratio preoperatively. Subsequently, Wright modified his formula to target the mean of the smallest deviation (distance with correction) and the largest deviation (near without correction).

Another method of formulating a surgical plan consists of the "prism adaptation test." Temporary membrane prisms

(Fresnel prisms) are pressed onto the patient's spectacle lenses to fully neutralize the esotropia on cover testing. The patient is then sent home wearing these prism spectacles and returns in 1–2 weeks to be rechecked. If the amount of esotropia has increased, the prism power is increased to match the new deviation, and the patient is again checked 1–2 weeks later. The process is repeated until the esotropia stops increasing. Surgery is then performed for the full "prism adapted" angle that is thus revealed. This increases the success rate of surgery from 75 to 85%. However, disadvantages include the increased number of visits and expense involved. The prisms can also blur vision and the process delays the time to the ultimate repair of the esotropia.

Follow-up

If a large overcorrection with reduced adduction is present within days of the surgery, the possibility of a slipped or lost muscle should be considered, requiring an early return to the operating room. If an esotropia >10 PD persists for weeks, the cycloplegic refraction should be rechecked and addressed if needed. If the persistent esotropia is only significant at near, bifocals should be considered (see high AC/A ratio section next). Otherwise, repeat surgery should be performed. If a consecutive exotropia is present, which is more likely in patients with continued amblyopia or higher hyperopia, reducing the plus power of the spectacles by up to 2.50 diopters may help control the exotropia. Reducing the spectacle power more than this is likely to make the strabismus becomes unstable and requires reoperation. Even if the surgery is successful, the prognosis for peripheral fusion and good stereopsis is lower than in fully AET.

High AC/A Ratio Accommodative Esotropia

If the esotropia at near fixation exceeds the esotropia at distance by >10 PD, while the full cycloplegic refraction is worn, the patient is said to have a high AC/A ratio (accommodative convergence to accommodation). These patients typically present at an earlier age than patients with a normal AC/A ratio, at approximately 2.7 years and have a lower mean amount of hyperopia, +2.25 diopters. However, patients may have any type of refractive state, including myopia or emmetropia. Most patients with a high AC/A ratio actually also have a refractive AET, that is, hyperopia with a distance esotropia that is fully or partly corrected with spectacles, rather than solely an esotropia at near. Therefore, as previously stated, referring to all cases of high AC/A ratio as "nonrefractive" AET is confusing and misleading.

As previously stated, accommodative effort is linked to convergence. The accommodation needed will depend on the refractive state of the eye, while the convergence needed will depend on fixation distance and interpupillary distance. In purely refractive AET, the problem is that there is excess accommodative "demand" due to uncorrected hyperopia, which leads to an excess amount of convergence. However, in purely nonrefractive cases, the problem is that an excess amount of convergence occurs despite normal accommodative demand.

Clinical Evaluation

A normal AC/A ratio is 3–5 depending on the method used to measure it. A strict calculation of the ratio is not needed in order to clinically manage the patient. Most clinicians simply consider a high ratio to be present if the near deviation exceeds the distance deviation by 10 PD or more while wearing the full cycloplegic refraction. This is sometimes called the "clinical method" of assessing the AC/A ratio. The other two methods quantify the ratio by comparing the change in the esodeviation that occurs when the fixation distance is changed (the heterophoria method) or when the accommodative demand is changed (the lens gradient method).

For the heterophoria method, the deviation is measured at distance and at near in single vision spectacle lenses (SVL), if glasses are applicable. The interpupillary distance is measured as well. The calculation for the heterophoria method is as follows:

$$AC/A = IPD + (D_n - D_d)/D$$

where IPD is the interpupillary distance in centimeters, D_n is the esodeviation in SVL at near in PD, D_d is that deviation at distance, and D is the fixation distance at near in diopters, which is the reciprocal of the distance in meters. For example, 33 cm = 0.3 m, which would be 1/0.3 = 3 diopters.

For the lens gradient method, also known as just the "gradient method," the deviation is measured at any fixed distance, first without additional lenses placed over the SVL, and then with additional lenses to change the accommodative demand. The patient can be measured at near or distance, as long as the same distance is used both times. Likewise, the additional lenses placed over the SVL can be plus power in order to relax accommodation, or can be minus lenses in order to stimulate accommodation.

The calculation for the gradient method is as follows:

$$AC/A = (D_0 - D_1)/P$$

where D_0 is the deviation at any fixed distance in SVL without extra lenses, D_1 is the deviation at that same distance with extra lenses, and P is the power of the additional lenses placed over the SVL.

Management

Several approaches have been used to treat the excess convergence at near in patients with a high AC/A ratio including observation, bifocal spectacles, and surgery.

Observation

Many clinicians do not feel additional intervention is warranted if the eyes are well aligned at distance, claiming this distance alignment protects binocular vision even if the eyes continue to cross at near. Supporting evidence consists of the following—the AC/A ratio usually improves spontaneously with age, partly due to an increasing interpupillary distance, and the binocular vision improves as well. Bifocals may improve the comfort of fusion but may not improve amblyopia, sensory fusion, or stereopsis. Bifocals may not prevent deterioration, and in fact may be associated with a greater need for surgery in the future and less improvement in the AC/A ratio over time, although other studies show the opposite (more information on the long-term effect of bifocals is provided here).

However, others believe that even if the eyes are straight at distance, excess convergence at near can cause amblyopia, loss of binocularity, asthenopia, a poor cosmetic appearance and sometimes diplopia, and therefore observation is not appropriate.

Bifocals

The majority of clinicians will prescribe bifocals for children with >10 PD of esotropia at near after they have worn any needed distance glasses for 4–6 weeks, although some prescribe bifocals at the first visit if marked convergence excess at near is observed, in an attempt to avoid having the parents purchase glasses twice in a row. The initial bifocal add prescribed is usually +2.50–+3.00 sphere, later titrated to the minimum add needed to keep the eyes aligned at near. A flat-top bifocal segment is preferred, and the prescription should specify that the segment be placed higher on the lens than what is customary for adults. Otherwise, the child may look over the segment at near rather than through it. Most clinicians feel the bifocal line should bisect the pupil but others feel it should be no higher than the lower edge of the pupil. The current author will start toddlers with the bifocal line in the center of the pupil, but move it progressively more inferiorly with increasing age, as older children will complain that the line interferes with downgaze at intermediate distances. Older children can also be successfully managed with "no-line" progressive bifocals. When prescribing progressive lenses, the optician should be instructed to start the transition zone several millimeters higher than customary for adults. If the child will not comply with bifocals, miotic drops may help as they do decrease the AC/A ratio, although the ratio does revert to pretreatment levels when the drops are discontinued. Other options in noncompliant children include observation in SVL alone, as stated above, or surgery in some cases.

After prescribing bifocals, the child is seen again in 4–6 weeks to determine whether the esotropia at near has decreased to <10 PD. If success is achieved, the child can then be followed every 3–6 months unless amblyopia requiring closer management is present. If bifocals fail to achieve the desired effect, or if a previously controlled esotropia at near decompensates, then surgery is considered after rechecking the cycloplegic refraction. Over time, the power of the bifocals can be slowly reduced to produce a small esophoria of 4–6 PD at near which may increase the fusional divergence amplitude, improving the AC/A ratio and allowing the bifocals to be weaned sooner. Usually, weaning can be started at age 7–8 and completed by age 10–12. Successful weaning has been reported to occur in 37–55% of patients. Inability to wean by the teen years can be an indication for surgery. If the patient also needs glasses for distance, switching to contact lenses often obviates the need for multifocal lenses, because less accommodation is required due to the optics of the reduced vertex distance. If not, bifocal contact lenses may also work.

There is conflicting information on which factors increase the chance of successful weaning. Some authors have found that the higher the initial AC/A ratio, the greater the chance, it will decrease over time, whereas others have found the opposite, and that a higher AC/A ratio increases the chance of decompensation over time. Similarly, some have concluded that a good initial response to bifocals improves the chances of normalization of the AC/A ratio over time, while others claim the opposite. Finally, some have found that wearing bifocals reduces the improvement in the AC/A ratio over time, whereas others have found that bifocals make no difference in this regard. There is a higher success rate of weaning from bifocals if good stereopsis is present.

Surgery

The indications for surgery in high AC/A ratio AET are somewhat controversial, if the eyes are well aligned at distance. Some clinicians will only recommend surgery if bifocals fail to align the eyes, while others prefer surgery to bifocals as the initial treatment. Many will also recommend surgery to eliminate the need for bifocals in older patients who cannot be successfully weaned.

Several different approaches to surgery have been used. If there is a significant distance esotropia as well (partially AET with a high AC/A ratio), operating for the distance deviation may also be adequate to correct the near deviation, given that bilateral medial rectus recession itself has been shown to markedly reduce the AC/A ratio. However, as this often results in an undercorrection at near, adding a scleral posterior fixation suture (Faden suture) has been advocated. Theoretically, a Faden suture only weakens a muscle in its field of action without affecting primary position alignment, reducing the risk of overcorrection at distance. However, Kushner et al., have found that operating for the near angle (while wearing distance correction) was more effective than a Faden suture, both in terms of postoperative alignment and ability to discontinue bifocal use. Furthermore, if the hyperopia was <+2.50 diopters, he advocated operating for the near angle without correction in order to allow glasses to be discontinued entirely. As previously mentioned, Wright recommends operating for the mean of the distance angle with correction (the smallest deviation) and the near angle without correction (the largest deviation) if there is a high AC/A ratio.

Newer approaches to surgery for the near-distance disparity include posterior pulley fixation sutures or the "Scott" procedure of performing a simultaneous recession and resection on the same muscle.

Long-term Sensory Outcomes

Patients with a high AC/A ratio have a worse prognosis for binocular vision than patients with refractive AET. As previously mentioned above (under Management-Observation), bifocals do not appear to improve long-term sensory outcome. Ultimately, only 5–12% of patients develop high-grade stereopsis.

INFANTILE ESOTROPIA

Infantile esotropia is a constant non-AET with onset before 6 months of age. It has also been called "congenital esotropia," although this is a misnomer as it is almost never present at birth. Although it is a fairly rare cause of childhood esotropia **(*see* Box 1)**, variously reported as occurring in 0.1–0.25% of children, it has been important to our understanding of the development of binocular vision and the timing of treatment. The risk of IET is well known to increase with any condition affecting neurodevelopment, including prematurity, low birthweight, hydrocephalus, cerebral palsy, chromosomal anomalies, and maternal smoking, alcohol, or drug abuse during pregnancy. The risk of esotropia may be as high as 44% in infants with neurodevelopmental issues. Many authors, however, exclude cases with neurological impairments from the category of IET itself. No specific genes for esotropia have been identified, but a positive family history has been noted in 34–45% of patients, although often for different types of strabismus such as AET, exotropia, or superior oblique palsy. The concordance rate for IET between monozygous (identical) twins is 81%, and 9% in dizygous twins, indicating a strong genetic component. Maumenee concluded that the trait was inherited in a Mendelian codominant pattern.

Pathophysiology

The cause of IET remains unknown. Historically, two competing theories have held sway. Worth believed the primary cause was a central congenital defect in sensory fusion, but Chavasse maintained that it was primarily a motor disorder and that the sensory abnormalities occurred secondarily as a consequence of the misalignment. The Chavasse theory was more widely accepted in America, notably by Costenbader and Parks, and gained further credence by the pioneering work of Ing, who showed that early surgical intervention improved the chance of attaining fusion and stereopsis. Hubel and Wiesel showed that inducing esotropia in infant animals produced changes in binocular cells in the lateral geniculate nucleus and striate cortex, which suggests that it is indeed the motor abnormality that causes the sensory abnormalities and not the converse. However, even with early successful realignment of the eyes, very few patients achieve high-grade stereopsis, indicating that elements of both theories may be correct. Other evidence supporting primary sensory abnormalities include the fact that orthotropic parents of children with IET are 11 times more likely to have primary monofixation syndrome (MFS) (a rare congenital absence of fine stereopsis without inciting factors), and the fact that a high-concordance rate of stereoacuity exists between orthotropic identical twins. Helveston believed there were two kinds of IET patients—those whose outcomes more closely reflected the Worth theory, and those who reflected the Chavasse theory.

Clinical Evaluation

Many newborns have transient strabismus in the first 2–3 months after birth, usually exotropia, but occasionally esotropia. The Congenital Esotropia Observation Study (CEOS) found that esotropia in the first 2–3 months of life was often small to moderate, variable, and intermittent. If the esodeviation was <40 PD and intermittent, up to 78% resolved spontaneously, whereas if a constant esotropia of 40 or more PD was present on two separate examinations at 10 weeks of age or older, with a cycloplegic refraction <+3.00 diopters, the chance of resolution without surgery was >3%.

Infantile esotropia usually presents as a large constant esotropia of 40 PD or more with full ductions (comitant) and normal refractive error **(Fig. 3)**. The angle of deviation

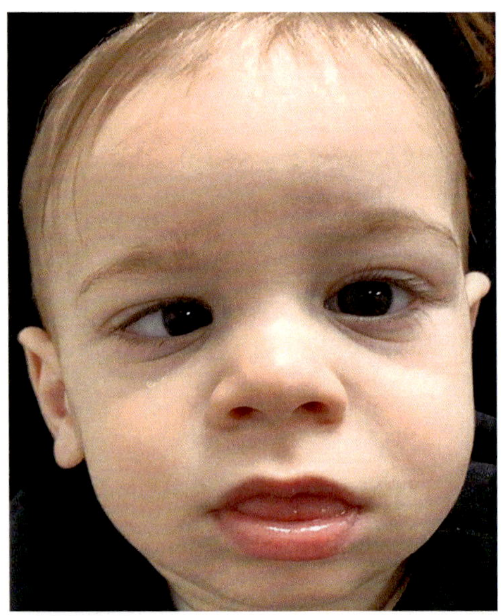

Fig. 3: Infantile esotropia. Infantile esotropia typically presents as a large angle constant esotropia by 6 months of age.
(*Courtesy:* Tamara Wygnanski-Jaffe, MD; Tel Aviv, Israel)

increases in the majority of IET patients over time, with 50% increasing by 20 PD or more.

Usually, patients with IET are seen when they are still preverbal, rendering parts of the examination more challenging. The child usually has equal visual acuity in each eye if there is no fixation preference between the two eyes. This can be confirmed by either observing spontaneous alternation occurring, or by briefly occluding the fixating eye to cause the deviating eye to take up fixation. After the occlusion is removed, the formerly deviating eye should maintain fixation through a blink, smooth pursuit (especially across the midline), and/or several seconds if no amblyopia is present. Many patients cross-fixate: that is, use the right eye in adduction to look at objects in the left field and the left eye to look at objects in the right field. Cross-fixation also usually indicates that no significant amblyopia is present, although sometimes mild amblyopia is still present. The CEOS found that the incidence of amblyopia was proportional to the duration of the esotropia, with an incidence of 19% at 2 months but 42% at 6 months. Other authors have reported amblyopia rates from 6 to 72%, somewhat dependent on length of follow-up.

Abduction of each eye should be full, but may show a pseudodeficit in a patient with a large esotropia and cross-fixation, because the contralateral eye will be used to regard the opposite visual field rather than abducting the ipsilateral eye. In this situation, abduction can usually be verified as normal by one of three methods. First, the fellow eye can be occluded to force fixation with the tested eye. Second, the examiner may use the oculocephalic reflex ("doll's head" maneuver) by gently turning the patient's head to the opposite side while having him fixate on an interesting target. Lastly, the vestibulo-ocular reflex (VOR) may be used by picking up the infant and spinning him horizontally both clockwise and then counterclockwise. This will induce a nystagmus with the fast phase (a saccade) opposite the direction of spin, confirming intact ductions to that side. The medial rectus muscle, one or both, can also be moderately restricted from contracture due to a large long-standing esodeviation, in which case observing a brisk abduction saccade will rule out a paresis. Forced duction testing immediately before surgery can confirm such restriction.

Monocular smooth pursuit asymmetry is normal in all infants <6 months of age, with pursuit in the temporal to nasal direction being better than pursuit from nasal to temporal. In 100% of children with IET, however, this asymmetric pursuit persists throughout life, regardless of successful treatment of the esotropia or amblyopia. It is best appreciated by having the patient observes an optokinetic drum rotating in each direction, with one eye patched. This can be a clinically useful marker for IET in a patient presenting at an older age in whom the date of onset is in doubt.

In very young patients, frequently the deviation can only be measured at near. In descending order of accuracy, the deviation can be measured by the prism alternate cover test, the Krimsky test or the Hirschberg test. The deviation is usually constant and large, averaging 50–60 PD.

If cycloplegic retinoscopy reveals 2.00 or more diopters of hyperopia, strong consideration should be given to the possibility of early-onset AET rather than IET, and a trial of glasses may be warranted.

Complete ocular evaluation including fundus examination should always be conducted on all new patients, as visually significant lesions including cataract and retinoblastoma can cause a sensory esotropia.

Additional findings in patients with IET include nystagmus, inferior oblique overaction (IOOA), and dissociated vertical deviation (DVD), but as these usually occur somewhat later than initial presentation, these will be discussed below under the "follow-up" section.

Ciancia Syndrome

Ciancia syndrome is a severe form of IET, with an esodeviation typically >60 PD with very limited abduction of both eyes. Nystagmus occurs on attempted abduction of either eye. Even the fixing eye remains in adduction, with a compensatory face turn toward the same side. Cross-fixation is consistently present. On forced duction testing, the medial rectus muscles are found to be tight. Undercorrection after surgery is common, and very large medial rectus recessions (7 mm or more) are needed.

Management

The treatment of IET is surgical. The goal of surgery is to restore normal alignment in order to improve binocular vision, amblyopia, and appearance.

Surgery usually consists of a bilateral medial rectus recession or a unilateral medial rectus recession combined with a lateral rectus resection/plication, which has been shown to be equally effective. If significant IOOA is present, it is addressed at the same surgery (see follow-up below). Larger amounts of esotropia may require operating on 3 or 4 horizontal muscles.

Classically, it has been taught that all amblyopia treatment should be completed prior to surgery, but differences of opinion exist (see also the section on management of partially AET above for further discussion). Lam found no change in motor or sensory outcome, if amblyopia therapy was postponed until after early surgery and some cases of amblyopia in older children resolved by surgery alone. Others have found no difference in outcome performing surgery first if the amblyopia was mild, but outcomes were worse if the amblyopia was moderate or severe. The benefits of completing amblyopia therapy before surgery probably need to be balanced against the benefits of performing surgery as early as possible.

The timing of surgery remains somewhat controversial. Historically, surgery has been performed early in the United

States, usually between age 6 and 24 months, while in parts of Western Europe, surgery has been deferred until age 2–4 years or later. This has been partly based on whether the Chavasse theory or the Worth theory has been more widely believed (see Infantile Esotropia: Pathophysiology section above).

Rationale for Early Surgery

As little as 3 weeks of prism-induced esotropia in infant monkeys has been shown to lead to a permanent decrease in binocularly driven cells in the visual cortex with a loss of stereopsis. Birch and others, using visual evoked potential (VEP) and forced preferential looking techniques in human infants, have shown that stereopsis develops abruptly beginning at 3–5 months of age and matures to an adult level by just 6–7 months. The critical period for susceptibility of stereopsis to disruption was found to peak at a mean of just 4.3 months.

In 1981, Ing reported that in a group of patients with IET, 80% developed at least peripheral fusion if aligned before 2 years of age. If surgery was delayed beyond 2 years, only 20% developed fusion. Ing later reanalyzed the data and found that the prevalence of stereopsis was greater if patients had surgery before 1 year of age. Wright operated even earlier, at age 13–19 weeks, in a small series of seven patients and found that five of them developed stereopsis, of which three had high-grade stereopsis. In a larger group of patients, Birch found that better fusion, stereopsis and fine stereopsis developed if surgery was performed before 6 months of age. However, only 38% developed any stereopsis, and only 20% had 200 seconds of arc or better on Randot testing. In a follow-up paper, she found that it was the duration of misalignment rather than the age of onset or the age at alignment that was the critical factor in determining stereopsis. If the duration of constant esotropia was >2 months, no patient had excellent stereopsis. If the duration was >12 months, only 4% had any stereopsis at all. The mean duration of esotropia before alignment in patients with measurable stereopsis was 9 ± 1.1 weeks versus 16 ± 0.7 weeks in patients with no stereopsis. Therefore, the window of time to intervene in these patients for the best sensory results seems to be very narrow indeed. The effect of age at surgery on stereopsis is summarized in **Figure 4**. Achieving some stereopsis was clinically relevant, Birch found that if stereopsis was absent, the risk of developing DVD was 2.5 times higher and the risk of needing reoperation on the horizontal muscles was 3.6 times higher.

Rationale for Later Surgery

There are several reasons, it may be better to delay surgery for IET. In very young patients, it may be difficult to measure the angle of esodeviation accurately. There may be a lack of stability in the angle, and it may increase or decrease over time, including undergoing complete spontaneous resolution in 34–48% of cases. Surgery in very small eyes may be more technically difficult, and anesthetic risk higher.

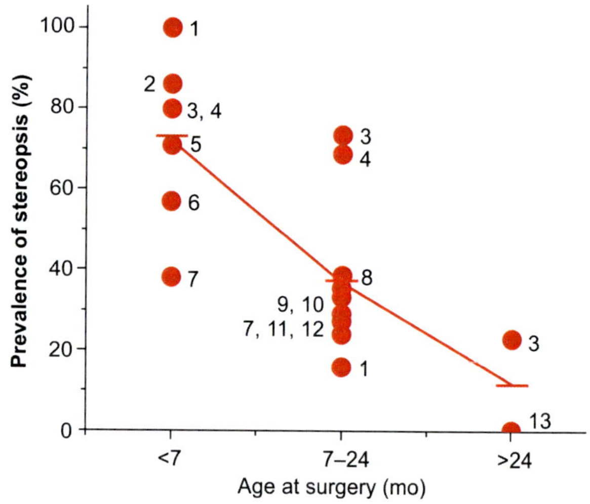

Fig. 4: Summary of stereopsis outcome by age at surgery. Each circle indicates the prevalence of stereopsis from each study cited. Short horizontal dashes represent mean prevalence of stereopsis for different age groups.

Source: Wong AMF. Timing of surgery for infantile esotropia: sensory and motor outcomes. Can J Ophthalmol. 2008;43:643-51. Reprinted by permission of Elsevier.

Ing found that the angle of esodeviation increases over the first few months if observed, with 50% of cases increasing by over 20 PD. The angle may not be stable until after 6 months. This may explain why Helveston found that if patients had surgery before age 6 months, they required on average one more surgery over long-term follow-up to 10 years. A meta-regression analysis of the Early versus Late Infantile Strabismus Surgery Study (ELISSS) and 12 other studies found that reoperation rates were 60–80% for children first operated around age 1 but only 25% for children operated around age 4. Birch found that even with early surgery, <0.5% had normal stereopsis and 60% had nil. Therefore, some authors have concluded that the benefits of early surgery for gross binocular vision may need to be balanced against a higher reoperation rate.

However, as already mentioned, other studies have found that the opposite: that the reoperation rate is lower if stereopsis is achieved through earlier surgery. Even subnormal stereopsis leads to improved sensorimotor developmental milestones in infancy. Also, as previously mentioned, the CEOS found that a constant esotropia of 40 PD or more was very unlikely to spontaneously resolve after age 10 weeks. A prospective study found that neither instability of the esotropia nor inaccurate measurements affected the long-term results after surgery, whether assessed by postoperative alignment, reoperation rate or attainment of stereopsis. Other studies have also found that the postoperative alignment was not affected by preoperative instability of the angle. Therefore, it seems that the concerns about operating early are unfounded, while the benefits are well-documented. The current author recommends operating as soon as 3 months of age for a constant esotropia of 40 PD or more in a neurologically intact child.

Follow-up

Patients require long-term follow-up after surgery for alignment, amblyopia, refractive error, and the development of late associations such as AET, nystagmus, IOOA, and DVD.

Transient small misalignments are common 1–2 weeks after surgery, but if a deviation >10 PD persists for 6 weeks, reoperation may be required. A larger incomitant postoperative deviation associated with a duction deficit should prompt an earlier return to the operating return to look for a slipped or lost muscle.

About 80% of patients are well-aligned 6 weeks after surgery, and 60–80% will develop the MFS. MFS is the best sensory outcome that most patients attain and consist of a small residual esotropia of 8 PD or less and peripheral sensory fusion without central fusion, which allows for gross stereopsis of 200 seconds of arc at best. High-grade stereopsis remains rare even with early surgery. The benefit of MFS is that the presence of at least peripheral fusion allows for the maintenance of normal fusional vergence amplitudes. The MFS has been associated with good stability even decades later. About 74% of postoperative patients with MFS maintained alignment 17.5 years later compared to only 45% of patients at 14 years who did not have MFS or better. Kushner found that all small residual horizontal deviations were not equal: long-term stability was much better with a small esotropia than with a small exotropia. An initial small postoperative exotropia for the first 1–2 weeks after surgery may be desirable in children <2 years old to allow for the development of fusional convergence amplitudes. However, if the child is over 2 years old, the exotropia usually increases over time due to a lack of peripheral fusion.

The reoperation rate has been variously reported as 25–69%, largely dependent on the length of follow-up. A reoperation rate of about 50% at 10 years rises as high as 66% at 20 years. Preoperative moderate amblyopia is a risk factor for reoperation. Surgery in patients with neurodevelopmental conditions such as cerebral palsy is associated with higher rates of overcorrection, and a variable and less predictable response to surgery. Parks recommended decreasing the amount of medial rectus recession by 0.5 mm in infants who had a premature birth at 30 weeks or less. Amblyopia, nystagmus, and poor stereopsis are also risk factors for requiring reoperation.

Even if amblyopia is completely treated preoperatively, it may be found postoperatively in 17–41% of patients, and therefore, patients require continued monitoring even with successful realignment of the eyes. Treatment of amblyopia is often successful, as <10% of patients have persistent amblyopia at 5 years, and it is usually mild if present.

The usual decrease in hyperopia during the first 9 months of life does not seem to occur in IET patients, and regular monitoring of the refractive error until age 8 years has been recommended. This may be related to the increased incidence of AET, which has been reported to occur in as many as 60% of former IET patients within 4 years (see also the introduction to AET above). Three risk factors for the development of AET in these patients include a duration of constant esotropia >3 months before repair, any increase of hyperopia by +0.50 diopters or more during follow-up, or poor stereopsis.

Latent nystagmus, IOOA, and DVD are frequent sequelae of IET, which usually do not appear until after 1 year of age.

Latent Nystagmus (Fusion Maldevelopment Nystagmus)

Latent nystagmus is now called fusion maldevelopment nystagmus syndrome (FMN or FMNS). While Lang reported an incidence of 50% in 1967, more recent reports indicate that it occurs in only 4–16% of patients. It is a jerk nystagmus that intensifies under monocular viewing conditions. Therefore, visual acuity testing in these patients may give an erroneously poor result, if total occlusion of the fellow eye is performed. Using a high plus lens (to "fog") rather than an opaque occluder over the untested eye can give a more accurate monocular visual acuity. In FMNS, the nystagmus is a jerk type with the fast phase toward the fixing eye. It is the only type of nystagmus that reverses direction with a change in fixation. If one eye is suppressed because of manifest strabismus, amblyopia, or other causes, the effect can be the same as occlusion and then the patient is said to have "manifest latent nystagmus" (MLN). The fixating eye in MLN often has a null point in adduction, causing the patient to adopt a compensatory head turn to the same side, which can be mistaken for a head posture due to incomitant strabismus. FMNS can be seen with any condition that disrupts binocular vision, not just IET.

Inferior Oblique Overaction

Inferior oblique overaction is seen in about 75% of patients after 1 year of age and may be unilateral or bilateral and symmetric or very asymmetric. It is characterized by over-elevation of the eye in adduction **(Fig. 5)**. Unlike IOOA secondary to a superior oblique palsy, it is not associated with a head tilt. Its occurrence appears to be independent of the sensory or motor status of the patient, that is, whether the primary esotropia was successfully treated or not. IOOA virtually never causes symptoms, but may be repaired to restore normal appearance. Treatment consists of an inferior oblique weakening procedure such as recession, myectomy, or anteriorization.

Dissociated Vertical Deviation

Dissociated vertical deviation is characterized by a slow upward drift of the nonfixating eye. It may also drift temporally and excyclotort. DVD may also be unilateral, bilateral, or asymmetric. It may only occur under monocular

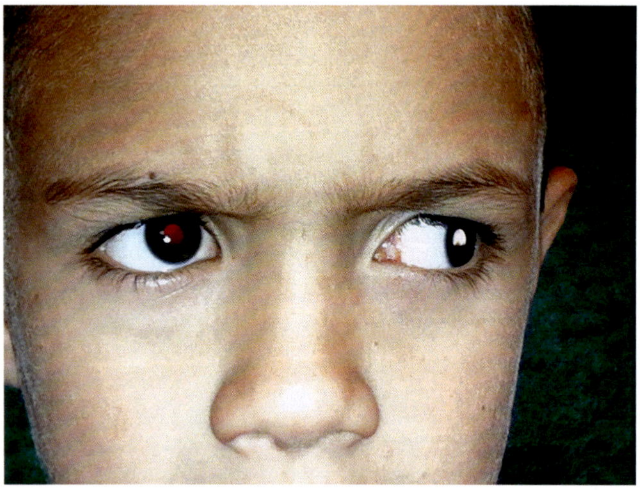

Fig. 5: Inferior oblique overaction of the right eye. The right eye overelevates in adduction.
(*Courtesy*: Miguel Paciuc-Beja, MD, Denver, Colorado, USA)

viewing conditions, in which case it is called "latent." Similar to FMNS, DVD can occur with any condition that disrupts early binocular development. The incidence of DVD is higher if surgery for esotropia is delayed beyond 2 years or in the absence of stereopsis. Occasionally, DVD is associated with an ipsilateral head tilt. DVD can be mistaken for IOOA, as the nose can occlude the vision of the adducting eye and trigger a latent DVD. DVD can be distinguished from IOOA by the following: unlike IOOA, DVD occurs in all directions of gaze, not just adduction. There is no corresponding hypotropia on alternate cover testing, no V-pattern, and the upward movement is a slow drift rather than a rapid swing up. The distinction is important as surgical treatment for DVD is different than IOOA. The superior rectus may be recessed, with or without a scleral posterior fixation suture (Faden suture), or the inferior rectus resected. Like IOOA, the indication for treatment is to restore a normal appearance.

About 59% of the time, IOOA and DVD coexist in the same eye, in which case an inferior oblique anterior transposition procedure addresses both issues.

OTHER FORMS OF COMITANT CHILDHOOD ESOTROPIA

Esotropia Associated with Neurodevelopmental Disorders

Mohney found that esotropia associated with neurodevelopmental disorders was actually the second most common type of esotropia after AET, representing 17.2% of all cases (***see* Table 1**). However, it is problematic to consider this esotropia as a separate category, as there is considerable overlap with the categories of infantile and AET. As previously mentioned, the risk of IET is well known to increase with any condition affecting neurodevelopment, reaching as high as 44% incidence. However, many authors exclude patients with neurological impairments from the category of IET. Patients with neurological disorders are also at higher risk for developing AET, and are more sensitive to smaller amounts of hyperopia, perhaps due to tenuous central fusion.

Compared to neurologically normal children, the esotropia in these patients may be more variable, intermittent, and follow a less predictable course, with some patients worsening over time, some spontaneously improving and some remaining stable. Surgery in such patients is associated with higher rates of overcorrection, and a variable and less predictable response to surgery. Therefore, some recommend avoiding surgery unless the deviation is reproducible over several visits, and the patient has sufficiently good visual acuity and cognitive status to benefit from improved alignment. Patients with Down syndrome appear to be an exception in that they respond well to treatment.

Sensory Esotropia

Severe visual impairment in one or both eyes, usually 20/100 or worse, can result in strabismus. Usually, this manifests as exotropia in adults, but in children under 2 years of age, esotropia is just as likely to occur. This difference may exist because children are more likely to be hyperopic and accommodative factors play a role. Surgery in such patients has a lower success rate compared to the more common causes of esotropia, likely due to a lack of binocular sensory feedback to maintain alignment postoperatively. Most authors recommend operating only on the worse seeing eye to avoid any risk to the better eye. Also, it is recommended to aim for a small undercorrection as exotropia (overcorrection) usually increases over time.

Consecutive Esotropia

Consecutive esotropia is an esotropia that develops after surgery for exotropia. An initial small 10–20 PD esotropia for the first 1–2 weeks after exotropia surgery is actually desirable, as the eyes usually drift further temporally during this period. A non-AET of over 10 PD that persists beyond 6 weeks requires reoperation.

Acquired Nonaccommodative Comitant Esotropia

Acquired nonaccommodative comitant esotropia is also known as acquired comitant esotropia (ACE), or if of acute onset, acute acquired comitant esotropia (AACE). As the name implies, this is esotropia that occurs after age 6 months and cannot be attributed to any accommodative, paretic, or restrictive etiology. Typically, a fairly large esotropia, 30–70 PD, develops acutely with diplopia, sometimes after a brief period of intermittency. Burian type 1 (or Swan type) occurs after prolonged occlusion (e.g., patching, hyphema, or severe eyelid edema occluding the visual axis). Type 2 (or Franceschetti type) has no apparent cause.

Most patients with ANAET have a good prognosis with surgery and recover binocular vision. It is the patients without apparent cause for their esotropia, i.e., type 2 that presents the most difficulty in management. If the onset is acute and an abduction deficit is present, then this may represent a sixth nerve palsy and neuroimaging is clearly warranted. However, if the deviation is comitant, the work-up is less clear. There have been scattered reports of brain tumors or Chiari malformation with horizontally comitant acquired esotropia, but most of these patients also had other signs such as nystagmus, developmental defects, A or V-patterns, divergence insufficiency, headache, ataxia, abnormal pupil responses, or papilledema. Therefore, in the absence of other signs, many authors have not recommended routine neuroimaging for these patients. Computed tomography (CT) or magnetic resonance imaging (MRI) scans do carry the risk of radiation or sedation, respectively. Others think it best to err on the side of caution. Failure to regain fusion and stereopsis after surgery or prism neutralization may increase the odds of an intracranial lesion being present.

Nystagmus Blockage Syndrome

Nystagmus blockage syndrome (NBS), also known as nystagmus compensation syndrome, is a condition in which accommodative convergence dampens an otherwise constant nystagmus. These patients have straight eyes and nystagmus at distance, but when viewing near targets, develops a variable large esotropia and the nystagmus decreases. Miosis occurs with the convergence. About 50% of all infantile nystagmus syndrome (INS) patients have an associated strabismus. What distinguishes NBS from other INS patients with esotropia is that the nystagmus increases in abduction of the fixing eye while the esotropia decreases. If prism is placed in front of the fixing eye, the fellow eye not only remains in adduction, but the esotropia actually increases. The patient is thus said to "eat" prism. While FMNS (manifest latent nystagmus) also has esotropia and a null point in adduction, the esotropia is constant and the patient does not "eat" prism. Surgery for the esotropia associated with NBS usually requires larger medial rectus recessions than anticipated.

Convergence Spasm

Convergence or accommodative spasm is an intermittent large esotropia at near caused by excessive accommodation, usually occurring in literate children. This leads to blurred vision, headache, asthenopia, and/or diplopia. Miosis and pseudomyopia are observed during the spasm. The condition is thought to be related to anxiety and stress. Reassurance and counseling may help. If not, sometimes a brief course of cycloplegic eye drops and/or reading glasses can prevent the episodes of excessive accommodation. Very rarely, the condition can be associated with organic lesions including intracranial tumors.

Cyclic Esotropia

Cyclic esotropia is a very rare condition in which a fixed repetitive period of orthotropia alternates with a period of comitant esotropia, usually on a predictable 48-hour cycle, although other time intervals do occur. The cause is unknown but is postulated to be related to the body's biological internal "clock" and circadian rhythm. It has been reported to rarely occur after surgery or trauma or to be associated with central nervous system disease. The condition most often occurs in preschool children (ages 2–6) and transforms into a stable noncyclical esotropia within months of onset. It responds well to standard surgery at any point in its evolution, with a good prognosis for binocularity.

Incomitant Childhood Esotropia

Incomitant esotropia in childhood is uncommon. It occurs due to paresis of the lateral rectus muscle, or restriction of the medial rectus muscle. The only somewhat common condition in this category is Duane's syndrome, which represents about 1% of all strabismus cases.

DUANE SYNDROME

Duane retraction syndrome (DRS) is the most common form of a group of disorders referred to as congenital cranial dysinnervation disorders (CCDD), in which abnormal innervation due to developmental defects of one or more cranial nerves leads to secondary fibrotic changes in the extraocular muscles. This group also includes Mobius syndrome and congenital fibrosis of the extraocular muscles (CFEOM).

Duane retraction syndrome is caused by agenesis of the sixth nerve nucleus, with misinnervation of the lateral rectus by a branch of the third cranial nerve. Huber described three types of DRS. In the most common form of DRS, type 1, which represents 85% of cases, decreased abduction is present with or without esotropia in primary position **(Figs. 6A to C)**. Type 2 (1% of cases) exhibits decreased adduction and exotropia, whereas the more common type 3 (15–25% of cases) exhibits both decreased abduction and adduction and may manifest as either esotropia or exotropia. In esotropic cases, a face turn toward the affected eye may be present. The esotropia is usually quite small, 30 PD or less, relative to the abduction deficit, especially when compared with other forms of sixth nerve palsy. In all types of DRS, adduction is associated with cocontraction of the medial rectus and lateral rectus muscles, leading to retraction of the globe into the orbit. This is most easily recognized as a narrowing of the palpebral fissure on adduction. The eye may also exhibit overelevation ("upshoot") or depression ("downshoot") on adduction. Most cases are unilateral, but about 20% are bilateral. DRS is usually an isolated finding, but about 30% are associated with systemic findings, especially Goldenhar syndrome.

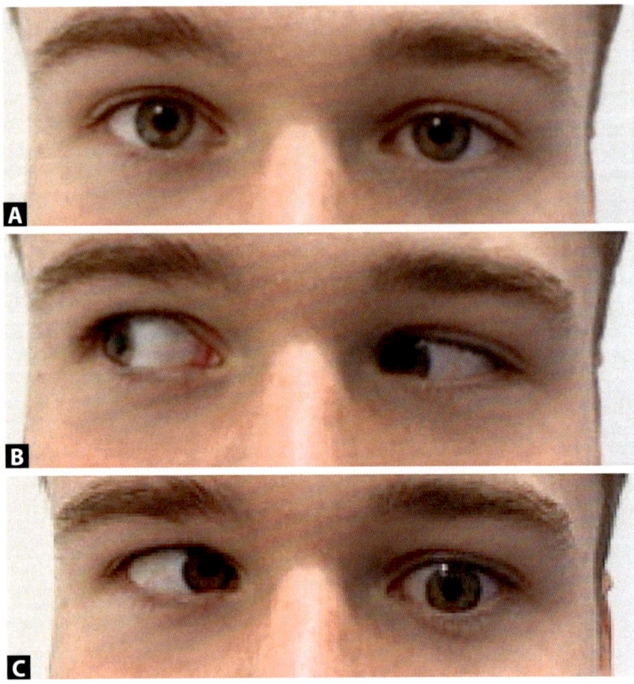

Figs. 6A to C: Duane syndrome type 1, left eye.
This patient's eyes are straight in primary position (A). On right gaze (B), the left palpebral fissure narrows due to globe retraction. On left gaze (C), the left eye is unable to abduct fully.
(*Courtesy*: Sophocles Sophocleous, OD, MD; Nicosia, Cyprus)

There is no procedure that can fully restore abduction in these patients. Many cases are simply observed, unless primary position strabismus, anomalous head posture, or cosmetically significant retraction, upshoot, or downshoot is present. The most commonly performed surgery for the esotropia is a unilateral medial rectus recession, although for larger esotropia, a bilateral medial rectus recession or an ipsilateral vertical rectus muscle transposition can be performed. Resections are avoided as they can worsen retraction.

Mobius Syndrome (Mobius Sequence)

Mobius syndrome is a heterogeneous group of CCDD (see Duane syndrome above) that has a combined sixth and seventh cranial nerve palsy in common. The cause is unknown but is postulated to include a vascular insult to the brainstem during embryogenesis and sometimes teratogens such as misoprostol and thalidomide. It is best referred to as a sequence rather than a syndrome, as a sequence, it is defined as a cascade of secondary events after an embryonic insult from heterogeneous causes. The facial nerve palsy gives these patients a mask-like facies, and they often present as neonates due to feeding problems from a weak suck reflex. Lagophthalmos may cause exposure keratopathy. Most commonly, the sixth nerve palsy is bilateral, but it can be unilateral or present as a gaze palsy due to the involvement of the sixth nerve nucleus or paramedian pontine reticular formation (PPRF). Other cranial nerves are often involved, and autism, developmental delay, distal limb, chest, and tongue anomalies can be present. About 50% are orthotropic and 50% have esotropia and may cross-fixate with spared convergence. In some patients, adduction may be weak as well and exotropia may result. The medial rectus muscles are often restricted on forced duction testing, and larger than average bilateral medial rectus muscle recessions may be required for correction.

Other Sixth Nerve Palsy in Childhood

Unilateral or bilateral sixth nerve palsy may rarely occur in neonates, probably due to transiently raised intracranial pressure during the birth process, and resolves within 6–10 weeks. More commonly, an apparent abduction deficit in infancy is actually IET with cross-fixation or Duane syndrome with indiscernible retraction. Unlike adults, relatively benign microvascular causes of acquired sixth nerve palsy such as diabetes or hypertension are very rare in children, and up to 45% of cases will have an intracranial neoplasm. Many cases are also associated with viral, postviral, or postvaccine inflammation and spontaneously resolve. Some idiopathic cases recur and resolve several times over childhood. MRI is mandatory in all cases without a clear-cut cause, or if other neurological signs are present, or if the palsy worsens or does not resolve within 10 weeks. Patching may be required for amblyopia if no compensatory head posture is present. For nonresolving sixth nerve palsy, surgery is approached as it is for adults, with a horizontal recess, resects procedure for partial palsy and vertical rectus muscle transposition for complete palsy.

Myasthenia Gravis in Childhood

Myasthenia gravis in childhood is rare and consists of three distinct forms. All are associated with initially variable and fluctuating ptosis and strabismus and can mimic virtually any other strabismus disorder. The first type is transient neonatal myasthenia which is caused by transplacental transfer of maternal antibodies. The second type, congenital myasthenic syndrome (CMS), usually presents before 1–2 years of age and is caused by structural or functional abnormalities at the neuromuscular junction. Since CMS is not autoimmune, antibodies are not detected on serology, and immunosuppressive therapy is not effective. The third form, juvenile autoimmune myasthenia gravis (AMG), is the most common and is similar to the adult form. It almost always occurs over 2 years of age, and in 75% of patients the onset is after age 4 years. Serological testing for antibodies is positive in 56–63% of patients. Edrophonium (Tensilon) or neostigmine testing and electromyography (EMG) can also help to confirm the diagnosis but are difficult to perform in young children. About 36–49% of AMG patients progress from ocular to systemic myasthenia gravis, usually within 2–4 years of onset. Anticholinesterase medication such as pyridostigmine (Mestinon) is often effective. Second-line treatments include immunosuppressive medications such as prednisone, azathioprine, and intravenous immunoglobulins.

Plasmapheresis and thymectomy are occasionally needed. The prognosis for AMG in children is better than it is for adults in terms of improvement, attaining remission and survival. Approximately 2 years of medication are required until lasting remission occurs. Strabismus surgery in both CMS as well as AMG can be successful if the deviation has been stable for at least 5 months.

Congenital Fibrosis of the Extraocular Muscles

Congenital fibrosis of the extraocular muscles is a rare congenital disorder, usually manifesting as severe non-progressive bilateral ptosis and restrictive external ophthalmoplegia. There are three primary phenotypes—(1) CFEOM1, (2) CFEOM2, and (3) CFEOM3. Severe bilateral hypotropia and exotropia are most common, but esotropia can also occur. Although the eye muscles are restricted and show fibrosis on histology, this is now known to occur secondary to cranial nerve dysgenesis primarily affecting the third and fourth cranial nerve, as part of the spectrum of disorders known as CCDD (see Duane syndrome above). It is usually autosomal dominant, although it can also be sporadic or autosomal recessive. It is rarely unilateral. Up to 95% of patients have amblyopia and 85% have astigmatism. CFEOM is difficult to treat given the severe restrictive abnormality of virtually all of the extraocular muscles. Gaining surgical exposure is difficult due to the severe restriction of rotation. Resections are not effective, and very large recessions or even tenotomies are needed.

SUGGESTED READING

1. Birch EE, Fawcett SL, Stager DR Sr. Risk factors for the development of accommodative esotropia following treatment for infantile esotropia. JAAPOS. 2002;6(3):174-81.
2. Birch EE, Stager DR Sr. Long-term motor and sensory outcomes after early surgery for infantile esotropia. JAAPOS. 2006;10:409-13.
3. Birch EE, Wang J. Stereoacuity outcomes after treatment of infantile and accommodative esotropia. Optom Vis Sci. 2009;86(6):647-52.
4. Christiansen SP, Chandler DL, Holmes JM, Bacal DA, Birch E, Donahue SP, et al. The relationship between preoperative alignment stability and postoperative motor outcomes in children with esotropia. JAAPOS. 2009;13:335-8.
5. Crawford ML, von Noorden GK. Optically induced concomitant strabismus in monkeys. Invest Ophthalmol Vis Sci. 1980;19(9): 1105-9.
6. Helveston EM, Neely DF, Stidham DB, Wallace DK, Plager DA, Sprunger DT. Results of early alignment of congenital esotropia. Ophthalmology. 1999;106(9):1716-26.
7. Hered R, American Academy of Ophthalmology, 2019-2020 BCSC (Basic and Clinical Science Course). Pediatric Ophthalmology and Strabismus. China: American Academy of Ophthalmology; 2019.
8. Hiles DA, Watson BA, Biglan AW. Characteristics of infantile esotropia following early bimedial rectus recession. Arch Ophthalmol. 1980;98(4):697-703.
9. Holmes JM, Mutyala S, Maus TL, Grill R, Hodge DO, Gray DT. Pediatric third, fourth, and sixth nerve palsies: a population-based study. Am J Ophthalmol. 1999;127:388-92.
10. Hutchinson AK. Refractive surgery for accommodative esotropia: past, present and future. Eur J Ophthalmol. 2012;22:871-7.
11. Ing MR, Roberts KM, Lin A, Chen JJ. The stability of the monofixation syndrome. Am J Ophthalmol. 2014;157:248-53.
12. Ing MR. Early surgical alignment for congenital esotropia. Trans Am Ophthalmol Soc. 1981;79:625-63.
13. Jacobs SM, Green-Simms A, Diehl NN, Mohney BG. Long-term follow-up of acquired nonaccommodative esotropia in a population-based cohort. Ophthalmology. 2011;118:1170-4.
14. Joint Writing Committee for the Multi-Ethnic Pediatric Eye Disease Study and the Baltimore Pediatric Eye Disease Study Groups. Risk factors associated with childhood strabismus: the Multi-Ethnic Pediatric Eye Disease and Baltimore Pediatric Eye Disease Studies. Ophthalmology. 2011;118(11):2251-61.
15. Kekunnaya R, Gupta A, Sachdeva V, Krishnaiah S, Rao BV, Vashist U, et al. Duane retraction syndrome: series of 441 cases. J Pediatr Ophthalmol Strabismus. 2012;49:164-9.
16. Kraft SP. A surgical approach for Duane syndrome. J Pediatr Ophthalmol Strabismus. 1988;25(3):119-30.
17. Kushner BJ, Fisher M. Is alignment within 8 prism diopters of orthotropia a successful outcome for infantile esotropia surgery?. Arch Ophthalmol. 1996;114(2):176-80.
18. Kushner BJ. Fifteen-year outcome of surgery for the near angle in patients with accommodative esotropia and a high accommodative convergence to accommodation ratio. Arch Ophthalmol. 2001;119:1150-3.
19. Lam GC, Repka MX, Guyton DL. Timing of amblyopia therapy relative to strabismus surgery. Ophthalmology. 1993;100:1751-6.
20. Lambert S, Lyons CJ. Taylor and Hoyt's Pediatric Ophthalmology and Strabismus, 5th edition. Netherlands; Elsevier: 2017.
21. Lembo A, Serafino M, Strologo MD, Saunders RA, Trivedi RH, Villani E, et al. Accommodative esotropia: the state of the art. Int Ophthalmol. 2019;39(2):497-505.
22. Miller MT, Strömland K. The Möbius sequence: a relook. JAAPOS. 1999;3(4):199-208.
23. Mohney BG. Common forms of childhood esotropia. Ophthalmology. 2001;108(4):805-9.
24. Mullaney P, Vajsar J, Smith R, Buncic JR. The natural history and ophthalmic involvement in childhood myasthenia gravis at the Hospital for Sick Children. Ophthalmology. 2000;107(3): 504-10.
25. Olitsky SE. High AC/A ratio esotropia: do we really need to be using bifocals? Am Orthopt J. 2016:66(1):5-9.
26. Oystreck DT, Engle EC, Bosley TM. Recent progress in understanding congenital cranial dysinnervation disorders. J Neuroophthalmol. 2011;31:69-77.
27. Park KA, Oh SY. The effect of reducing hyperopic correction in patients with accommodative esotropia. JAAPOS. 2013;17:363-6.
28. Pediatric Eye Disease Investigator Group. Spontaneous resolution of early-onset esotropia: experience of the Congenital Esotropia Observational Study. Am J Ophthalmol. 2002;133(1):109-18.
29. Prism Adaptation Study Research Group. Efficacy of prism adaptation in the surgical management of acquired esotropia. Arch Ophthalmol. 1990;108(9):1248-56.
30. Simonsz HJ, Kolling GH. Best age for surgery for infantile esotropia. Eur J Paediatr Neurol. 2011;15(3):205-8.
31. Sondhi N, Archer SM, Helveston EM. Development of normal ocular alignment. J Pediatr Ophthalmol Strabismus. 1988;25(5):210-1.
32. von Noorden, GK. Binocular Vision and Ocular Motility: Theory and Management of Strabismus, 5th edition. St. Louis, Mo: CV Mosby; 1996.
33. Wallace DK, Christiansen SP, Sprunger DT, Melia M, Lee KA, Morse CL, et al. Esotropia and Exotropia Preferred Practice Pattern®. Ophthalmology. 2018;125(1):P143-83.
34. Wong AM. Timing of surgery for infantile esotropia: sensory and motor outcomes. Can J Ophthalmol. 2008;43(6):643-51.
35. Wright KW, Bruce-Lyle L. Augmented surgery for esotropia associated with high hypermetropia. J Pediatr Ophthalmol Strabismus. 1993;30:167-70.
36. Wright KW, Edelman PM, McVey JH, Terry AP, Lin M. High-grade stereo acuity after early surgery for congenital esotropia. Arch Ophthalmol. 1994;112(7):913-9.
37. Wright KW, Strube YNJ. Pediatric Ophthalmology and Strabismus, 3rd edition. New York: Oxford University Press; 2012.

22

CHAPTER

Exotropia

Srijana Adhikari

INTRODUCTION

Exotropia is a common form of strabismus in children. The estimated global prevalence of exotropia in pediatric age group is 1.07%. The prevalence ranges in different countries and regions. It is more common in Asian and African regions than in Europe and North America where esotropia is reported to be more common.

ETIOLOGY

The etiology of exotropia is still unclear. Small exodeviations are common in the normal population. Transient exotropias may be observed in the newborn which usually resolve by 2–4 months. There are various theories on the etiology of exotropia. Duane stated that exotropia occurs because of the innervational imbalance between the convergence and divergence mechanism. Neuroanatomic substrate including the area of tegmentum of brain stem in humans has been suggested as possible site of divergence. No true divergence nucleus, however, has been discovered as yet. Bielschowsky stated that there is an abnormal position of rest in exodeviation related to anatomic factors, interpupillary distance, the shape and size of the orbit, properties of extrabulbar tissues, and orbital depth. Some authors suggested that horizontal muscle length and insertion affects the equilibrium of passive forces between medial and lateral rectus (LR) muscle leading to exotropia.

The newer theories believe that exodeviations are governed by both the mechanical and innervational factors. The static position of rest is the relative position of visual axis when there is no stimulus for fusion. There exists a dynamic interplay between the ocular convergence and divergence mechanism. Any imbalance favoring divergence results in development of exodeviation.

Genetic Factors

Heredity plays an important role in the development of exotropia but genetics may be multifactorial. There may be positive family history in many cases. Maternal smoking during pregnancy and low birth weight is significant and independent risk factors for the development of horizontal deviations.

CLASSIFICATION

Exotropia in children is broadly classified as comitant and incomitant. Comitant strabismus is more common than the incomitant **(Box 1)**.

PRIMARY INTERMITTENT EXOTROPIA

Intermittent exotropia is the most common form of divergent strabismus. It is the condition when deviation occurs intermittently with periods of good alignment or orthophoria in between. There can be suppression or diplopia when eye deviates. Intermittent exotropia accounts for half of all cases of exotropia. Some studies suggest female preponderance of intermittent exotropia. It has a wide spectrum of manifestation ranging from straight eye almost all the time to constant deviation **(Figs. 1A to C)**.

BOX 1: Classification of exotropia.

Comitant:
- Primary
- Consecutive
- Residual
- Sensory
- Accommodative
- *Primary*:
  - Intermittent
  - Constant
- Decompensated intermittent exotropia
- Congenital or infantile exotropia
- Exotropia associated with craniofacial anomalies, systemic diseases, and syndromes

Incomitant:
- Third N palsy
- Duane retraction syndromes
- Congenital fibrosis syndrome, strabismus fixus, and dissociated horizontal deviation (DHD)

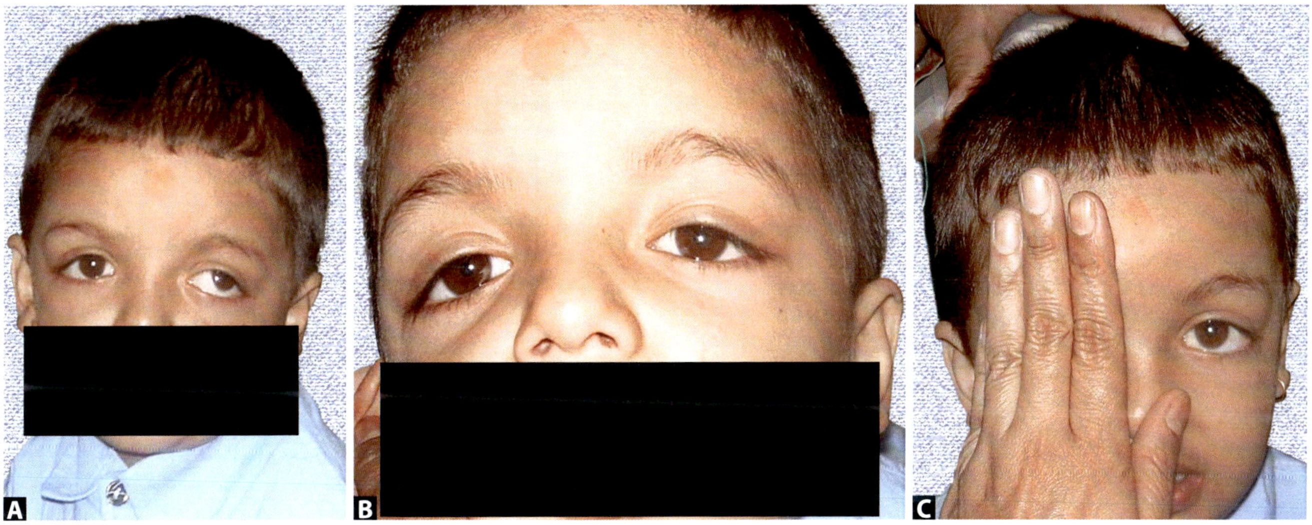

Figs. 1A to C: Intermittent exotropia for distance.

Classification

The classification is based on the measurement of the angle of deviation in near and distance fixation. It is classically divided into three types (Burian classification):

1. Basic type
2. Convergence insufficiency
3. Divergence excess (true divergence and pseudo or simulated divergence).

- *Basic*: When distance deviation is within 10 prism diopter (PD) of near deviation. This group of patients has normal fusional convergence (tenacious proximal fusion), normal accommodative convergence by accommodation (AC/ A) ratio, and normal proximal convergence **(Fig. 2)**.
- *Convergence insufficiency*:
  - The near deviation is >10 PD of distance deviation. Patients have either a low AC/A ratio or decreased fusional convergence amplitude. This condition needs to be distinguished from patients with pseudoconvergence insufficiency.
  - In pseudoconvergence insufficiency, monocular occlusion or the fixation at distance causes increase in distance deviation. In the early stages of convergence insufficiency, patients have asthenopic symptoms, visual fatigue, blurring, and intermittent diplopia. As the condition progresses, the exophoria develops into frank exotropia with near deviation more than the distance deviation. Orthoptic exercises are helpful in these conditions.
- *Pseudodivergence excess*:
  - A larger deviation is present for distance, compared to near of >10 PD.
  - The causes can be:
    - *Tenacious proximal fusion*: After 30–60 minutes of monocular occlusion, the near deviation is equal to the distance deviation. This presentation is due to increased tonic fusional convergence.
    - *High AC/A ratio*: After near addition of +3.0 D, the near deviation equals to the distance deviation. However, the +3 D test should be done after the prolonged occlusion test. Such patients are prone to postoperative overcorrections, if operated on their full distance deviation. These would then need bifocals with +3.0 D near add.
    - *True divergence excess*: A larger exotropia for distance compared to near of >10 PD, which persists even after 60 minutes of occlusion and with +3.00 D lenses. The AC/A ratio is normal. It is important to document these as they have bearing on the surgical planning.

Natural History

Natural history of intermittent exotropia is still not clear as there is lack of prospective longitudinal studies. Some retrospective studies revealed that majority of intermittent exotropia progresses to constant deviation, few remains the same and very few improves. This may be the cause of controversies and wide variation of practice in surgical intervention of intermittent exotropia. In a study, Von Noorden found that 75% of 51 untreated patients showed progression over an average follow-up period of 3.5 years, whereas 9% worsened and 16% improved. Hiles et al., in their study of 48 patients found no significant change in the deviation after an average of 11 years follow-up. Similar results were found in studies done by Pediatric Eye Disease Investigator Group (PEDIG) and Romanchuk et al.

Sensory Adaptation in Intermittent Exotropia

Intermittent exotropia in initial phase exhibits excellent fusion and stereopsis. This is because eyes were aligned during the development of binocular single vision. When exotropia starts to manifest, then patients start to show suppression of

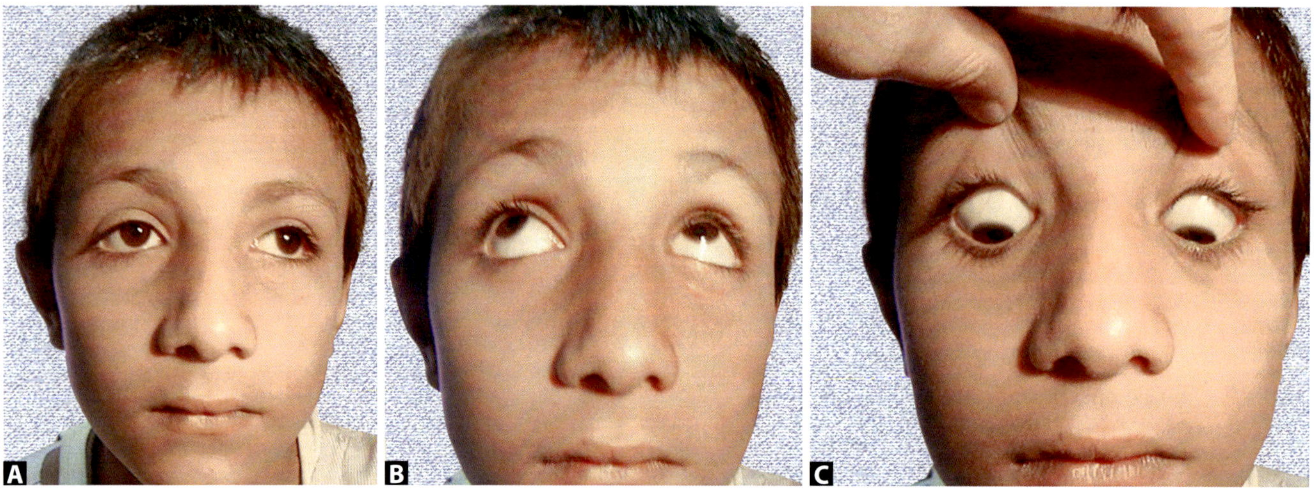

Figs. 2A to C: Exotropia with "V" pattern.

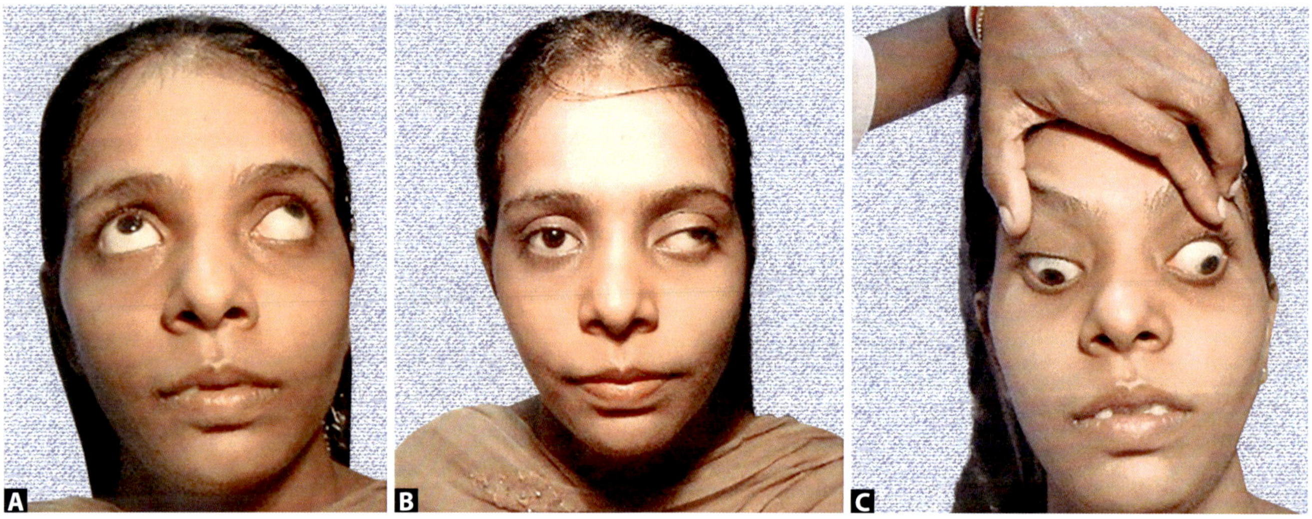

Figs. 3A to C: Constant unilateral exotropia-left eye. No pattern.

temporal retina. In older children with late onset manifest exotropia, diplopia occurs due to cortical plasticity and lack of suppression. The retinal correspondence is normal during the aligned state and may be abnormal in deviated state. Amblyopia in intermittent exotropia is rare. It occurs, if there is associated anisometropia or if the constant exotropia develops in early infancy.

Clinical Characteristics of Intermittent Exotropia

Age at Onset

The age of onset in intermittent exotropia is mostly during early childhood, in the second or third year of life. Burian and Spivey reported 63% of their patients having an age of onset <5 years of age. With rare exceptions, exodeviations usually begin as an exophoria that may deteriorate into intermittent and then constant exotropia as suppression develops.

Mode of Presentation

The symptoms of intermittent exotropia can start in early infancy. It starts at first as exophoria which progressively increases to intermittent deviation. The symptoms usually worsen when the child is tired, sick, soon after waking up from sleep, inattention, or gazing at far distance. There may be symptoms of blurred vision, asthenopia, visual fatigue, and intermittent diplopia in older children. One of the common initial presentations of intermittent exotropia in children is photophobia and squinting (closure of one eye) in bright light especially in sunlight. It is not clear why bright light entering the squinting eye causes photophobia. There is an assumption that bright light dazzles retina and disrupts fusion leading to deviation. Monocular eye closure may be an attempt to avoid diplopia and confusion.

Refractive Error

Patients with intermittent exotropia commonly have associated refractive error. It may have a role in development of intermittent exotropia. Patients with uncorrected myopia use less than normal accommodative effort during near vision thus causing decreased accommodative convergence. This constant under stimulation of convergence may cause an exodeviation to develop. Similarly, patients with high degree of uncorrected hypermetropia do not make any effort to attain clear vision and, hence, the convergence mechanism is less active leading to low AC/A ratio. Jampolsky et al., stated a distinct relationship of anisomyopia and anisoastigmatism with exodeviation. Anisometropia with unequal vision in two eyes may cause an obstacle to fusion, facilitate suppression, and therefore contribute to the pathogenesis of exotropia.

Clinical Evaluation of Intermittent Exotropia

Assessment of Control of Deviation

Control of deviation in intermittent exotropia is crucial in subsequent management and decision for surgery. The measure of control is the amount of time, the eye becomes aligned and the frequency at which the eye drifts out. The observation by parents at home is very important in assessment. Some older children and adults complain of diplopia or awareness of their own deviation. There are two popular scoring scales—(1) Mayo clinic score and (2) the Newcastle control score.

The Mayo score is mainly based on timed observation **(Table 1)**. An average of three scores is recommended to provide reliable measure. The Newcastle control score **(Table 2)** is based on the score popularized by Rosenbaum to decide the time for surgical intervention. This is a subjective assessment and is divided into two parts—(1) the home control based on the parental observation and (2) office control based on cover test examination in clinic. Surgery is advised if the deviation is present >50% of time and poor control in clinic examination.

TABLE 1: Intermittent exotropia control scale (Mayo control score).

Score	***Criteria***
5	Constant exotropia
4	Exotropia >50% of examination before dissociation
3	Exotropia <50% of examination before dissociation
2	No exotropia unless dissociated recovers in >5 seconds
1	No exotropia unless dissociated recovers in 1–5 seconds
0	No Exotropia unless dissociated recovers in <1 second (phoria)

Note: This scale is applied to each patient for both distance and near fixation which, when combined, yields an overall control score ranging from 0 to 10. Levels 5–3 are assessed during an initial 30-second period of observation. Levels 2–0 are graded as the worst of three rapidly successive trials. An occluder is placed over the *right* eye for 10 seconds and then removed; measuring the length of time, it takes for fusion to become reestablished. The *left* eye is then occluded for a 10-second period and the time to refusion is similarly measured. A third trial of 10-second occlusion is performed, covering the eye that required the longest time to refuse. The worse level of control observed following the 3, 10-second periods of occlusion should be recorded for that visit. If the patient has a microesotropia by simultaneous prism and cover test, but exodeviation by alternate cover test, the scale applies to the exodeviation.

TABLE 2: The revised Newcastle control score for intermittent exotropia.

Criteria	***Score***
Home control (right exotropia or monocular eye closure seen)	
Never	0
<50% of time fixing in distance	1
>50% of time fixing in distance	2
>50% of time fixing at distance + seen at near	3
Clinic control (Scored for near and distance fixation)	
Immediate realignment after dissociation (exophoria)	0
Realignment with the aid of blink	1
Remains manifest after dissociation or prolonged fixation	2
Manifest spontaneously	3
Total score n/9	

Objective Measurement

This includes both sensory and motor evaluation in clinic. Before any measurement, visual assessment and refraction are very important. There should be full correction of refractive error as this influences the deviation measurements. The hypermetropia should be given the maximum tolerable correction and the myopia the least acceptable correction.

Sensory Evaluation

This includes distance and near stereoacuity test.

Measuring distance stereoacuity in children is challenging. However, it is more important than the near stereoacuity as loss of control of deviation in distance starts earlier than control in near (except for the convergence insufficiency type). Mentor B Vat II BVI is the device that measures distance stereoacuity using both contour circles and random dot stereograms from 240 to 15 seconds of arc disparity. Poor control in distance deviation correlated well with changes in clinic control. The newer devices are Frisby Davis Distance (FD2) test and Distance Randot (DR) test. The FD2 performance only deteriorates when the patient is constantly tropic whereas DR performance deteriorates at the earliest stages of intermittency. Clinical decisions based on measured stereoacuity thresholds should account for the test method used **(Fig. 4)**.

Another option is a red-green filter that splits the Snellen chart into red and green halves may be a useful tool in assessing level of distance control. The worth four dot test in

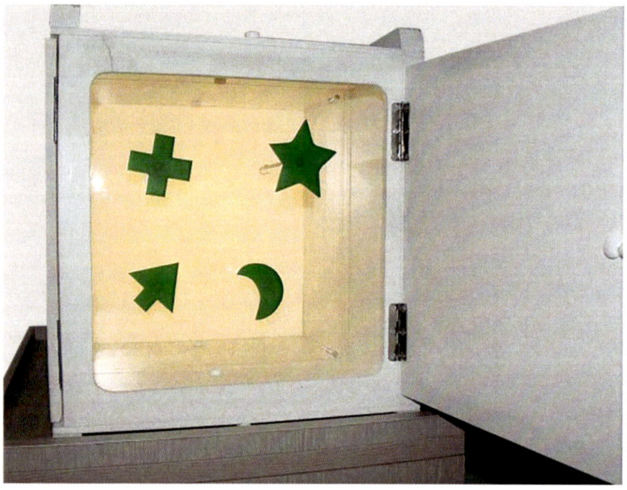

Fig. 4: Frisby–Davis test.

Snellen acuity chart can also be used for this purpose to find distance fusion and suppression.

Near stereoacuity is easier to measure in children with easy availability of charts with good sensitivity. However, near stereoacuity does not correlate well with the early loss of control of an intermittent exodeviation, as the deviation at distance has deteriorated to a significant degree by the time near stereoacuity is affected. The Titmus Fly test is a good, reliable test for children to measure near stereoacuity.

Motor Evaluation

Measurement of angle of deviation in intermittent exotropia is a big challenge especially in smaller children. The angles are variable because of nature of deviation or poor attention span in children for fixation target. It also varies with the timing of examination. If it is done late in the afternoon, patients are tired with poor tonic fusional convergence. Hence, deviation is easily elicited. On the other hand, if the examination is done early in the morning, then the patient's tonic fusional convergence is active with good control of tropia. The proper refractive correction is important before starting measurement. Repeat measurements may be needed if there is large variation.

The Prism Cover Test

The prism cover test should be done for both in near and distance. The distance target should be at 20 feet. Sometimes the fixation target can be in true infinity; at the end of hallway or outside window. This eliminates accommodation and reduces variability. The measurement should be done with prolonged alternate cover testing to suspend tonic fusional convergence. If there is significant disparity in near-distance measurement, then patch test is required.

Monocular Occlusion or Patch Test

The patch test is used to reduce tonic fusional convergence to differentiate true divergence excess from the pseudodivergence excess and reduced angle variability. One eye is covered for 30 minutes–1 hour and the deviation is measured without allowing binocular fusion. Eyes are closed till the prism cover test is done. The patch test should be done before +3 D lens test for near deviation to avoid misdiagnosing AC/A ratio. Combining the patch test and far distance measurement can greatly reduce undercorrections and has improved the overall result.

Measurement of deviation with +3 diopter lens: This test is done to measure the AC/A ratio and to find out whether the divergence excess is due to high AC/A ratio or not. After the patch test, when the distance deviation is still more than the near deviation, +3 D test is done. If the near measurement with +3.0 D lens, after patch test, equals the distance measurement, then it is pseudo-divergence excess due to high AC/A ratio. These are the group of patients who develop near-distance disparity even after surgery and would need bifocal glasses.

Prism Adaptation Test

Prism adaptation to measure total preoperative exodeviation has been reported to improve surgical success for patients with intermittent exotropia. In this test, preoperative add-on prisms are applied to a patient's spectacle correction, with amount of surgery decided by the amount of prisms required to neutralize the deviation.

- *Measurement of fusional convergence amplitude*: This test is particularly important in patients with convergence insufficiency. Convergence amplitudes are measured using loose prisms or prism bars for both distance and near. With both eyes open, base-out prisms are gradually added until a blur point followed by diplopia is reported by the patient. Patients with suppression do not appreciate diplopia. In these circumstances, the break point is noted when one eye starts to deviate outward under binocular viewing conditions. Normal convergence amplitudes are 20 PD for distance and 30–35 PD for near. After the break point, base-out prisms are reduced until single vision is reported or motor fusion observed. This recovery point is normally 2–4 PD less than the actual break point. In some patients with intermittent exotropia, this difference is large. In these patients, it is very difficult to regain fusion once it is disrupted.
- *Measurement of near point of convergence*: This is another important test in convergence insufficiency type of intermittent exotropia. While measuring the near point of convergence, a fixation target at 30–40 cm is gradually brought closer to the eyes. The near point of convergence is the point at which one eye starts to lose fixation and drifts out. It should normally be 5–7 cm from the tip of the nose. Any deficiency in convergence amplitudes (near amplitudes <20 PD) or a large near point of convergence (exceeding 10 cm) constitutes convergence insufficiency. This test is particularly important in patients complaining of asthenopic symptoms related

to near work. Reduced convergence amplitudes may precede an exodeviation measured by cover test. These types of patients benefit from orthoptic exercises.

Treatment of Intermittent Exotropia

Nonsurgical Treatment

Nonsurgical treatment most of the time is a temporary measure. It is indicated in some situations where surgery cannot be undertaken or not indicated. Patients should be kept in close observation with periodic assessment of deviation and stereoacuity. In children, the nonsurgical therapies may prevent or reverse the deterioration of deviation by preserving binocular vision. Nonsurgical treatments may be indicated in following circumstances:

- *Small angle deviation with good control and normal distance stereoacuity*:
  - Young children in which the risk of developing monofixation syndrome weighs out the surgical intervention. Surgery can be delayed till the age for foveal suppression passes out.
  - Children who are not fit for general anesthesia.
  - These children can be kept under "observation", as many studies have shown that in quite a number of these children either do not progress, remain exophoric or even outgrow their tropia.
- *Refractive error and amblyopia management*: Blurring of vision in one or both eyes due to refractive error causes obstacle to fusion and can lead to suppression and amblyopia, contributing to progressive loss of control of an intermittent exotropia. Correction of refractive errors often helps control the frequency of deviation and may lead to phoric state in some children. Full correction in myopic patients will promote active accommodative convergence. Hypermetropia in intermittent exotropia poses a unique challenge. Special consideration should be given to the age of the patient, the extent of hypermetropia and the AC/C ratio, as correcting even small amounts of hyperopia may decrease the accommodative convergence and worsen the exodeviation. Some studies have shown good control of deviation with hyperopic correction, may be due to the fact that improved visual acuity is required for good fusion and good ocular alignment. If surgery is planned in children with hypermetropia, maximum tolerated plus or full cycloplegic correction should be worn at least 4–6 weeks before surgery to yield full exotropic deviation. Amblyopia if any present should be treated. This improves vision and good control in deviation.
- *Over minus correction*: This is based on the principle that overcorrecting the prescription of patient with minus lens induces accommodative convergence and can reduce the exodeviation. Overminus correction of 1–3 D can be given to children. Patients should be closely monitored. The minus correction can be reduced after stabilization of deviation. Studies have shown that minus lenses improved fusion quality and in some instances also the angle of deviation. Overminus lens therapy can be considered as a primary short-term treatment. They may be particularly useful in those patients with a high AC/A ratio.
- *Occlusion therapy*: This is used in young children as antisuppression therapy. Patching is done either in dominant eye or alternate patching in children with equal fixation preference. Studies show good control of exotropia with less chance of progression with patching therapy. It is a good temporary measure to delay surgery. Follow-up should be done in 3–4 months. If the angle of deviation is decreased or patient develops good control, occlusion can be continued with regular follow-up.
- *Orthoptic exercises*:
  - Orthoptic exercises are helpful in smaller deviation and especially for convergence insufficiency type intermittent exotropia. Small base in prism can be used to relieve diplopia and asthenopic symptoms. Base-out prism is also in practice which is believed to increase the accommodation effort and, hence, decrease deviation.
  - The result of convergence insufficiency treatment trial is supported orthoptic therapy for the treatment of convergence insufficiency. At the same time, it also has been shown to be effective in the treatment of convergence insufficiency type X (T) with a maximum deviation of 25 PDs. A recent retrospective study of 74 patients utilized office and home-based therapy with prism exercises, pencil push-ups, 3D tests, and dominant eye occlusion and showed improvement in 88% of patients with basic-type of right exotropia (XT), 88.8% of patients with divergence excess-type XT, and 100% of convergence insufficiency-type XT. There are now computer-based orthoptic programs that are easily accessible and can be used at home by patients. However, it is still unclear as which type of orthoptic exercises are most effective, for how long and at what frequency to be prescribed. In authors' clinical experience, exodeviations up to 25 PD, should be given a fair trial of orthoptic exercises. Even, well-explained and well-complied "pencil-push-ups" have shown good results.
- *Botulinum toxin*: This is one of the effective temporary measures for treatment of intermittent XT. However, it remains unlikely to replace surgery. One study showed satisfactory alignment in 50% of patients for up to 12 months following the initial injection of botulinum. It is a reasonable alternative in patients with small angle intermittent exotropia, small postoperative over or under corrections, or anesthetic or medical contraindications to surgery.

Surgery for Intermittent Exotropia

Indications for Surgery

The goal of strabismus surgery is to preserve or restore binocular vision and cosmesis. There is no common consensus on indication of surgery, age at which intervention is needed and the type of surgery. However, following conditions warrant for the surgical intervention in most of the patients.

- *Poor control of deviation*: Both control at home and in the clinic as described earlier may be used and correlated to assess control of the deviation. If the deviation occurs >50% of all waking hours, it indicates poor control of exotropia.
- *Increasing angle of deviation*: Documenting the size of deviation in each follow-up is very important in intermittent exotropia. If the angle of deviation increases, then surgery is indicated.
- *Deterioration of stereoacuity*: Distance stereoacuity is important in intermittent exotropia. Probably this is the most important objective evaluation for surgical intervention. Distance stereoacuity deterioration precedes near loss. Younger children may not reliably perform distance acuity and any deterioration in near stereoacuity is a definite sign of intervention. In older children, bothersome diplopia or visual confusion is an indication for surgical correction.
- *Severe asthenopia*: In patients with smaller deviation but severe asthenopia or diplopia that hinders day-to-day activities, and not relieved by conservative nonsurgical measures, need surgery.
- *Age of surgical intervention*:
  - The timing of surgery in intermittent exotropia has always remained controversial. Early intervention poses risk of monofixation syndrome and amblyopia if there small, consecutive, and postoperative esotropia. This hinders the development of good fusional potential in these children as they are in their formative age of visual development. Some studies have suggested small under correction to prevent monofixation syndrome. The need for repeat surgery is an issue in deciding about the timing of surgery. Parental decision is an important factor for surgical intervention. A retrospective study of 106 children reported that children with XT whose accompanying parent reported poorer "health-related quality of life" (HRQOL) were more likely to undergo surgery than those who reported better HRQOL. Parents' concern about the child's ability to function and psycho-social concern about their child can be associated with the decision to perform surgery. As there is no guideline for the time of surgery, the criteria for good surgical outcome also vary among the practitioners. Any strabismus surgery in children should have binocular single vision as a primary goal followed by cosmetic alignment. The good sensory outcome mainly depends on the preoperative stereoacuity. And the good motor outcome depends on good postoperative alignment.
  - In a nutshell, the timing of surgery should not be dependent on a single parameter, as operating on too young patient, has abovementioned risks. Small exodeviations with good fusion can wait and simply observed. Breaking of fusion and deterioration of stereoacuity are important indications for intervention. Prolongation in periods of deviation, most of waking hours, initiates decrease in stereoacuity and risk of amblyopia. Proper refractive correction is mandatory. All these factors have to be carefully looked into before surgical intervention. And it is prudent, to defer surgery, for as long as possible. Some patients with very infrequent deviations, with normal vision in both eyes, may continue with such situation life long and are not keen for any intervention.

Type of Surgery

The type of surgery in intermittent exotropia is again a subject of debate. There are many studies comparing the outcome of unilateral recess resect versus bilateral LR recession surgery in intermittent exotropia with mixed results.

- *Bilateral LR recession*: This is the surgery of choice in children with intermittent exotropia. This is preferred in children with divergence excess type. Symmetric surgery is usually preferred over resect recess procedure as latter may cause lateral incomitance with esotropia in side gaze and sometimes intractable diplopia in older children and adults.
- *Monocular resect procedure*: This is the procedure of choice for many surgeons with good outcome especially in cases with basic type and convergence insufficiency type. This is also the procedure of choice in patients with amblyopia. The deviation >50 PD should consider undergoing bilateral LR recession with one eye medial rectus (MR) resection.
- *Bilateral MR resection*: This procedure is of choice in convergence insufficiency type. However, this may cause narrowing of lid fissure. >5 mm of MR resection should be avoided.
- *One muscle LR recession*: Recession of unilateral LR gives good outcome in in small angle exotropia.
- *Augmented bilateral LR recession*: The augmented formula may be preferable to the standard formula for patients undergoing symmetric surgery to correct intermittent exotropia.

The Surgery Doses

Preoperative deviation measurement is very important in deciding the dose for surgery. Near distance disparity is

TABLE 3: Bilateral surgery.

Exotropia (prism diopter)	*LR OU recession*	*MR OU resection*
15	4 mm	3 mm
20	5 mm	4 mm
25	6 mm	5 mm
30	7 mm	5.5 mm
35	7.5 mm	6 mm
40	8 mm	6.5 mm
50	9 mm	

(LR: lateral rectus; MR: medial rectus)

TABLE 4: Unilateral surgery.

XT (prism diopter)	*Recess LR*	*Resect MR*
15	4	3
20	5	4
25	6	4.5
30	6.5	5
35	7	5.5
40	7.5	6
50	8	6.5

(LMR: lateral rectus; MR: medial rectus; XT: right exotropia)

common. Patch test is useful in revealing the maximum latent deviation. The repeat examinations may be needed in children if there is variable measurement. The dose of surgery should depend on the amount of distance deviation in basic and pseudodivergence excess. However, in cases of true divergence excess, the decision making is difficult. In these situations, target angle for surgery should be average of near and distance deviation. However, parents should be well informed that there may be the need of bifocal correction for near or reoperation.

The surgical doses for exotropia surgery have been derived from Marshal M Parks table with modification by Kenneth Wright. These numbers are a guide and should be modified as necessary **(Tables 3 and 4)**.

Three-muscle Surgery

For large horizontal deviations, surgery on three muscles may be planned for the primary operation. The amount of surgery can be judged from the above tables. For XT of >50 PD, three-muscle surgery is preferred, with one of muscles on adjustable suture, gives added advantage.

Some Special Considerations in Planning Surgery

- *Lateral incomitance*: Lateral incomitance is sometimes associated with intermittent exotropia. Patients whose primary position deviation exceeds right and left lateral gazes by 20% or at least 10 PD have significant horizontal incomitance. They may benefit from reducing the intended surgical weakening procedure on the LR muscle. This modification prevents overcorrection on lateral gazes but risks under correction in primary position.
- *Vertical deviation and pattern strabismus*: Small amount of vertical strabismus, of 10 PD or less, associated with intermittent exotropia can be ignored. This usually gets fixed with the horizontal surgery. The other way is to do a small transposition of horizontal muscle at the time of surgery. For example, the recessed LR and the resected MR muscle may be displaced superiorly one-half to a whole tendon width in the hypotropia (directions are reversed for a hyperdeviation). This acts as an additional upward vector assisting in the control of the vertical deviation. The surgery for "A" pattern exotropia with superior oblique overaction, the preferred procedure is a posterior three-quarters tenectomy of the superior oblique tendon. In "V" pattern deviations **(*see* Fig. 2)** with inferior oblique overaction, the patients will benefit from an inferior oblique weakening procedure. Alternatively, transposition procedures can be adopted. In "V" pattern, the MR is shifted downwards and LR is shifted upwards. In "A" pattern, reverse procedure is adopted. In simple terms, the MR is always shifted toward the "closed" end and LR shifted toward the "open" end. Half tendon to full tendon width can be transposed, which roughly gives 10–20 PD correction, respectively. In cases where "No" pattern is present, i.e., deviations are same in up gaze and down gaze, the surgical nomogram for straight gaze is maintained **(*see* Figs. 3A to C)**.

Postoperative Outcomes in Intermittent Exotropia

The successful surgery is measured in terms of both motor and sensory alignment. Immediately after surgery, a small consecutive esotropia of 8–10 PD is desirable. Even a large consecutive esotropia up to 20 PD may resolve without further surgery. Parents and patients should be warned of possible postoperative diplopia. Postoperative diplopia associated with the initial overcorrection usually resolves by 1-2 weeks. In smaller children, alternate part-time patching of each eye helps prevent suppression and amblyopia and may facilitate straightening of the eyes. If the exotropia is not congenital and has become obvious after the binocular mechanism has been in place, no permanent diplopia will occur. The child and parents can be well assured.

In case of uncertainty, a prism neutralization of tropia test is a good way of predicting the postoperative diplopia. As soon as the deviation is neutralized and the two foveas are conjugate, the child will complain of diplopia of the target. No diplopia shows that binocularity is good with bifoveal fixation, and no postoperative diplopia is likely to occur. Worrisome postoperative diplopia usually occurs in manifest strabismus of long standing. But this also clears by maximum 1 month.

Overcorrection

Overcorrection that persists beyond the immediate postoperative period is less common than undercorrection, even when surgery for the largest measured angle of exodeviation is performed. Postoperative overcorrection can be managed initially with prism or orthoptic exercises. In smaller children, alternate patching can prevent amblyopia. Plus lenses (+2.50 - +3.00 D), as near addition in bifocals will preserve fusion in patients with esotropia for near targets. Base-out prisms also serve to preserve fusional status and are tapered gradually. If significant esotropia persists even after 6 weeks, then reoperation should be considered. Rarely, a large overcorrection following an over-recessed or slipped LR muscle may occur. In this situation, immediate intervention may be needed. Advancing the previously recessed LR muscle is the surgery of choice in reoperation. If esotropia persists for near, weakening of the MR, through a recession and/or a faden operation, may be indicated.

Undercorrection

It is more common than the overcorrection. Under correction after initial bilateral LR recession is common, requiring a second surgical intervention in about one-third of patients. Under correction, usually 15 PD or more needs reoperation. It is advisable to wait for 8–12 weeks before planning reoperation. Factors contributing under corrections can be:

- Increasing deviation in viewing distant objects especially beyond 6 m
- Small amounts of coexisting vertical misalignment
- Failure to identify oblique muscle dysfunction and "A" or "V" pattern exotropia
- Failure to reveal the total amount of distance exotropia in preoperative measurements
- Uncorrected refractive error, especially significant hyperopia.

Orthoptic exercises, minus lens therapy or prisms can be tried in initial period of under correction. If no improvement, then reoperation can be performed between 6 and 8 weeks postoperative period. Re-recession of LR has limited outcome. MR resection is a good option. If unilateral recess-resect procedure was the initial surgery, then reoperation can be planned on the other eye.

The Prognosis

Long-term (5–10 years) prognosis of surgical outcome in intermittent exotropia is around 60%. Short-term outcome is good (80%) within 6 months–1 year. Orthoptic exercises and prism therapy in postoperative period for under correction or overcorrection can improve surgical outcome and long-term prognosis.

The success rate, as in most types of strabismus, is dependent on the length of follow up. In one of the longest follow-up studies, Richard and Parks found a 56% success rate with one surgery, defining success as a postoperative deviation >10 PD. 38% of their patients were under corrected and 6% were overcorrected. An additional surgery improved their success rate to around 80%. Another study reported 80% success rate after two surgeries with a 10-year follow-up. Hardesty attributed the long-term success to the aggressive use of postoperative prisms for both over and under corrections to maintain constant fusion to prevent suppression.

INFANTILE EXOTROPIA

Infantile exotropia is a rare condition. It is defined as idiopathic, large-angle, and constant exotropia appearing in the first 6 months–1 year of life. Based on the literature, it is reported to affect about 1 per 30,000 infants in the general population.

Exodeviations appear in over one-third of healthy neonates. Mostly, they are transient and resolve by 6 months as the vergence system matures. Therefore, primary infantile exotropia is likely caused by arrested development of the convergence system in this sensitive early period **(Figs. 5A and B)**.

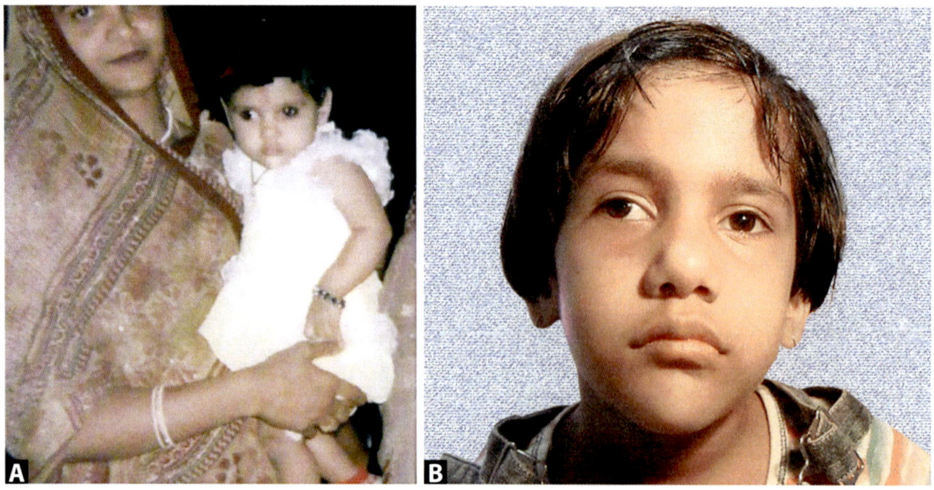

Figs. 5A and B: Infantile exotropia.

Primary infantile exotropia usually occurs in otherwise healthy children without any systemic or ocular abnormalities. Most of the time the disease is sporadic, however, familial cases have also been reported. Secondary infantile exotropia occurs due to systemic anomalies such as cerebral palsy, hydrocephalus, generalized developmental delay, and chromosomal anomalies. Other causes of incommitant infantile exotropia can be sensory due to poor vision, innervational anomalies such as Duane syndrome and congenital third nerve palsy. Strabismus is common in craniosynostosis, with rates from 39 to 90.9% in Crouzon, Apert, Pfeiffer, and Saethre-Chotzen syndromes. Infantile exotropia may be familial with variable penetrance, as was suggested in one case report, and it may be more common in Asians and Africans than in Caucasians.

It can have a wide range of angles, from 30 to 90 PDs, and almost always exceeds 30 PD. Distance and near deviations are almost equal, but sometimes near deviation may be more. The angle is usually stable initially, increasing slowly. Amblyopia occurs in up to 25%, usually strabismic amblyopia. Some authors classify "early onset intermittent exotropia" as a subclassification. This is important because intermittent deviations can wait intervention, but a constant large angle deviation needs early surgery.

Positive angle kappa, where the eye seems to be deviated out, should also be distinguished. But the deviation is small, not >10–15 PD, and the eye will have no "refixation" movement on alternate cover test. Age of onset of strabismus, as in infantile esotropia, is more important and should be determined by photographs of children, if history is not convincing.

Treatment

- *Nonsurgical*: Refractive errors and amblyopia should be addressed first, with occlusion or penalization of the dominant eye. Difficulty arises in wearing specks in infants. This helps in stabilizing the deviation, but unlikely to resolve exotropia. Those who improve with occlusion or penalization therapy are more likely to have early onset intermittent exotropia rather than true infantile exotropia. In the absence of amblyopia or eye preference, alternate occlusion therapy, as an antisuppression therapy can be instituted.

  Botulinum toxin injection to both lateral muscles in doses of 2.5–5.0 units can be offered as an alternative therapy. There are few studies on botulinum toxin in infantile exotropia, and the results are short lived. This can be tried only as a temporary measure to buy more time for surgery especially in cases of cerebral palsy.
- *Surgical procedure*: Infantile exotropia requires surgery. Although the angle of the deviation is generally stable, the strabismus angle may reduce with occlusion. Patients with infantile exotropia should be approached in the same manner as those with infantile esotropia—surgery should align the eyes preferably before the age of 24 months to achieve optimal motor and sensory results. Once the diagnosis of infantile exotropia is confirmed and any refractive error or amblyopia is corrected, the child should be followed for a few weeks to be sure that the angle of the strabismus is stable.

  Bilateral LR recession or monocular recess resect is the surgery of choice. However, if the angle is large, then three-muscle surgery may be required. Ocular or systemic disorders are more common in infantile exotropias than in esotropias. Also, infants with constant exotropia have a much stronger chance than those with intermittent exotropia of having a coexisting problem. Thorough systemic examination is needed. The magnetic resonance imaging (MRI) scan helps in localizing extraocular muscles in cases of craniosynostosis or congenital fibrosis syndromes. The pattern strabismus is common and should be addressed accordingly.
- Postoperative surgical outcomes appear to be influenced more by the duration of misalignment, rather than the age at surgery.

SENSORY EXOTROPIA

The term sensory exotropia refers to a unilateral exodeviation that develops as a result of loss of vision in one eye. Children under age 5 or 6 years who develop strabismus due to vision loss in one eye have an equal chance of developing esotropia or exotropia. After 6 years of age, exotropia is more common to develop. Sensory exotropia occurs in children as a result of a wide range of congenital and acquired ocular disorders. In compromised vision development, normal binocular vergence reflexes cannot develop which results in strabismus. The causes include congenital cataracts, ptosis, trauma, intraocular tumors, corneal opacities, eyelid hemangiomas, retinal detachments, and most importantly anisometropic amblyopia. These conditions should be treated as soon as possible. If the problem is present early in childhood then exotropia can be prevented, if vision can be restored by vigorous treatment, especially of amblyopia. Irrespective of an early or later onset, if exotropia has already developed, it may still reduce, if vision can be recovered **(Fig. 6)**.

Measuring the angle of the exotropia can be tricky when the vision is poor in one eye. The prism and alternating cover test may not be accurate because of poor fixation. The angle is better measured with the modified prism and light reflex (Krimsky) test. Sensory exotropia is usually over 30 PD. If the cause of the vision deficit persists then the angle can increase progressively. Sometimes in long-standing cases, LR contracture develops and the overlying soft tissues may shorten, creating a tight LR syndrome.

Several adaptations can occur in sensory exotropias. If the vision is very poor, there may be deep suppression and

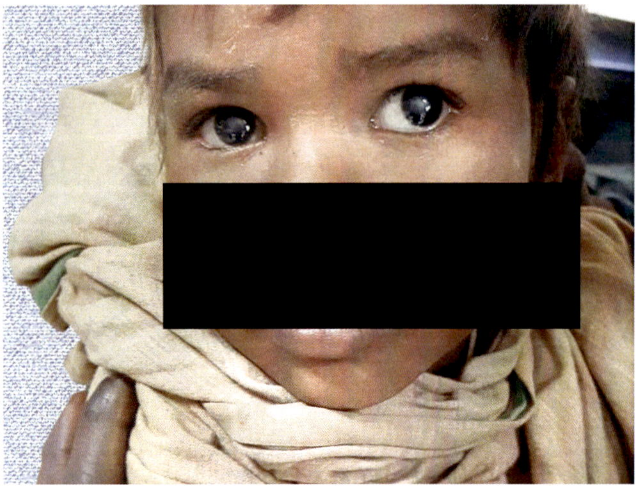

Fig. 6: Sensory exotropia (Bil cataracts).

no binocular responses. Children whose vision is not severely reduced and who have exotropia not exceeding 40 PD may develop ARC. Children with anisometropic amblyopia and exotropia may retain NRC. Young children can avoid diplopia by suppressing the displaced image. Older children who develop sensory exotropia may experience diplopia because they cannot develop anomalous retinal correspondence (ARC). Surgery of choice is the unilateral resect recess procedure. Patients with preoperative measurement under 40 PD tend to have a 75% chance of achieving a stable small angle heterotropia. Over the angle of 45 PD, the results decrease dramatically to 40–50% of long-term success. Monocular recess resect is the procedure of choice in sensory exotropia. The surgical dose should be modified from the normal table and should be decided according to deviation, the severity of amblyopia and potential of regaining vision. The maximum amount of recession or resection may be required. The postoperative overcorrection of 10–15 D should be the target.

CONSECUTIVE EXOTROPIA

It occurs following surgery of esotropia, as an overcorrection, after a variable period of time.

It may intermittent or constant. In small amounts of exodeviations, orthoptic exercises or prism addition can be tried. For larger consecutive deviations, surgery on LR can be contemplated.

MANIFEST CONSTANT EXOTROPIA

Constant primary exotropia usually manifests as infantile exotropia. Late onset manifest "constant" exotropia chronologically results from "decompensation" of intermittent exotropia, where the effort of fusion wanes. The transition from intermittent to constant type depends upon a number of factors already discussed in intermittent type. If these factors, particularly refractive errors and amblyopia, are not addressed timely and properly, would result in constant exotropia. Cases of true-divergence excess, without any AC/A abnormality, are more prone to develop constant exodeviation sooner. Once the deviation becomes constant, it may remain uniocular or alternating.

In case, the deviation becomes uniocular and persists for longer duration, strabismic amblyopia may result. In children, who continue with intermittent variety and manifest only during special circumstances, continue to have good vision and good binocularity. Such patients in this situation continue well into adulthood. The author has witnessed number of such patients who have intermittent exodeviation without any complaints. And the deviation occurs very infrequently, usually during far gazing or drowsiness. These are such examples where surgery may never be required and the patient may not give consent.

In other situations, where the deviation has become constant and quite large, surgery is required to avoid amblyopia and loss of stereopsis, and chances of eccentric fixation in children. Patients, who develop constant exotropia late into teenage or early adulthood, mostly come for cosmesis. Refractive error, if present should be first corrected, and presence of any amblyopia noted, and patient should be warned of prolonged postoperative diplopia.

As far as type of surgery is concerned, if deep amblyopia has already set in, then monocular recess-resect can be done, otherwise bilateral LR recession is procedure of choice.

ACCOMMODATIVE EXOTROPIA

Accommodative exotropia is a relatively uncommon disorder resulting from uncorrected myopia. As accommodation is less required in such patients for near work, the normal convergence is also minimized (near reflex) and the eyes tend to turn outward. Presentation is usually after 5–6 years when myopia tends to progress. In cases of high uniocular myopia, one eye is not used for distance as well as near, and therefore drifts outward. Correction of myopia by spectacles and high uniocular myopia by contact lenses usually resolves the deviation. The deviation is intermittent to begin with and then becomes constant.

Studies have revealed that there may be a small group of patients of exotropia associated with "accommodative dysfunction" in an emmetropic person. We have understudied and underrated the accommodative dysfunctions. Clinical testing indicated exotropia existed in patients who had severely reduced amplitudes of accommodation and difficulty in sustaining accommodation. It is recommended that in intermittent exotropic patients, careful evaluation of accommodation for adolescent and young adults should be done to rule out an accommodative defect as a contributing cause. In situations of decompensated intermittent exotropia, where a major drive to accommodation is lost via the "'convergence-accommodation to convergence (CA/C) linkage, loss to any attempt for fusion, makes the exotropia to progress further.

SUGGESTED READING

1. Bielschowsky A. Lectures on motor anomalies II. The theory of heterophoria. Am J Ophthal. 1938;21:1129.
2. Biglan AW, Davis JS, Cheng KP, Pettapiece MC. Infantile exotropia. J Pediatr Ophthalmol Strabismus. 1996;33:79-81.
3. Buckley EG, Seaber J, Tsironis E. Success of motor alignment in exotropia treated with botulinum toxin versus surgery. Am Orthopt J. 1996;46:127-32.
4. Burian HM, Franceschetti AT. Evaluation of diagnostic methods for the classification of exodeviations. Trans Am Ophthalmol Soc. 1970;68:56-71.
5. Burian HM, Spivey BE. The surgical management of exodeviations. Am J Ophthalmol. 1965;59:603-20.
6. Chen X, Fu Z, Yu J, Ding H, Bai J, Chen J, et al. Prevalence of amblyopia and strabismus in Eastern China: results from screening of preschool children aged 36-72 months. Br J Ophthalmol. 2016;100(4):515-9.
7. Chew E, Remaley NA, Tamboli A, Zhao J, Podgor MJ, Klebanoff M. Risk factors for esotropia and exotropia. Arch Ophthalmol. 1994;112:1349-55.
8. Chia A, Dirani M, Chan Y, Gazzard G, Eong KGA, Selvaraj P, et al. Prevalence of amblyopia and strabismus in young Singaporean Chinese children. Invest Ophthalmol Vis Sci. 2010;51(7):3411-7.
9. Chia A, Seenyen L, Long QB. A retrospective review of 287 consecutive children in singapore presenting with intermittent exotropia. JAAPOS. 2005;9(3):257-63.
10. Clark MP. Intermittent Exotropia. In: Taylor D, Hoyt C. Pediatric Ophthalmology and Strabismus, 5th edition. Netherlands: Elsevier; 2016.
11. Cotter SA, Mohney BG, Chandler DL, Holmes JM, Repka MX, Melia M, et al. A randomized trial comparing parttime patching with observation for children 3 to 10 years of age with intermittent exotropia. Ophthalmology. 2014;121:2299-310.
12. Cotter SA, Mohney BG, Chandler DL, Holmes JM, Wallace DK, Pediatric Eye Disease Investigator Group, et al. Three-year observation of children 12 to 35 months old with untreated intermittent exotropia. Ophthalmic Physiol Opt. 2020; 40(2):202-15.
13. Dadeya S, Kamlesh, Naniwal S. Usefulness of the preoperative prism adaptation test in patients with intermittent exotropia. J Pediatr Ophthalmol Strabismus. 2003;40:85-9.
14. Donahue SP, Chandler DL, Holmes JM. A randomized trial comparing bilateral lateral rectus recession versus unilateral recess and resect for basic-type intermittent exotropia. Ophthalmology. 2019;126(2):305-17.
15. Duanne A. A new classification of the motor anomalies based upon physiological principles together with their symptoms, diagnosis and treatment. Am Ophthalmol Otolaryngol. 1897;6:84.
16. Good WV, Hoyt CC. Exotropia. In: Good WV, Hoyt CS (Eds). Strabismus Management. Boston: Butterworth Heinmann; 1996. p. 93.
17. Haggerty H, Richardson S, Rhisos S. The Newcastle Control Score: a new method of grading the severity of intermittent distance exotropia. Br J Ophthalmol. 2004;88(2):233-5.
18. Hardesty H. Management of intermittent exotropia. Binocul Vis Q. 1990;5:145.
19. Hashemi H, Pakzad R, Heydarian S, Yekta A, Aghamirsalim M, Shokrollahzadeh F, et al. Global and regional prevalence of strabismus: a comprehensive systematic review and meta-analysis. Strabismus. 2019;27(2):54-65.
20. Hatt SR, Leske DA, Liebermann L, Mohney BG, Brodsky MC, Yamada T, et al. Association between health-related quality of life and the decision to perform surgery for childhood intermittent exotropia. Ophthalmology. 2014;121:883-8.
21. Holmes JH, Birch EE, Leske DA, Fu VL, Mohney BG. New tests of distance stereoacuity and their role in evaluating intermittent exotropia. Ophthalmology. 2007;114(6):1215-20.
22. Hunter DG, Kelly JB, Buffenn AN, Ellis FJ. Long-term outcome of uncomplicated infantile exotropia. J AAPOS. 2001;5:352-5-6.
23. Kenneth WW, Spiegel PH. Pediatric Ophthalmology and Strabismus, 2nd edition. New York: Springer-Verlag, Inc.; 2003.
24. Kim H, Yang HK, Hwang JM. Long-term surgical outcomes of augmented bilateral lateral rectus recession in children with intermittent exotropia. Am J Ophthalmolol. 2016;163:11-7.
25. Kushner BJ, Richard G. Scobee Memorial Lecture: Exotropic deviations: a functional classification and approach to treatment. Am Orthopt J. 1988;38:81-93.
26. Lee SY, Hyun Kim J, Thacker NM. Augmented bilateral lateral rectus recessions in basic intermittent exotropia. JAAPOS. 2007; 11(3):266-8.
27. Moheny B, Holmes J. Office based scale in control of intermittent exotropia. Strabismus. 2006;14;147-50.
28. Moheny B. Common form of childhood strabismus in an incidence cohort. Am J Ophthalmolog. 2007;144;465-67.
29. Mohney BG, Cotter SA, Chandler DL, Holmes JM, Wallace DK, Yamada T, et al. Three-year observation of children age 3 to 10 years old with untreated intermittent exotropia. Ophthalmology. 2019:126(9):1249-60.
30. Noorden GK von. Exodeviations. In: Binocular Vision and Ocular Motility. Theory and management of strabismus. 5th edition. St Louis: Mosby; 1996. p. 341.
31. Pediatric Eye Disease Investigator Group. A randomized trial evaluating short-term effectiveness of Overminus lenses in children 3 to 6 years of age with intermittent exotropia. Ophthalmology. 2016;123(10):2127-36.
32. Rosenbaum A, Stathacoupulos R. Subjective and objective criteria for recommending surgery in intermittent exotropia. Am Orthopt J. 1996;42:46-51.
33. Santiago AP, Ing MR, Kushner BJ. Intermittent exotropia. In: Rosenbaum AL, Santiago AP (Ed). Clinical Strabismus Management: Principles and Surgical Techniques, 1st edition. Philadelphia: Saunders; 1999. pp. 163-75.
34. Schiemann M, Rouse M, Kulp MT, Cotter S, Hertle R, Mitchell GL. Treatment of convergence insufficiency in childhood: a current perspective. Optom Vis Sci. 2009;86:420-8.
35. Velez G. Surgical treatments of exotropia with poor vision. In: Reinecke RD (Ed). Strabismus II: Proceedings of the Fourth Meeting of the International Strabismological Association. Orlando: Grune and Stratton; 1984. pp. 263-7.
36. Von Noorden GK. Binocular Vision and Ocular Motility, 6th edition. St Louis: Mosby; 2002. pp. 340-5.
37. Von Noorden GK. Binocular Vision and Ocular Motility: Theory and Management of Strabismus. St. Louis: Mosby; 1985.
38. Wiggins R, Noorden GV. Monoocular eye closure in sunlight. J Ped Ophthal. 1990;27:16.
39. Zou D, Casafina C, Whiteman A. Predictors of surgical success in patients with intermittent exotropia. JAAPOS. 2017;21(1):15-8.

23

CHAPTER

Complex Forms of Strabismus

Edward Kuwera, Mireille Jabroun

BRIEF HISTORY

The old Greeks first defined "*strabismus*" as a disorder of eye movements and position. By today's standards, their treatment options would be seen as bizarre, but it was a start in the treatment of amblyopia. More than a thousand years later, in the Byzantine Empire, around the year 900 AD, there was the first mention of occlusion for the treatment of strabismus in history. In the 13th century, the first eye hospital was established in France, and in the 16th century, a German physician designed special hoods to put them over one's head to treat strabismus. In the year 1722, a French ophthalmologist Charles de Saint-Yves wrote in his book that by covering the non-strabismic eye, the strabismic eye will immediately look straight ahead—something that we now know as a cover test. He also proposed that the non-strabismic eye should be covered in order to restore the correct eye position of the deviated eye. A few years later, in 1743, George Comte de Buffon, another French physician described that the weak eye regains all its strength by occluding the good eye, which is why he is considered as a beginner of the occlusion therapy in amblyopia. The first idea of treating strabismus (and amblyopia) surgically came in the 18th century by John Taylor, although his surgical techniques on eye muscles were later recognized as a fraud. Roughly 100 years later, Germans Stromeyer and Dieffenbach, and Belgian Cunier were the first to have performed a proper surgery for treating strabismus. It was also then noted by Ludwig Boehm that the surgery to correct strabismus also improved amblyopia.

INTRODUCTION

Strabismus is a misalignment of the eyes, also referred to as *squint* (though a misnomer) that may affect 1–3% of children. It is seen more commonly in patients with a history of prematurity, systemic or genetic diseases, and those with a family history of strabismus. Although it may also be referred to as *lazy eye*, this term is not specific to strabismus alone, so we recommend against using this description. There is typically a dominant, or fixating eye, but this may alternate depending on the type of strabismus and level of acuity in each eye. Common forms of strabismus are usually in the horizontal axis and are comitant, or the same in all directions of gaze, while the more complex forms of strabismus tend to have incomitance and can vary significantly depending on the direction of gaze. This chapter will focus on the latter forms of strabismus.

All children should have periodic visual screenings, as the potential for successful treatment of strabismus and amblyopia is greatest in young children. If not promptly recognized or treated, a plethora of functional deficits may result and persist into adulthood, with far reaching impacts on productivity and quality of life. The resulting morbidities include:

- *Psychosocial repercussions*: Interference with social contact and cosmetic distress. Children begin to develop a negative attitude toward classmates with strabismus as early as the age of 6 years. This attitude adversely affects interpersonal relationships, self-image, schoolwork, and participation in sports, and only intensifies in the teenage and adult years. In adults, it can affect their ability to find a partner, job, and may even manifest as a more serious psychiatric disorder.
- *Increased risk of impairment of the sound eye (if there is amblyopia)*: The lifetime risk of impairment to the sound eye is estimated to be 1:100–1:1,000 from accidental trauma or other etiologies such as macular degeneration and retinal vein occlusion.
- *Impaired binocular function*: There is reduced, or absent, stereopsis, which can affect visual-motor skills, and even restrict careers such as aviation.
- Most adult strabismus represents deterioration of childhood strabismus, which can occur even after decades of good ocular alignment. Recurrence is more common in adults who lack binocular vision and stereopsis, or those who had partially treated, or untreated amblyopia.

Current standards of care in the treatment of strabismus and amblyopia are largely based on the work of two study groups that conducted randomized clinical trials to define treatment protocols. There is the UK-based Monitored Occlusion Treatment of Amblyopia Study (MOTAS), and the US-based Pediatric Eye Disease Investigator Group (PEDIG).

The strengths of these studies include a large cohort, broad age groups, different types of amblyopia in a wide range of acuities, certified examiners, and standardized acuity testing protocols. The primary limitation in both studies is the lack of control subjects.

When dealing with complex forms of strabismus, it is important to emphasize the significantly increased chance of requiring multiple operations, along with the near impossible nature of achieving perfect results. There will likely be residual diplopia in some, or in many directions of gaze, but the goal is to optimize the "sphere" of single vision to primary and down-gaze, as these are the most important directions of gaze for the average person. There are exceptions to consider in patients who have specific visual needs, such as boxers who require single vision in upgaze to protect their chin by keeping a chin-down posture.

LANCASTER RED-GREEN TESTING

The Lancaster red-green (LRG) test is an invaluable diagnostic tool of which we strongly recommend its use in complex strabismus. It is a binocular, dissociative, and subjective test that is particularly useful in paralytic or restrictive strabismus. It has the advantage of providing a measure of comitance, primary and secondary deviations, and subjective torsion in the nine diagnostic directions of gaze. These results facilitate patient understanding of the problem and plan of care by allowing them to also see a direct graphical representation of their pattern of misalignment.

The test consists of a calibrated screen with a linear grid of black spots mounted, or directly drawn, onto a wall. More information about set-up and interpretation of this test can be found in the 2006 edition of the American Orthoptic journal in an article by David Guyton, MD and Alex Christoff, CO—*The Lancaster Red-Green Test*.

The primary limitations of the test are that it requires the user to be precise in documentation in order to have accurate results, and the test cannot be done if a patient suppresses vision in the deviated eye. Alternatively, a photo of each position can be taken to maximize accuracy.

Briefly Summarizing the LRG Test

- Red lines correspond to the right eye, and green lines to the left eye.
- The lines are to be superimposed in a vertical fashion, with any deviation indicating displacement and/or torsion.
- The distance between each dot on the grid corresponds to 15 prism diopters (PD) of displacement.
- The plot is presented such that it is through the perspective of the patient. For example:
  - Orthotropia would be represented by superimposed vertical red and green lines.
  - Exotropia would be represented by a vertical red line displaced to the right of a vertical green line.
  - Esotropia (ET) would be represented by a vertical red line to the left of a vertical green line.
  - A right hypertropia would be represented by a vertical red line above a vertical green line.
- Torsion is indicated by tilting of the vertical line either to the left, or right, and is interpreted as the same direction that eye is torted.
  - For example, a red vertical line that has the top of the line rotated 45° clockwise would indicate a right eye that is extorted by a similar, but not exact amount. This is because there is sensory adaptation to torsion, such that what is experienced by the patient may not be as much as what is measured objectively.

We will use some examples of this test throughout the chapter as a supplement to the standard evaluation of strabismus.

CONGENITAL CRANIAL DYSINNERVATION DISORDERS

Congenital cranial dysinnervation disorders (CCDD) are a broad spectrum of congenital disorders that affect the extraocular muscles, resulting in various forms of incomitant strabismus. Our focus will be on congenital fibrosis of the extraocular muscles (CFEOM), Duane syndrome, and Moebius syndrome.

Congenital Fibrosis of the Extraocular Muscles

Congenital fibrosis of the extraocular muscles is a congenital, nonprogressive ptosis and ophthalmoplegia characterized by the abnormal development of the extraocular muscles' innervation, primarily from cranial nerves III and IV. Its prevalence is 1:250,000. Initially thought to be a developmental abnormality of extraocular muscle tissue, it was only recently found to be a secondary process.

Pathophysiology

The fibrosis of the extraocular muscle is now known to be secondary to an innervational abnormality rather than a primary muscle process. Clinically, resulting in incomitant vertical strabismus and variously incomitant horizontal strabismus.

Examination Findings

Patients with CFEOM often present with a chin-up head posture, ptosis, and difficulty with supraductions and sometimes also restriction to the horizontal movement. Other ocular phenotypic associations are Marcus Gunn jaw-winking phenomenon and retinal dystrophy. CFEOM can be classified into three major types based on the presenting phenotype and associated genetic cause.

1. CFEOM1, an autosomal dominant disorder, is characterized by severe bilateral ptosis and limitation to elevation

in both eyes secondary to a heterozygous mutation in KIF21A1, whose function involves the microtubules of neuronal axons.
2. CFEOM2 is primarily autosomal recessive and results from homozygous mutations in PHOX2A2. Patients typically have severe bilateral ptosis and horizontal deviation similar to bilateral third nerve palsies.
3. CFEOM3 has a more complex genetic background and can be associated with heterozygous mutations in TUBB3 and rarely in KIF21A or TUBB2B. It is primarily an autosomal dominant disorder, but autosomal recessive mutations have been described to be associated. Phenotypic presentation varies even within the same family and can have unilateral involvement. We will now review the management of a case of CFEOM.

Case

A 16-year-old female was noted to have down-turning of both eyes since birth, more pronounced on the left. She underwent bilateral inferior rectus recession of 5 mm in the right eye (OD) and 8 mm in the left eye (OS) at 1 year of age. At 4 years of age, she had a second surgery—left inferior rectus (LIR) disinsertion and bilateral medial rectus recessions of 4 mm, along with a sling of the left upper eyelid for ptosis correction.

Postoperatively, her alignment improved, but the more hypotropic left eye continued to bother her. There was no diplopia. Ductions showed limitation of elevation worse in abduction (–4 OU) than adduction (–2 OD and –3 OS). There was some limitation of depression in OS more than OD, where both eyes appear to intort on attempted depression and extort on attempted elevation. Her distance and near deviations were exotropia (XT) of 10 PD and a left hypotropia of 10–12 PD. There were no significant changes with head tilt. She had 2+ fundus extorsion of both eyes.

The initial limitation of elevation was due to fibrosis of the inferior rectus muscles. However, its recurrence in the left eye postoperatively, combined with the fundus extortion, is likely a result of reattachment of the LIR with progressive tightening over time, even after the disinsertion procedure. Since she never had surgery on her left superior rectus (LSR), some success may be obtained by tightening the inactive muscle, which is the LSR in this case. It is possible that she will benefit from a rerecession of the LIR and resection of the LSR. It is important to consider eyelid position with any surgery on the superior rectus (SR). The left upper lid might become slightly more ptotic with a resection. Therefore, careful dissection of the perimuscular connective tissue from the SR and the levator muscle is important to minimize this risk.

At time of surgery, forced ductions showed moderately tight LIR and LSR muscles. The LIR was explored, recessed 4 mm and transposed nasally 4 mm. The SR was resected 5 mm and nasally transposed 4 mm, later adjusted to 8-mm resection.

Postoperatively, she had a small overcorrection of 5 PD of a left hypertropia. This is generally desirable in her case as her LSR resection is expected to relax over time, especially against an already tight LIR, which may also progressively tighten. The nasal transposition here serves to improve her small angle exotropia to decrease the number of muscles operated on. This transposition procedure was not enough to fix the XT, so she underwent an additional 6 mm advancement of the left medial rectus (LMR). She was happy with her final alignment.

Treatment Recommendations

Neuroimaging is recommended in rare cases of unilateral disease, and in the presence of neurological, or developmental delay. Although not essential for the diagnosis, the absence or hypoplasia of cranial nerve III would be confirmatory, and reviewing the extraocular muscles would be beneficial in surgical planning and excluding other causes such as congenital orbital fibrosis.

A thorough genetic evaluation and counseling is essential as CFEOM can also be associated with systemic findings such as facial weakness, intellectual disabilities, and anosmia with hypogonadotropic hypogonadism (Kallmann syndrome) in TUBB3-associated disease. Hence, the importance of obtaining a specific genetic diagnosis.

Surgical management is often needed given the severity of the restriction and associated exposure keratopathy with the lack of a Bell's phenomenon. Surgical approach varies and should be individualized and guided by forced duction testing at the time of surgery. Muscle recessions are often performed given the restrictive nature of this disease, and large amounts are needed in some patients. Rectus muscle myectomy and superior oblique tenotomy can be performed and reserved for severe or recurrent cases. Resections of the antagonist muscle can be safely used. Fixation of the lateral rectus (LR) to lateral orbital wall might also be needed in some cases of CFEOM3. It is crucial to explain to patients that there is a high risk of needing additional surgery, and most patients will require more than one. The goal of surgery is to alleviate any restriction with a minimal number of muscles, given the need for subsequent surgeries and risk of anterior segment ischemia. Patients should be counseled appropriately. There is a high risk of associated keratopathy, and if eyelid surgery is required, it is best to leave the lids at 1–2 mm above the center of the pupil.

Duane Syndrome

This was first described in 1887 by Stilling, but later popularized by Alexander Duane who published a case series of patients with the condition. Duane syndrome is a congenital, nonprogressive limited horizontal eye movement associated with globe retraction on adduction and subsequent palpebral fissure narrowing, with, or without up or downshooting of the eye. It is more commonly seen unilaterally, usually the left eye, and mostly in females, but bilateral involvement is well recognized.

Treatment Recommendations

At the time of surgery, or if a sedated MRI is warranted, exaggerated forced duction testing typically confirms the passive limitation of elevation in adduction with a restricted superior oblique tendon. This has even been described to be curative in some cases (Squirrell D, 2005)! In other cases of acquired Brown syndrome, a steroid injection into the trochlear region can be attempted.

If surgery is required, several approaches have been described. Superior oblique tenotomy (Berke RN, 1949) or tenectomy has been widely used in the past, but led to overcorrection by creating an iatrogenic superior oblique palsy. As a result, Parks recommended simultaneous inferior oblique weakening with those procedures. Other surgeons prefer tendon lengthening by split tendon elongation or Z tenotomy. Silicone spacers are also an option; however, they can cause a foreign body reaction in some patients. Undercorrection is expected after silicone spacers and typically improves over time. Our preferred procedure is the adjustable suture spacer. It allows for intraoperative adjustment guided by fundus torsion and forced ductions as well as postoperative adjustment fine-tuned to the patient's actual deviation or subjective experience.

THYROID EYE DISEASE

Thyroid eye disease (TED), also known as *Grave's ophthalmopathy*, is an autoimmune condition that affects retrobulbar tissue. There is no specific age of diagnosis, but it is most prevalent in females in their 3rd to 5th decade, although it is usually more severe in males. It tends to present within 18 months of other endocrine manifestations in 80% of patients in a biphasic course with a progressive phase lasting up to 3 years, and a stable or inactive phase.

Pathophysiology

Thyroid eye disease is caused by inflammatory infiltration of the extraocular muscles with subsequent restrictive myopathy and progressive fibrosis. There is activation of autoantibodies to thyroid stimulating hormone (TSH) receptors, leading to an overexpression of these receptors, inducing proliferation of fibroblasts and secretion of proinflammatory cytokines and hyaluronan. These substances collect in the interstitial space, increasing the osmotic gradient, with subsequent accumulation of fluid between muscle fibers. Most patients are hyperthyroid (80%) while 15% are hypothyroid and 5% are euthyroid.

Examination Findings

Patients with restrictive strabismus secondary to TED can have associated eyelid retraction, proptosis, lateral flare, and exposure keratopathy. Patients should be also monitored for compressive optic neuropathy. Although usually not necessary for diagnosis and management, enlargement of the involved muscles can be detected on orbital MRI and CT scan, and is characterized by tendon sparing. The most common muscles involved are the inferior rectus, followed by the medial rectus, and then the SR. The LR can uncommonly be involved, though oblique muscle involvement has been well described and is often overlooked. Multiple muscle involvement is commonly seen and often needs to be addressed. Patients should be counseled that smoking can exacerbate the disease and cessation decreases the risk of diplopia and exophthalmos.

Case

Figures 5 and 6 illustrate the postoperative motility and LRG plot, respectively, of a 39-year old female with a history of TED secondary to Grave's disease. She developed a left hypotropia after undergoing an LSR recession of 9 mm, and a left inferior oblique recession that was performed to correct a left hypertropia thought to be caused by TED affecting the SR, superimposed on old left 4th nerve palsy. Her LRG illustrates the left hypotropia present in all directions of gaze, greatest on left gaze and in upgaze across the board. She has a limitation of elevation of her left eye worse in abduction. No significant torsional misalignment was found. This postoperative pattern is suggestive of either having a slipped SR muscle, or overcorrection. Intraoperatively, her SR muscle was not found to be slipped, so it was advanced to the insertion. This illustrates the high risk of overcorrection in cases of TED, and was certainly increased by weakening of both elevators—the SR and inferior oblique.

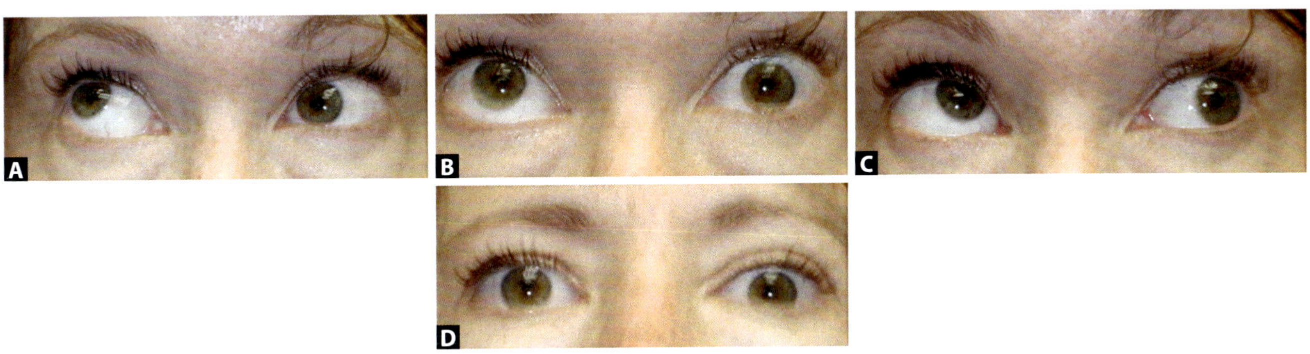

Figs. 5A to D: Postoperative overcorrection of a left superior rectus recession.

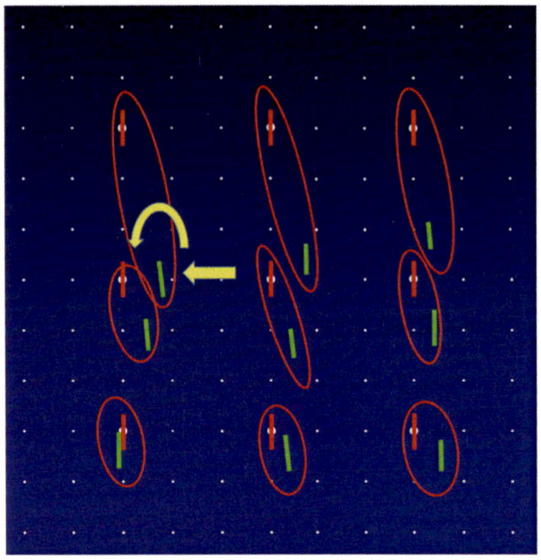

Fig. 6: Lancaster red–green plot of a postoperative overcorrection of a left superior rectus recession. Note the hypotropia and extorsion of the eye.

Treatment Recommendations

Thyroid eye disease associated with restrictive myopathy is often challenging to treat. In mild cases, patients can be managed with prisms. However, surgery is needed in most patients to restore fusion and enlarge the range of binocular single vision. It is crucial to delay surgery in cases of active disease and treat with temporary solutions like prism, or occlusion. At least 6 months of stable strabismus measurements and nonactivity are needed before considering any surgical intervention. If orbitopathy is planned, it should precede strabismus as the alignment often changes, with strabismus surgery preceding eyelid surgery.

Muscle recessions are the standard approach, though resections have been described in select cases, but with risk of worsening strabismus and motility. Because of the fibrotic muscle tissue, surgical tables often over correct and numbers should be reduced. We prefer using adjustable sutures as they allow for postoperative refinement. Using the resting position of the eye has been described and is guided by ductions, but often involves very large recessions on both eyes, and on several muscles to be successful.

There is a risk of worsening proptosis with muscle recessions, especially when recessing two consecutive recti muscles. Eyelid position may also change, and these are important considerations. Patients should be counseled accordingly. When recessing the inferior rectus, we typically place the lower lid retractors on adjustable sutures to minimize any changes to the position of the lower eyelid. Adjustment of the lid retractors should be done after finalizing the adjustment of the inferior rectus.

In cases of equally restricted infraduction in both eyes, and a small, or no ocular misalignment in primary position, patients tend to have significant lid retraction and use a chin-up posture to compensate. Fixation duress can be differentiated from other causes of abnormal head posture, and lid retraction as it persists under monocular occlusion. Management should include bilateral inferior rectus operations rather than unilateral. Care should be taken not to induce intorsion in downgaze in large bilateral recessions.

Evaluation of any vertical misalignment should include the evaluation of torsion before any surgical intervention, even if the patient is not symptomatic for torsion, as most people are able to adapt to small torsional deviations. Most people can adapt and fuse around 7–10° of torsion, but care should be taken in cases of preexisting ocular torsion. Assessing fundus torsion is always important, but not always revealing as in cases of superior oblique muscle involvement; intorsion can be minimized by the simultaneous extorsional effect of the restricted inferior rectus muscles. Both contribute to the hypotropia. If not simultaneously addressed, and very large recessions of the inferior rectus muscles are done, postoperative intorsion and A-pattern strabismus can develop, despite correction of the vertical strabismus. LRG testing is our preferred method to evaluate torsional misalignment as it allows for its evaluation in all directions of gaze. In some instances, forced duction testing at the time of surgery will be needed to help differentiate simultaneous involvement of the ipsilateral superior oblique versus the contralateral SR. Surgical planning should proceed accordingly.

Late overcorrection in TED has been well recognized, so many surgeons prefer undercorrections at the immediate postoperative period. However, final alignment is not achieved until 1-year postoperative. Some speculate that the inferior rectus has a higher tendency for slippage, especially on adjustable sutures. For this reason, some surgeons use a semiadjustable technique. This limits the adjustment to the central muscle fibers and can allow for only a few millimeters of adjustment, resulting in central sagging of the muscle. We prefer using nonabsorbable suture materials to decrease the risk of slippage and optimize the adjustment process. In some cases, late overcorrection is not due to inferior rectus muscle slippage. A concomitant ipsilateral restricted SR often pulls the eye up against a weakened inferior rectus. Forced ductions and careful assessment of ductions preoperatively can elucidate this finding.

ANESTHETIC MYOTOXICITY

Strabismus may develop from retrobulbar or peribulbar anesthetic injections for both anterior and posterior segment eye surgery. This is attributed to myotoxicity as a result of local anesthetic infiltration into any of the extraocular muscles. Diplopia subsequently occurs in patients who have otherwise binocular vision. The incidence of strabismus from local anesthetic myotoxicity is approximately 1 in 200 (0.5%). Evidence for local anesthetic as the culprit, rather

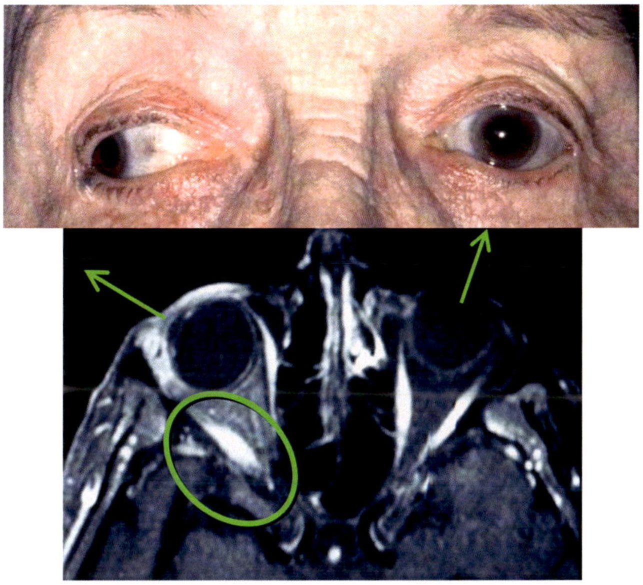

Fig. 7: Local anesthetic myotoxicity to the right lateral rectus and the corresponding axial MRI.

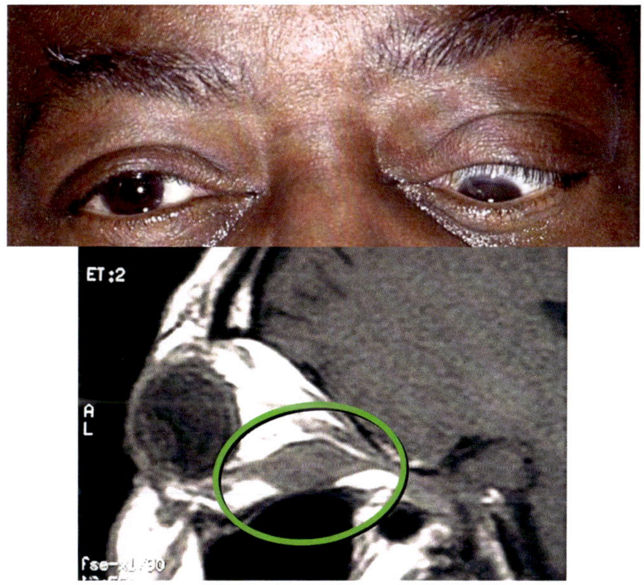

Fig. 8: Local anesthetic myotoxicity to the left inferior rectus and the corresponding sagittal MRI.

than scarring or mechanical effects from procedures such as scleral buckling are:

- Higher risk of strabismus after local than general anesthesia
- Poor correlation between the affected muscle and location of the buckle
- Similar distribution of affected muscles when compared to cataract surgery
- Finding tight muscles at the time of surgery with significant improvement from a large recession of the affected muscle alone.

In 1985, Rainin reported experimental injections of 0.75% of bupivacaine into extraocular muscles prior to cataract surgery caused strabismus in four out of six patients with ptosis in the remaining two. Similar experiments were carried out on primates using local anesthetic injections of either 2% lidocaine or 0.75% bupivacaine directly into intraocular muscles. This resulted in widespread damage over most of the cross-sectional area of the muscle fibers. Regeneration of muscle tissue was found in younger, but not older monkeys. MRI early in the course of injury has shown swelling consistent with edema **(Figs. 7 and 8)**. All of the anesthetics studied were found to be myotoxic, with bupivacaine causing the most damage, and procaine the least.

Pathophysiology

Many authors have contributed to the proposed mechanism of injury described as localized muscle fibrosis and hypertrophy, most notably by David Guyton, MD and Alan Scott, MD. Initially, during the acute phase, there is a temporary paresis of the involved muscles as the fibers degenerate. This is followed by a progressive and segmental fibrosis with hypertrophy of the muscle, especially in older individuals.

TABLE 1: Muscles involved in anesthetic myotoxicity in 30 patients over 4 years by David Guyton, MD.

Muscle(s) involved	***Number of patients***
Inferior rectus	16
Superior rectus	4
Inferior oblique	3
Superior oblique	2
Medial rectus	2
Lateral rectus	2
Inferior and medial rectus	1

Source: Guyton DL. Strabismus complications from local anesthetics. Semin Ophthalmol. 2008;23(5):298-301.

Lastly, there is reversal and worsening of the initial diplopia in what appears to be "overaction" of the affected muscle. Although the inferior rectus muscle is most often involved, all of the extraocular muscles can be affected. The extraocular muscles that are most frequently affected, as experienced by Dr Guyton, are listed in **Table 1**.

Examination Findings

The manifestation of strabismus will depend on what muscle(s) is affected. As discussed earlier, there tends to be an initial paresis of the muscle, followed by progressive fibrosis and restriction of the same muscle, reversing the strabismus over a period of 2 weeks to a month.

Here we will review a case of postcataract surgery strabismus in which the right inferior rectus muscle was affected.

Case

A 76-year-old female with a noncontributory medical history presents with vertical diplopia immediately following cataract

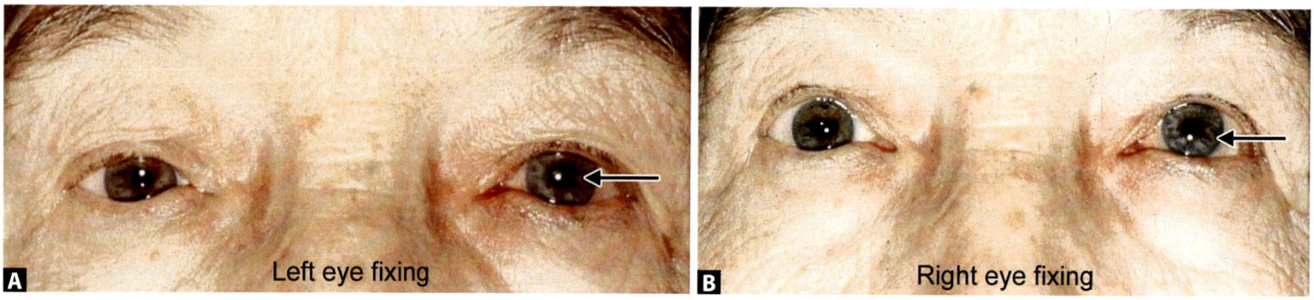

Figs. 9A and B: Restriction of the right inferior rectus with a hypotropia on fixation with the left eye.

Prism and alternate cover test

Near$_{cc}$ ET 15 RhypoT 20		
	ET 12 RhypoT 27	
ET 17 RhypoT 27	ET 15 RhypoT 22	ET 20 RhypoT 25
	ET 17 RhypoT 30	
Fundus torsion 1+ extorsion right eye None left eye		

Motility

Right eye		
0	0	0
0	0	0
0	0	–2

Left eye		
0	0	0
0	0	0
0	0	0

Fig. 10: Motility and strabismus examinations showing and esotropia and right hypotropia.

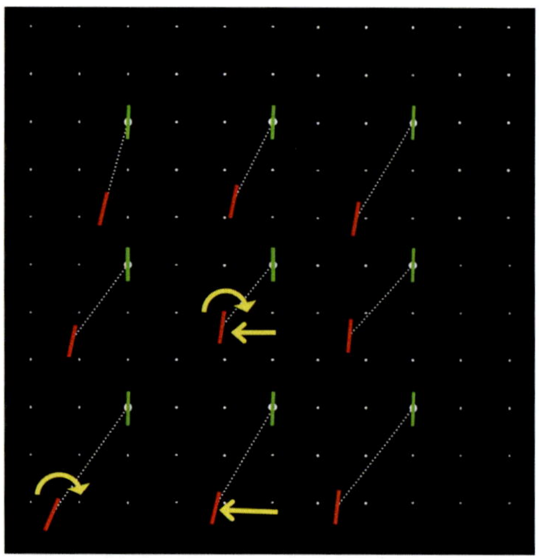

Fig. 11: Left eye fixating. Preoperative Lancaster red–green plot showing and esotropia worse in downgaze and right eye extorsion worse in down- and ingaze.

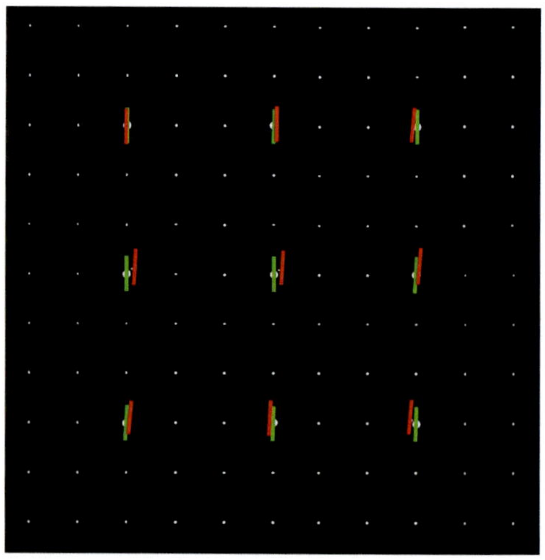

Fig. 12: Six weeks post right inferior rectus recession 16 mm.

surgery with intraocular lens implantation of the right eye. The surgery was done with a retrobulbar injection mixture of 2% lidocaine and 0.75% bupivacaine. Patient describes progressively worsening vertical diplopia over 2 months, along with a torsional component.

Her motility and strabismus examination are shown in **Figures 9 to 12**. It is evident, especially on the LRG plot, the type of misalignment and torsion, she is experiencing and where it is worst.

There is an ET and right hypotropia that is worse on downgaze. Furthermore, there is significant extorsion of the right eye compared to the left eye that worsens on down- and ingaze, which can only be due to a tight right inferior rectus muscle. No other muscle can cause extorsion on depression and adduction. A tight inferior oblique would cause a hypertropia of the right eye, and a tight superior oblique would cause intorsion.

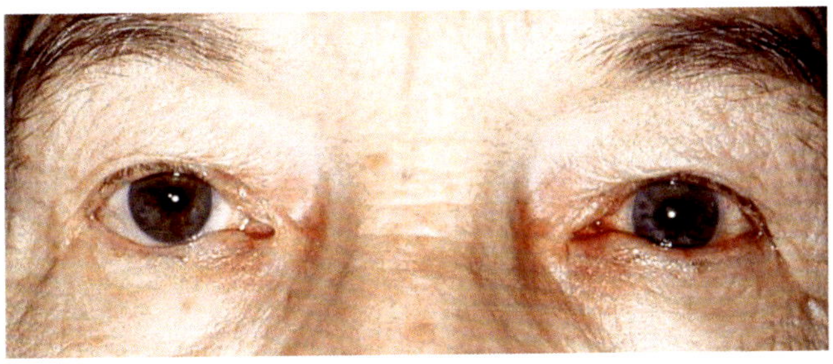

Fig. 13: Six weeks postoperative right inferior rectus recession 16 mm.

During surgery, she was found to have a very tight right inferior rectus on forced duction testing and subsequently underwent a large inferior rectus recession. **Figures 12 and 13** show her alignment 6 weeks postoperative with excellent results.

Treatment Recommendations

It is important to elicit any history of a reversal of diplopia over time (usually over 2–4 weeks), as this is essentially pathognomonic for anesthetic myotoxicity. The inferior rectus is most frequently affected, but any of the extraocular muscles can be involved.

Use hyaluronidase, if a retrobulbar or peribulbar injection must be given. Brown et al., found that during a period of unavailability of hyaluronidase in 1998, there was a threefold increase in myotoxicity after cataract surgery. Hyaluronidase has been shown to have a protective role by allowing the anesthetic to rapidly dissipate from the injection site. This allows for lower volumes and concentrations of the agent to be used while still maintaining efficacy.

Consider administering sub-Tenon's local anesthetic using blunt cannula techniques. This lessens the risk of retrobulbar hemorrhage and direct injection into muscle tissue. Simply bathing the muscle in anesthetic has not been shown to cause significant myotoxicity. If a patient experiences significant pain during the injection, it may be a result of direct infiltration into muscle tissue, and this should signal the provider to stop. Shift toward topical anesthesia whenever possible. **Figure 14** shows the position of a retrobulbar needle when advanced into the orbit—it is self-evident that any of the extraocular muscles can be injured in this manner.

Remember that the strabismus will be at its greatest deviation when looking away from the field of action of the involved muscle. Torsion is extremely important and the authors have found LRG testing to be most helpful in its evaluation.

Use forced ductions to guide the surgical plan and use adjustable sutures whenever possible. Plan for large recessions of a single muscle and advise patients on the increased risk of recurrence, or need for repeat surgery when compared to patients with normal extraocular muscles. Explain that once a muscle has been damaged, it can no longer function in the same way, and thus, the surgical outcome is no longer as predictable.

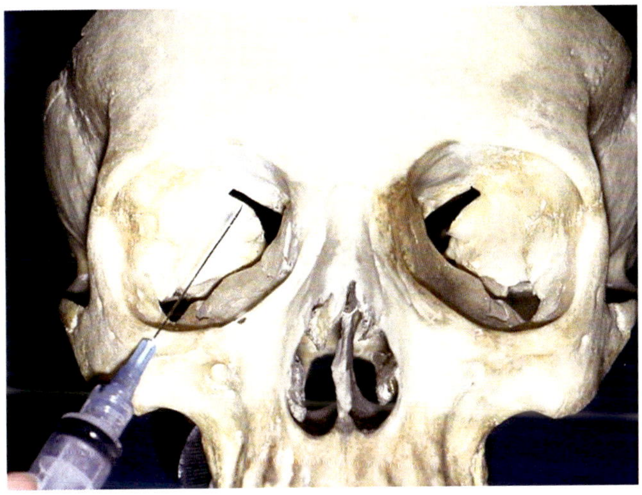

Fig. 14: Location of a retrobulbar needle during retrobulbar injections.

HEAVY EYE SYNDROME

First described in 1966 by Dr Bagshaw (J, 1966), heavy eye syndrome (HES), also known as *myopic strabismus fixus* and *convergent strabismus fixus*, is typically induced by axial myopia that results in painless, progressive large angle ET, and hypotropia with resultant limitations to elevation and abduction. This is most common in high myopia, usually around 18 diopters, but there have been case reports of this condition in the absence of high myopia, and in the presence of high myopia with exotropia.

This should be differentiated from sagging eye syndrome, which typically occurs in elderly patients in the absence of high myopia. Demer et al., describe a typical presentation with additional findings of ptosis and superior sulcus abnormalities. There is degeneration of the LR-SR band, a ligament which suspends the LR pulley, which leads to a similar pathophysiological process as HES, but with more pronounced hypotropia. Its association with ptosis is a result of the similar degenerative change found in age-related dehiscence of the levator aponeurosis.

Pathophysiology

The mechanism of dysfunction has been evaluated using orbital imaging via CT and MRI. Krzizok and Schroeder found displacement in the paths of all extraocular muscles, particularly inferior displacement of the LR. This inferior displacement and compression against the orbital wall from posterior "bulging" of the globe are what was thought to be the cause of the abduction weakness. However, this theory alone does not explain why there would be an elevation deficit, and as such, have continued to be elucidated further.

The leading theory is from Yamaguchi et al., who believe that there is superotemporal prolapse of the posteriorly elongated globe which results in herniation between the superior and LR muscles, displacing the LR inferiorly and SR medially. Inferior displacement of the LR pulls the eye

Refraction

Wearing Rx

	Sphere	Cylinder	Axis
Right	–9.72	+0.75	105
Left	–9.50	+1.00	080

Age: 5 yrs
Type: DVO

A

Strabismus Exam

Method: Alternate cover / Fixing eye: Right / Correction cc	Distance	Near	Near +3DS	N Bifocals
	ET 25 RHT 20	ET' 23 RHT' 18		

	0	0	0	ET 30 RHT 24	–3	–3	–4	
ET 16 RHT 16	0	○	0	ET 25 RHT 20	0	○	–2	ET 30
	0	0	0	E 2 LH 1	+2	0	0	

R Tilt	L Tilt
E(T) 26	ET 30
RHT 16	RHT 20

B True hypotropia OS

AHP: Chin up

Figs. 15A and B: (A) Patient's prescription showing high myopia; (B) Strabismus and motility examination.

inferiorly, and medial displacement of the SR pulls the eye nasally, resulting in limitations of abduction and elevation.

Examination Findings

Patients typically present with progressive diplopia in both the horizontal and vertical meridians, and may exhibit features of pseudoptosis, pseudoproptosis (from the axial elongation), and may have an abnormal head posture to compensate for the diplopia. High-resolution MRI is useful to confirm the diagnosis and guide surgical planning, but may not be necessary if all the clinical criteria for HES are met:

- Severe myopia > –6.00 D or axial length > 27 mm
- Esotropia or hypotropia > 4 PD
- Limitation in abduction or supraduction.

Next, we will discuss the management of a difficult case of HES.

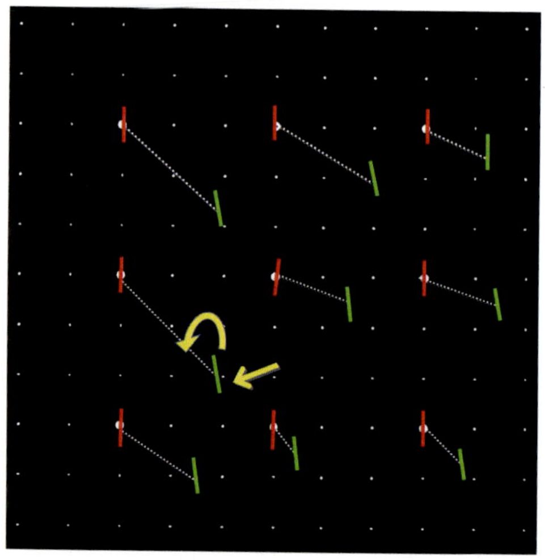

Fig. 16: Left hypotropia with extorsion, worse in left gaze and upgaze.

Case

A 57-year-old male with a history of high myopia presents with ET and diplopia. Patient has had diplopia for 15–20 years, described with a torsional component, and is worse at distance. Patient adopts a chin-up posture to maintain some form of single vision. Examination of his MRI of the orbits showed a greater distance between the left superior and LR muscles than between the same muscles of the right eye. The left LR muscle was also displaced farther downward on the left eye, wrapping around the temporal part of the globe at about 4:15 o'clock, whereas the right LR muscle wrapped around 8:30 o'clock, helping to confirm the diagnosis.

His refraction, motility, and strabismus exams are shown in **Figures 15A and B**.

The preoperative LRG plot **(Fig. 16)** shows a left hypotropia with extorsion. The ET in this case was >30 PD, and would not be corrected by operating only on the LMR muscle. It would be necessary to operate on both medial rectus muscles for the ET, as well as to do the Yokoyama procedure (unification, or anastomosis of the lateral and SR muscle bellies) on the left superior and LR muscles, suturing the muscles together with a permanent suture, about 14 mm posterior to their insertions. Adjustable sutures were to be used on both medial rectus muscles, but one cannot adjust

Strabismus Exam

Method: Alternate cover	Distance	Near	Near +3DS	N Bifocals
		Ortho		

	Distance			Near	Near +3DS			N Bifocals
	0	0	+1	LHT 25	0	−1	−2	
ET 16 RHT 12	0	○	0	XT 7 RHT 20	0	○	0	RHT 22
	0	0	0	Ortho	+Tr	0	0	

R Tilt	L Tilt
RHT 20	RHT 20

The Lancaster red–green test today shows significant improvement in the alignment in downgaze, and he does not have to hold his chin up as high now to see singly as he did before

Fig. 17: Patient's postoperative strabismus examination.

the Yokoyama procedure, so there was a chance that further surgical procedures may be necessary in the future.

Procedure 1

- Yokoyama of the left eye with union of the left superior and LR muscles 14 mm from their insertions.
- Bilateral medial rectus recessions of 8 mm, later adjusted to 4 mm in both eyes.

Postoperative month 1: Patient continues to have diplopia, but only in the vertical meridian with slight torsion. Horizontal diplopia was present on side gazes. The strabismus examination is shown in **Figure 17** and LRG plot on **Figure 18**.

Lancaster red–green test showed significant improvement in the alignment in downgaze, and he did not have to hold his chin up as high to see singly as before. The remaining problem was limitation of the left eye in moving upward on left gaze. Surgery on a vertical rectus muscle on either eye to help to compensate for this limitation of movement of the left eye would interfere with the good fusion, which he now had in slight downgaze. The pattern of remaining misalignment is similar to that of an apparent overaction of the RIO muscle, complete with some remaining extorsion, especially on downgaze. Weakening the RIO muscle would help to balance the remaining limitation of the left eye looking upward, likely increasing the range of gaze over which he can see singly with comfort.

Procedure 2

Right inferior oblique large myectomy of 18 mm

10-weeks postoperative: Patient no longer had diplopia on primary gaze and could see singly over a wide range. Diplopia was only present from a small right hypertropia on far left gaze, and far upgaze. His strabismus examination and LRG plot are shown in **Figures 19 and 20**, respectively.

Treatment Recommendations

Heavy eye syndrome typically requires surgical intervention to allow for single vision. For extremely mild cases, observation and/or refractive correction may be all that is necessary.

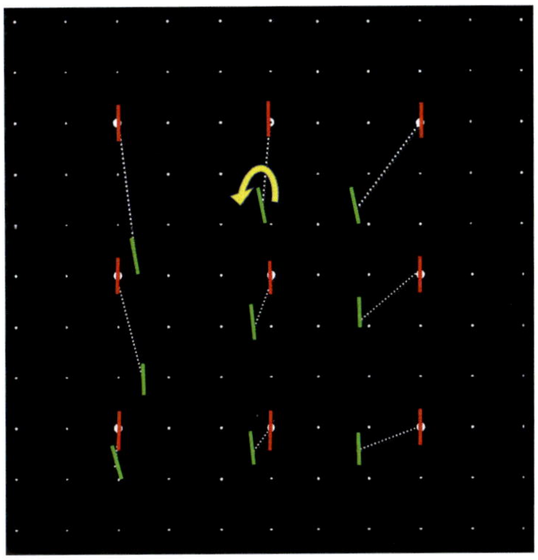

Fig. 18: Left hypotropia worse in up and left gaze, but significantly improved on downgaze.

For mild-to-moderate cases where fusion is possible without an overly large amount of prism, prism spectacles may be attempted.

There are several surgical options available in the treatment of HES, and all derive from the principle of correcting the displaced paths of the extraocular muscles. The authors have had good success with the Yokoyama procedure, specifically.

We have recreated a similar table **(Table 2)** referenced from Hennein and Robbins which nicely reviews the different techniques and their corresponding advantages/disadvantages.

Always use forced ductions to guide the surgical plan, and use adjustable surgery as much as possible. Consider the vessel-sparing techniques for multiple muscle surgeries, elderly patients, or those with coagulopathies to prevent anterior ischemic syndrome. Avoid techniques that use scleral passes in very high myopia or with findings of thin sclera to avoid perforation.

Explain clearly to patients that multiple surgeries are highly probable in this condition, and that single vision in all directions of gaze is near impossible to achieve. The goal is to provide as much single vision as possible in primary and

TABLE 2: Surgical techniques in the treatment of heavy eye syndrome.

Name	*Technique used*	*Advantages*	*Disadvantages*
Yokoyama	Create an anastomosis of the superior and lateral rectus muscle bellies (Yamaguchi M, 2010)	Supports the eye by reinforcing the area of prolapse and improves the path of the muscles	May not address the esotropia sufficiently without involving the medial rectus muscles
Yamada	Hemitransposition of the superior and lateral rectus muscles together, combined with medial rectus recessions (Yamada M, 2002)	Corrects the path of muscle displacement	May not sufficiently correct supraduction and abduction Requires scleral passes in a highly myopic eye
Partial Jensen	Superior half of the lateral rectus is sutured to the lateral half of the superior rectus without disinsertion of the muscle (Larsen PC, 2004)	Vessel-sparing procedure with no scleral passes	May be limitation to supraduction and abduction in the early postoperative stage
Silicone band loop myopexy	A silicone band is used to join the lateral and superior rectus muscles using a scleral tunnel (Shenoy BH, 2015)	Vessel-sparing procedure	Only corrects up to 40 PD of esotropia

Strabismus Exam

Method: Alternate cover | Distance | Near | Near +3DS | N Bifocals

Fixing Eye: Left | | X' 6

Correction cc

	–2	–2	–2	ET 30 RHT 24	0	---	---	
XT 10 RHT 6	–1	○	0	ET 25 RHT 20	–1.5	○	–1	RHT 5
	---	---	0	E 2 LH 1	0	---	---	

Heterophoria—Residual small angle 8 weeks following right inferior oblique muscle large myectomy. A Lancaster Red–green test was performed

Fig. 19: Second postoperative alignment showing significant improvement.

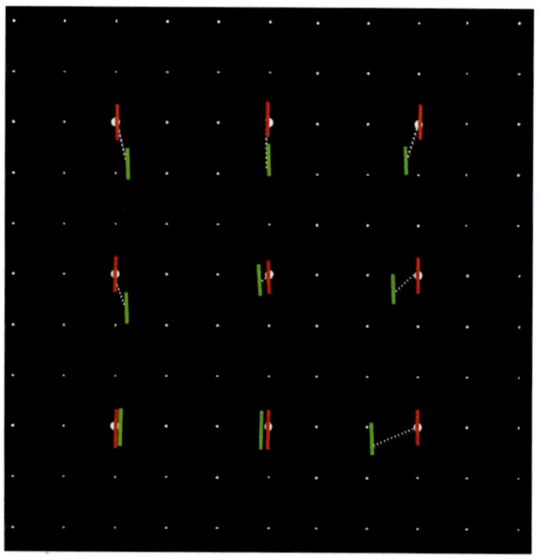

Fig. 20: Only a left hypotropia remaining in far left gaze and far upgaze.

downgaze, as they are the most important directions of gaze for the average person.

STRABISMUS FROM ORBITAL FLOOR FRACTURE

Orbital fractures are one of the most common types of facial fractures and were first described by Lang in 1889 (W, 1987). They consist of 3–45% of all pediatric facial fractures and can have significant long-term sequelae if not managed appropriately. Children, particularly, have unique characteristics on presentation when compared to their adult counterparts. When very young, the roof may be involved more frequently as a result of the larger skull and lack of sinus pneumatization.

Pathophysiology

Children may present with "*trapdoor*" fractures due to immature, elastic, cancellous bone with resilient periosteum—a type of fracture caused by increased intraorbital pressure which displaces a flap of bone that immediately returns to its original position, trapping any contents that may have herniated into the defect. These are considered surgical emergencies. Adult bones are more brittle and less elastic, thus, tend to stay open. Strabismus results from the altered motility of the affected extraocular muscle and surrounding soft tissue, whether by restriction (through impingement or compression by a bony structure), injury and paresis, or change in muscle pathway.

Strabismus may also persist, or develop after repair of a floor fracture. The incidence of diplopia after surgical repair is estimated to be 10–37%. Silbert et al. report the most common causes of diplopia following orbital fracture repair:

- Incomplete removal of the extraocular muscle and/or soft tissue from the herniation site prior to placement of the implant
- Incorrect placement of the implant, causing more tissue entrapment
- Neuromuscular trauma
- Orbital adherence syndrome.

Examination Findings

Children may present with minimal signs when compared with adults, only complaining of diplopia on history and limited extraocular motility on examination—termed a "*white-eyed*" blowout fracture. As a result of this entrapment, though, children may also present with the oculocardiac reflex—consisting of bradycardia, nausea, vomiting, and possibly syncope. Adults will typically also have periorbital edema, ecchymoses, and subconjunctival hemorrhage.

Management of orbital floor fractures is similar in children and adults. Indications for surgery include:

- Muscle entrapment or muscle restriction causing diplopia or the oculocardiac reflex
- Enophthalmos > 2 mm
- Orbital floor defect >50% of the floor or medial wall.

In children, it is recommended to intervene earlier due to the high incidence of trapdoor fractures. Otherwise, observing closely for 1–2 weeks in adults may be appropriate, watching for new signs to develop as edema resolves, and fibrosis develops.

Here, we present an atypical case of complicated strabismus status post repair of an orbital floor fracture in an adult male. We chose this case to illustrate the usefulness of the LRG test, importance of fundus torsion, and how muscles other than the inferior rectus can be affected.

Case

A 31-year-old male who presents with double vision, primarily on downgaze, after sustaining a right orbital floor fracture that was repaired twice using a MEDPOR implant. The inferior rectus had been found to be herniating through a posterior portion of the fracture prior to repair. Forced ductions were free after orbital surgery. **Figures 21 and 22** showing head posture and eye positions.

Patient's motility and strabismus exams are shown in **Figure 23**.

Lancaster red-green plot shows a right hypertropia in all directions of gaze, increasing significantly on downgaze, more on down-and-right gaze than to the left. There is slight intorsion of one eye compared with the other. There is extorsion of the right eye that worsens on downgaze.

The key to understanding the problem is extorsion of the right eye. If there was only weakness of the right inferior rectus, then the right eye should show intorsion. Extorsion indicates that most surely the inferior oblique muscle is tight and extorting the eye, as well as preventing it from moving down fully. This is known as an "*inverted Brown pattern*",

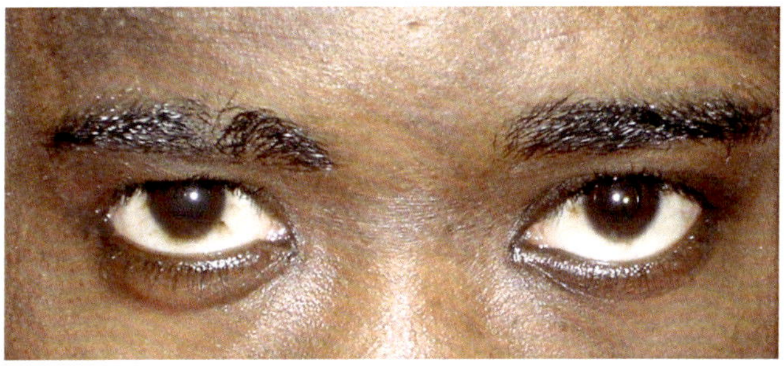

Fig. 21: Patient adopts a chin-down head posture to avoid diplopia.

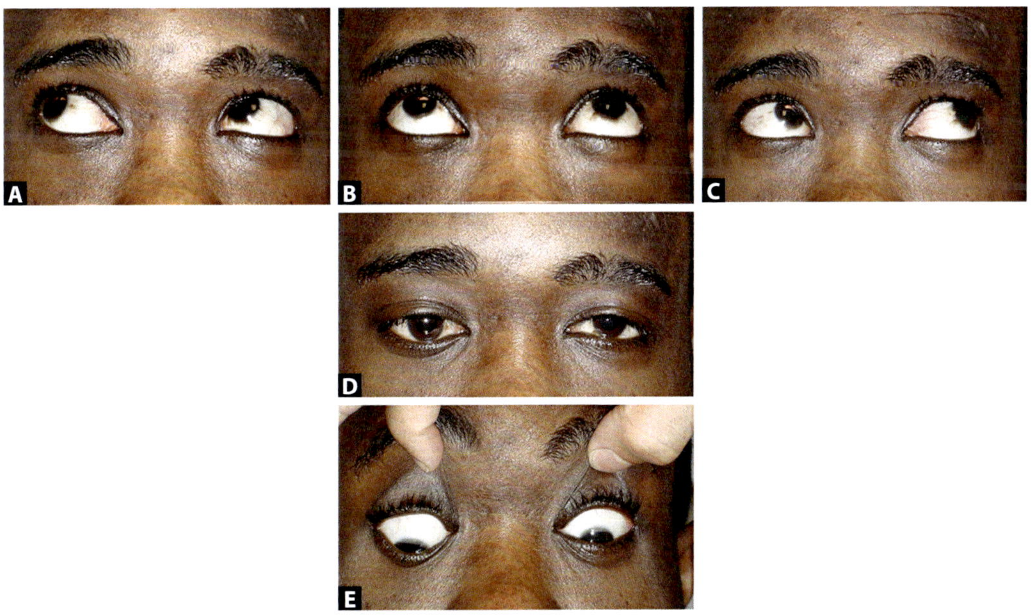

Figs. 22A to E: Eye positions in different directions of gaze.

Prism and alternate cover test

Near$_{cc}$ RHT 18		
	RHT 25	
ET 5 RHT 25	RHT 35	RHT 9
	RHT 50	
Fundus torsion 2+ extorsion right eye Trace extorsion left eye		

Motility

Right eye		
0	0	0
0	0	0
–3	–2	–2

Left eye		
0	0	0
0	0	0
0	0	0

Fig. 23: Preoperative alignment showing a right hypertropia and limited infraduction of the right eye.

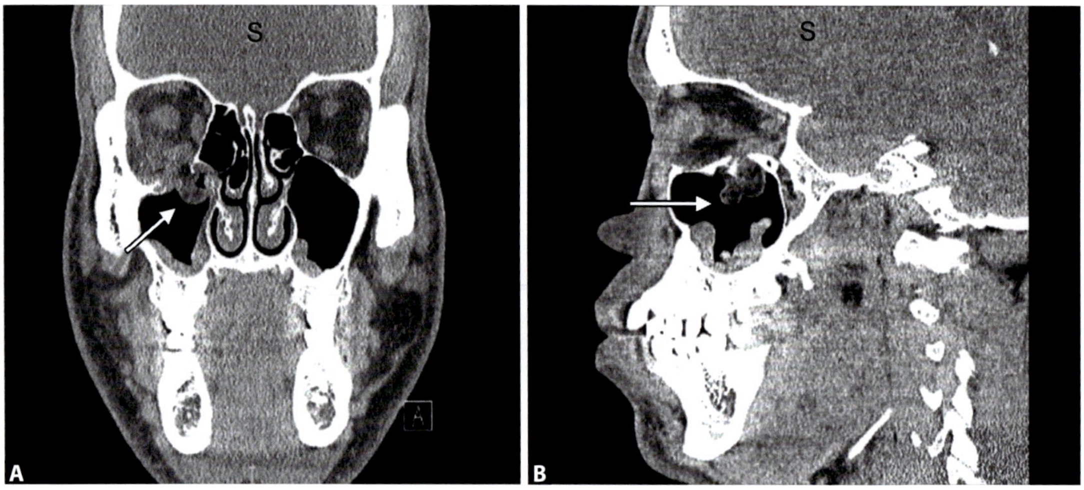

Figs. 24A and B: Coronal and sagittal CT showing a right inferior orbital floor fracture with herniation of contents into the maxillary sinus.

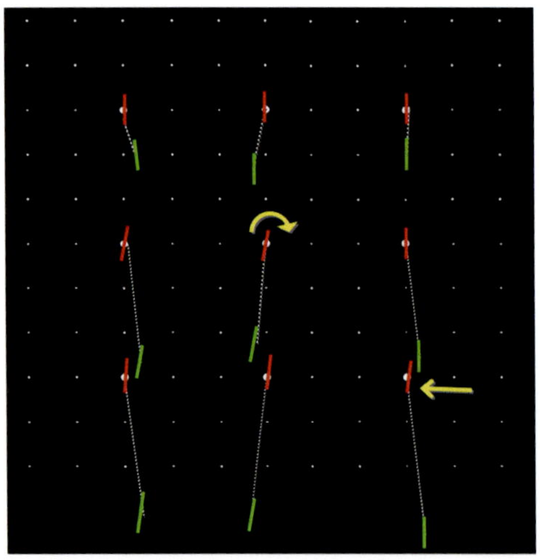

Fig. 25: Preoperative Lancaster red–green plot showing extorsion of the right eye with worsening right hypertropia on downgaze.

coined by David Guyton, MD. This problem best responds to a weakening procedure of the inferior oblique. In this case, a denervation and extirpation were recommended based on the severity of the problem.

It is important to note that with long-standing strabismus, sensory adaptation may change the subjective experience of diplopia, and torsion may not show up as much on the LRG plot when compared to fundus ophthalmoscopy. Here, the objective fundus torsion significantly guides the plan of treatment, indicating the problematic muscle as the RIO.

Figures 24A and B show orbital floor fracture with herniation of orbital contents. **Figure 25** shows LRG plot of the same patient.

Nine weeks postoperative, the patient has significant improvement to straight ahead and upgaze, with some remaining diplopia on downgaze, especially down-and-right. See **Figure 26** for his postoperative motility and strabismus examinations.

Postoperative LRG plot **(Fig. 27)** shows good alignment except for a small residual right hyperdeviation in primary position, increasing in right gaze, and especially in down-and-right gaze. Patient experiences diplopia beyond 10° of straight downgaze.

No further surgery was recommended at this time since the patient was happy with the results and tolerated any residual strabismus well. Additional, but minor,

Prism and alternate cover test

Near$_{sc}$ X2, RH 4		
	Ortho	
Ortho	RHT 3	Ortho
	X10 RHT 25	

Motility

Right eye		
–2 to –3	0	0
0	0	0
0	0	0

Left eye		
0	0	0
0	0	0
0	0	0

Fig. 26: Postoperative alignment showing significant improvement.

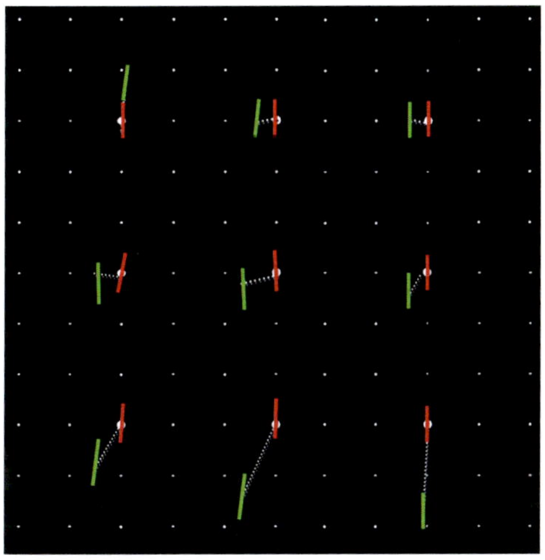

Fig. 27: Nine weeks of postoperative Lancaster red–green plot showing significant improvement.

improvements over time were expected. Any further procedure to treat the remaining hypertropia (such as a right inferior rectus resection) could worsen the alignment in upgaze, which would be unlikely to improve.

Treatment Recommendations

Strabismus, which develops from orbital floor fractures, can be challenging to treat. For mild cases, observation, or prism spectacles may be all that is necessary. If the fracture needs to be repaired, whether diplopia develops before, or after its repair, consider speaking directly with the primary surgeon. Obtain as much information as possible regarding the anatomical findings, or consult a colleague in the oculoplastic department to decide if orbital, strabismus, or combination surgery is necessary. Careful planning of strabismus surgery guided by imaging is crucial in most of these cases. Do not hesitate to obtain additional imaging as indicated. Use adjustable sutures when possible, and remember to check for torsion, whether through direct visualization, or diagnostic tools like the LRG test, as it can drastically change management.

REOPERATIONS/ADHERENCE SYNDROME/SLIPPED MUSCLE

There is little more feared by the strabismologist than reoperations. They are fraught with difficulty as a result of scar tissue, fat adherence, often unknown muscle locations, and low reliability of standard surgical tables. Repka et al., report the rate of strabismus surgery to be approximately 1 in 750 patients over a 4-year-period, with a 1 year reoperation rate of 6.72% for children aged 6–9 years, increasing up to 11.5% for adults 65 years and older. Another group found an average reoperation rate of 8.5%, while adjustable sutures were associated with significantly lower reoperation rates in horizontal surgery, but increased reoperations in vertical surgery.

Careful examination, diagnosis, and planning of the surgery go without question. Use caution when there are no prior medical records available, including what is reported by the patient, as findings frequently do not correlate with self-reported history. Use forced ductions to guide treatment. We cannot emphasize enough the importance of adjustable sutures to maximize options. Explain to patients that the chances of needing additional surgery are significantly higher in reoperations, and that perfection is usually not possible.

To the authors' best knowledge, literature on the management of reoperations is sparse, as the need for additional surgery is predicated on many factors, and is usually tailored to each patient on an individual basis. Here we will review some general guidelines and review a case to offer advice on how to approach these complicated forms of strabismus.

General Guidelines

It is generally recommended to wait for 6–8 weeks before reoperating. Kushner reports that exceptions include a slipped muscle, lost muscle, large overcorrection after a superior oblique tuck, or hypertropia >5 PD the day after a vertical transposition. These should be explored within 1–2 days after surgery.

Careful examination, looking for patterns of incomitance, paresis, and restriction are required for successful management.

Look for scar tissue and location of ciliary vessels on the slit lamp. Ask for old photographs if the history is unclear.

When dealing with an undercorrection, it is important to consider whether the initial surgery is near, or at, its maximum recession, as any further surgery may cripple the function of the muscle. In these circumstances, it is better to tighten the antagonist muscle.

When dealing with overcorrections such as consecutive deviations (exotropia or ET) and surgery is planned, look for signs of muscle underaction, as in convergence insufficiency pattern after ET surgery, or divergence insufficiency after exotropia surgery. These are clues that the now weakened muscles may need to be advanced. At the time of surgery, it may also be useful to make a small incision to hook each muscle that was previously operated on, testing for laxity versus normal tightness. If these muscles are lax, advancing them on adjustable sutures is the recommended course of action. If the muscles are not lax, then operate on fresh muscles. Forced ductions also guide planning concordantly.

Example: A patient who underwent bilateral LR recessions for an exotropia develops a consecutive ET 6 months of postoperative. During the reoperation, first check the laxity of the LR muscles. If they are found to be lax, advance them; if they are normal in tightness, recess the medial rectus muscles instead.

Lateral gaze is an important variable to consider in reoperations, particularly incomitance. In situations where there is less strabismus on lateral gaze, correcting primary gaze could lead to an overcorrection on side gaze, with narrowing of the field of single vision. One may need to tighten the antagonist muscle, rather than weaken the agonist causing the deviation.

Example: A patient underwent bilateral rectus recessions for exotropia and was found to be undercorrected, but with less deviation on lateral gazes. Consider tightening the medial rectus in this case, as presumably any further weakening of the lateral recti will only worsen the incomitance, while tightening the medial recti will maintain their strength.

Treat any new vertical misalignment from prior surgery as a fresh vertical case, provided there is no evidence of a restrictive process that would first warrant exploration.

In the operating theater, forced ductions should be performed to assess for tightness of all extraocular muscles, including the obliques. For the obliques, we use a single-handed, modified version of Guyton's exaggerated traction test also used by Kushner. To test for inferior oblique tightness in the right eye, one would grasp the nasal limbus using forceps and push the eye into the inferonasal quadrant, rolling the eye back and forth between the 6 o'clock and 3 o'clock positions to feel its tightness. This is done in the superonasal quadrant to assess tightness of the superior oblique. If restrictions are found using forced ductions, recheck them after clearing the suspected area of adhesions. If there is still a restriction remaining, consider a *reverse-leash* effect and explore the quadrant in the area of limitation. A reverse leash is a restriction typically caused by fibrosis of the globe against the orbital wall, preventing movement into that field of gaze.

Adherence Syndrome

With prior operations that violate Tenon's capsule or expose extraconal fat, significant scarring and adherence may occur. The authors prefer a fornix approach in most cases, even with significant conjunctival scarring, but others may choose to approach this using a limbal incision. Careful dissection of underlying scar tissue is important, but avoids excessive lysis of adhesions, as this may result in a significant rebound effect and even worsen scar formation. We have had little experience with mitomycin C, but there are numerous reports in literature that support its use of 0.2 mg/mL for 5 minutes as effective and safe in the treatment of restrictive strabismus and reduction of adhesions. Amniotic membrane transplantation has also been used successfully to help prevent recurrence of fibrosis and adhesion formation.

Hooking the muscle may not be simple. Muscles in a reoperation may be adherent to the underlying sclera, and blunt, combined with sharp dissection may be necessary to free up space, or to hold space for a muscle hook to enter. The hook may also need to be cleared of any scar tissue as it comes out the other side.

In recessions, a pseudotendon **(Fig. 28)** may form between the insertion and the recessed muscle. Suspect this when similar tissue is thought to be found much anterior than expected. It is typically more "springy" in feel when compared to muscle tissue, which is typically more firm and less elastic. Excise any pseudotendon to reduce bulk when advancing a muscle, and be sure to secure the muscle and not pseudotendon with sutures.

Reoperations can be marred by similar appearing tissues and alterations in anatomy, making it even more difficult to

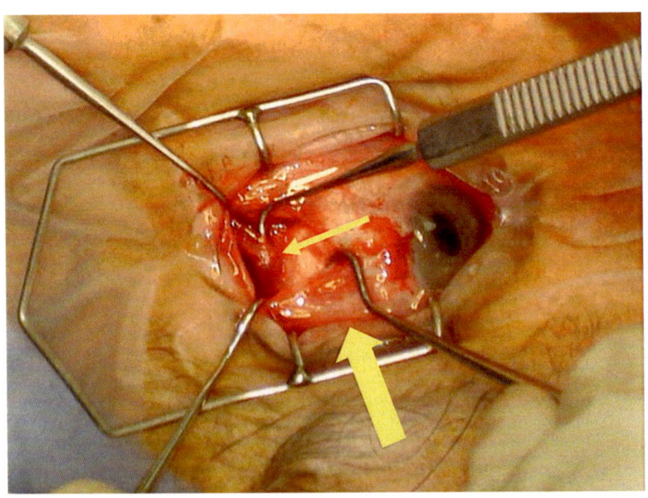

Fig. 28: Difference in appearance between stretched scar (thin arrow) and muscle tendon (thick arrow).

properly identify structures. Shokida et al., report using 0.1% Trypan blue dye to help contrast tissues, specifically staining muscle sheath, tendons, and fibrotic tissues, but not sclera or muscle fibers.

Slipped Muscle

Slipped muscles should be differentiated from stretched scars. Stretched scars are connective tissue bridges that form between the end of the cut muscle and sclera, causing the muscle to have an indirect attachment to sclera that elongates over time when under tension. This causes a postoperative underaction and overcorrection with recessions, or an undercorrection after a resection. The etiology of this problem is impaired wound healing. These typically take months to appear, unlike slipped muscles, which occur early after surgery, and may be bilateral when bilateral surgery is done. Since the nature of the problem is with healing, it will affect both sides. Stretched scars tend to appear similar to muscle tissue, but when traced far back enough to true muscle, a change in interface is usually seen.

A slipped muscle refers to a phenomenon that occurs when the muscle slips backward into its own capsule, presumably as a result of improper suture placement, securing only the muscle capsule and not the tendon itself. As a result, the muscle does not attach to sclera and slides posteriorly. This can be seen on dynamic orbital imaging, revealing a fusiform enlargement of the muscle belly on attempted gaze in its field of action, indicating contractility, with no corresponding thickening of the empty anterior capsule. Lost muscles will already show this fusiform enlargement on primary gaze. Lastly, slipped muscles will typically show some force generation, unlike lost muscles.

Treatment is similar for both of these conditions, but appropriate suspicion and careful discernment of the problem is crucial. The goal is to resect any tissue leading up to the muscle, effectively advancing the muscle toward the insertion. For a stretched scar, permanent sutures are recommended as one cannot rely on the patient's wound healing to change. For a slipped muscle, traditional sutures can be used as long as it is certain that the true muscle tendon is properly secured during the reoperation. On examination, scar tissue tends to be firmer and more opaque than muscle capsule, and a distinct bump may be felt in the transition between muscle and stretched scar. An example of a stretched scar and its similarity of muscle tendon is shown in **Figure 28**. Note that the stretched scar is slightly more translucent and thinner in comparison, with the foot of the hook nearly visible. A slipped muscle capsule will look even more translucent.

Now we will review a case of a lost muscle and its management.

Case

A 69-year-old female presented with double vision and the inability to abduct her right eye immediately following bilateral endoscopic anterior and posterior ethmoidectomies, sphenoidectomies, maxillary anastomoses, and mucous membrane removal. She also had intraorbital bleeding postoperatively.

Patient was seen and found to have a 55–60 right exotropia, with a very small, but apparent adduction motion, only from the exodeviated position. This was masquerading as a partial oculomotor nerve palsy. Her eyes, motility and strabismus examination can be seen in **Figures 29 and 30**, respectively.

The patient's MRI showed significant disruption of the medial rectus muscle in its mid portion, with scarring to the disrupted right orbital wall, making it very unlikely that the medial rectus could be located and advanced in any meaningful way to hold the eye inward. There was no thickening of the muscle on attempted adduction on the MRI.

The plan was to attempt to try and free the medial rectus muscle, but more likely the right superior and inferior rectus muscles would need to be transposed nasally.

Procedure

The right medial rectus muscle was identified in its anterior 15 mm—secured and followed backward to clear it from surrounding tissues. The muscle was tightly tethered to the nasal orbital wall approximately 15–20 mm posterior to its insertion and was nonelastic in the portion of its length. It was isolated, but then eventually amputated for fear of creatIng increased restriction by reattaching it to the globe.

The right superior and inferior rectus muscles were both cleared far backward, and resected 7 mm using a vessel-sparing technique—1 bundle of small vessels reflected temporally before the muscle was secured, along with resection made of

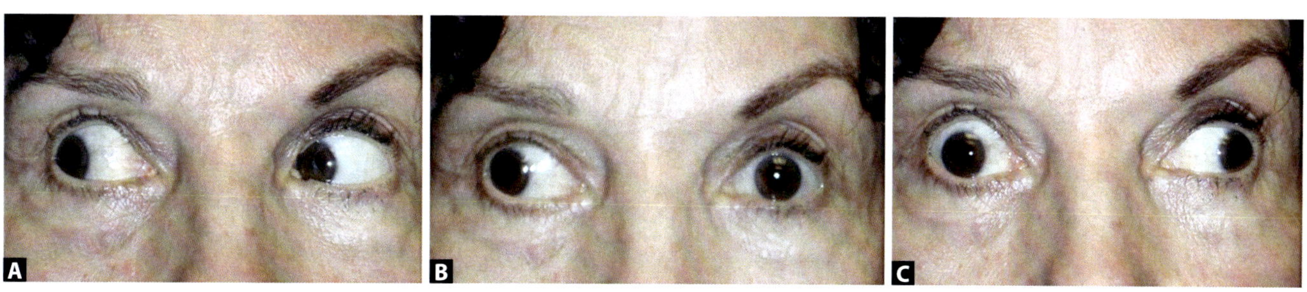

Figs. 29A to C: Primary and side gazes. Note the significant adduction deficit of the right eye.

Prism and alternate cover test

Near$_{sc}$ RXT 65–70		
	RHT 75	
RXT 50	RXT 75	RXT 85
	RHT 75	

Motility

Right eye		
0	0	0
0	–6	–6
0	0	0

Left eye		
0	0	0
0	0	0
0	0	0

Fig. 30: Preoperative examination.

Prism and alternate cover test

Near$_{sc}$ Ortho		
ET 10	Ortho	RXT >50

Motility

Right eye		
0	0	0
–3.5	0	–1
0	0	0

Left eye		
0	0	0
0	0	0
0	0	0

Fig. 31: Postoperative examination.

each muscle, leaving some portion of the muscle at the original insertion site to receive the bundle of retained vessels.

The adjustable sutures from each vertical rectus muscle were fished beneath the nasal conjunctiva and attached at the opposite corner of the original medial rectus muscle insertion. This pulled the eye nasally significantly with a slightly overcorrected position.

Postoperatively in the recovery area there was a very small right hypertropia. The right inferior rectus muscle was tightened 1–2 mm further, leaving a small ET in primary gaze.

Her 6-week postoperative examination is shown in **Figure 31**. This was deemed to be an extremely good result by all parties.

ACKNOWLEDGMENT

We thank Dr Guyton for contributing images and cases for this book chapter. We also thank him for his contributions to ophthalmology, ophthalmic optics, strabismus, and most importantly, to humankind, for which we are eternally grateful.

The Zanvyl Krieger Children's Eye Center, The Wilmer Eye Institute, The Johns Hopkins University School of Medicine, Baltimore, Maryland.

SUGGESTED READING

1. Bagshaw J. Heavy eye phenomenon. A preliminary report. Br Orthopt J. 1966;23:75-8.
2. Barh A, Swaminathan M, Mukherjee B. Orbital fractures in children: clinical features and management outcomes. J AAPOS. 2018;22(6):415.e1-415.
3. Bleik JH, Zaatari GS, Cherfan GM. Inferior oblique muscle injury after peribulbar anesthesia presenting as ipsilateral superior oblique palsy: a clinicopathologic report. J AAPOS. 2018;10:178-9.
4. Brown SM, Brooks SE, Mazow ML, Avilla CW, Braverman DE, Greenhaw ST, et al. Cluster of diplopia cases after periocular anesthesia without hyaluronidase. J Cataract Refract Surg. 1999;25:1245-9.
5. Capo H, Guyton DL. Ipsilateral hypertropia following cataract surgery. Ophthalmology. 1996;103:721-30.
6. Capo H, Roth E, Johnson T, Muñoz M, Siatkowski RM. Vertical strabismus after cataract surgery. Ophthalmology. 1996;103:918-21.
7. Carlson BM, Emerick S, Komorowski TE, Rainin EA, Shepard BM. Extraocular muscle regeneration in primates. Local anesthetic-induced lesions. Ophthalmology. 1992;99:582-9.

8. Carlton J, Kaltenthaler E. Amblyopia and quality of life: a systematic review. Eye. 2011;25(4):403-13.
9. Chen PL, Chen WY, Lu DW. Evaluation of mitomycin C in reducing postoperative adhesions in strabismus surgery. J Ocul Pharmacol Ther. 2005;21(5):406-10.
10. Christoff A, Guyton DL. The Lancaster red-green test. Am Orthopt J. 2006;56:157-65.
11. Durnian JM, Noonan CP, Marsh IB . The psychosocial effects of adult strabismus: a review. Br J Ophthalmol. 2011;95(4):450-3.
12. Engle EC. The genetic basis of complex strabismus. Pediatr Res. 2006;59(3):343-8.
13. Gaur N, Sharma P. Management of Duane retraction syndrome: a simplified approach. Indian J Ophthalmol. 2019;67(1):16-22.
14. Güçlü ES, Sarı AA, Dinç E, Metin TÖ, Yılmaz BÇ, Taşdelen B. Efficacy of mitomycin-C and infliximab in reducing adhesion and fibrosis following strabismus surgery. Turk J Med Sci 2016;46(5):1401-6.
15. Gunton KB, Wasserman BN, DeBenedictis C. Strabismus. Prim Care. 2015;42(3):393-407.
16. Guyton DL. Exaggerated traction test for the oblique muscles. Ophthalmology. 1981;88(10):1035-40.
17. Guyton DL. Strabismus complications from local anesthetics. Semin Ophthalmol. 2008;23(5):298-301.
18. Hamada SD, Devys JM, Xuan TH, Ganem S, Sahel JA, Héran F, et al. Role of hyaluronidase in diplopia after peribulbar anesthesia for cataract surgery. Ophthalmology. 2005;112:879-82.
19. Hayashi T, Iwashige H, Maruo T. Clinical features and surgery for acquired progressive esotropia associated with severe myopia. Acta Ophthalmol Scand. 1999;77(1):66-71.
20. Hennein L, Robbins SL. Heavy eye syndrome: myopia-induced strabismus. Surv Ophthalmol. 2021;66(1):138-144..
21. Hsu CK, Hsieh MW, Chang HC, Tai MC, Chien KH. Anatomic factors predicting postoperative strabismus in orbital wall fracture repair. Sci Rep. 2019;9(1):14785.
22. Hunter DG, Lam GC, Guyton DL. Inferior oblique muscle injury from local anesthesia for cataract surgery. Ophthalmology. 1995;102(3):501-9.
23. Injuries and diseases of the orbit. Traumatic enophthalmos with retention of perfect acuity of vision. By William Lang, 1889. Adv Ophthalmic Plast Reconstr Surg. 1987;6:3-6.
24. Kim WJ, Kim MM. Subsequent strabismus surgeries in patients with no prior medical records. Indian J Ophthalmol. 2018;66(10):1451-5.
25. Koide R, Honda M, Kora Y, Ozawa T. Diplopia after cataract surgery. J Cataract Refract Surg. 2000;26:1198-204.
26. Koltai PJ, Amjad I, Meyer D, Feustel PJ. Orbital fractures in children. Arch Otololaryngol Head Neck Surg. 1995;121:1375-9.
27. Krzizok TH, Schroeder BU. Measurement of recti eye muscle paths by magnetic resonance imaging in highly myopic and normal subjects. Invest Ophthalmol Vis Sci. 1999;40:2554-60.
28. Kushner BJ. Re-operation strategies in strabismus-Cooper's dictum amended. J Binocul Vis Ocul Motil. 2018;68(2):45-53.
29. Larsen PC, Gole GA. Partial Jensen's procedure for the treatment of myopic strabismus fixus. J AAPOS. 2004;8(4):393-5.
30. Lee SC, Park SH, Han SK, Yoon EK, Dhong ES, Jung SO. Prognostic factors of orbital fractures with muscle incarceration. Arch Plast Surg. 2017;44(5):407-12.
31. Leffler CT, Vaziri K, Cavuoto KM, McKeown CA, Schwartz SG, Kishor KS. Strabismus surgery reoperation rates with adjustable and conventional sutures. Am J Ophthalmol. 2015;160(2):385-90.
32. Ludwig IH, Chow AY. Scar remodeling after strabismus surgery. J AAPOS. 2000;4(6):326-33.
33. Mahindrakar A, Tandon R, Menon V, Sharma P, Khokhar S. Effectiveness of mitomycin C in reducing reformation of adhesions following surgery for restrictive strabismus. J Pediatr Ophthalmol Strabismus. 2001;38(3):131-5.
34. Marsh JD, Yilmaz PT, Guyton DL. Deficiency of depression in adduction: clinical characteristics and surgical management of the "inverted Brown pattern". J AAPOS. 2016;20(1):7-11.
35. McKean-Cowdin R, Cotter SA, Tarczy-Hornoch K, Wen G, Kim J, Borchert M, et al. Prevalence of amblyopia or strabismus in Asian and non-Hispanic white preschool children: multi-ethnic pediatric eye disease study. Ophthalmology. 2013;120(10):2117-24.
36. Mendonca TM, Tiberwala S, Sachdeva V, Kekunnaya R. Convergent strabismus fixus without high myopia. J AAPOS. 2016;20(1):83-5.
37. Monga S, Kekunnaya R, Sachdeva V. Exotropia-hypotropia complex in high myopia. J Pediatr Ophthalmol Strabismus. 2013;50(6):340-6.
38. Nakao Y, Kimura T. Prevalence and anatomic mechanism of highly myopic strabismus among Japanese with severe myopia. Jpn J Ophthalmol. 2014;58(2):218-24.
39. Noorden GK. The History of Strabismology. Belgium: JP Wayenborgh; 2002.
40. Oh SY, Clark RA, Velez F, Rosenbaum AL, Demer JL. Incomitant strabismus associated with instability of rectus pulleys. Invest Ophthalmol Vis Sci. 2002;43(7):2169-78.
41. Ohta M, Iwashige H, Hayashi T, Maruo T. Computed tomography findings in convergent strabismus fixus. Nippon Ganka Gakkai Zasshi Soc. 1995;99:980-85.
42. Olusanya BA. Brown syndrome with severe amblyopia: a case report from Africa. Pan Afr Med J. 2015;20:56.
43. Peragallo JH, Pineles SL, Demer JL. Recent advances in clarifying the etiologies of strabismus. J Neuroophthalmol. 2015;35(2):185-93.
44. Posnick JC, Wells M, Pron GE. Pediatric facial fractures: evolving patterns of treatment. J Oral Maxillofac Surg. 1993;51:836-44.
45. Rahi J, Logan S, Timms C, Russell-Eggitt I, Taylor D. Risk, causes, and outcomes of visual impairment after loss of vision in the non-amblyopic eye: a population-based study. Lancet. 2002;360:597-602.
46. Rainin EA, Carlson BM. Postoperative diplopia and ptosis. Arch Ophthalmol. 1985;102:1337-9.
47. Repka MX, Lum F, Burugapalli B. Strabismus, strabismus surgery, and reoperation rate in the United States: analysis from the IRIS registry. Ophthalmology. 2018;125(10):1646-53.
48. Rutar T, Demer JL. "Heavy eye" syndrome in the absence of high myopia: a connective tissue degeneration in elderly strabismic patients. J AAPOS. 2009;13(1):36-44.
49. Scott AB, Alexander DE, Miller JM. Bupivacaine injection of the eye muscles to treat strabismus. Br J Ophthalmol. 2007;91(2):146-8.
50. Sharma TK, Grewal JS, MacDonald M. Divergent strabismus fixus-a case report. Eur J Ophthalmol. 2005;99(1):36-40.

24

CHAPTER

Alphabet Patterns and Primary Oblique Muscle Dysfunctions

Fatma Yülek

INTRODUCTION

Alphabetical patterns of strabismus denote significant difference in size of the horizontal strabismic deviations in defined positions of upgaze and downgaze. Mostly A- or V-pattern strabismus has been described under this title. However other forms such as X, Y, arrow, and lambda patterns have also been recently involved in this term. About 12–50% of the patients with horizontal strabismus may have coexisting A- and V-patterns. Therefore, recognizing and treating these patterns are critical to increase the effectiveness of horizontal strabismus surgery.

BRIEF HISTORY

The earliest description of V-pattern strabismus in a patient with bilateral superior oblique (SO) palsy and esotropia in downgaze was done by Duane in 1897. After publication of a series of papers emphasizing the importance of performing measurements of strabismic patients with the eyes in the straight upward and downward positions of gaze by Urrets-Zavalia in 1948, Urist introduced the concept in 1951, and consequently Albert proposed the worldwide accepted descriptive terms: A- and V-patterns.

The causes and treatment of A- and V-patterns was denoted by Knapp in 1959 who also recommended treatment of A- and V-patterns by operating on the dysfunctional oblique muscle causing pattern deviation. Unless oblique dysfunction is present, vertically displacing and transposing the horizontal rectus muscles was the proposed approach similar to current management.

CLASSIFICATION AND CLINICAL FEATURES

In V-pattern esotropia **(Figs. 1A to I)**, the deviation increases in downward gaze and decreases in upward gaze. On the other hand, in V-pattern exotropia, the deviation increases in upward gaze and decreases in downward gaze **(Figs. 2A to I)**. The esodeviation increases in upward gaze and decreases in downward gaze in A-pattern esotropia **(Figs. 3A to I)**, while in A-pattern exotropia, the exodeviation increases in downward gaze and decreases in upward gaze. The difference between upgaze and downgaze as 10 prism diopters (PD) for A-pattern and 15 PD for V-pattern, usually does not require treatment, and is corrected automatically with the correction of horizontal deviation. Authors generally advocate treatment of deviations greater than what is stated.

The properties and associated clinical conditions of the other relatively rare alphabet patterns are summarized in **Table 1**.

ETIOPATHOGENESIS

Several etiological mechanisms have been proposed so far; basically mechanical (peripheral) and neural (central). On the other hand orbital and pulley anomalies and ocular torsion are also important factors in pathogenesis.

Mechanical Factors

Two mechanical theories have been proposed, i.e., horizontal muscle overaction (OA) and oblique muscle OA/underaction.

Horizontal Muscle Overaction

This theory proposes an imbalance between actions of rectus muscles. For example, A-pattern with underacting medial rectus (MR) muscle in downgaze and underacting lateral rectus (LR) muscle in upgaze whereas V-pattern with overacting MR in downgaze and overacting LR in upgaze. Some electromyographic studies do not approve this theory. On the contrary Demer et al. have revealed that superior and inferior compartments of horizontal rectus muscles have distinct and separate innervation, which may also explain the A- or V-pattern if these compartments are recruited separately during upgaze and downgaze.

Oblique Muscle Dysfunction

This is basically the result of tertiary action of oblique muscles: Abduction that is produced with primary or secondary oblique OA. According to the cyclovertical muscle imbalance theory which was first introduced by Knapp in

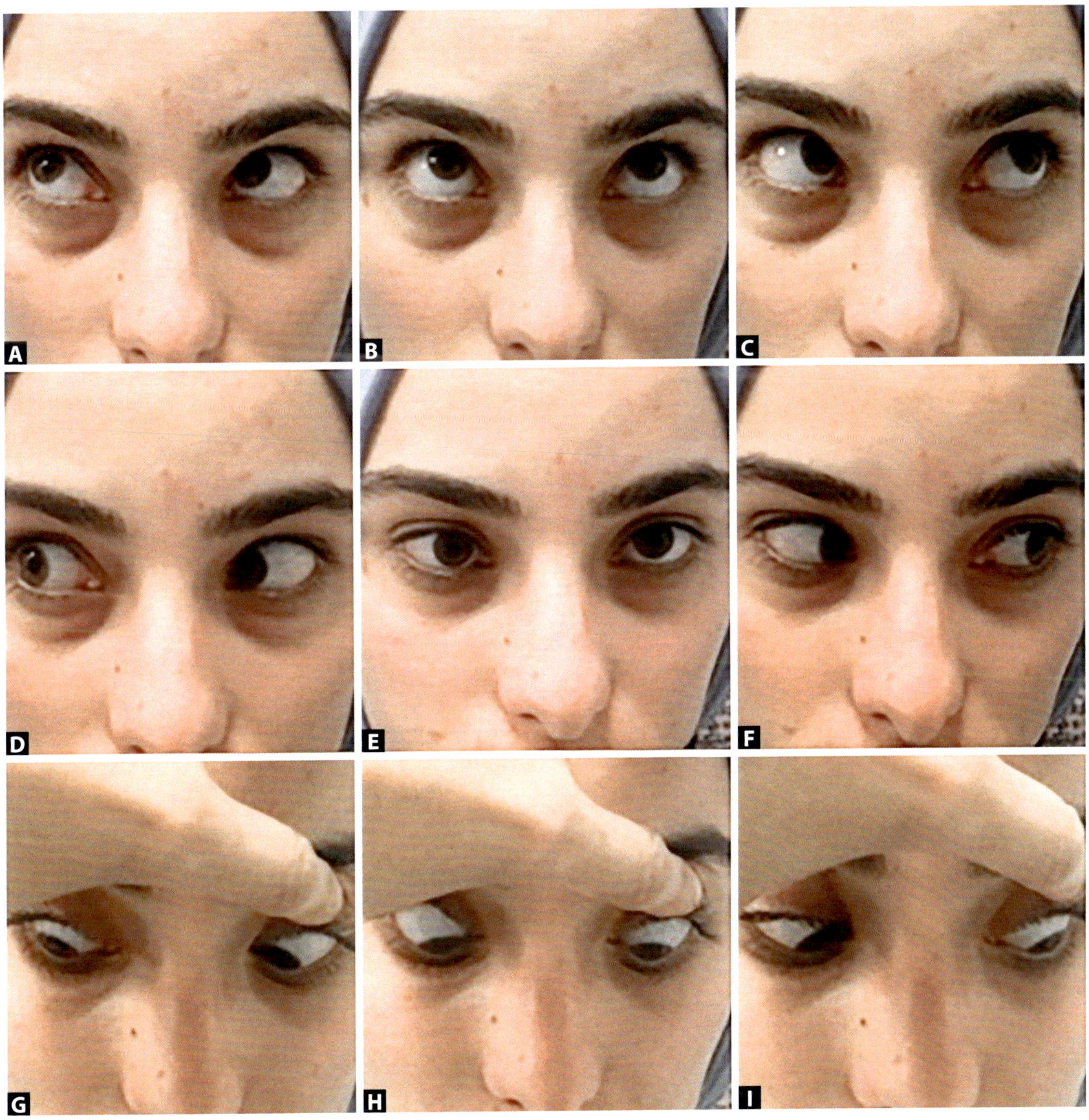

Figs. 1A to I: In V-pattern esotropia, the deviation increases in downward gaze and decreases in upward gaze.

1959, inferior rectus (IR) underaction and superior oblique overaction (SOOA) was the cause of A-pattern. Superior rectus (SR) underaction and inferior oblique overaction (IOOA) was the cause of V-pattern. However some cases may not follow these rules. A-pattern esotropia may be accompanied by paradoxical IOOA.

Anomalies of Orbital Structures

The orbital anatomy may cause pattern strabismus by abnormal vector forces. The angle between the visual axis and the insertion of the IO and SO tendon is increased in shallow orbits in some syndromes such as Crouzon and Apert. Thus, the abducting ability of the SO and IO muscles decrease in downgaze and upgaze, respectively.

In patients with craniosynostosis, magnetic resonance imaging (MRI) studies have revealed that increased excyclorotation of the muscles have been found to be associated with increased V-pattern.

Anomalies of the external facial configuration are also related to pattern strabismus.

Downward slanting of lateral canthus (antimongoloid) palpebral fissures, malar hypoplasia, and an S-shaped contour of the lower eyelid have been found to be correlated with IOOA. On the other hand, malar hypoplasia and esotropia have been reported to present a tendency for IO underaction.

The mongoloid palpebral fissures, prominent cheek bones and upward displaced lateral canthus are related to SOOA. Patients with mongoloid slant have A esotropia and V exotropia, whereas patients with antimongoloid slant have V esotropia and A exotropia. On the contrary, malar hypoplasia was reported to be associated with overacting IO muscles and exotropia while if there is malar hypoplasia and esotropia together, an inclination toward underaction of the IO muscles may be present. Possibly facial and orbital anthropometric data may not always be consistent.

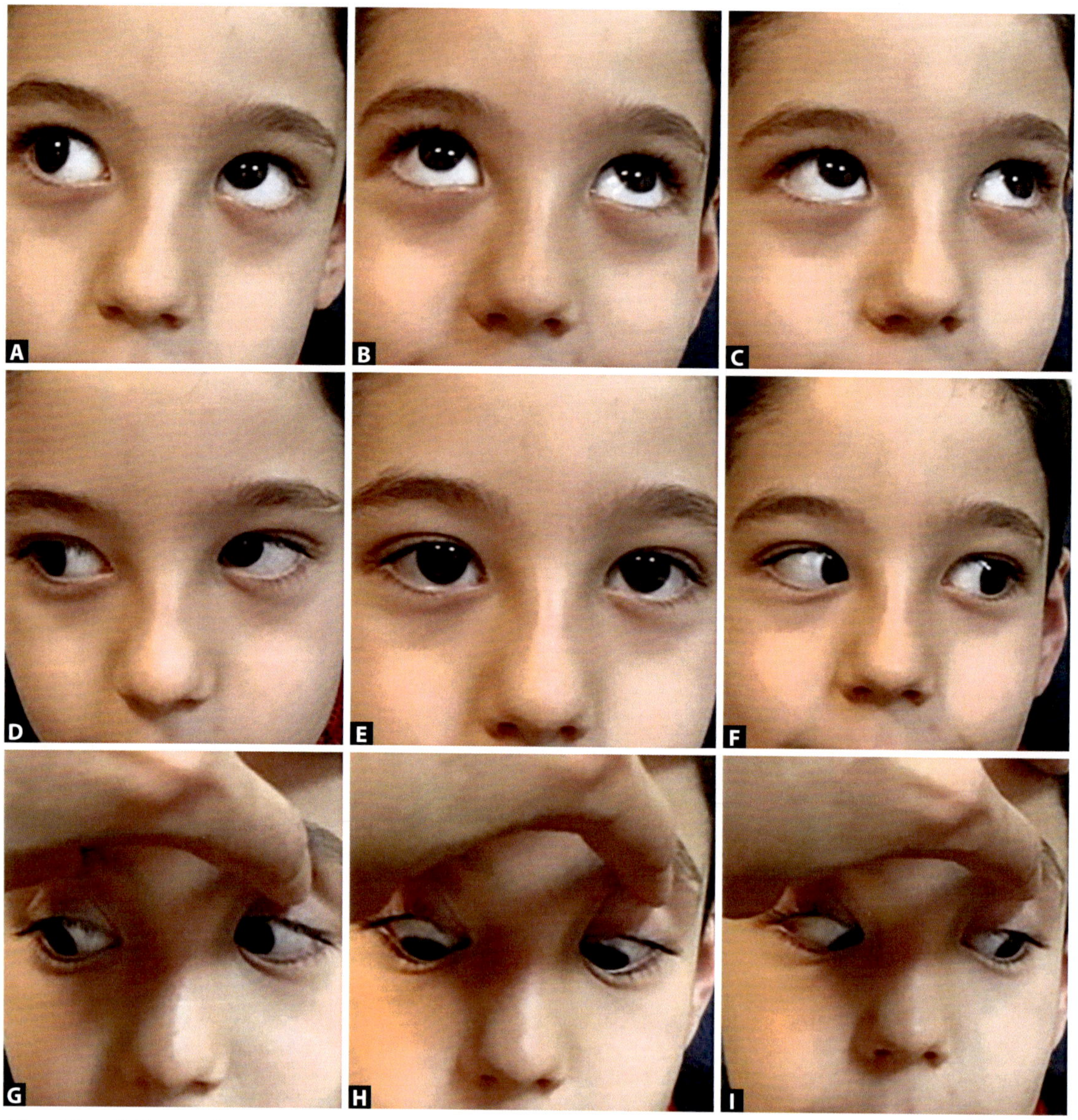

Figs. 2A to I: The exodeviation increases in upward gaze and decreases in downward gaze in V-pattern exotropia.

Some acquired conditions such as hydrocephalus and neurological anomalies like spina bifida may be associated with A-pattern.

Abnormalities of Extraocular Muscle Pulleys

Coronal computed tomography or MRI gives important clues regarding the relationship of horizontal and vertical rectus muscles in patients with pattern deviations. Rotations of the globe and rectus muscles and a displaced orientation of the position of the rectus muscle insertions may cause pattern deviations, vertical and horizontal strabismus. Clark et al., have proposed that upward or downward displacement of pulley system around LR may be related to V-and A-pattern, respectively. Small mislocations of rectus muscle pulleys can produce incomitance in vertical gaze. Inferior displacement of the LR pulley is associated with apparent overelevation in adduction, while superior displacement with overdepression in adduction. Thus, pulley heterotopy can itself cause incomitance without dysfunctional oblique muscles, hence resulting in A- or V-pattern strabismus.

Torsion Causing A-or V-patterns

The effect of torsion of the globe on horizontal rectus function in upgaze and downgaze has been studied by Kushner. With excyclorotation, the MR becomes a partial elevator and the SR has a reduced elevating function. As a result of several observations he concluded that torsion is only a minor contributing cause for pattern strabismus for several reasons:

- In primary oblique muscle overaction OA the elevation or depression of the eye was curvilinear as the eye was moved from abduction to adduction.
- Harada–Ito procedure for torsional diplopia could not abolish the significant IOOA.
- Horizontal muscle transposition for pattern strabismus increased the fundus torsion.

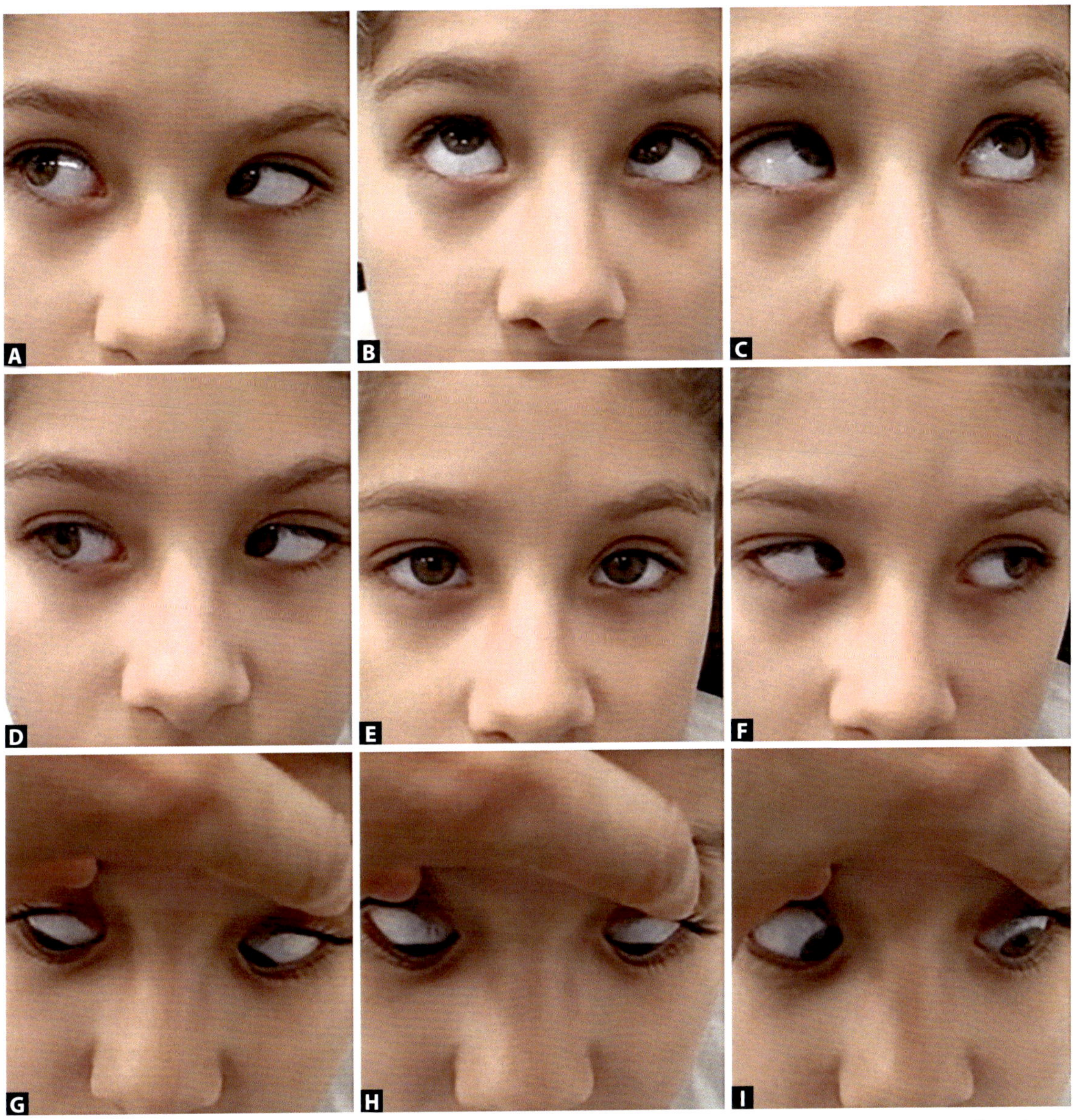

Figs. 3A to I: The esodeviation increases in upward gaze and decreases in downward gaze in A-pattern esotropia. There is also marked superior oblique overaction.

TABLE 1: Summarizing various types of pattern strabismus and associated conditions.

Type of pattern deviation	*Description*	*Associated conditions*
Y-pattern	Deviation is minimal between primary and downgaze, and occurs only in upgaze	• Bilateral inferior oblique overaction (OA) seen in congenital esotropia or exotropia • Duane retraction syndrome (DRS) • Brown's syndrome • Rarely congenital aberrant innervation of lateral rectus (LR) muscle with superior rectus nerve
Lambda-pattern	Minimum or no deviation difference in primary deviation and upgaze. Maximum divergence occurs between primary and downgaze	• Bilateral superior oblique (SO) OA • Inferior rectus underaction (over-recessed or slipped muscle)
Arrow-pattern	Maximum convergence occurs in between the primary and downgaze	Bilateral SO palsy
X-pattern	Increased divergence in both up and downgaze	• OA of all four oblique muscles Or • Tight LR muscle causing a leash effect in long-standing exotropia **(Figs. 4A to I)** and type 3 DRS

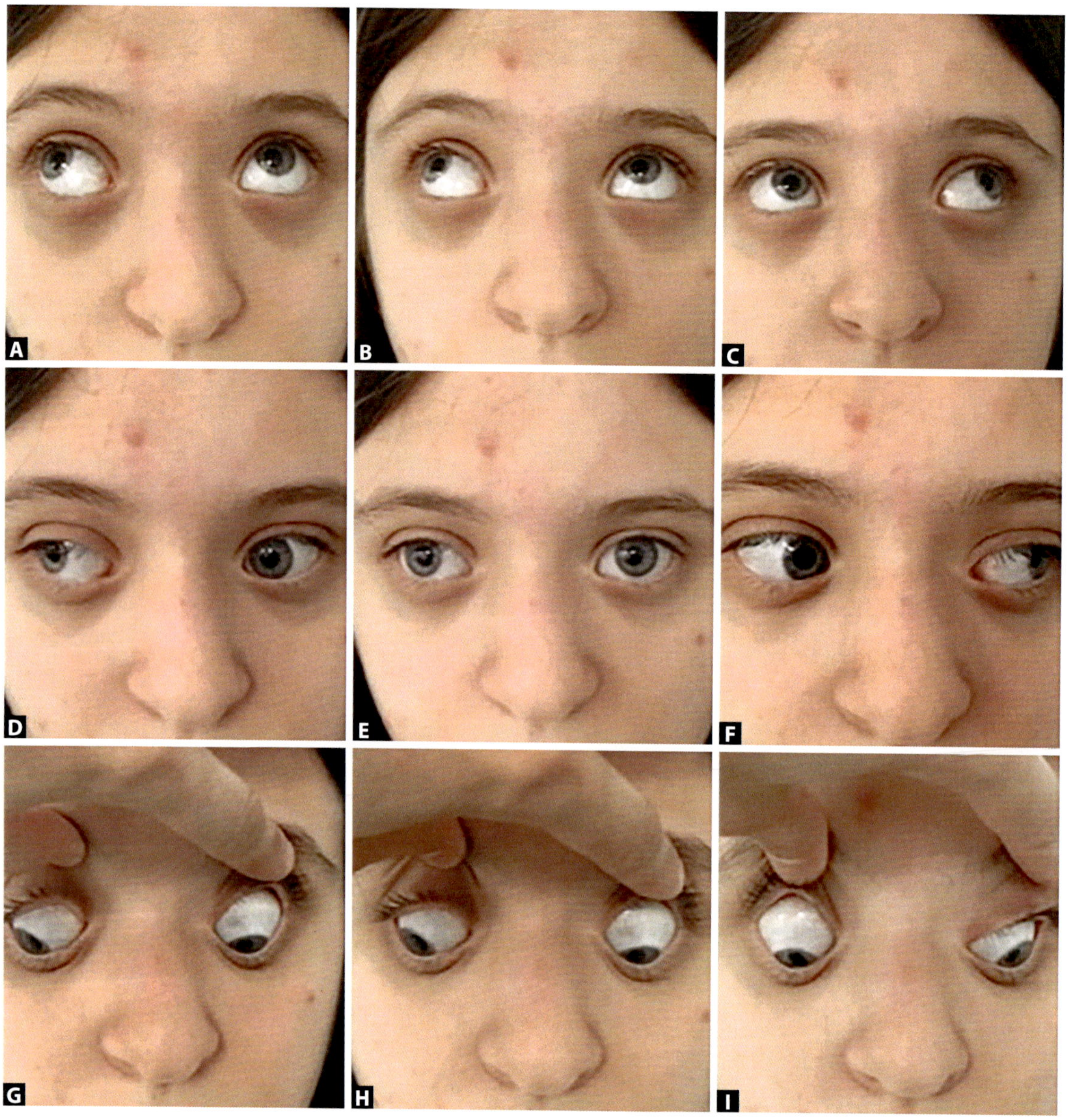

Figs. 4A to I: X-pattern with tight lateral rectus muscle causing a leash effect in long-standing exotropia.

So they conclude that torsion is only a minor contributing cause for pattern strabismus.

Neural Mechanisms and Sensory Deprivation

According to Guyton and Weingarten, poor binocular function may cause some forms of A and V syndromes. Deficient or absent fusion is often associated with asymmetric and bilateral excyclotorsion of the globe. Excyclorotation results in a partial elevator function in MR and reduced elevating function in the SR thus producing the clinical appearance of IOOA. Reduced sarcomeres and secondary shortening of IO muscle with time may produce OA of the muscle.

Loss of fusional control leads to torsional drift, which is similar to exotropic drift seen in sensory strabismus.

Das and Mustari showed in animal models that innervation to extraocular muscles (EOMs) from motor nuclei produce the inappropriate cross-axis eye movements, resulting in pattern strabismus and dissociated vertical deviation (DVD) supporting abnormal supranuclear circuits as one of the neural causes for pattern strabismus.

DIAGNOSIS AND EVALUATION

The presentation depends on the underlying strabismus and size of deviation. According to the size of deviation in different gaze positions, head positions like chin up or down may be assumed by the patient. Some head positions may cause symptoms at presbyopic ages with use of progressive bifocals. Reading difficulties may be noted in children also. Diplopia, asthenopia, unusual eye movements in extreme positions of gaze, head posture, and trauma history should be inquired.

It is important to be aware of the clinical conditions that are associated with pattern deviation: craniofacial anomalies, craniosynostosis, abnormally oriented eyelid fissures, fourth nerve palsy, spina bifida, thyroid eye disease with large IR recessions (A-pattern with increased activity of the yoke SO muscle), aberrant regeneration of third cranial nerve (V-pattern with aberrant innervation of IO muscle with fibers to MR).

Sensory evaluation includes best corrected visual acuity and evaluation of fusion. Amblyopia and anisometropia should be treated. Patients may have fusion depending on the orthotropia in any gaze. Suppression and abnormal retinal correspondence (ARC) may be present with tropia in all positions of gaze.

An abnormal head posture (AHP) to maintain fusion may sometimes be observed in pattern strabismus such as chin elevation in V-pattern exotropia. Asthenopia and double vision may be common complaints, especially if more deviation with downgaze. Cyclotorsion is both an etiological factor and a common feature of pattern strabismus.

For accurate diagnosis and management, motor examination should include:

- Measurement of deviation in 9 gaze positions. In practice, measurement in primary position, right gaze, left gaze, upgaze, and downgaze is done.
- Evaluation of overelevation and overdepression in adduction.
- Objective assessment of fundus torsion.

Lack of cooperation and a short attention span may lead to variable measurements in young children. Evaluations on several occasions are necessary to document the magnitude and nature of the deviation in upgaze and downgaze. Pseudo-V-pattern may be observed with increased accommodative convergence/accommodation (AC/A) ratio. Measurements at distance and near will be the same in primary gaze in patients with V-pattern without abnormal AC/A ratio. An increased AC/A may be simulated if the fixation target is below primary gaze at near. Distance correction should be used to view the fixation target. Versions should be tested beyond the recommended limits into the extreme positions of gaze. The oblique over/underactions should be evaluated.

Y-patterns may be more common in patients with IOOA without corresponding SO underaction since normal SO provides the abducting force keeping the eyes aligned in downgaze. Similarly lambda patterns may represent SOOA in the absence of corresponding IO underaction.

Superior oblique paresis produces a V-pattern and an "arrow subtype" in downgaze owing to the lack of abducting effect of paretic SO in downgaze. IOOA also produces a V-pattern with a Y subtype because of increased abduction in upgaze as the field of action of IO is upgaze and acts also as abductor. "Lambda" subtype is typically associated with SOOA with increased abduction in downgaze, the field of action of SO.

Imaging of the orbit may be considered in some unusual selected cases.

TREATMENT

Approach to the patient should follow regular rules in strabismus. Refractive errors should be corrected and amblyopia must be treated with the goal of achieving equal vision in both eyes. Usually deviations >10 OD in downgaze and 15 PD in upgaze, and those that may interfere with the development of binocular function needs surgical correction.

Deviations detected early in life can be treated to promote the development of some degree of binocular function. Young patients with spina bifida and A-pattern may be corrected safely before 8 years of age without causing diplopia and even with some chance of binocularity in patients.

Careful patient selection is important, especially during treatment of A-pattern exotropia that may cause torsion and disturbing cyclodiplopia.

The first step in the management of A- and V-patterns is to determine if there is associated oblique muscle OA or paresis. If significant dysfunction is detected, then oblique muscles should be surgically addressed. Primary A-V-patterns with normal oblique muscle function can be managed by "offsetting" the horizontal rectus muscles.

The main surgical goals are aimed at:

- Correcting horizontal and vertical alignment in important positions of gaze.
- Achieving single binocular vision.
- Correcting any head posture.

There are several surgical options that should be weighed considering several clinical positions: oblique muscle surgery, horizontal muscle transpositions, and slanting horizontal muscle recessions.

The surgical strategy should also consider coexisting orbital anomalies, lid fissure anomalies, abnormal structure of horizontal and oblique muscles, pulley anomalies, and defects in eyelid position, which are critical in surgical decisions.

The MR is always transposed toward the apex of the V (infraplaced) or the apex of A (supraplaced), while LR is transposed to bottom of the pattern (supraplaced to correct V-patterns and infraplaced for A-pattern) **(Figs. 5 and 6)**.

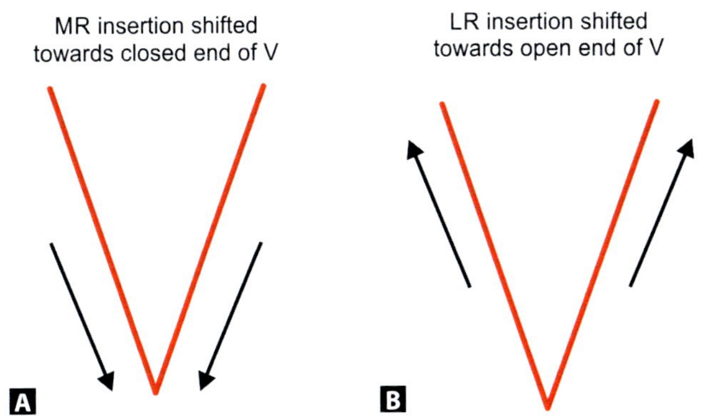

Figs. 5A and B: The medial rectus (MR) is transposed toward the apex of the V (infraplaced) and the lateral rectus (LR) to the open end of V (supraplaced) for V-pattern deviations.

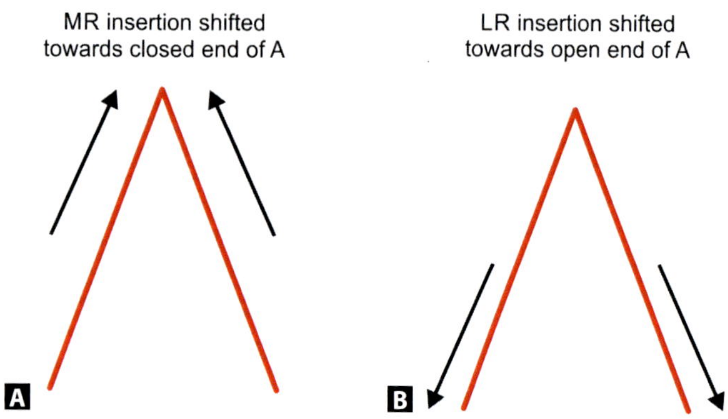

Figs. 6A and B: The medial rectus (MR) is transposed toward the apex of the A (supraplaced) and the lateral rectus (LR) to the open end of V (infraplaced) for A-pattern deviations.

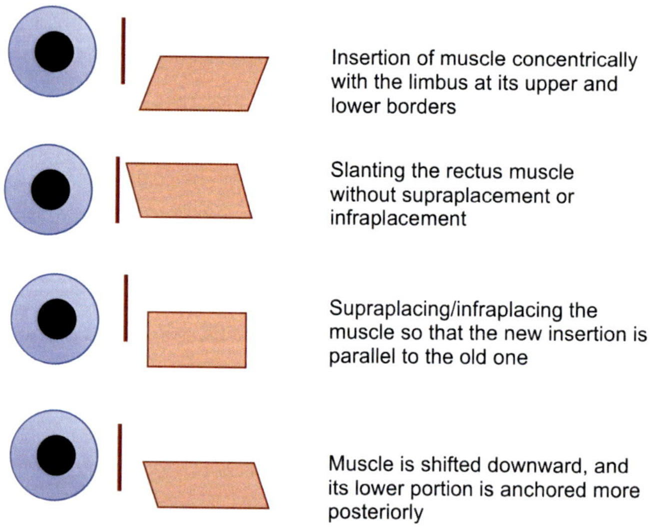

Fig. 7: Techniques for horizontal muscle transposition. The variations of the horizontal muscle transpositions according to the location and configuration of the new insertion.

The type of surgery and involvement of muscles depends upon the amount of A–V-patterns and the amount of OA or underaction of the oblique muscles.

Horizontal Muscle Transposition

The horizontal rectus transpositioning procedure works by moving the rectus muscle up (supraplacement) or down (infraplacement) to change the vector of the muscle force. For example, if the MR muscles were infraplaced, they would tighten in upgaze and loosen in downgaze, which would correct a V-pattern. Conversely, supraplacement would loosen the MR in upgaze and tighten in downgaze, thus correcting a A-pattern. Vertically shifting the horizontal muscles does not change the muscle's force in primary position.

In horizontal strabismus associated with A-pattern, the MR is shifted towards the apex while the LR is shifted towards the open end. Displacement of "one-half" of tendon width corrects about 10–15 PD of pattern while "full tendon" displacement corrects around 20 PD of pattern. In deviations larger than these figures, the OA of oblique muscles should be assessed and surgery planned accordingly.

Also slanting the muscle without supra/infraplacement has been recommended. The upper or lower border of the horizontal rectus muscle may be slanted more posteriorly during recession: For V-pattern esotropia, MR muscle may be recessed with its lower portion being fixed more posteriorly than the superior part on the sclera. This may reduce the adducting force of MR in downgaze. The schematic diagrams of these techniques are summarized in **Figure 7**.

Before planning vertical shift of horizontal muscles, ruling out significant oblique muscle dysfunction is critical. If the oblique over action is not noticed and horizontal muscle vertical displacement is done, the oblique muscle dysfunction may be exacerbated.

Oblique Muscle Weakening

In patients with overacting IO muscles, weakening procedures may eliminate >20 PD of V-pattern. The effect on horizontal alignment in primary gaze after weakening the IO is usually not remarkable.

On the other hand, the effect produced by weakening (tenotomy) of the SO tendon may vary depending on the amount of pattern present and whether the tenotomy is performed nasal (more effect: 25–45 PD) or temporal (less effect: 20–40 PD) to the lateral border of the SR muscle. The effect of SO tenotomy on the size of the horizontal deviation in primary gaze may be more prominent. A temporal tenotomy may lead to 8 PD of esoshift while nasal tenotomy may produce 3 PD of esoshift. Taking into consideration this point in horizontal surgery is important for predictable results. In patients with fusion, SO tenotomy should be used cautiously according to some authors in order to avoid disturbing diplopia. During SO tenotomy dividing the tendon nasally and cutting the attachments with SR may increase the weakening effect. Iatrogenic SO palsy also may result. Therefore, partial tenectomy of the posterior fibers of the SO tendon is another option for A-pattern strabismus.

Some complications may be observed with oblique muscle surgery. Failure or inability to identify all the fibers of oblique muscles may cause asymmetric weakening of oblique muscles that may cause vertical diplopia, torsion, and new head postures.

The suggested surgical algorithm for different patterns is summarized in the **Table 2**.

OBLIQUE MUSCLE DYSFUNCTION

This section would deal with only primary oblique muscle dysfunctions.

OVERELEVATION IN ADDUCTION (INFERIOR OBLIQUE OVERACTION)

The general term, IOOA may sometimes be misleading. In fact the term "overelevation in adduction" instead may be more appropriate to use most of the time. However, for

TABLE 2: Suggested surgical algorithm for different patterns.

Pattern	*Suggested surgery*
A-pattern with SO overaction	Horizontal muscle surgery and SO weakening
A-pattern without SO overaction	For esotropia—bimedial rectus recession with upshift or bilateral LR recession with downshift—for exotropia
V-pattern with IO overaction	Horizontal muscle surgery and IO weakening
V-pattern without IO overaction	Bimedial recession with downshift (for esotropia) or bilateral LR recession with upshift (for exotropia)
Y-pattern with IO overaction	Bilateral IO weakening
Y-pattern with SO underaction	SO graded tuck (horizontal muscle surgery if esotropia >10 PD)
Lambda-pattern with SO overaction	Bilateral SO tenotomy

(IO: inferior oblique; LR: lateral rectus; SO: superior oblique)

defining some definitions like "primary inferior oblique overaction (PIOOA)" we will use initial terminology also. PIOOA is usually of unknown etiology. The term "secondary IOOA" refers to IOOA secondary to SO palsy. Primary IOOA is usually associated with congenital esotropia, sometimes with congenital exotropia or an isolated entity without other strabismus. PIOOA is present in 70% of infantile esotropes, 35% of accommodative esotropes, and 30% of intermittent exotropes. About 25% cases of PIOOA are unilateral, but most of them eventually become bilateral.

Clinical Features

Primary inferior OA is usually bilateral but can be very asymmetric. The main clinical signs include an upshoot of adducting eye on versions, a V-pattern, and extorsion on indirect ophthalmoscopy. If the OA is symmetric, there may be no significant hypertropia in the primary position. Children with congenital PIOOA do not experience subjective extorsion because they have learned to sensorially adapt to it. Hence, no torsion is admitted by the patient on Maddox rods, Bagolini striated glasses, or Lancaster red-green testing. Bilateral IOOA produces a "left hypertropia on right gaze and a right hypertropia on left gaze" and little or no hypertropia on primary gaze. The hyperdeviation in the affected may manifest with only a few degrees of adduction, on full adduction or only in the field of action of the IO. Distinguishing a primary cause from secondary OA due to SO paresis largely depends on the head-tilt test. A negative head-tilt test indicates primary IOOA, whereas a positive test (increasing hypertropia with head tilt towards the side of the IOOA) indicates SO palsy. Differentiating the V-pattern is also helpful. A "Y" pattern subtype indicates primary IOOA, whereas an "arrow" subtype indicates a SO paresis.

Unilateral primary IOOA is unusual and many cases may actually represent very asymmetric bilateral IOOA. Unilateral PIOOA is associated with an ipsilateral hypertropia, usually 10–15 PD, in primary gaze that increases in gaze opposite to the overacting muscle, i.e., a right hypertropia in primary gaze would increase with gaze directed to left side. A "V" pattern may be present but is not the rule.

Differential Diagnosis

An upshoot of adducting eye on versions can be present in some other conditions also. (1) DVD can become manifest on adduction as that eye vision is blocked by the nasal bridge, which acts as an occluder. (2) A tight LR muscle can also cause elevation on attempted adduction of that eye, as in Duane's syndrome, due to a leash effect as the eye is adducted. (3) Differentiating from secondary IOOA due to SO palsy.

Several grading systems have been derived for the OA quantification, but none of them is accurate. A method stated is as follows: OA of +1 is 10 PD; +2 IS 20 PD; +3 is 30 PD; +4 is 45 PD (PD is prism diopters).

Treatment

In general, surgery is suggested for IOOA of +2 or more. If the IOOA is bilateral but asymmetric, bilateral IO weakening procedures are advised. The procedure can be performed even when one eye displays only +1 OA to prevent unmasking of the minimally overacting IO. If amblyopia is present, it may be appropriate to restrict surgery to the amblyopic eye.

The surgical management of IOOA is based on either weakening the IO muscle by diminishing the muscle tension (force) or changing the vector of mechanical force of the muscle by moving the insertion site. To decrease muscle force techniques such as myectomy and recession may be used.

Inferior oblique recession with anteriorization diminishes muscle tension by changing the functional insertion. The more the IO muscle is anteriorized, the more it becomes a depressor. I personally rarely suggest full anteriorization to the IR insertion with a "J" deformity of the new insertion because of the risk of antielevation syndrome. IO recession with placing the IO not anterior to the 5 mm back from the IR insertion and bunching up the insertion IO may be safer for preventing antielevation syndrome.

PRIMARY SUPERIOR OBLIQUE OVERACTION

Primary SOOA is usually of unknown etiology. It may usually be associated with a paresis of the contralateral IR muscle causing the yoke SO to overact, or rarely an ipsilateral IO paresis.

Clinical Features

Downshoot of the adducting eye on versions and divergence in downgaze with the characteristic A-pattern (usually a lambda-pattern) and intorsion, which increases in downgaze are main clinical properties. The subjective torsion is absent since primary SOOA is congenital and patients adapt to the intorted position, and do not show on subjective tests but objective torsion on indirect ophthalmoscopy is usually obvious.

Bilateral SOOA is usually associated with a small or no hypertropia in primary position, since the bilateral deviations cancel each other, but reversing hypertropias on side gaze are typical with right hypertropia to right gaze and a left hypertropia to left gaze. The lambda type of pattern is often quite large (>20 PD). If the bilateral SOOA is asymmetric, this may cause a hypertropia in primary position. Like IOOA, most cases of SOOA are bilateral with varying degrees of asymmetry. There may be some limitation to elevation in adduction of both eyes related to tight SO.

Unilateral cases will result in a hypertropia contralateral to the overacting SO with a small A pattern <10 PD and some limitation to elevation in adduction associated with a tight SO. Primary SOOA can be seen with esotropia or exotropia, and occasionally without any horizontal strabismus. The IO action is usually normal. One important condition in differential diagnosis is Brown's syndrome which can usually be differentiated from primary SOOA on a clinical basis, by hypertropia that is greatest in upgaze and a Y-pattern with an exotropia in upgaze. Forced duction testing, rotating the eye up and in, shows restriction in Brown's syndrome and no restriction in SOOA.

In IO paresis, a rare entity that may also be confused with a positive head-tilt test and a hypertropia in the contralateral eye that is greatest when the patient looks up, also helps to differentiate it from primary SOOA.

Unilateral SOOA causes hypertropia contralateral to the overacting SO muscle. The hypertropia increases on horizontal versions to the opposite side of the overacting muscle. A small "A" pattern of around 10 PD is typical of unilateral SOOA. Later there may be some limitation to elevation in adduction, due to tight SO muscle.

Treatment

In patients with binocular fusion, especially those with high-grade stereopsis (i.e., patients with intermittent exotropia and A-pattern) there is considerable risk for developing postoperative diplopia, if a consecutive SO paresis occurs following SO weakening procedures such as tenotomy and tenectomy. If the amount of SOOA is relatively small in comparison to the amount of A-pattern, supraplacement of the MR or infraplacement of the LR muscles in addition to weakening the SO muscles is more reasonable. OA of SO of +2 or more can be dissociating and SO surgery can be considered. In associated horizontal strabismus with SOOA, horizontal muscle surgery can be performed in the same sitting as SO weakening procedure, as SO surgery does not change the horizontal alignment in primary position.

If SOOA and "A" is present in a fusing patient, it is advisable to do vertical offsets of horizontal muscle or the Wright's tendon expander surgery, rather than tenotomy or tenectomy of SO muscle, to avoid postoperative SO palsy.

Superior oblique weakening procedures run a risk of exacerbating DVD. If DVD and SOOA coexist, the following options should be taken into account. With significant DVD (>10 PD) and significant SOOA (+2 or +3) and large "A" pattern, simultaneous large SR recession and Wright's SO expander procedure should be considered. If there is small DVD (5–7 PD) and +2 SOOA, only SO expander procedure will suffice but the lengthening should be reduced by 1 mm to avoid precipitation of DVD. If exotropia coexists with mild SOOA and mild DVD, only horizontal muscle surgery with vertical transpositioning should be planned, and SO should be left alone.

Bilateral SOOA is usually associated with large "A" pattern and bilateral SO weakening procedures are advised. Either SO tenotomy or Wright's silicone expander procedure will correct the OA and the "A" pattern. If OAs are "asymmetric", then larger tendon expander should be used on the side of larger OA. Tendon expanders do not correct >10 PD of vertical deviation; for larger deviation, a vertical muscle surgery will have to be added.

Patients with secondary SOOA due IO palsy will show ipsilateral SOOA and a large contralateral hypertropia in primary position. The hypertropia increases when the patient looks up and in with the affected eye. In such cases, ipsilateral SO weakening and contralateral SR recession is the best choice.

Differential Diagnosis

Differentiating SOOA from some mimicking disorders is important in view of management.

- Brown's syndrome, the hypertropia is greatest in upgaze in contralateral eye, while in SOOA the hypertropia is more in upgaze. Also Brown's syndrome is associated with a "Y" pattern and exotropia in upgaze. Finally, the standard forced duction test, rotating the eye up and in, will be positive, showing restriction, in case of Brown's syndrome.
- IO paresis is another entity that can be confused with primary SOOA. Primary IO palsy is rare. Patients with IO palsy show ipsilateral OA of SO, but present with a positive head-tilt test and a contralateral hypertropia that is greatest when patient looks up and in.

For completion sake, **Table 3** depicts salient features for diagnosis of disorders of oblique muscles.

TABLE 3: Clinical pictures that may be observed with over/underelevation/depression in adduction.

	Clues for diagnosis	***Overelevation in adduction***	***Overdepression in adduction***	***Underelevation in adduction***	***Underdepression in adduction***
Craniofacial syndromes	• Dysmorphic appearance • Imaging helpful	+			+
Duane syndrome	• Limited abduction • Lid fissure narrowing	+	+		
SO palsy	• Hypertropia with excyclotropia • Three-step test helpful, if congenital, presence of facial asymmetry	+			+
IO contracture	Exaggerated forced duction	+			+
Pseudo IOOA	No elevation in side gaze, no SOUA	+			
DVD	Hypotropia of adducted eye	+			
Antielevation syndrome	Prior surgery, lower eyelid bulging on upgaze	+			
Contralateral eye inferior restriction	Prior surgery, abnormal forced ductions	+			
SO tendon incarceration syndrome (Demer, 2002)	Prior surgery, hypertropia with incyclotropia	+			
Pulley heterotopia	Orbital imaging for anomalous pulley position	+			
SOOA	A-pattern, fundus excyclotropia, association with spina bifida, horizontal strabismus		+		
IO palsy	Three-step test, underelevation in adduction, incyclotropia, A-pattern		+	+	
Brown's syndrome	Underelevation in adduction, V-pattern, positive forced duction		+	+	
IO adherence syndrome	Prior surgery, hypotropia with excyclotropia	+		+	

(DVD: dissociated vertical deviation; IO: inferior oblique; IOOA: inferior oblique overaction; SO: superior oblique; SOOA: superior oblique overaction; SOUA: superior oblique underaction)

SUGGESTED READING

1. Biglan AW. Ophthalmologic complications of meningomyelocele: a longitudinal study. Trans Am Ophthalmol Soc. 1990;88:389-462.
2. Clark RA, Demer JL. Lateral rectus superior compartment palsy. Am J Ophthalmol. 2014;157(2):479-87.e472.
3. Clark RA, Miller JM, Rosenbaum AL, Demer JL. Heterotopic muscle pulleys or oblique muscle dysfunction? J AAPOS. 1998;2(1):17-25.
4. Das VE, Mustari MJ. Correlation of cross-axis eye movements and motoneuron activity in non-human primates with "A" pattern strabismus. Invest Ophthalmol Vis Sci. 2007;48(2):665-74.
5. Demer JL. The orbital pulley system: a revolution in concepts of orbital anatomy. Ann N Y Acad Sci. 2002;956:17-32.
6. Demer JL. Should we require evidence about the etiology of A-pattern strabismus? J AAPOS. 2010;14(1):4-5.
7. Diamond GR, Parks MM. The effect of superior oblique weakening procedures on primary position horizontal alignment. J Pediatr Ophthalmol Strabismus. 1981;18(1):35-8.
8. Donahue SP, Itharat P. A-pattern strabismus with overdepression in adduction: a special type of bilateral skew deviation? J AAPOS. 2010;14(1):42-6.
9. Kekunnaya R, Mendonca T, Sachdeva V. Pattern strabismus and torsion needs special surgical attention. Eye (Lond). 2015;29(2):184-90.
10. Knapp P. Vertically Incomitant horizontal strabismus: the so-called "A" and "V" syndromes. Trans Am Ophthalmol Soc. 1959;57:666-99.
11. Kushner BJ. Effect of ocular torsion on A and V patterns and apparent oblique muscle overaction. Arch Ophthalmol. 2010;128(6):712-8.
12. Miller MM, Guyton DL. Loss of fusion and the development of A or V patterns. J Pediatr Ophthalmol Strabismus. 1994;31(4):220-4.
13. Rubin SE, Nelson LB, Harley RD. A complication in weakening the superior oblique muscle in A-pattern exotropia. Ophthalmic Surg. 1984;15(2):134-5.
14. Sharma P, Halder M, Prakash P. Torsional changes in surgery for A-V phenomena. Indian J Ophthalmol. 1997;45(1):31-5.
15. Urist MJ. The etiology of the so-called A and V syndromes. Am J Ophthalmol. 1958;46(6):835-44.

25

CHAPTER

Paralytic Strabismus

Birsen Gökyiğit, Rebika Dhiman

INTRODUCTION

The three pairs of cranial nerves (3rd, 4th, and 6th) innervate the six extraocular muscles, the levator palpebral superioris, and carry the parasympathetic fibers for pupillary innervation bilaterally. Any interruption in the nerve supply of one or more of these cranial nerves will cause motor imbalance and result in paralytic strabismus. It may be a "paresis", which is partial loss of muscle action, or a "paralysis" implying complete loss of muscle activity.

The paralytic strabismus in acute case is characterized by the presence of "incomitance", i.e., varying ocular deviation in different gazes, and "limitation of movement" which is greatest in the direction of action of the paralyzed muscle.

STAGES OF PARALYTIC STRABISMUS

A paralytic strabismus usually evolves in three stages. Initially, the primary feature is weakness of the paralyzed muscle which is closely followed by the over action of the direct antagonist. During this phase, the deviation is greatest in the direction of movement of the affected muscle due to loss of contractile function of the muscle. Over time, this leads to over action and subsequent contracture of the direct antagonistic muscle in the ipsilateral eye resulting in the deviation becoming maximum in the field of action of this muscle.

In the final stage, the deviation becomes similar in all gazes termed as a "spread of comitance". However, not every patient may go through all these stages and the patient can remain in the first stage with the maximum deviation in the direction of the movement of the affected muscle.

Workup in Paralytic Strabismus

History related to the onset, duration, and associated ocular and systemic features are important. In acute cases, patients commonly present with complains of binocular diplopia and/or ocular deviation.

Clinical Features

Diplopia and Abnormal Head Posture

In patients of paralytic strabismus who had binocularity before being affected, diplopia is very disturbing. To avoid diplopia, patients develop the abnormal head position (AHP) in the direction of movement of the affected muscle to avoid the action of the paretic muscle. It is best to observe for the head posture when the patient is comfortable and unaware of being examined, as sometimes the patient may purposely try to conceal the AHP. So, one must look for the head posture as soon as the patient enters the clinician's room and it may be the first sign that the clinician can appreciate. AHP can be in the form of face turn, head tilt, or chin-up or chin-down. This is called ocular torticollis. In horizontal rectus palsy, the face turn is in the direction of action of the paralyzed muscle and in cyclovertical muscle palsy, the head is tilted to the side of the hypotropic eye and the chin moves in the direction of action of the paralytic muscle. Thus, the horizontal, vertical, or torsional diplopia is eliminated and single binocular vision is maintained. The head turn toward the side of the paralyzed eye will compensate for a right lateral rectus (LR) paralysis, and a head tilt to one shoulder (ocular torticollis) with chin depression is characteristic of a superior oblique (SO) paralysis on the opposite side. In 15% of patients, paradoxically, the head may be in the opposite direction to what is expected. This is done to increase the gap between the diplopic images so that one of the images can be easily ignored and this is called "reverse AHP". It is important to distinguish between congenital ocular and nonocular torticollis. When evaluating the paralytic head position, other reasons for AHPs should always be kept in mind. A common cause of torticollis is congenital muscular torticollis and this should be differentiated from ocular torticollis as seen in SO palsy **(Table 1)**. Regardless of the reason, prolonged head tilt can cause facial asymmetry as in congenital palsies. This asymmetry may be from the restriction of normal facial growth caused by persistent muscle pull on the facial bone toward one side or less arterial supply on the affected side. The facial asymmetry caused by head tilt must be differentiated from plagiocephaly.

Past-pointing

Past-pointing is the anomaly of the egocentric localization. This occurs as excessive innervation is required to stimulate the paretic muscle to bring about the ocular movement to look

TABLE 1: Differential diagnosis congenital muscular versus ocular torticollis.

	Congenital muscular	*Ocular*
Age	Onset in first 6 months after birth	Generally, onset around 18 months of age
Head position	Strengthening the head, either voluntary or passive, is difficult	Strengthening the head is easy in anyway and can tipped opposite side
Neck position	In palpation there is hardness in sternocleidomastoid muscle	There is normal muscle in palpation
Vision	There is no visual problem	Noticeable diplopia on strengthening of head or during tilting it opposite side
Effect of occlusion	Torticollis never change by occlusion of either eye	If there is no secondary skeletal problem, head strengthen after occlusion the eye

at the object of regard. This excess innervation is perceived as though the object of regard is lying further away than the actual position, leading to past-pointing. This is tested by asking the patient to briskly point at any object kept in the field of action of the paralyzed muscle and a board kept over the hands to avoid direct visualization of hand movements by the patient. In recent onset extraocular muscle paralysis, the hand overshoots. This may be useful to distinguish between congenital and acquired paralysis.

Amblyopia

Amblyopia in paretic strabismus may develop in children during the critical period of visual development who are unable to maintain simultaneous binocular vision in any gaze leading to suppression of one eye. Mostly suppression develops in the paretic eye. Rarely, patient may fixate with their paralyzed eye either due to increased separation of the images by using secondary deviation that allows the distant image to be ignored easily, or due to preexisting mild amblyogenic factors in the fellow eye like anisometropia. Such cases develop amblyopia in the unaffected eye.

Paralytic Workup

Extraocular Movements

The paralytic workup includes careful assessment of the extraocular movements, both binocular (versions) and uniocular (ductions), to identify the paralyzed muscle(s). Limitation of deviation is greatest movement is greatest in the direction of action of the paralyzed muscle. The amount of deviation corroborates with the extent of limitation in paralytic squints. While in restrictive squint like Duane's retraction syndrome, the limitation of movement is out of proportion to the amount of deviation.

Amount of Deviation

Besides evaluating the ocular motility, measuring the angle of deviation in diagnostic positions of gaze with either eye fixating is an essential part of the workup. These measurements can be obtained objectively or subjectively. Objective methods for measuring ocular deviation are prism and cover test and synoptophore. Subjective methods include diplopia charting and Hess screen, Lees screen, etc. Prism and cover test must be performed with either eye fixing. At first, measurements should be done when fixating with the unaffected eye (primary deviations), and then repeated while fixating with the affected eye (secondary deviations). The secondary deviation is always larger than the primary deviation in paralytic strabismus **(Figs. 1A and B)**. This is because the eyes will have equal innervation as per the Hering's law and the fixing eye governs the amount of innervation. For example, in left sixth nerve palsy, when the patient fixates with the healthy right eye, a certain amount of left esodeviation is seen because of the insufficient innervation to the left LR. But, if the patient attempts to fixate with the affected left eye, the left LR requires excessive effort to keep the eye on the object of regard. So, the brain sends equal excessive innervation to its yoke muscle, i.e., the right medial rectus (MR) and therefore the eye deviates more. The measurements should be repeated in nine positions of gaze.

Parks' Three-step Test and Bielschowsky Head Tilt Test (Figs. 2A and B)

The evaluation is challenging, especially in vertical strabismus where one has to differentiate between a pair of elevators or depressors in each eye. Parks' three-step test and Bielschowsky head tilt test are useful in identifying the affected cyclovertical muscle.

In the Parks' three-step test, each step answers one of the following questions:

- Does the patient have right or left hypertropia in the primary position?
- Does this deviation increase in dextroversion or levoversion?
- Does the hypertropia increase with head tilt to right or left shoulder?

A paretic oblique or vertical rectus muscle can be identified in most cases by using this three-step method.

However, these tests are valid only if paralysis involves one cyclovertical muscle. It can be misleading if more than one muscle is affected. In these cases, Hess screen, Lees screen,

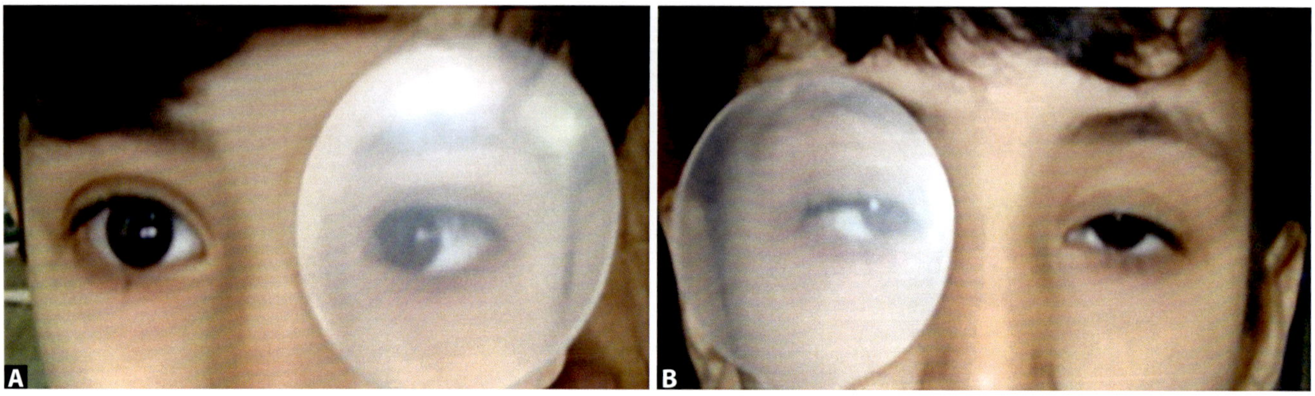

Figs. 1A and B: Primary deviation is seen behind the occlude on the left and secondary deviation is seen behind the occlude on the right in a child with left abducens palsy.

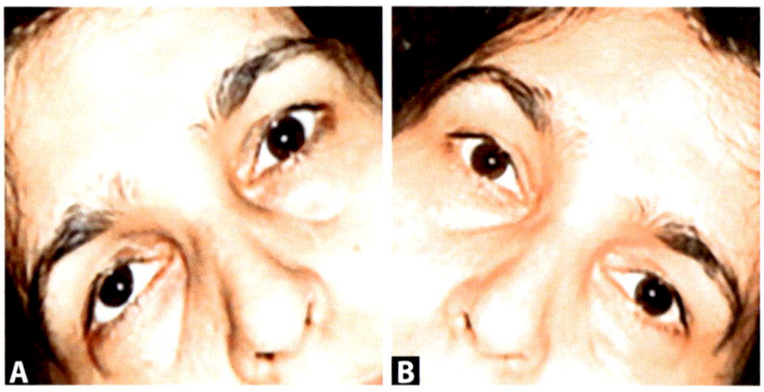

Figs. 2A and B: Bielschowsky head tilt test is diagnostic for a right superior oblique paralysis with increase of the right hypertropia on tilting the head to the right shoulder.

and similar examinations are more valuable both in diagnosis and follow-up.

Torsion

Torsional change may occur in palsy of any cyclovertical muscle. Torsion can be documented subjectively using double Maddox rod test or synoptophore. In double Maddox rod test, we place two different colored Maddox rods (e.g., red and white) in front of each eye in a trial frame. Vertically placed Maddox rods will create two horizontal lines. In torsional diplopia, the line perceived by the paretic eye will appear tilted. One Maddox rod is rotated till the two lines become parallel and the amount of rotation can be measured on the trial frame in degrees. Objective methods to assess torsion are by noting the position of the fovea with respect to the optic disk on indirect ophthalmoscopy or fundus photography. The horizontal line drawn through the fovea cuts the disk midway between the center of the disk and the lower pole in normal individuals. This line cuts the disk at a higher level in incyclotorsion and at a lower level in excyclotorsion.

Forced Duction Test

The forced duction test (FDT) is a simple and most useful method for distinguishing the mechanical restriction of ocular motility from palsy. Mechanical restriction of extraocular movements may be seen in orbital blow out fracture, thyroid eye disease or other structural anomalies of the extraocular muscles, conjunctiva, Tenon's capsule, etc. During the FDT, the eye is held with two toothed-forceps near the limbus; at 6 and 12 o'clock to check for horizontal recti and, at 3 and 9 o'clock to check for the vertical recti. The eye is then passively rotated in the direction opposite to the action of the muscle to be tested, e.g., to distinguish between a LR palsy and mechanical restriction of the MR, the eyeball is passively abducted. If resistance is encountered, it is noted as tight or positive FDT implying contracture of MR or restriction in the adjacent medial conjunctiva or Tenon's capsule. If no resistance is felt, then the FDT is negative implying that the limitation of movement is due to LR palsy. Occasionally, FDT tightness may be noted in the direction of the action of the muscle being tested. This is due to retroequatorial adhesion of the recti and is described as the "reverse leash effect". Although FDT can be performed using topical anesthesia, performing the test under general anesthesia can give more accurate results. It is important to avoid the use of succinylcholine for general anesthesia because it may change the tension in the muscles and thereby alter the results. One must note that while performing FDT for recti muscles, the globe should be lifted and for oblique muscles, the globe should be depressed into the orbit (**Figs. 3A and B**).

Active Force Generation Test (Fig. 4)

The active force generation test (AFGT) evaluates the strength of the paretic muscle in the presence of secondary restriction, i.e., when the FDT is positive. It can be done only under topical anesthesia. Perilimbal fixation is used and the patient is asked to look or make an attempt to look in the direction of action of the paralyzed muscle. Any tug felt during the attempt is indirect evidence of the contraction of the paretic muscle and thus implies some residual muscle strength. No tug indicates complete paralysis of the muscle. Force generation test indicates the severity of paralysis and differentiates between complete and partial paralysis, and between the paralytic and restrictive components of strabismus. Therefore, it guides the

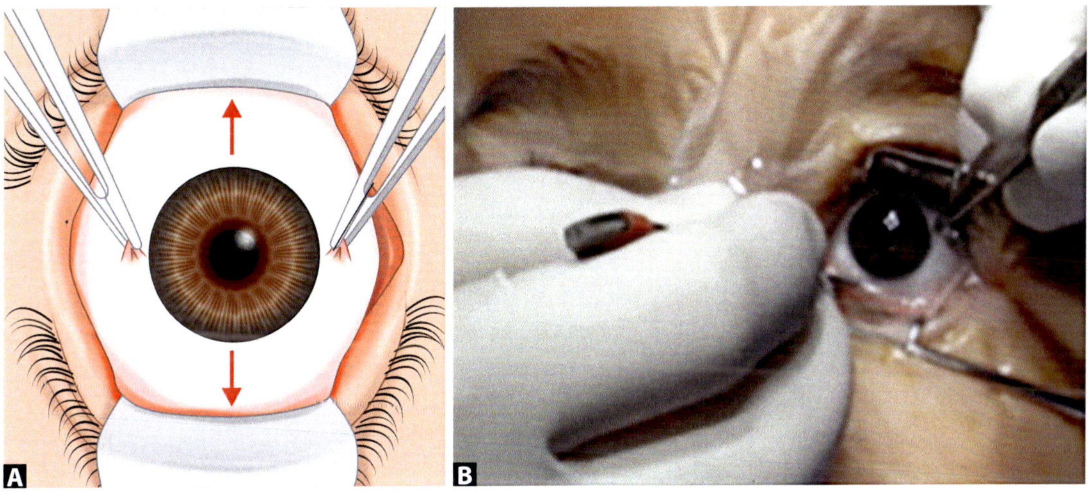

Figs. 3A and B: Forced duction test being done for vertical recti (A) and for oblique muscles (B).

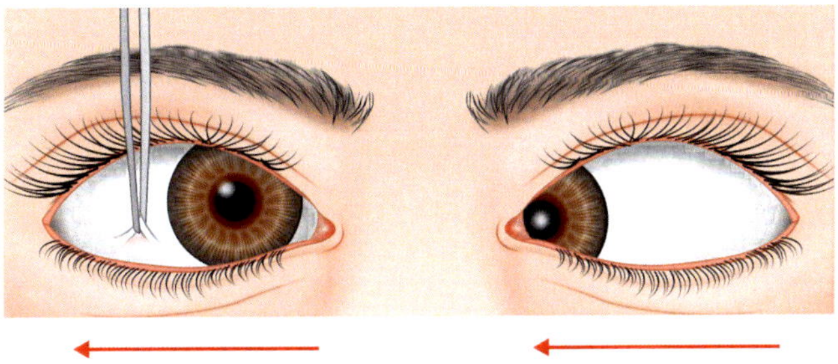

Fig. 4: Forced generation test for right abducens palsy. When the patient attempts to right gaze, try to feel the right lateral rectus force with gentle pressing against the muscle activity direction.

surgical planning between recess-resect versus transposition procedure.

Imaging

Imaging is an essential part of the workup in acquired palsies. Neuroimaging helps in identifying the underlying cause and becomes absolutely indicated in all acute onset palsies.

Contrast-enhanced magnetic resonance imaging (CEMRI) is the investigation of choice in most cases. Computed tomography (CT) scan is useful in trauma or bony pathologies. In suspected cases of aneurysms, fistulas or venous sinus thrombosis, magnetic resonance (MR) angiography or MR venography may be indicated. Orbital imaging not only has a specific place in the diagnosis of paralytic strabismus but also aids in surgical planning. In long-standing cases of palsy, denervation atrophy of the affected extraocular muscle is evident in the form of reduction in muscle size. It can help diagnose rare cases of muscle agenesis, muscle slip, etc. It can discriminate paralytic from restrictive causes of squint such as myositis, orbital inflammation, myocysticercosis, and thyroid eye disease. Dynamic magnetic resonance imaging (MRI) is a new technique that picks up muscle contractility in various gazes and thereby gives the idea about the functional state of the muscle. This is especially useful in paralytic squint with aberrant regenerations.

Other Investigations

The eye movement velocity is markedly decreased in the paralyzed muscle's action area. While it can be noted by observation, electromyography provides an objective measurement. Electromyography can be used to differentiate whether the pathology belongs to the muscle or the nerve.

Binocular visual field charting gives the idea about the diplopia-free field or the field of binocular single vision in palsy. One can use it to document the change on follow-up regarding the progression or improvement of the paralyzed muscle.

Evaluation of underlying etiology may require various laboratory investigations such as complete hemogram, erythrocyte sedimentation rate (ESR), C-reactive protein (CRP), renal function, and liver function tests. In elderly, blood sugars including hemoglobin A1c (HbA1c), lipid profile, blood pressure, etc., should be assessed to rule out ischemic or microvascular etiology. Hyperhomocystinemia has been associated in young onset ischemic ocular motor palsy and therefore requires testing for serum homocysteine levels. Thyroid function test and tests for myasthenia gravis may be indicated in suspected cases. Additional workup may include serology for infectious causes such as Lyme's disease and syphilis and autoimmune workup. Lumbar puncture for cerebrospinal fluid (CSF) analysis including cell count, protein, glucose, and cytology may be indicated in certain cerebral infectious and inflammatory conditions.

Differentiation between Paralytic and Restrictive Strabismus

The motor imbalance caused by paralytic strabismus must be clearly distinguished from comitant and/or restrictive forms of strabismus. **Tables 2 and 3** summarize the differentiating features between these entities.

TABLE 2: Differential diagnosis between paralytic and nonparalytic strabismus.

	Paralytic strabismus	*Nonparalytic strabismus*
Onset and progress	Acute, slowly, congenital	First 6 months of age, slowly
Age	Any age	Generally, in childhood
Head trauma	Common	Rare
Secondary deviation > primary deviation	Characteristic	Absent
Diplopia	Common	Uncommon
Anomalous retinal correspondence (ARC)/ amblyopia	Unusual	Common
Comitance	Late stage	Common
Abnormal head posture	Often	Rare
Torsion	Common (cyclovertical strabismus)	Rare (A and V pattern)
Neurogenic findings/systemic disease	Possible	Very rare
Past pointing	Common (in acute faze)	Very rare

TABLE 3: Differential diagnosis between paralytic and restrictive strabismus.

	Force duction test	*Force generation test*	*Saccadic velocity*
Restriction (+) paralysis (–)	+	+	Normal
Restriction (+) paralysis (+)	+	–	Decreased/absent
Paresis	–	+	Decreased
Paralysis	–	–	Absent

OCULOMOTOR OR 3RD CRANIAL NERVE PALSY

Nerve Anatomy

The third nerve nucleus complex consists of six subnuclei located in the mesencephalon in the midbrain that supply the superior rectus (SR), inferior rectus (IR), medial rectus MR, inferior oblique (IO), and levator palpebrae superioris (LPS). In addition, the third nerve carries the parasympathetic preganglionic fibers arising from the paired Edinger–Westphal nucleus to the ciliary ganglion for the control of pupillary constriction and accommodation. While the subnuclei for the MR, IR and IO innervate the ipsilateral muscles, the fibers from the SR subnuclei cross at the lower end of the nuclear complex and innervate the contralateral muscle. The central lower core of the nuclei complex bilaterally innervates the levator palpebral superioris muscle. The fascicular part of the nerve travels ventrally through the red nucleus and the cerebral peduncles. The basilar part exists the midbrain at the interpeduncular fossa and runs in between the superior cerebellar and posterior cerebral arteries and then parallel to the posterior communicating artery **(Fig. 5)**. Here the fibers supplying the IR, MR, SR, and IO run in a medial-to-lateral arrangement. It enters the cavernous sinus, runs along its lateral wall and into the orbit through the superior orbital fissure **(Fig. 6)**. The nerve then divides into superior and inferior branches immediately before entering the anterior cavernous sinus or in the orbit. While the superior part of the nerve innervates the SR and levator palpebral superioris, the inferior branch innervates the MR, IR, IO, and sphincter pupillae. Pupillary fibers are located superficially along the superomedial aspect of the nerve being supplied by the pial blood vessels. In contrast, the main trunk of the fibers is supplied by the vasa vasorum.

Causes

The causes for oculomotor paralysis can be evaluated under following headings:

- Vascular ischemia (diabetes mellitus, atherosclerosis, hypertension, and giant cell arteritis)
- Compression [aneurysms, neoplasms, hydrocephalus, arteriovenous (AV) fistulas, etc.]
- Trauma (open/closed head traumas)
- Hemorrhage (orbital/intracranial)
- Inflammation/demyelination (viral, postviral, and multiple sclerosis)
- Idiopathic
- Congenital.

Vascular ischemia or microvasculopathy is the most common cause of acquired third nerve palsy. Aneurysm, especially of the posterior communicating artery, may be seen in around 10% cases. Therefore, all acquired third-nerve palsy cases should be investigated thoroughly with neuroimaging. In children, congenital anomaly (43%) and trauma (20%) are the two most frequent causes.

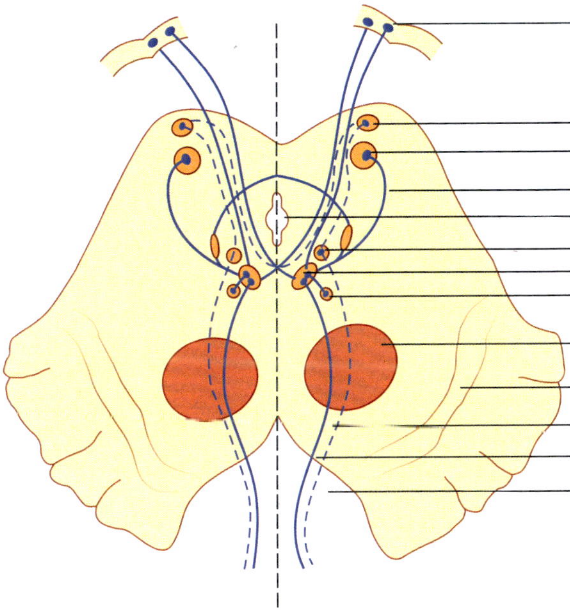

Fig. 5: Oculomotor nuclear complex.

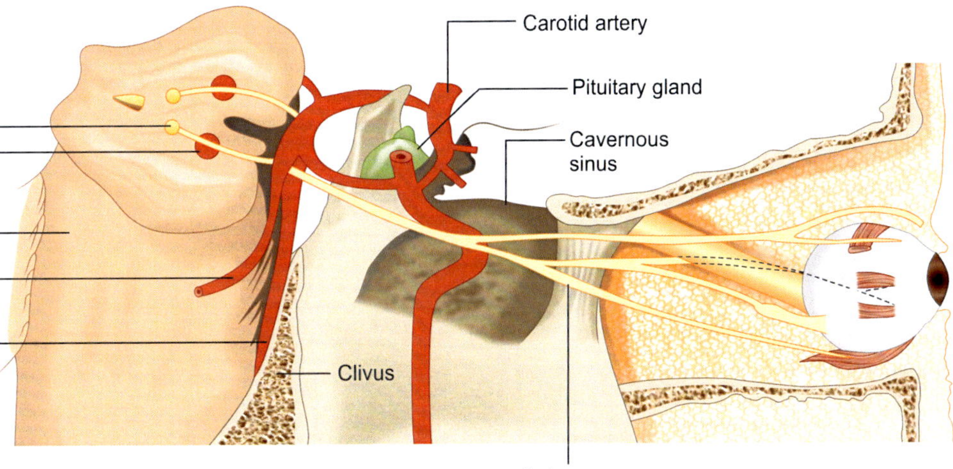

Fig. 6: Course of oculomotor nerve (lateral view).

Clinical Features

Depending upon the site of involvement and the underlying cause, third nerve palsy could be partial or complete, pupil-sparing or involving, and isolated or associated with other neurological symptoms. Therefore, precise knowledge of the nerve origin and course along with associated clinical symptoms or signs helps in localizing the site of lesion.

A supranuclear lesion causes conjugate paresis. A complete third nerve palsy with nuclear involvement presents with ipsilateral mydriasis, bilateral ptosis, contralateral elevation deficit, and ipsilateral adduction and depression deficits. Infarction, tumor, metastasis, demyelination, etc., are some important lesions affecting the nerve at nuclear and supranuclear levels. Wall-eyed bilateral internuclear ophthalmoplegia (WEBINO) is a rare presentation characterized by dissociated abducting nystagmus, impaired convergence, and supranuclear vertical gaze palsy. It is caused by midbrain lesion damaging the bilateral medial longitudinal fasciculus (MLF) and pretectum.

As the fascicular part of third nerve passes in close relation to brainstem structures, its involvement is associated with other neurological deficits as described in **Table 4**. The involvement of the basilar part of the nerve in the subarachnoid space is usually isolated. Aneurysms of the posterior communicating artery or the posterior cerebral artery and extradural/subdural hematoma are the common causes of third nerve palsy in the subarachnoid space. Severe trauma causes extradural or subdural hematoma that leads to downward herniation of the temporal lobe, which then compresses the third nerve as it passes over the tentorial edge. Third nerve palsy following a minor trauma should raise the suspicion of an underlying aneurysm. Pupillary involvement is a common phenomenon in these compressive lesions (due to compression of superficial pupillary fibers from outside). There may be associated pain also.

TABLE 4: Various syndromes noted in fascicular third nerve involvement.

Syndrome	*Site of involvement*	*Clinical features*
Benedikt's syndrome	Red nucleus	Ipsilateral 3rd nerve palsy + contralateral tremors
Weber's syndrome	Cerebral peduncle	Ipsilateral 3rd nerve palsy + contralateral hemiplegia
Nothnagel's syndrome	Superior cerebellar peduncle	Ipsilateral 3rd nerve palsy + cerebellar ataxia
Claude's syndrome	Red nucleus + Superior cerebellar peduncle	Combined features of both Benedikt's and Nothnagel's syndromes

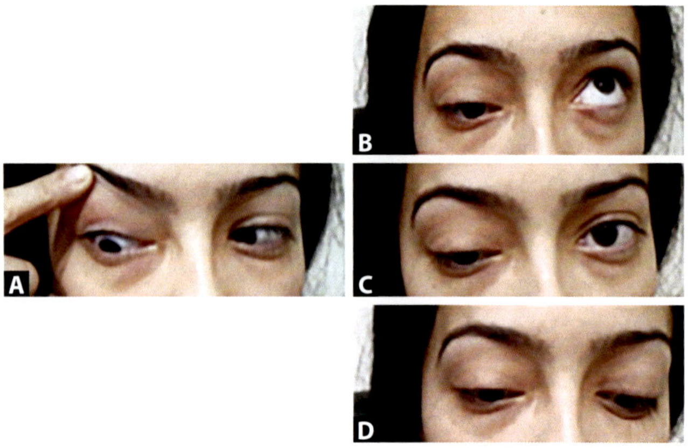

Figs. 7A to D: Right 3rd cranial nerve superior division paralysis.

Multiple cranial nerve palsies are common in the cavernous involvement due to close proximity of 3rd, 4th, 5th, and 6th cranial nerves in this region. Cavernous sinus thrombosis, carotid-cavernous fistula, pituitary apoplexy, Tolosa-Hunt syndrome, neoplasms (pituitary tumors, craniopharyngioma, meningioma, nasopharyngeal carcinoma, and metastasis), and aneurysm of internal carotid artery are some common causes affecting the cavernous region.

Orbital lesions may involve the superior division **(Figs. 7A to D)**, inferior division, or both the branches of the third nerve. Superior division involvement causes ptosis and limitation of upgaze. Limitation of downgaze, adduction, and pupil dilatation are seen in inferior division involvement. Types of orbital involvement can be inflammatory, infiltrative, metastatic, etc. It may be associated with orbital features such as proptosis and chemosis. Orbital apex syndrome is characterized by features of ophthalmoplegia and vision loss due to involvement of the ocular motor nerves and optic nerve at the orbital apex or superior orbital fissure.

Compressive versus Medical Lesions

One must note that compressive lesions such as aneurysm and tumor compress the nerve from outside. This involves the superficial pupillomotor fibers and its blood supply and therefore causes pupil-involving third nerve palsy. On the other hand, medical lesions like microangiopathy associated with diabetes mellitus or hypertension affect the vessel supply of the main nerve trunk, i.e., vasa vasorum, and thus spare the pupillary fibers. However, exceptions may be there. If pupillary involvement is seen in third nerve palsy caused by microvascular ischemia, then typically the anisocoria is <1 mm and the pupils remain reactive. But these findings may also be seen in early cases of compressive third nerve palsy where the palsy is still evolving.

Individual Extraocular Muscle Palsy of Abducent Nerve

Superior Rectus Muscle Paralysis

Superior rectus palsy is mostly congenital or traumatic. In acute cases, there is defective elevation in abduction with ptosis. In long-standing cases, the elevation deficit extends in all gazes—abduction, adduction, and primary position. Overaction of ipsilateral IR and contralateral IO muscles with mild excyclotropia may be noted. The affected eye is hypotropic with the absence of the Bell's phenomenon. The chin is elevated and the head is inclined toward the healthy eye. Ocular torticollis and pseudoptosis are some other characteristics that may be seen. To discriminate pseudoptosis from true ptosis, patients are made to fixate using the affected eye while unaffected eye is covered. In case of pseudoptosis, the drooping of the upper lid improves while in true ptosis it does not. Monocular elevation deficiency, heavy eye syndrome in high myopia and restrictive causes involving the IR like endocrine orbitopathy, orbital floor blow out fracture, myositis, etc., are some important differentials. These restrictive causes can be differentiated from SR palsy using FDT. FDT is positive in restrictive squint while it is negative in palsy. But sometimes, long-standing SR palsy may develop secondary ipsilateral IR fibrosis leading to positive FDT.

Medial Rectus Muscle Paralysis

Isolated MR paralysis without the involvement of other muscles supplied by the inferior division of 3rd nerve is very rare. There is exotropia with an adduction deficit. A face turn is noted toward the healthy eye. Differential diagnoses include internuclear ophthalmoplegia (INO) (deficient adduction of the ipsilateral eye and nystagmus of the contralateral abducting eye caused by lesion of MLF), synergistic divergence (simultaneous paradoxical abduction in both eyes on attempted abduction in one eye), Duane's retraction syndrome type 2, and supranuclear disorders.

Inferior Rectus Muscle Paralysis

There is a downgaze limitation in IR palsy, especially in abduction, with incyclotorsion and hypertropia. Isolated IR palsy is rare and is mostly congenital but may also be seen following orbital floor fracture or inferior peribulbar injections.

Inferior Oblique Muscle Paralysis

Inferior oblique muscle paralysis is also very rare and needs to be differentiated from Brown syndrome. There is elevation deficit in adduction with ipsilateral SO overaction. In IO palsy, FDT is negative with A-pattern strabismus.

Complete Oculomotor Nerve Palsy

In complete cranial third nerve or oculomotor nerve palsy, all extraocular muscles except the LR and SO are affected. In addition, sphincter pupillae, ciliary muscle, and levator palpebrae superior are also paralyzed. There is exotropia, incyclotorsion, mild hypotropia, ptosis, and accommodation loss in the paralyzed eye **(Figs. 8A to E)**. Pupil is dilated and there is absence of light reflex. General relaxation of the tonus of four out of six extraocular muscles may produce a small degree of proptosis. Abnormal head posture (AHP) may not develop in complete palsy due to ptosis. This also increases the risk of amblyopia in congenital or young-onset cases. Due to extensive limitation of extraocular movements, generally patients have no binocular visual field. In long-standing cases, LR and SO muscles may go in contracture. Aberrant regeneration may occur during the recovery of acquired third nerve palsy (discussed below). In complete third nerve palsy, it is difficult to determine the involvement of the trochlear nerve. One must note the incyclotorsion by observing the movement of a prominent nasal limbal vessel or specific point in nasal iris on biomicroscopic examination while the patient attempts to adduct or look down in abduction. The presence of incyclotorsion confirms the intactness of SO action.

Aberrant Regeneration

Aberrant regeneration or oculomotor synkinesis is characterized by misdirection of the regenerating axons that leads to paradoxical co-contraction of muscles. This happens following the breach of the endoneural sheath as may occur in trauma and slowly growing tumors or aneurysms. Rarely, it may be seen in congenital cases of third nerve palsy. Various types of aberrant regenerations have been described.

- Inverse Duane's retraction sign is the elevation of the eyelids during attempted adduction.
- Pseudo-Von Graefe's sign is the elevation/retraction of the upper eyelid on downward gaze or adduction **(Figs. 9A to C)**.
- Pseudo-Argyll Robertson pupil is characterized by greater response to accommodation reflex than light reflex.
- Czarnecki's sign is the segmental contraction of the sphincter on eye movements.
- Adduction of the eye on attempted upward or downward gaze.
- Limitation of elevation and depression of the eye with globe retraction on attempted vertical movement.

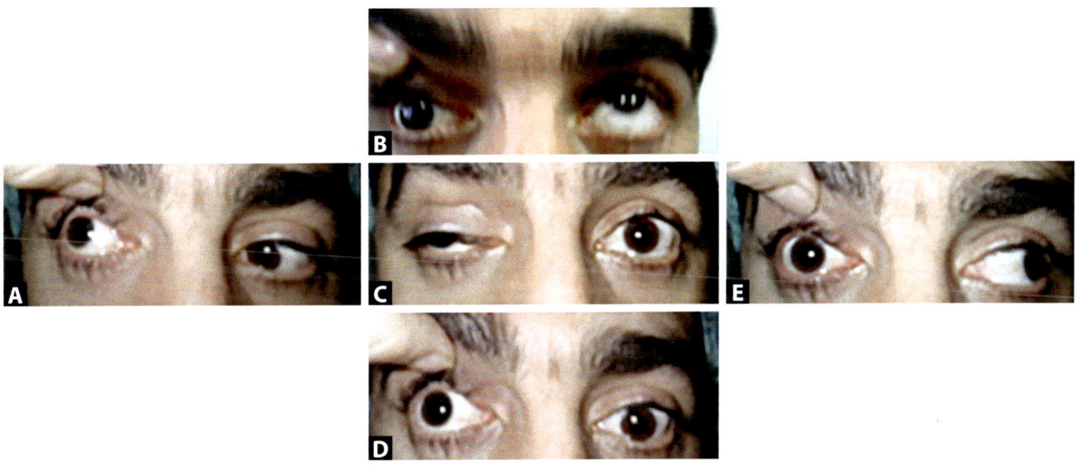

Figs. 8A to E: Right complete 3rd cranial nerve paralysis.

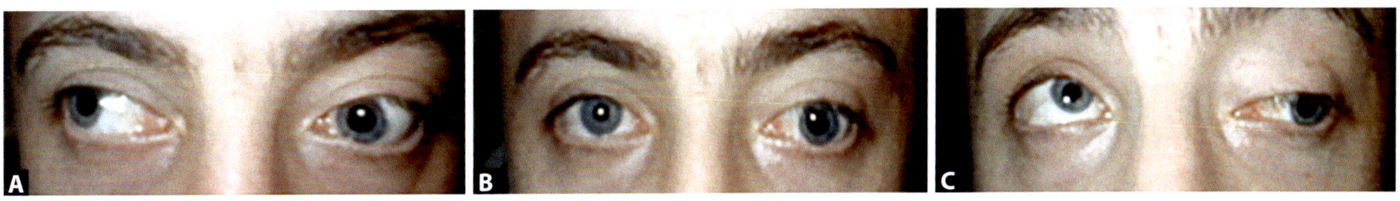

Figs. 9A to C: Aberrant medial rectus to LPS innervation following left 3rd cranial nerve palsy showing correction of ptosis on adduction (pseudo-Von Graefe's sign).

Management

Nonsurgical

Management of any ocular motor nerve palsy requires thorough evaluation to identify the underlying cause followed by the treatment or appropriate referral for the treatment of the same. Prompt neuroimaging is indicated in third nerve palsy with acute onset, young onset (<40 years) cases, cases with minor trauma (may be seen in aneurysms), pupillary-involvement, aberrant regeneration, multiple cranial nerve involvement, in the presence of other neurological features, and nonresolution of symptoms within 6–8 weeks of onset. In suspected cases of aneurysms, MR angiography and CT angiography becomes necessary. Rarely, catheter angiogram may be needed to look for small aneurysms that may be missed on noninvasive imaging studies. Congenital and presumed ischemic cases (pupil-sparing complete third nerve palsy) with underlying risk factors showing resolution on follow-up may not necessarily need neuroimaging.

As many cases may recover spontaneously or with treatment of the underlying cause, especially ischemic and traumatic cases, observation with regular follow-up should be done in the first 6 months of acute palsy. In ischemic neuropathies, the underlying risk factors such as diabetes and hypertension should be adequately controlled and managed. If some recovery is noted, then the observation period can be extended to 1 year. But waiting longer in patients with no positive course in the initial 6 months may negatively impact the treatment outcome. During this period, occlusion, prismatic glasses, and Fresnel prisms can be used in one eye to eliminate diplopia. In cases with complete third nerve palsy, ptosis acts as a natural patch for relieving diplopia. Precautions should be taken to avoid amblyopia in children by giving refractive correction and occlusion therapy. Botulinum toxin A (BTX-A) injection is a temporary measure that can be used in complete or partial acute third nerve palsies. The injection is given in the antagonist muscle like the LR. This helps in maintaining the ocular alignment during the acute phase and prevents the LR from going into contracture from secondary fibrosis. In older cases, BTX injection in the antagonist may help enlarge the binocular visual field.

Surgical

Surgery is considered when no further improvement is noted and the ocular misalignment remains stable for 6–12 months after onset. Surgical management of a third nerve palsy is often challenging due to involvement of most of the extraocular muscles resulting in simultaneous horizontal, vertical, and torsional misalignment. The ultimate goal of surgery is to align the eyes in primary position. This would expand the binocular diplopia-free field and establish binocular single vision in the primary position. However, limitation of movement may still persist in other gazes. Multiple surgeries might be needed in a staged manner. Therefore, appropriate patient counseling should be done regarding the surgical outcome setting realistic expectations for the same.

The choice of surgery is governed by several factors such as the type of involvement (partial or complete), number of extraocular muscles affected, and the presence or absence of aberrant regeneration **(Flowchart 1)**. Differentiation between paresis and complete palsy can be done using the parameters given in **Table 5**.

Planning the surgery for partial third cranial nerve palsy involves the basic rules of weakening the strong muscle, strengthening the weak muscle, and using transposition procedures if there are ineffective muscles. And if there is ptosis, ptosis surgery should be planned after the strabismus surgery. However, it is best to avoid ptosis surgery in patients with poor Bell's phenomenon.

In SR palsy, various choices available for treatment include IR recession, SR resection, IR Faden, Knapp's procedure involving the transposition of medial and LR adjacent to the insertion of SR muscle, and rarely nasal transposition of SO. IR recession may be associated with undesirable effect of lower lid retraction, especially where >4 mm recession is indicated. Therefore, it has been suggested to combine additional procedures on other vertical muscles when it is necessary to exceed this amount. Or, a modified technique of IR recession that involves recessing the 90% deeper fibers of the IR muscle while keeping the approximate 10% surface fibers attached can be done.

In isolated MR paralysis, LR recession and/or MR resection is the preferred treatment option in cases with some residual MR function. Vertical recti transposition (to MR insertion) and LR disinsertion with periosteal anchoring can be done in complete involvement of MR. If there is associated aberrant regeneration, then other procedures like tenotomy of the SO, myectomy of the IO muscle, or medial transposition of split LR can also be attempted.

In isolated IR palsy, procedures such as SR recession, inferior muscle resection/plication, reverse Knapp's procedure, and anterior transposition of IO muscle can be done.

In isolated IO muscle paralysis, the surgical plan is decided according to the amount of hypertropia. If hypertropia is <10 prism diopter (PD) in primary position, ipsilateral SO tendon expander or SO split tendon elongation is performed. If hypertropia is >10 PD in the primary position, contralateral SR recession might be added to the previous operation choice.

Management of complete oculomotor palsy remains a formidable challenge as all the extraocular muscles except the LR and SO are affected. If FDT is tight on adduction suggesting restriction in the LR muscle, then maximal or supramaximal LR recession is planned. This can be combined with MR resection, if MR has some residual action as noted by the duction past the midline or a tug felt on AFGT. In cases where the SO muscle is intact, the transposition of this muscle to the superior border of MR insertion provides

Flowchart 1: Algorithm for surgery in oculomotor nerve palsy.

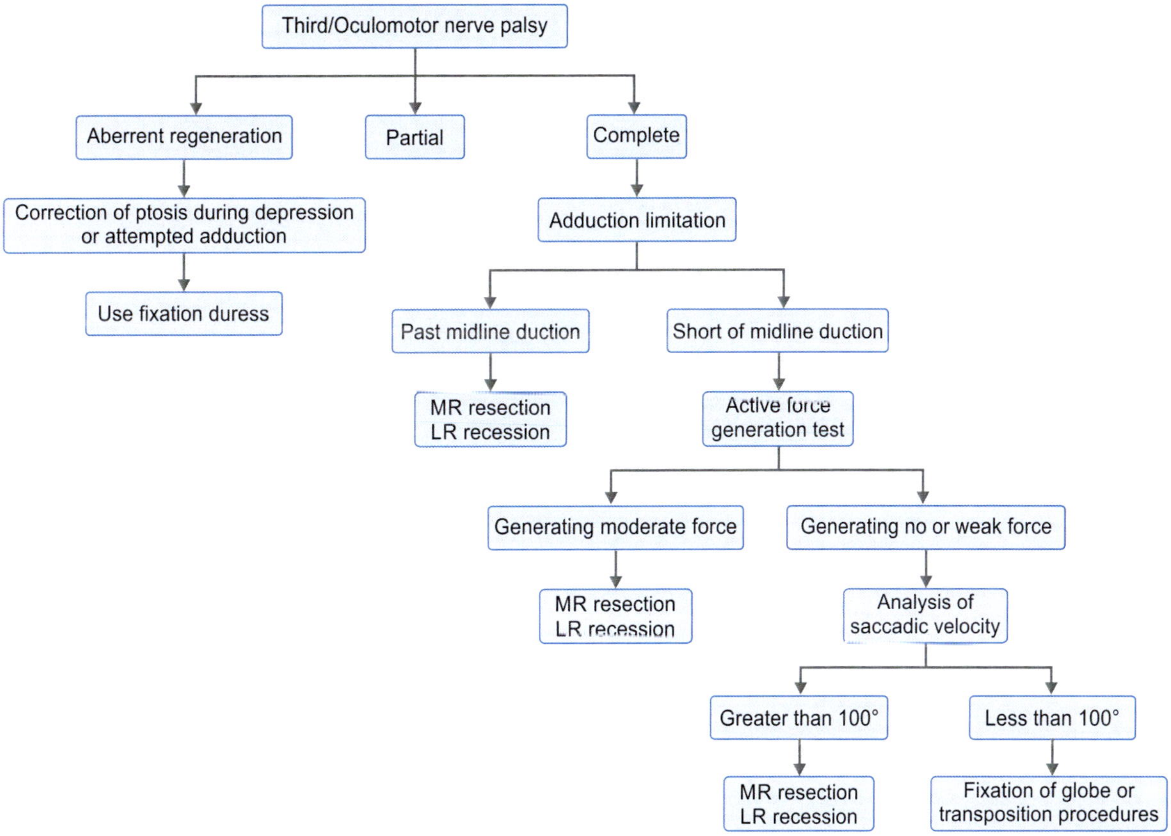

(LR: lateral rectus; MR: magnetic resonance)

TABLE 5: Differentiation between complete and partial ocular motor palsy.

Parameters	*Complete oculomotor (3rd nerve) palsy*	*Partial oculomotor (3rd nerve) palsy*
Ductions	Does not cross midline	Crosses midline (usually); ductions may be reduced if antagonist muscle contracts
Saccadic velocity (agonist)	Reduced to <100° per second	Greater than 175° per second
Difference of saccadic velocity of agonist-antagonist	Less than 40%	40%
Force generation	Not present	Decreases
Forced duction	Contraction of only antagonist muscle causes restriction	Contraction of only antagonist muscle causes restriction

a slight reduction in the deviation. This may or may not be combined with trochleotomy. However, the procedure is not very effective and may be associated with paradoxical movements of the globe and induced hypertropia.

Nasal transposition of the LR either the whole muscle or by splitting and reattaching the arms superior and inferior to the insertion of the MR is one of the most effective management described for complete third nerve palsy. Gokyigit's method and its modifications published with very successful results and with nonserious mild and transient complications.

This procedure can be augmented by the application of posterior fixation sutures to the transposed ends as described by Saxena et al., using nonabsorbable sutures (e.g., Ethibond).

Further refinement of postoperative outcomes can be done using adjustable technique of split nasal LR transposition with crossed action insertion.

Medial globe anchor is the last resort technique where the eyeball is fixated to the medial orbital wall at the anterior lacrimal crest. This can be achieved by using 5-0 nonabsorbable polyester suture, fascia lata, orbital periosteal flap, SO tendon or silicon bands through a skin incision or through a precaruncular approach.

Therefore, in complete third nerve palsies, we either completely eliminate the effect of the LR and mechanically pull the globe medially, or transpose the strength of the lateral muscle, the only muscle remaining intact into MR area.

TROCHLEAR OR 4TH CRANIAL NERVE PALSY

Nerve Anatomy

The fourth nerve nucleus is located in the anterior mesencephalon under the inferior colliculus (ventral to Sylvian aqueduct), at the lower end of the third nerve nucleus. The fascicular part of the nerve passes posteriorly around the aqueduct and completely decussates to the contralateral side in the anterior medullary velum. It emerges from the dorsal aspect of the midbrain, turns around the superior cerebellar peduncle and the cerebral peduncle, passes in between the posterior cerebral artery and the superior cerebellar arteries, and emerges ventrally to enter the cavernous sinus **(Fig. 10)**. The cavernous part of the nerve passes along the lateral wall between the oculomotor nerve above and the first division of the trigeminal nerve below. It enters the orbital cavity through the superior orbital fissure to supply the contralateral SO muscle.

The trochlear nerve is the thinnest and longest among the cranial nerves and therefore most easily affected by trauma. For this reason, SO muscle paralysis is the most common isolated extraocular muscle paralysis seen in clinical practice that typically presents with hypertropia in the affected eye. In fact, SO palsy should be the first diagnosis to consider in cyclovertical deviations.

Etiology

Superior oblique palsy can be congenital or acquired. Helveston et al. observed that almost 75% cases of all 4th nerve palsies were congenital. Congenital palsy could be due to tendon anomalies such as redundant, misdirected or absent tendon, abnormality in muscle structure or insertion, or due to trochlear nerve palsy caused by nucleus hypoplasia, and birth trauma. However, the exact cause is still debatable. It can also be seen in association with other congenital anomalies like craniosynostosis or plagiocephaly. In plagiocephaly, retrograde placement of trochlea leads to desagitallization of SO and hence its underaction. A common cause of acquired SO palsy is head trauma, including relatively minor trauma. The involvement can be bilateral and asymmetric in traumatic cases and therefore mandates careful evaluation of both eyes. Other causes can be microvascular (hypertension, diabetes, and atherosclerosis), aneurysms, tumor, hydrocephalus, orbital or intracranial infection, inflammation and following intracranial or sinus surgery. Despite advanced imaging and diagnostic methods, etiology may not be detected in about a third of the cases.

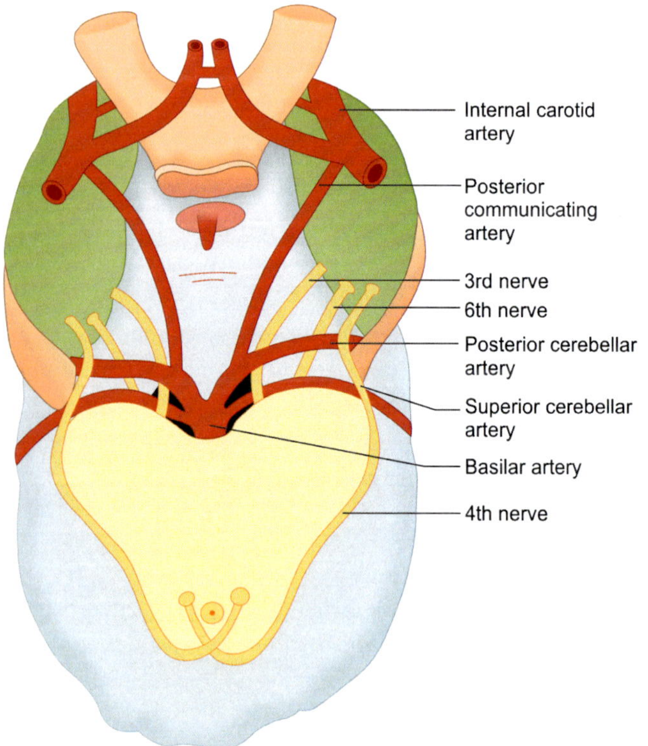

Fig. 10: 4th cranial nerve (dorsal view).

Clinical Features

In children, the cause is mostly congenital. Usually, the palsy remains well compensated and unrecognized in childhood. They may suddenly manifest in adulthood or in advanced age due to decompensation. In these patients, diplopia is subtle (than acquired cases) and the predominant complaint is asthenopia. It can be inferred that the etiology is congenital based on the facial asymmetry or the detection of the characteristic AHP from old photographs. Facial asymmetry in congenital SO palsy is characterized by midfacial hypoplasia between the lateral canthus and the edge of the mouth on the side of the head tilt **(Figs. 11A and B)**.

In acquired cases, vertical or torsional diplopia is the chief complaint, especially when reading books and descending stairs. To avoid diplopia, the patient takes the abnormal head posture towards the action of the affected SO, i.e., face slightly turned towards the opposite side, chin is depressed, and the head is tilted towards the opposite side. In bilateral cases, there may not be any deviation in primary position but there is a distinct V-pattern and chin-down head position.

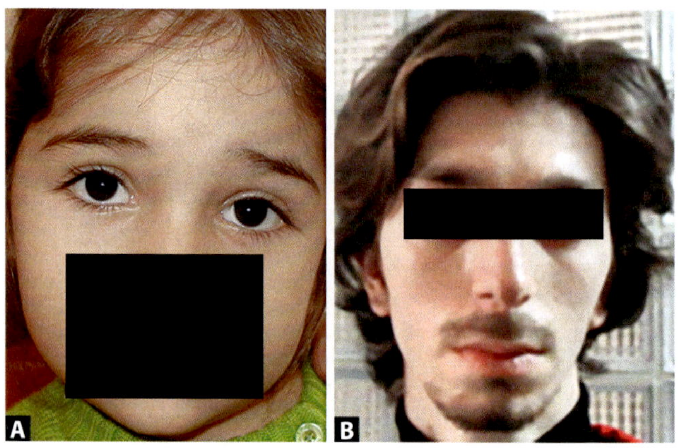

Figs. 11A and B: Marked facial asymmetry and head tilt in the right congenital trochlear nerve palsy.

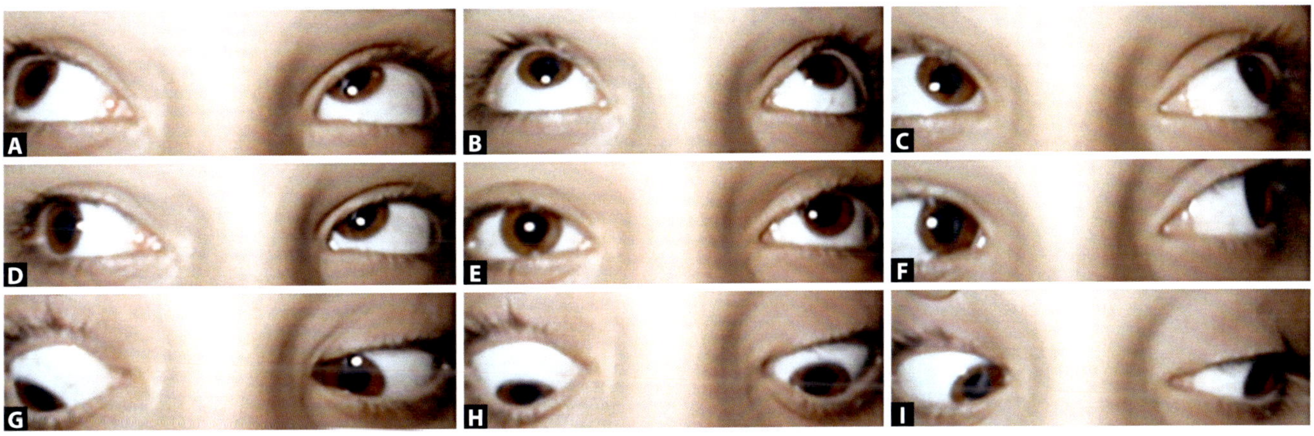

Figs. 12A to I: Nine gaze clinical photograph with noticeable hypotropia in left eye in primary position with inferior oblique overaction and superior oblique underaction suggestive of left cranial nerve fourth palsy.

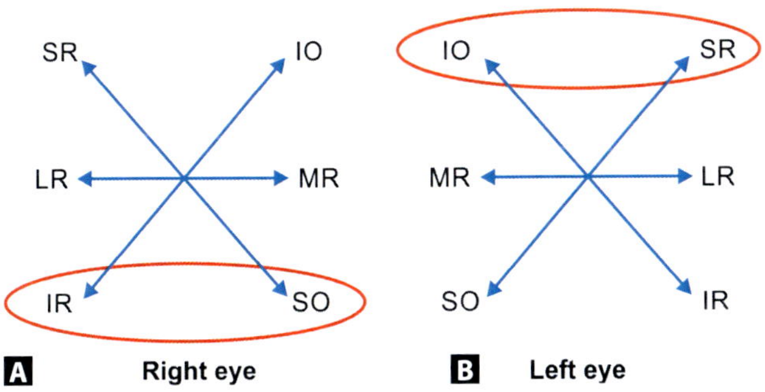

Figs. 13A and B: Evaluation of first question "which eye has hypertropia in primary position" of Parks', for diagnosis of the paretic muscle in the patient with right hypertropia. It may be caused by paresis of right superior oblique, right inferior rectus, left superior rectus, or left inferior oblique.

(IO: inferior oblique; IR: inferior rectus; LR: lateral rectus; MR: magnetic resonance; SO: superior oblique; SR: superior rectus)

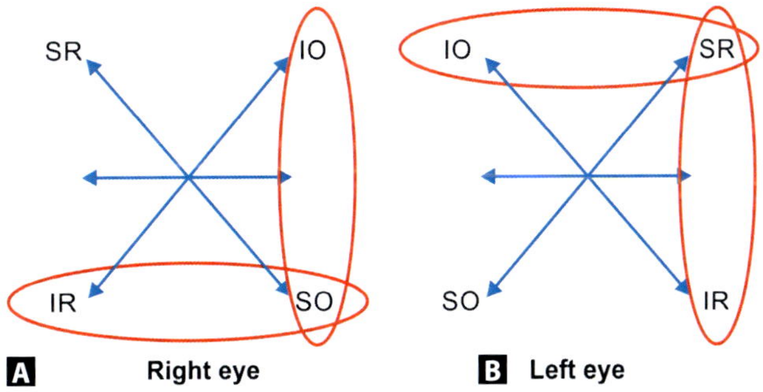

Figs. 14A and B: Inference of step 2 of Park test. If right hypertropia increases inleft gaze (levoversion) , it may be due to paresis of right SO or left SR. It may be caused by paresis of right superior oblique or left superior rectus.

(IO: inferior oblique; IR: inferior rectus; SO: superior oblique; SR: superior rectus)

On examination, hypertropia and excyclotorsion are evident. Maximum limitation is noted in the direction of action of the affected SO muscle (down and in) with overaction of the ipsilateral IO **(Figs. 12A to I)**. On Parks' three-step test and Bielschowsky head tilt test following findings would be noted:

- *Step 1*: Ipsilateral hypertropia in primary gaze can be due to weak depressors in the same eye (IR and SO) or weak elevators in the contralateral eye (SR and IO) **(Figs. 13A and B)**.
- *Step 2*: Increased magnitude of hypertropia in contralateral than ipsilateral gaze can be due to underacting SO in the same eye or underacting SR in the contralateral eye (of the four muscles identified in the first step) **(Figs. 14A and B)**.
- *Step 3*: Greater hypertropia on tilting the head towards the affected side than the contralateral side can be due to underacting SO in the same eye or underacting IO in the contralateral eye (of the four muscles identified in the first step) **(Figs. 15A and B)**.

As SO is the only muscle that fulfills all three steps in this case scenario, therefore this is a case of SO palsy. Hypertropia

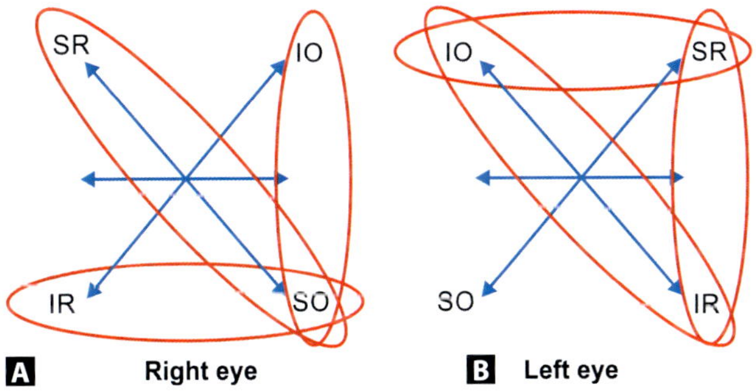

Figs. 15A and B: Inference of 3rd step of Park test. If right hypertropia increases during head tilt to right shoulder , then right SO paresis should be suspected. It may be caused by paresis of the right superior oblique.

(IO: inferior oblique; IR: inferior rectus; SO: superior oblique; SR: superior rectus)

is worse on opposite gaze due to unopposed activity of the palsied SO muscle's antagonist, the IO that increases hypertropia in adduction. Hypertropia is worse on head tilt towards the affected side as the defective incyclotorsion from the palsied SO is compensated by the hyperactivity of the other incyclotorter, i.e., the ipsilateral SR. The hyperactivity

TABLE 6: Differentiation between congenital and acquired superior oblique palsy.

Parameters	*Acquired SO palsy*	*Congenital SO palsy*
Etiology	Can acquire at any age	Present since birth
Fusional amplitude	Within normal limits (2–3 diopters)	Increased by 16–30 diopters
Diplopia	Present (usually)	Absent
Facial symmetry	Absent	
Head tilt	Any time after onset	Since infancy (can be seen in old photographs)
Subjective torsion	Present (usually)	Absent
Amblyopia in affected eye	Absent (usually)	May or may not be present
Therapeutic effect of occlusion	Occlusion of paretic eye straightens the head	No effect on either eye
Neuroimaging	Volume of respective muscle (SO) may be decreased	Normal/mildly decreased muscle volume

(SO: superior oblique)

of the ipsilateral SR causes not only increased incyclotorsion but also increased magnitude of hypertropia.

In long-standing cases, the hypertropia may be similar in all gazes due to "spread of comitance". The spread of comitance is characterized by contracture of the ipsilateral antagonist (ipsilateral IO), overaction of the contralateral yoke muscle (contralateral IR), and secondary inhibitional palsy of the contralateral antagonist (contralateral SR).

Bilateral SO palsy will have alternating hypertropia, i.e., left hypertropia in right gaze and right hypertropia in left gaze and larger degree of excyclotorsion than in unilateral cases (>10°). Excyclotorsion can be documented using double Maddox rod test or synoptophore. When the Maddox rods are placed in front of the eyes with the lines oriented vertically, the patient with trochlear nerve palsy will perceive the horizontal line seen through the hypertropic or the affected eye as tilted downwards nasally due to excyclotorsion of the affected eye.

Vertical fusional range is higher than normal in congenital SO palsy (>10 PD; normal values—2-3 PD) to compensate for the vertical ocular misalignment. If this is documented, then no further investigation is needed, as this is suggestive of benign congenital paralysis. Exaggerated FDT (FDT for SO) may reveal tendon laxity in congenital SO palsy associated with tendon anomalies. **Table 6** enumerates the differentiating points between the congenital and acquired cases of SO palsy.

Orbital or neuroimaging may be required in acquired cases for evaluation of the underlying cause.

Differential Diagnosis

The common differentials for SO palsy include skew deviation, myasthenia gravis, thyroid eye disease, Brown syndrome, and orbital blow out fractures.

Management

Nonsurgical

Acquired 4th cranial nerve palsy may improve spontaneously over time. Spontaneous recovery may be noted in as high as 82% cases with 50% cases showing nearly complete recovery. Patients with trauma or microvascular etiology are more likely to recover. For this reason, a 6-12 month waiting period with close follow-up of patients is advised. If this group of patients does not recover spontaneously, neurological imaging becomes mandatory to investigate an alternative etiology. Nonsurgical measures can be used meanwhile to obviate the symptoms of diplopia and deviation. Occlusion of one eye alleviates the diplopia. Prisms may be used in small and comitant deviations for compensating for diplopia in the primary position. However, management with prisms may not be very effective, because the deviation is mostly incomitant accompanied by a torsional component. Injection of BTX into the IO muscle has been attempted with variable success rates to reduce hypertropia and may help alleviate diplopia during recovery.

Surgical

The primary indications for strabismus surgery in trochlear nerve palsy are removing the troublesome diplopia and torsion, reducing AHP, and expanding the diplopia free binocular visual fields in primary position. In congenital cases, timely correction of head posture may also correct the facial asymmetry that has just begun.

The choice of surgery is governed by factors such as the gaze of the highest deviation, amount of hypertropia in primary position, associated IO overaction or SR contracture, result of the traction test, and whether the involvement is unilateral or bilateral. Knapp's has given the classification based on the gaze of maximum hyperdeviation and the preferred surgical treatment for the same **(Table 7)**.

Surgical procedures applied can be summarized as strengthening of the hypofunction muscle (SO tuck, folding, and advancement), weakening of the ipsilateral antagonist muscle with overaction (IO weakening procedures), the recession of the ipsilateral SR muscle (in long-standing cases with SR contracture), or weakening of the contralateral synergist (IR weakening in the contralateral eye).

TABLE 7: Knapp's classification for superior oblique palsy based on the gaze of maximum hyperdeviation and the preferred surgical treatment.

Class	Measurements obtained as shown above	Diagnosis	Surgery
I	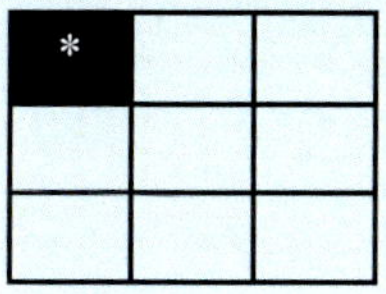	Class I Paresis of LSO	Weakening of LIO
II	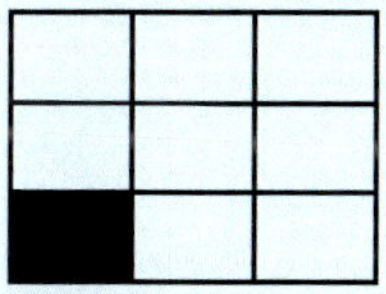	Class II Paresis of LSO	Tucking/strengthening of LSO
III	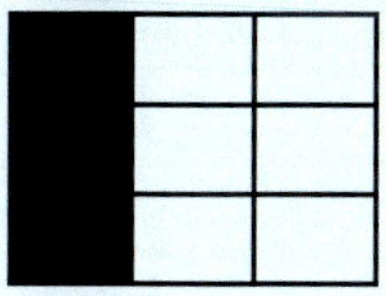	Class III Paresis of LSO	If LH is <25 prism diopters then tuck LSO, if >25 prism diopters then tuck LSO and weaken LIO
IV	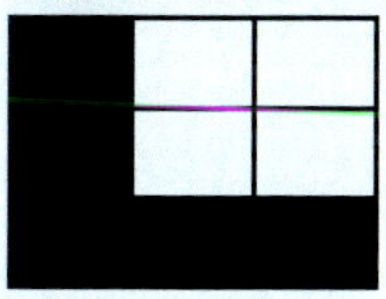	Class IV Paresis of LSO	• First surgery • Tuck LSO • Weaken LIO <25 prism diopters • Second surgery • Strengthening of LIR
V	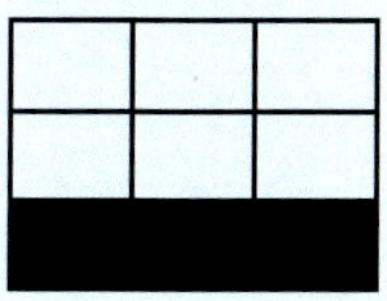	Class V Paresis of LSO	Recess RIR or tuck LSO
VI	1. Underaction SO and OU 2. Overaction IO and OU 3. V pattern 4. Bilaterally positive Bielschowsky test	Bilateral SO SO paresis	Tuck SO bilaterally
VII	"Canine tooth syndrome". Underaction inferior oblique (acquired Brown syndrome), underaction superior oblique. Usually due to trauma in the area of trochlea		

* Shaded area represents field of greatest vertical deviation.

(IO: inferior oblique; LIO: left inferior oblique; LIR: left inferior rectus; LSO: left superior oblique; OU: oculus uterque; RIR: right inferior rectus; SO: superior oblique)

- *Inferior oblique weakening procedures*:
  - Elliot and Nankin's recession with anteropositioning where both the ends of the muscle are inserted adjacent to the lateral border of IR. In contrast to true recessions, anteropositioning alters the path of the muscle by anteriorizing it. Therefore, it is a stronger weakening procedure. But it may be associated with the postoperative limitation of elevation during abduction resulting in an apparent IO overaction in the contralateral eye accompanied with a Y-pattern exodeviation. This has been described as antielevation syndrome (AES) by Kushner.
  - Modified Elliot and Nankin's recession with anteropositioning where the anterior end of IO is placed adjacent to lateral border of IR (like in Elliot and Nankin's technique), but the posterior end is inserted 5 mm posterior along the lateral border of the IR muscle. This technique is weaker than the Elliot and Nankin's recession.
  - IO recession with 1+ and 2+ (clarify station) (total anteropositioning) where the muscle is inserted 1 mm and 2 mm anterior to the lateral border of IR, respectively. This provides a greater weakning effect.
  - Anteronasal transposition (ANT) of IO where the muscle is brought nasal to IR and inserted 2 mm nasal and posterior to the nasal border of IR. This is an effective technique for torsional diplopia in the absence of significant vertical deviation in primary position. This procedure converts the IO muscle from an extorter and elevator to an intorter and tonic depressor in adduction. It is recommended in severe and recurrent SO palsies. Extreme ANT may induce

exotropia in the primary position. Adjustable ANT has also been described.
- *Myectomy*: It involves the surgical removal of a segment of IO muscle. It cannot be graded and not a preferred surgery for IO.

- *Superior oblique strengthening procedures*:
    - Superior oblique tuck or tenoplication is performed in congenital SO palsy with tendon laxity on traction testing. The amount of tuck is titrated based on intraoperative tension of the SO muscle with an end point of inducing mild postoperative Brown syndrome, which is expected to become better over time. Yet, many surgeons have reported iatrogenic Brown syndrome postoperatively. The tenoplication is preferably done through a transconjunctival route in the upper temporal quadrant to avoid the risk of trochlear damage. Selective strengthening of the intorsion action can be achieved by the selective plication of only the anterior fibers of the SO tendon.
    - Harada-Ito procedure is employed for the correction of excyclotorsion, especially in bilateral SO palsy. The original method was to anteriorize the anterior half of the SO tendon (responsible for intorsion) without disinsertion. This technique has been modified whereby the anterior half of the tendon is disinserted and moved forward and laterally. Adjustable sutures can also be used with this procedure. It corrects around 10° of excyclotorsion in primary gaze and 15–20° in downgaze.

ABDUCENT NERVE OR CRANIAL 6TH PALSY

Nerve Anatomy

The nucleus of the abducent (also called abducens) lies in the lower pons, at the base of the fourth ventricle, in close association with the facial nerve nuclei. The fascicle of the facial nerve loops around the abducent nuclei to create facial colliculus. Horizontal gaze center, i.e., paramedian pontine reticular formation (PPRF) also lies in close proximity with the abducent nucleus. Each abducent nucleus consists of large motor cells that stimulate the ipsilateral LR muscle, and smaller groups of cells that relay in the oculomotor nucleus via the MLF and supply the contralateral MR muscle. The fascicular part traverses the medial lemniscus and the pyramidal tract to emerge at the pontomedullary junction ventrally **(Fig. 16)**. The basilar part of the nerve travels in the subarachnoid space from posterior cranial fossa to the middle cranial fossa where it takes two bends. First bend occurs as it exits the pons. Then the nerve courses vertically along the clivus, pierces the dura, and then takes the second bend where it turns anteriorly and enters the Dorello's canal under the petroclinoid (Gruber's) ligament. Of all cranial nerves, abducent nerve has the longest subarachnoid course. The cavernous part of the nerve travels horizontally lying lateral to the internal carotid artery and finally enters the orbit through the superior orbital fissure to supply the ipsilateral LR.

Etiology

Abducent nerve palsy is the most commonly affected ocular motor nerve and a common cause of acquired horizontal diplopia. Nuclear and fascicular involvement may occur due to infarction, infection, demyelination, tumor, or metabolic disease like Wernicke disease. In subarachnoid space, the causes include acoustic neuroma, nasopharyngeal tumor, and raised intracranial pressure. Raised intracranial pressure leads to downward displacement of the brainstem that causes traction on the abducent nerve at the point where it is tethered in the Dorello's canal. Otitis media, mastoiditis, and fracture of the base of the skull can involve the nerve as it courses over the petrous apex. Cavernous involvement can be due to cavernous sinus thrombosis, carotid-cavernous

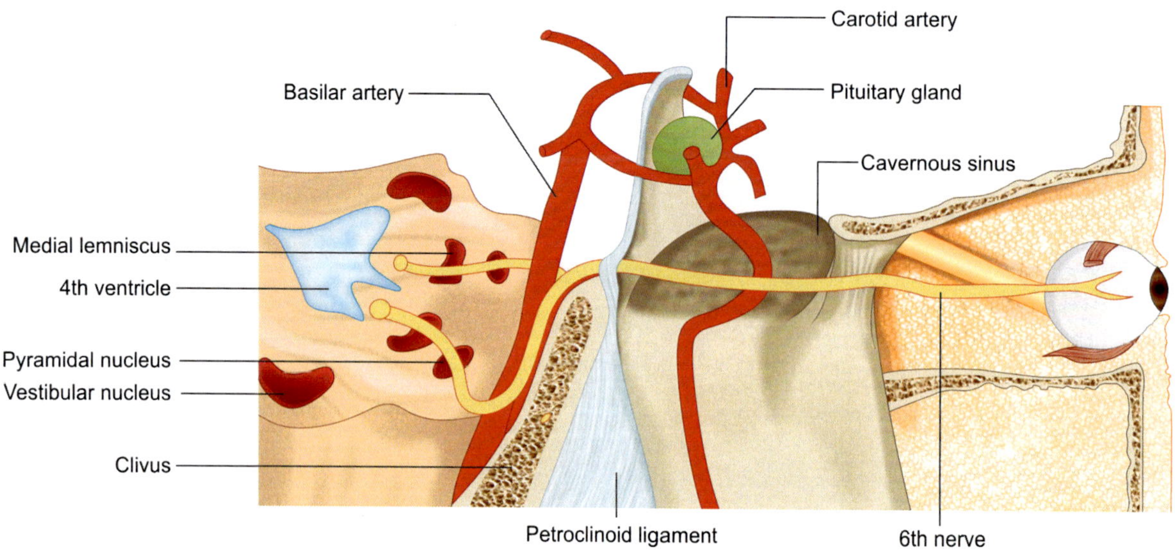

Fig. 16: Course of 6th crania nerve (lateral view).

fistulas, internal carotid artery aneurysm, inflammation like Tolosa-Hunt syndrome, etc. Orbital involvement can be inflammatory, infectious, traumatic, or neoplastic (myositis, orbital cellulitis, orbital pseudotumor etc.).

Isolated palsies over the age of 40 years are usually due to microvascular ischemia leading to infarction of the nerve fibers. In children, apart from congenital abducent nerve palsy, trauma, neoplasm, and raised intracranial pressure are important acquired causes. In trauma, the shearing forces damage the nerve as it passes over the petrous apex or Dorello's canal. Tumors are mostly posterior fossa tumors, such as brainstem glioma, medulloblastoma, ependymoma, and cystic cerebellar astrocytoma. Tumor removal surgeries can also attribute to 6th nerve palsy. Benign 6th nerve palsy usually develops following a viral infection or a vaccine. Bilateral involvement is mostly related to trauma, vascular lesions, or tumor.

Clinical Features

A case of abducent nerve palsy presents with a noticeable esodeviation **(Figs. 17A to C)**. In acute onset cases, patients complain of binocular horizontal diplopia and may adopt a compensatory face turn in the direction of the paralyzed muscle. The diplopia is typically worse at distance. The esodeviation and the limitation of movement are greatest on attempted abduction on the affected side **(Figs. 18A to C)**.

Nuclear and fascicular involvement of the nerve is never isolated due to close association with other cranial structures. Similarly, the basilar and the cavernous part of the nerve are in proximity with other cranial nerves such as facial nerve and trigeminal nerve. Several syndromes have been described in association with abducent nerve palsy due to involvement of these structures **(Table 8)**. Therefore, a complete neurological examination and assessment of various cranial nerves should be done in abducent nerve palsy.

If the involvement is due to raised intracranial pressure, others features such as headache, nausea, and vomiting will be present. This may or may not be accompanied with papilledema. Therefore, a fundus evaluation is mandatory in every case of abducent nerve palsy. Gradenigo's syndrome has classically been described with the infection of the petrous temporal bone (petrous apicitis) seen in otitis media. Sometimes, cerebellopontine angle tumors and nasopharyngeal carcinomas may present with similar picture referred to as pseudo-Gradenigo's syndrome. Nasopharyngeal carcinoma commonly present in fourth to seventh decade of life with other symptoms such as nasal obstruction, rhinorrhea, epistaxis, and serous otitis media secondary to obstruction of the Eustachian tube. A carotid-cavernous fistula is mostly seen following trauma (75%) or may occur spontaneously (25%). This causes the arterialization of the sinus and ocular/orbital veins and presents with features of pain, proptosis, chemosis, ocular congestion, bruit, ocular pulsation, or diminution of vision. Tolosa-Hunt syndrome is an idiopathic condition characterized by chronic granulomatous inflammation that affects the cavernous sinus and typically presents with "painful ophthalmoplegia". Orbital involvement may be associated with proptosis, decrease in vision, etc.

Differential Diagnosis

Duane retraction syndrome, essential infantile esotropia with crossed fixation, Möbius syndrome, myasthenia gravis, thyroid eye disease, ethmoidal blow out fracture (medial orbital wall trauma with MR entrapment), divergence insufficiency, and functional convergence spasm are some of the important differentials. Myasthenia gravis is a common mimicker of ocular motor palsy. Evaluation for diurnal variation, ice test, rest test, Tensilon test may help differentiate it from palsy.

Management

Nonsurgical

In acute palsy, the foremost goal is to identify the underlying cause through proper evaluation and manage the same.

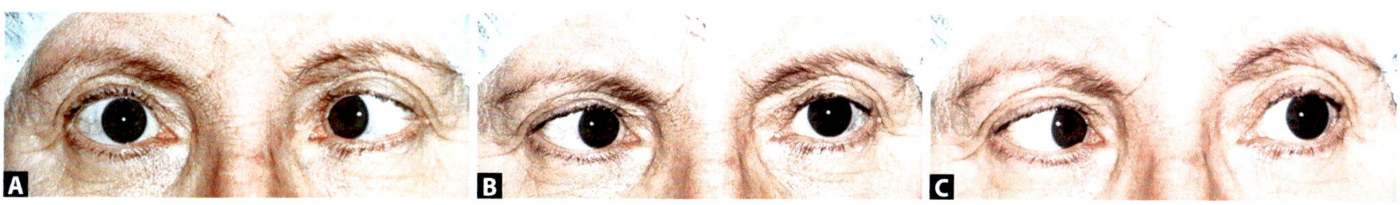

Figs. 17A to C: A case of right 6th cranial nerve palsy following brain surgery.

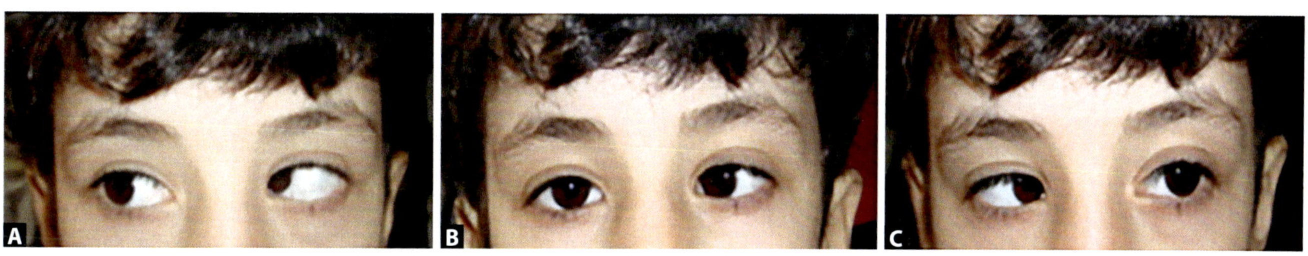

Figs. 18A to C: Left abducens palsy in a child after trauma.

TABLE 8: Various syndromes seen with abducent nerve palsy.

	Site of involvement	***Clinical features***
Nuclear involvement	Inferomedial pons (6th and 7th nerve nuclei + PPRF)	• Ipsilateral abducent nerve palsy (limitation of abduction) • Ipsilateral lower motor neuron facial palsy • Ipsilateral horizontal gaze palsy
Fascicular involvement		
Raymond's syndrome	Pyramidal tract	• Ipsilateral 6th nerve palsy • Contralateral hemiparesis
Millard–Gubler syndrome	Pyramidal tract	• Ipsilateral 6th nerve palsy • Ipsilateral 7th nerve palsy (lower motor neuron type) • Contralateral hemiparesis
Foville syndrome	Inferomedial pons + PPRF + long tract (corticospinal tract + medial lemniscus + descending sympathetic fibers)	• Ipsilateral 5th nerve palsy (loss of facial sensations) • Ipsilateral 6th nerve palsy (lateral rectus palsy) • Ipsilateral 7th nerve palsy (lower motor neuron type) • Ipsilateral 8th nerve palsy (sensorineural hearing loss) • Ipsilateral gaze palsy • Contralateral hemiparesis • Contralateral hemisensory loss • Ipsilateral Horner's syndrome
Basilar/subarachnoid part		
Petrous apex syndrome or Gradenigo's syndrome	In Dorello's canal under the petroclinoid ligament	• Ipsilateral 6th nerve palsy (lateral rectus palsy) • Ipsilateral 7th nerve palsy (lower motor neuron type) • Ipsilateral 8th nerve palsy (sensorineural hearing loss) • Ipsilateral 5th nerve palsy (facial pain)
Intracavernous part Cavernous sinus syndrome	Cavernous sinus	3rd + 4th + 6th + ophthalmic and maxillary division of 5th nerve + internal carotid artery + carotid sympathetic plexus (optic nerve, optic chiasma, and pituitary gland may or may not be affected)

(PPRF: paramedian pontine reticular formation)

Careful and close follow-up is necessary. Isolated acquired abducent palsy in adults presumably due to microvascular ischemia may resolve spontaneously. Meanwhile, patching and prisms can be advised along with the control of risk factors namely diabetes, hypertension, arteriosclerosis, hypercholesterolemia, etc. Some advocate the use of BTX in the ipsilateral MR in the acute phase to temporarily decrease the ocular misalignment and to prevent secondary MR contracture. But it carries the risk of ptosis, induced hypertropia, subconjunctival hemorrhage, and globe perforation. In pediatric 6th nerve palsy, the management is more aggressive. Precautions should be taken to prevent amblyopia in very young children. Neuroimaging is absolutely indicated in pediatric palsies. Other indications for imaging are acute onset cases, young-onset cases, associated neurological (nausea, vomiting, hemiparesis, etc.), or orbital signs and multiple cranial nerve involvement. Imaging should be specifically directed to the suspected area of involvement such as the brainstem, cavernous sinus, and nasopharynx. Lumbar puncture may be done in suspected cases of raised intracranial pressure. The workup can be supplemented by other laboratory studies to rule out vascular, infectious, or inflammatory pathology.

Surgical

In cases where no improvement is observed at 6 months, surgery should be performed to eliminate diplopia and to correct the esodeviation and abnormal head posture in the primary position. The type of surgery will be governed by the amount of esodeviation, residual LR function, and presence or absence of MR contracture. If the duction of the paretic eye on lateral gaze is beyond the midline or if the LR muscle shows some tug on AFGT, it suggests that the affected LR muscle has residual action. Maximum recession of the MR and resection of the LR can be planned in the same eye in such cases. If the palsy is complete with no duction beyond the midline or no tug felt on AFGT, then transposition procedure with or without MR recession is the procedure of choice **(Flowchart 2)**.

Vertical rectus transposition can be single tendon or double tendon transposition. Double tendon transposition can be partial or full tendon transposition. Transposition procedure can be augmented with additional procedures like MR recession or Foster sutures applied to the transposed muscles **(Flowchart 3)**. But it is safer to perform these surgeries stepwise. Combining too many procedures may result in overcorrection. Transposition procedures may provide some useful abduction as well. Some of the transposition procedures described are:

- Full tendon vertical recti transposition carries the "risk of anterior segment ischemia" ± Foster sutures (applied to the transposed tendon 8 mm posterior to the insertion)
- *Hummelsheim procedure*: This is the partial vertical rectus muscle transposition to LR. The effect can be increased by applying Foster augmentation sutures on the transposed part of the muscles.

Flowchart 2: Surgical management algorithm of 6th nerve palsy.

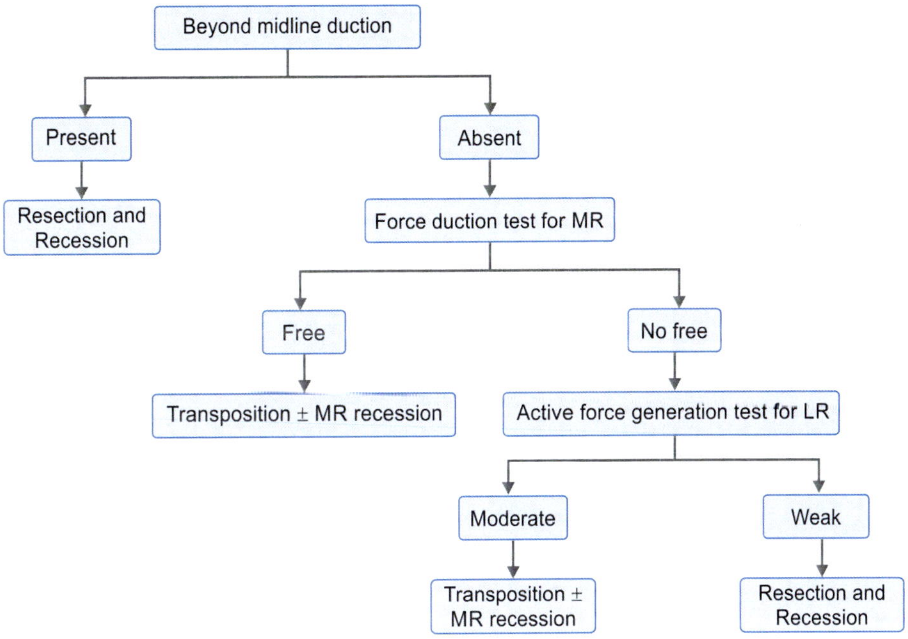

(LR: lateral rectus; MR: magnetic resonance)

Flowchart 3: Surgical options for 6th nerve palsy.

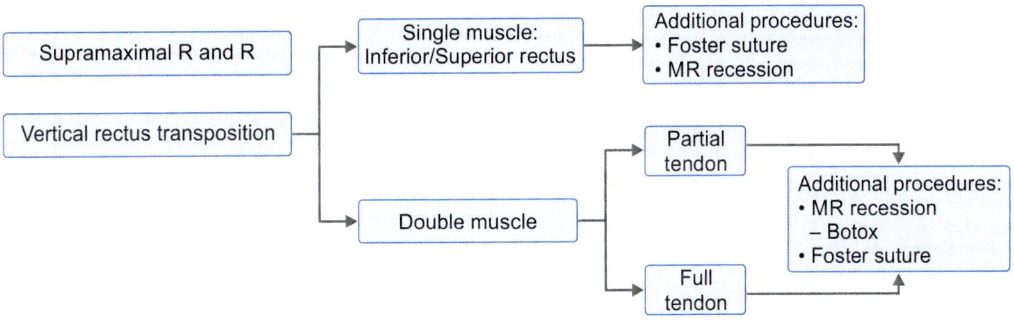

(MR: magnetic resonance; R and R: recession and resection)

- *Jensen's procedure*: This is the split-tendon transfer of superior and IR to LR without disinsertion. Superior, inferior recti, and the LR are split into half. The upper half of the LR and the lateral half of the SR are brought together with a nonabsorbable suture. Similarly, the lower half of the LR and the lateral half of the IR are brought together and secured with a nonabsorbable suture. This procedure has the advantage of preserving the anterior ciliary vessels and therefore reduced risk of anterior segment ischemia. But it can still occur due to strangulation of vessels by the sutures.
- *Nishida's procedure*: This is a popular technique and preformed where the two halves of vertical recti are sutured onto sclera near LR insertion without tenotomy.
- *SR transposition*: As this is a single tendon transposition, there is lesser risk of anterior segment ischemia and therefore can be safely supplemented with MR recession. Although there is risk of inducing vertical and torsional diplopia, but clinically this has not been commonly observed.
- IR transposition is rarely advocated.

As per a systematic review, partial tendon vertical rectus transposition or SR transposition augmented with Foster sutures or MR recession has shown better results than augmented full tendon vertical recti transpositions achieving a correction of around 40–50 PD.

MÖBIUS SYNDROME

This syndrome was first described by Paul J Möbius in 1888. This is a rare neurological disorder characterized by multiple cranial nerve involvement with orofacial and limb deformities such as cleft palate, micrognathia, microphthalmia, syndactyly, absent phalanges, digital hypoplasia, scoliosis, and pectoral hypoplasia. Although any cranial nerve from 5th to 12th can be affected, abducens and facial nerve paralysis involvement is the most common **(Fig. 19)**. It is mostly congenital and bilateral. Various degree of esotropia may be present in the primary position according to the severity of abducens paralysis. In some cases, paralysis may be incomplete or asymmetric.

A multidisciplinary approach involving the pediatrician, ophthalmologist, otolaryngologist, neurologist, dental specialists, etc., is needed in the management of Möbius syndrome. Corrective surgery for large esotropia in the primary position requires bilateral large MR recession. A combined recession-resection procedure for incomplete cases and vertical recti transposition for complete palsies are also very useful for treatment.

DOUBLE ELEVATOR PALSY

Double elevator palsy is characterized by upgaze limitation in all gazes and hypotropia with pseudo or true ptosis. It has been named as double elevator palsy by Dunlop because the clinical appearance is compatible with the palsy of the two elevators of the eye, SR, and IO. However, both muscles are affected in only 30% of the cases. For this reason, the term "monocular elevation deficit" is more appropriately used.

Its etiology is usually congenital. Rarely, lesions affecting the third nerve nucleus may be acquired. SR palsy, IR restriction, and supranuclear lesions are the causes for the upgaze limitation. Neuroimaging is useful determining the etiology.

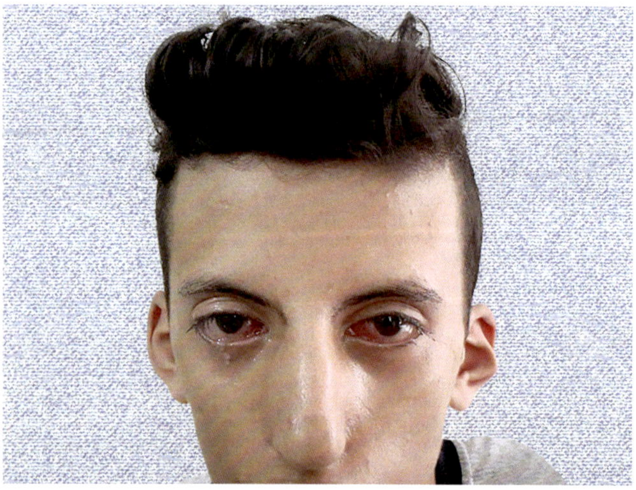

Fig. 19: A 13-year-old boy with Möbius syndrome.

Clinical Diagnosis

When fixing with the unaffected eye, the affected eye will have hypotropia with upgaze limitation in adduction, primary position and abduction upgaze restriction and pseudoptosis or ptosis. In case of pseudoptosis, it disappears on switching fixation to the affected eye. In unilateral disease, eye movements are normal in the horizontal and the downward gazes in general **(Figs. 20A to I)**.

Differential diagnosis includes congenital IR fibrosis, orbital floor blowout fracture, thyroid eye disease, Brown syndrome, agenesis of SR, and old acquired SR palsy.

Treatment

If there is no abnormal head posture or hypotropia in primary position, treatment is not necessary. Primary indications for surgery are significant head posture and hypotropia in the primary position. Treatment aims to correct the above and gain binocularity and enlarge the binocular visual field in primary position. In surgical planning, strabismus surgery should be performed before ptosis surgery.

As IR fibrosis may be present in 70% of cases, thus, a FDT at the beginning of the procedure is a guide for the selection of proper procedure. In cooperative cases, forced generation test also beneficial to discriminate IR fibrosis from SR palsy. If IR contracture is present, then the first step is to perform IR recession. If IR recession is not adequate, then transposition surgery may be done as a second stage surgery.

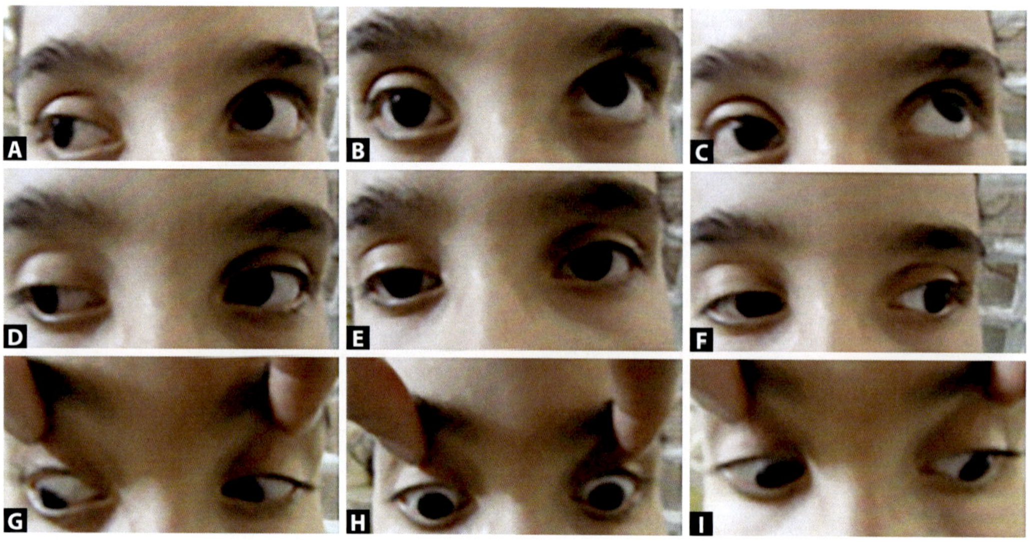

Figs. 20A to I: Nine gaze clinical photograph of a case of right monocular elevation deficiency (double elevator palsy).

Horizontal recti transposition to the SR area, with or without augmentation is also a preferred operation. During transposition, the horizontal recti are sutured adjacent to the nasal and temporal edge of SR insertion. This is the Knapp's procedure. If the deviation is not very large, partial transposition is preferred. Full muscle tendon transposition is usually done if the vertical deviation is >25 PD and partial tendon transposition is preferred if the deviation is <25 PD.

In some cases, which have large angle deviation, both IR recession and horizontal recti vertical transposition may be combined in one go. If operating in more than two muscles, one should prefer doing a vessel protecting surgery or the treatment should be divided into two sessions.

Botulinum toxin A injection to the IR has been used by some for insufficient results obtained following both transposition and recession operations. Some authors have even tried vertical recess-resect procedure for vertical deviation and horizontal recess-resect procedure for horizontal deviation. Here, the surgery is performed on the ipsilateral eye for vertical deviation and on the fellow eye for horizontal deviation. SR recession on the unaffected eye is also feasible following insufficient results for vertical deviation on effected eye.

DOUBLE DEPRESSOR PALSY

Paralysis of both depressors of the eye (IR and SO) is rare as both are innervated from different nerves. It might be the result of secondary SR contracture following long-standing IR palsy. In congenital cases, MRI has shown normal volume in IR and a positive FDT for depression. In such cases the cause can be the contracture of the SR or the adjacent tissues.

When the patient is fixating with normal eye, the affected eye is hypertropic. On switching fixation to the affected eye, the normal eye becomes hypotropic. Ductions are restricted in the entire lower field of gazes.

Reverse Knapp's procedure and SR recession are the recommended treatment modalities.

SUPRANUCLEAR EYE MOVEMENT DISORDERS

The most common supranuclear movement disorders are INO and skew deviation, which has been discussed in this section. Dorsal mid-brain syndrome (Parinaud's syndrome), and horizontal and vertical paralysis of the gaze may also be seen.

Horizontal Gaze Disorders

Horizontal Gaze Palsy

The PPRF is the horizontal gaze center. So, if PPRF is involved, then the patient will have ipsilateral horizontal gaze palsy.

Wall-eyed Bilateral Internuclear Ophthalmoplegia

Wall-eyed bilateral internuclear ophthalmoplegia is a rare disorder in which bilateral INO is associated with bilateral exotropia. Exotropia is believed to occur due to the disruption of the input from otolithic organs.

Internuclear Ophthalmoplegia (INO)

Internuclear ophthalmoplegia is caused by the lesion involving the MLF. MLF is a paired white matter tract through the center of the brainstem, lying ventral to the cerebral aqueduct in the midbrain and the fourth ventricle in the pons and medulla. It is the final common pathway for different types of conjugate eye movements such as saccades, smooth pursuit, and vestibulocochlear reflex. Saccades are initiated by the frontal eye field (FEF), which then sends signals to the contralateral PPRF for horizontal saccades and the rostral interstitial nucleus of the medial longitudinal fasciculus (riMLF) for vertical saccades. The PPRF is the horizontal gaze center that activates the ipsilateral abducens nucleus and sends signals to the LR muscle of the same side and via abducent excitatory interneurons (after decussation) to the contralateral MR subnucleus of the oculomotor nucleus through the MLF, thus resulting in horizontal gaze opposite to the initiating FFF.

If there is interruption of MLF due to any cause such as demyelination, inflammation, trauma, tumors, etc., it will block the connection between the contralateral 6th nerve nucleus and the ipsilateral 3rd nerve nucleus, thus resulting in INO. INO is characterized by impaired adduction on the ipsilateral eye and ataxic nystagmus in the abducting eye. But convergence is intact. This helps in differentiating INO from 3rd nerve palsy and myasthenia.

One-and-a-Half Syndrome

A combined lesion of MLF and PPRF manifests with combination of signs of both, and is referred to "one-and-a-half-syndrome" as it is characterized by loss of all horizontal movements other than abduction in the contralateral eye. So, a left-sided lesion will cause left gaze palsy, adduction deficit of the left eye and ataxic nystagmus on abduction in the right eye.

The diagnosis can be made clinically in the above cases. Often, the symptoms are minimal and spontaneous recovery may occur. Neuroimaging helps in identifying the etiology. A Fresnel prism can be given for residual deviation in the primary position. Strabismus surgery may be done for exotropia in WEBINO.

Vertical Gaze Disorders

The vertical gaze center is believed to be the rostral interstitial nucleus of the MLF in the midbrain.

Parinaud's Dorsal Midbrain Syndrome

It is also known as convergence retraction syndrome, pretectal syndrome, or the Sylvian aqueduct syndrome. The syndrome is characterized by one or more of the following signs: limitation of the upward eye movements such as saccade and pursuit (Parinaud's sign), limitation of downward eye movements, light near dissociation, convergence retraction nystagmus, lid retraction (Collier's sign), skew deviation, etc. This is associated with the affection of the dorsal midbrain by various causes such as hydrocephalus, meningitis, pineal gland tumors, and demyelination. In hydrocephalus, the dilatation of the third ventricle, aqueduct or the suprapineal recess causing stretching/compression of posterior commissure leading to Parinaud's syndrome.

Progressive Supranuclear Palsy

Progressive supranuclear palsy is a late-onset neurodegenerative disease that occurs in sixth decade. It is characterized by postural loss of balance and vertical supranuclear paralysis. As the disease progresses, all vertical saccades deteriorate, so they experience difficulty in daily life functions such as reading, eating, and develop total ophthalmoplegia over time. The prognosis is poor with high mortality.

Skew Deviations

Skew deviation is a vertical strabismus caused by supranuclear lesions. It is often associated with ocular torsion and head tilt, which together constitute the 'ocular tilt reaction'. Skew deviation is often the initial manifestation of diseases that affect the brainstem, cerebellum or peripheral vestibular system. Since some skew deviations may mimic trochlear nerve palsy, differentiating these two conditions can be challenging. Trochlear nerve palsy is commonly diagnosed clinically by 'Park Three-Step' test. In contrast, the vertical misalignment in skew deviation does not follow any set pattern; it may be comitant, incomitant or may alternate with change of gaze direction.

Further, in trochlear nerve palsy the excyclotorsion is present in hypertropic eye only; whereas in skew deviation, it is present in both eyes and is conjugate.

In cases of bilateral trochlear nerve palsy, excyclotortion is present in both hypertropic eyes and is disjunctive.

Clinical Features

The vertical strabismus may be comitant, incomitant. Rarely, it may alternate with eye position, i.e., right hypertropia in right gaze and left hypertropia in left gaze. Skew deviation is mostly associated with other neurologic signs and ocular tilt reaction comprising triad of skew deviation, ocular torsion and head tilt. The pathologic head tilt is ipsilateral to the hypotropic eye and ocular torsion is such that the 12 o'clock position of both eyes rotate in the same direction as that of the head tilt (i.e., the hypotropic eye is excyclotorted and the hypertropic eye incyclotorted). In acute cases, tortional nystagmus is commonly present. Skew deviation and ocular tilt reaction are commonly caused by ischemia, infarction, multiple sclerosis, tumors, trauma, intracranial hemorrage, syringobulbia, neurosurgical procedures, and raised intracranial pressure.

A new test to differentiate between trochlear nerve palsy and skew deviation is the decrease by more than 50% of hypertropia from upright to supine position of head in skew deviation.

Management (Flowchart 5)

In cases of suspected skew deviation, congenital causes of DVD, or pseudostrabismus should excluded. If upright-supine test is positive and Park-three step test negative, other neurological signs should be looked for and an enhanced MRI is indicated to look for brainstem or cerebellar lesions.

Gaze Palsies

Gaze palsy, as the name implies, affects the conjugate movements of eyes. There are different types of conjugate eye movements, including saccades, pursuit, optokinetic, and vestibulo-ocular. The anatomic systems that control these, diverge and converge at various levels, and it is possible for some lesions to impair some eye movements and spare others. Hence, a left saccadic palsy is a selective gaze palsy affecting only leftward saccades but not leftward pursuit or vestibular-ocular movements. The terms "partial" or 'complete' when applied to gaze palsy indicate whether some movement across mid-line is present in the paretic direction.

Horizontal Gaze Palsy

Horizontal gaze palsy is a limitation of conjugate movement of eyes in horizontal direction. It may be unilateral or bilateral. It may be congenital or acquired.

Congenital horizontal gaze palsy is a rare disease. It is autosomal recessive and results from abnormal development of brainstem. It emerges from defective "horizontal gaze palsy-associated" gene on chromosome 11q23-q25. Congenital gaze palsy may be associated with Mobius syndrome and pendular nystagmus with scoliosis.

Acquired supranuclear gaze palsies may occur with stroke, head injury, tumors, seizures, and rarely with metabolic disorders. In hemiplegia, the eyes are deviated towards the side of lesion, which usually resolves within a week. In irritative lesions such as seizures, the eyes deviate away from the site of damaged hemisphere.

The horizontal gaze center lies in the midbrain (pontine reticular formation, PPRF). Incomplete lesions of PPRF result in difficulty in maintaining eccentric gaze and produces gaze-evoked nystagmus. Bilateral lesions of the PPRF may cause complete loss of voluntary horizontal gaze (bilateral gaze palsy) **(Fig. 21)**. Large lesions may extend into "ventral pons" injuring the corticospinal tracts, and rendering the patient quadriplegic, creating a "locked-in syndrome". Such patients appear unconscious, but voluntary vertical and lid movements are spared, importantly differentiating locked-in syndrome from coma. Ocular bobbing can occur in this situation.

Flowchart 5: Management of skew deviation.

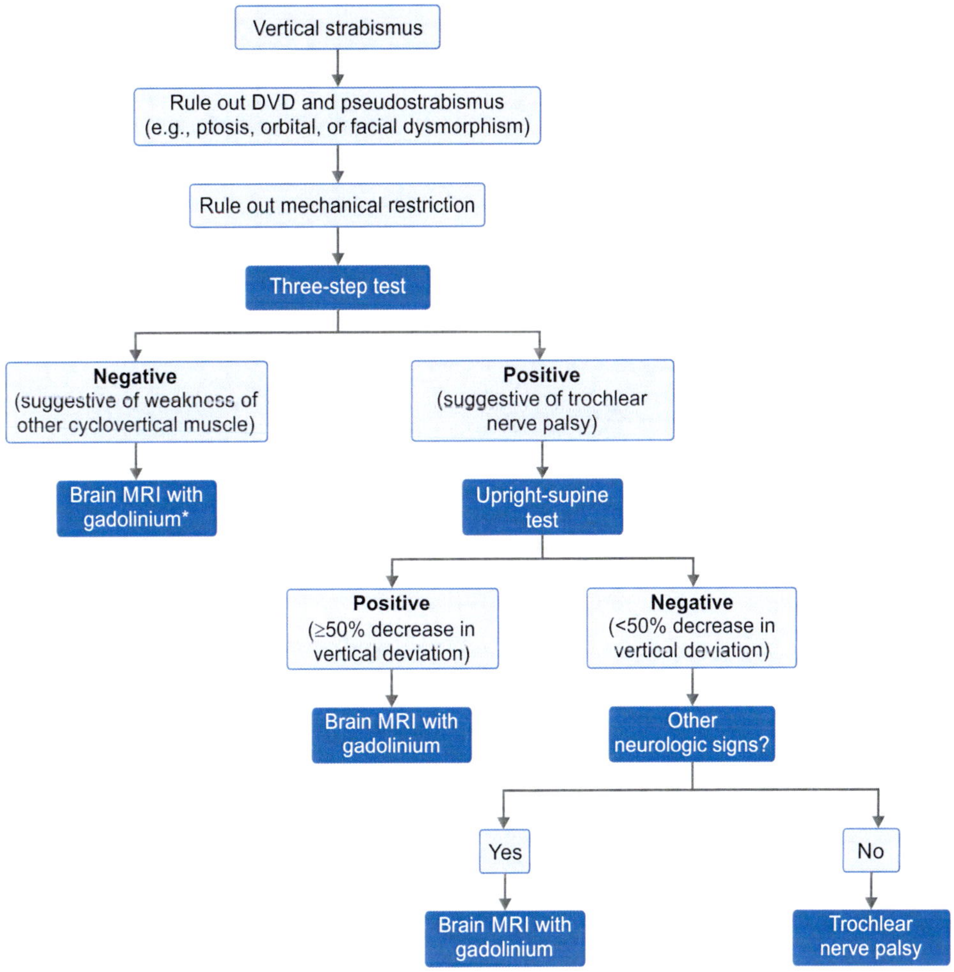

*Also consider myasthenia gravis if typical signs are present

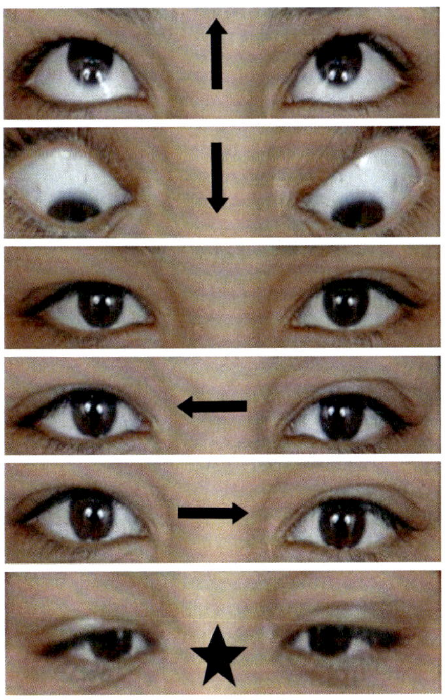

Fig. 21: Bilateral horizontal gaze palsy.
Source: sciencedirect.com

Vertical Gaze Palsy (Fig. 22)

Vertical gaze palsy is limitation of conjugate, bilateral, limitation of eye movements in upgaze or downgaze. Rostral interstitial nucleus of MLF, interstitial nucleus of Cajal, and posterior commissure, all located in rostrum midbrain, are the brainstem centers of vertical eye movement. The most common causes for vertical gaze palsies are stroke, tumors, trauma, ischemia, hydrocephalus, metabolic (Neiman-Pick-C; Tay-Sachs; Wilson disease; kernicterus) and congenital midbrain disorders like progressive supranuclear palsy.

Vertical gaze palsy can present as partial or complete bilateral impairment of upward or downward gaze. Upgaze palsy is most common, then combined up and down gaze, followed by downgaze palsy. If MLF (medial longitudinal fasciculus) is extensively affected, other signs include pupillary defects, oculomotor signs of 3rd nerve involvement, impaired convergence, and skew deviations. In thalamic damage, behavioral disturbance, apathy and slowness of thought can occur. If the posterior commissure is affected, pathologic lid retraction (Colliers' sign), semi-dilated pupils, and light-near dissociation can be seen.

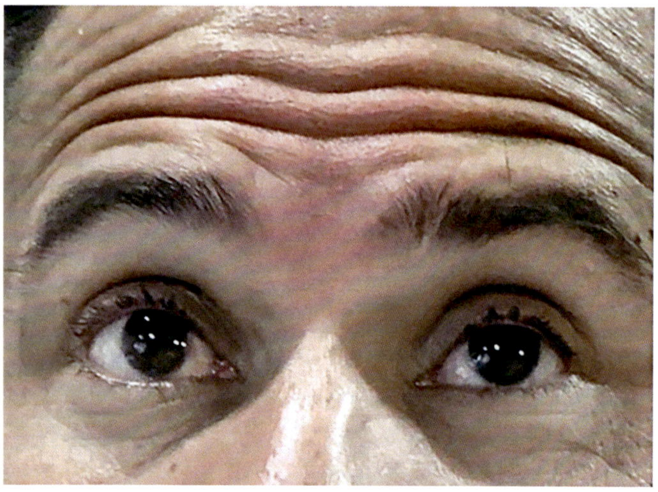

Fig. 22: Vertical gaze palsy.

In diagnostic procedures, neuroimaging (MRI) is the mainstay in establishing midbrain lesions. If infection is suspected, CSF testing is indicated, and tests for metabolic disorders.

The main diseases to differentiate in children are myasthenia gravis and skew deviations.

Management is directed to diagnosing the underlying cause and symptomatic treatment of ocular complaints.

CONCLUSION

In conclusion, detailed workup is important to differentiate ocular motor palsy from concomitant and restrictive paralysis. Clinical workup aided by laboratory and imaging studies help identify the underlying cause. The management of the underlying disease process is of prime importance. Observation and follow-up is recommended in initial phase of acute palsy awaiting spontaneous recovery. Surgical intervention can be planned for stable deviation with no further recovery. The choice of the surgery should be made from case to case basis after proper patient counseling.

SUGGESTED READING

1. Akar S, Gokyigit B, Yılmaz OF. Graded anterior transposition of the inferior oblique muscle for V-pattern strabismus. J AAPOS. 2012;16(3):286-90.
2. Aygit ED, İnal A, Ocak OB, Celik S, Fazıl K, Yildiz BK, et al. Simplified approach of Gokyigit's technique for complete cranial nerve third palsy. Int Ophthalmol. 2019;39(1):111-6.
3. Gokyigit B, Akar S, Kaynak P, Demirok A, Yilmaz OF. Long-term results of deeper muscle fibers recession of an inferior rectus operation. J Pediatr Ophthalmol Strabismus. 2014;51(1):17-26.
4. Gokyigit B, Akar S, Satana B, Demirok A, Yilmaz OF. Medial transposition of a split lateral rectus muscle for complete oculomotor nerve palsy. J AAPOS. 2013;17(4):402-10.
5. Gokyigit B, Akar S, Yilmaz OF. A Novel Technique for inferior rectus recession. Clin Ophthalmol. 2014;8:263-9.
6. Gokyigit B, Celik S, Inal A. Surgical Technique for Palsy of Superior Division of Oculomotor Nerve. Beyoglu Eye J. 2017;2(2): 67-70.
7. Gokyigit B, Inal A, Ocak OB, Aygit ED. Sliding shape extraocular muscle transposition with plication: a novel method. Beyoglu Eye J. 2019;4(2):120-2.
8. Kushner BJ. Restriction of elevation in abduction after inferior oblique anteriorization. J AAPOS. 1997;1:55-62.
9. Ocak OB, Inal A, Aygit ED, Celik S, Ocak SY, Gurez C, et al. Comparison of different ten-don transposition techniques for the treatment of monocular elevation deficiency type 2. J AAPOS. 2020;24(1):8.e1-8.e4.
10. Ocak OB, Inal A, Aygit ED, Celik S, Ocak SY, Karabulut GO, et al. Surgical management in type 1 monocular elevation deficiency. J Pediatr Ophthalmol Strabismus. 2018;55(6):369-74.
11. Phuljhele S, Dhiman R, Sharma M, Kusiyait SK, Saxena R, Mahalingam K, et al. Acquired ocular motor palsy: current demographic and etiological profile. Asia Pac J Ophthalmol (Phila). 2020;9(1):25-8.
12. Prasad S, Volpe NJ. Paralytic strabismus: third, fourth, and sixth nerve palsy. Neurol Clin. 2010;28(3):803-33.
13. Saxena R, Sethi A, Dhiman R, Sharma M, Sharma P. Enhanced adjustable nasal transposition of split lateral rectus muscle for surgical management of oculomotor nerve palsy. J AAPOS. 2020;24(3):183-6.
14. Saxena R, Sharma M, Singh D, Dhiman R, Sharma P. Medial transposition of split lateral rectus augmented with fixation sutures in cases of complete third nerve palsy. Br J Ophthalmol. 2016;0:1-3.
15. Saxena R, Singh D, Chandra A, Sharma P. Adjustable anterior and nasal transposition of inferior oblique muscle in case of torsional diplopia in superior oblique palsy. Indian J Clin Exp Ophthalmol. 2015;1:104-6.
16. Saxena R, Sinha A, Sharma P, Pathak H, Menon V, Sethi H. Precaruncular periosteal anchor of medial rectus, a new technique in the management of complete external third nerve palsy. Orbit. 2006;25:205-8.
17. Saxena R, Sinha A, Sharma P, Phuljhele S, Menon V. Precaruncular approach for medial orbital wall anchoring of the globe in oculomotor nerve palsy. J AAPOS. 2009;578-82.
18. Sharma P, Prakash P. Degsagittalisation of obliques: a case report of plagiocephaly with inferior oblique overaction. Indian J Ophthalmol. 1993;41:32-4.
19. Sharma P1, Gogoi M, Kedar S, Bhola R. Periostal fixation in third nerve palsy. J AAPOS. 2006;10:324-7.
20. Singh A, Bahuguna C, Nagpal R, Kumar B. Surgical management of third nerve palsy. Oman J Ophthalmol. 2016;9(2):80-6.
21. Stager DR Jr, Beauchamp GR, Wright WW, Felius J, Stager D Sr. Anterior and nasal transposition of the inferior oblique muscles. J AAPOS. 2003;7:167-73.
22. von Noorden GK, Campos EC. Paralytic strabismus. In: von Noorden GK (Ed). Binocular Vision and Ocular Motility, 6th edition. St Louis: Mosby; 2002. pp. 414-451.

26

CHAPTER

Techniques in Strabismus Surgery

Shivanand J Sheth, Syed Faraaz Hussain

INTRODUCTION

Surgical management of strabismus is often considered as a definitive solution to achieving successful ocular alignment in patients, and as a result, improve their social appearance, self-confidence, and often eliminate troublesome diplopia. It can also help achieve or restore higher grades of binocular function, and in patients with nystagmus, help improve their visual acuity.

Strabismus surgery can also be used as a stepping stone to improve ocular alignment so that other forms of binocular vision management such as exercises, prisms, and optical corrections can then be brought into play, which was not possible prior to surgery, as the misalignment was too large, too complex, or multi-planar.

Ideally, our objective is to provide binocular single vision (BSV) with stereopsis in all gazes for distance as well as near, with a normal head posture. If that is not possible, the hope is to achieve BSV with stereopsis at least in primary position and down gaze, where maximal daily work is done. If binocular sensory outcomes are not achievable, at least the motor component, i.e., satisfactory ocular alignment should be achieved. The goals are often divided into sensory and motor outcomes, but practically they overlap as sensory mechanisms improve motor alignment and motor alignment is a must for optimum sensory outcome. The psychosocial benefits of improved alignment have been well documented and it must be stressed that it is not to be considered just a "cosmetic" surgery.

ANATOMY

In order to learn the art of strabismus surgery, a basic working knowledge of the embryology, ocular anatomy, and ocular neurophysiology is a must. Detailed anatomy of the extraocular muscles (EOMs) is out of the scope of this chapter.

The conjunctiva should be respected, not because of aesthetics alone, but also because its scarring and inappropriate handling can cause alteration of outcomes. Incisions and closure of the conjunctiva must be meticulous **(Fig. 1)**. There is some redundancy of the bulbar conjunctiva, which is what strabismus surgeons usually incise. A fold of conjunctiva, the plica, present medially must not be accidentally incised or incorporated into closure with sutures, as it can lead to unsatisfactory healing.

The scleral thickness varies with age and area, being thinnest in neonates. Location wise, scleral thickness is 1.1–1.7 mm at the posterior pole, 0.6–0.7 mm at the limbus and thinnest just behind the insertion of the EOMs, i.e., 0.3–0.45 mm. This is extremely relevant to the operating surgeon, as this is the area where scleral sutures are passed and pull exerted.

The Tenon's capsule (fascia bulbi) is a condensation of fibrous connective tissue forming the facial system which suspends the globe in the orbit, separating it from the orbital fat **(Fig. 2)**. Its inner or global surface is smooth and shiny, separating it from the sclera by a potential episcleral or sub-Tenon's space. The potential area above it is the subconjunctival space lined by conjunctiva anteriorly. About 1–1.5 mm from the limbus, the Tenon's layer, conjunctiva, and sclera fuse, forming a complex insertion just posterior to which the conjunctiva and Tenon's can be separated. It should be handled with care, especially posteriorly as breach can result in orbital fat prolapse and adherence, which can be difficult to manage. It also serves as a protective mechanism against mechanical and infective assault. Many structures pierce the Tenon's capsule to approach the eyeball, including optic nerve, EOMs, vortex veins, and other neurovascular tissues.

The recti beyond their orbital course pierce Tenon's capsule about 8–10 mm from their scleral insertion to enter the sub-Tenon's space, where usually most of the manipulation is performed. After entering this space, the EOMs have no sheath, but are covered by connective tissues loosely fused with the muscle. These expand laterally along the edges of muscle to form the intermuscular membrane persisting up to the insertion of adjacent muscles.

The sheath of superior rectus (SR) in its orbital aspect is adherent to the inferior surface of the sheath of levator palpebrae superioris (LPS) muscle. The global portion of the SR sheath is associated with the superior oblique (SO) tendon sheath.

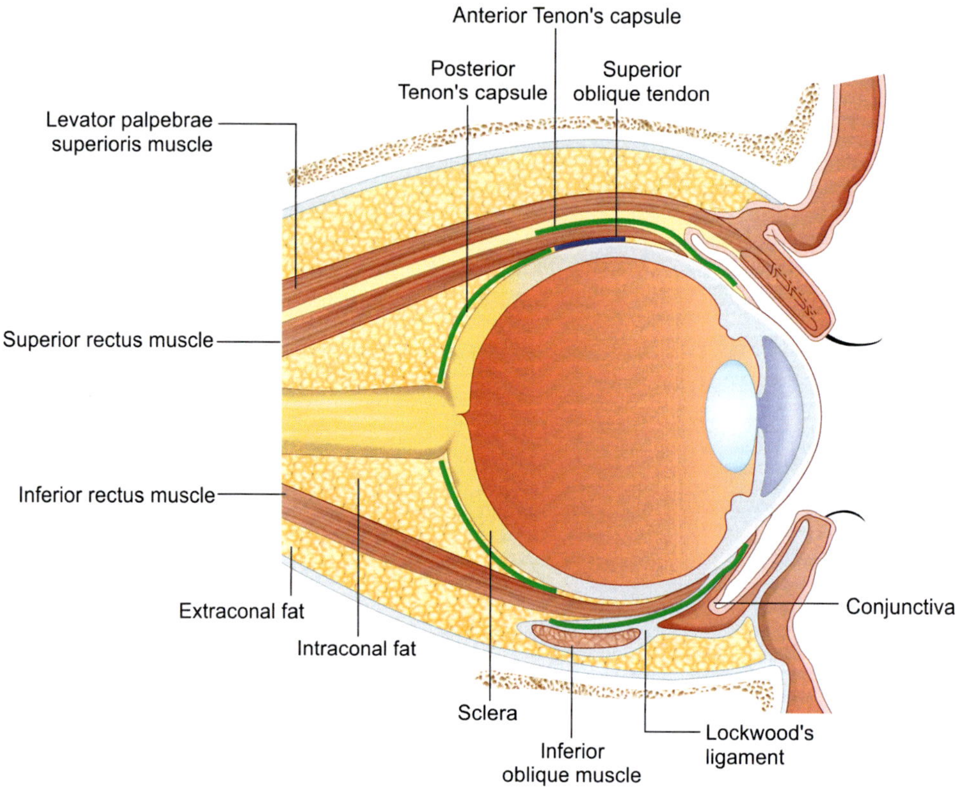

Fig. 1: Anatomy of extraocular muscles along with orbital facial structures.
Source: Coats DK, Olitsky SE. Strabismus Surgery and its Complications. Berlin/Heidelberg: Springer-Verlag Berlin Heidelberg; 2007.

The fascia surrounding the inferior rectus (IR) is thicker than other recti. The global portion of its sheath fuses with the Tenon's capsule orbital part and contributes to the formation of *Lockwood's ligament.* Surgically, it should be remembered that any vertical rectus manipulation can result in palpebral fissure changes.

The sheath of inferior oblique (IO) is continuous from origin to insertion, becoming thicker near its insertion. It is tightly adherent to the orbital aspect of the sheath of the IR. Small extensions also exist near the insertion to the sheath of the lateral rectus (LR) and optic nerve posteriorly.

Each rectus muscle has a unique distance of insertion from limbus, anterior to equator of globe and this also varies in infants and changes as one ages.

APPROACH AND CONJUNCTIVAL INCISIONS

After appropriate anesthesia, the eye is prepared by cleaning with 10% povidone iodine for the skin and 5% for the conjunctival sac. Appropriate draping should be done and the marking of the eye/s on which surgery is to be performed should be clearly visible even after draping is done. Presurgical timeout should be done prior to commencement of surgery, to ensure that the correct eye and muscles are being operated on and that the surgical plan is appropriate.

Some surgeons prefer to instill phenylephrine (2.5%) or brimonidine (0.1%) to cause vasoconstriction in order to have a "cleaner" operative field. Before beginning with the conjunctival incision, it is recommended that the operative field be inspected (especially note any unique landmarks, prior surgical or trauma scars, identify plica and caruncle medially).

The forced duction test (FDT) is performed to rule out any restriction or tightness. It is recommended before and after conjunctival incision, after dissection of check ligaments and Tenon's capsule, after hooking of muscle, after muscle disinsertion, after scleral suturing, and after conjunctival closure.

After appropriate anesthesia, a self-retaining speculum is applied, conjunctiva with episclera is held close to limbus with fixation forceps (usually two diagonally opposite ends) and the patient (if under topical) is asked to look in the opposite direction of testing to relax the muscle. The globe is passively rotated in the direction opposite to the suspected restriction site being tested [rotated laterally, if medial rectus (MR) area is being tested] while maintaining a slight lift on the globe for recti (slight propulsion) to keep muscles stretched and to retro-pulse slightly for obliques (during exaggerated FDT). Any restriction is physically felt, noted, and graded.

Conjunctival incisions can have multiple approaches **(Fig. 3)**.

Limbal incisions are generally preferred for beginner surgeons, and in certain difficult situations such as for reoperations due to the excellent exposure it provides. The conjunctiva is grasped just behind the limbus, rotating the globe to expose the area of the muscle of interest, usually

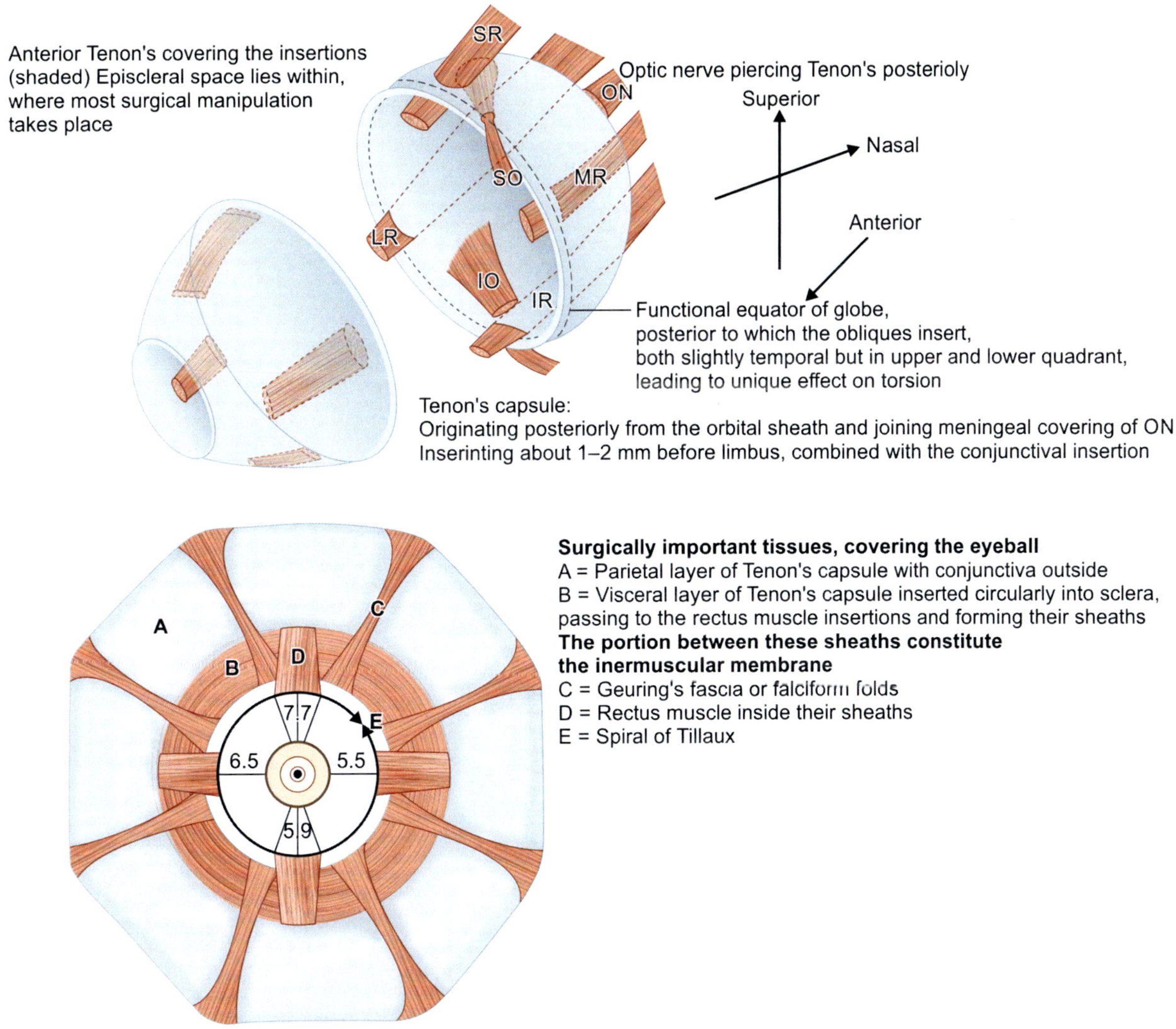

Fig. 2: Relationship of Tenon's capsule to extraocular muscles.
(IO: inferior oblique; IR: inferior rectus; LR: lateral rectus; MR: medial rectus; ON: optic nerve; SO: superior oblique; SR: superior rectus)

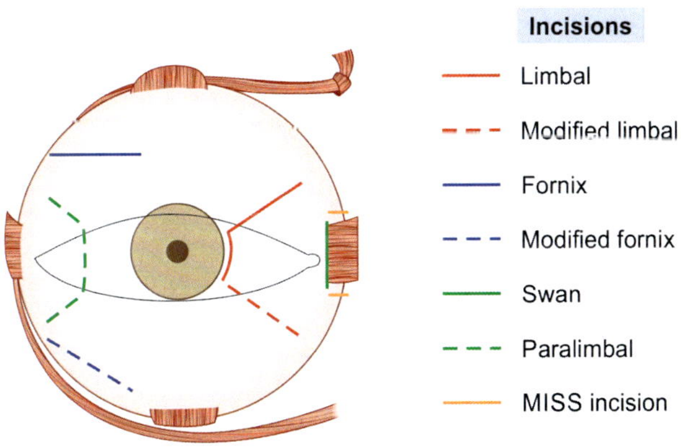

Fig. 3: Different conjunctival incisions.

achieved with a curved locking forceps or a fixation suture. Sharp dissection is used to first create a conjunctival opening at one end which is then extended to create a 2–3 clock hour with the fornix as the base. A blunt tipped Westcott scissors is used to dissect further and radial extensions on either side can be made and extended to 6–8 mm. The free corners of the conjunctival opening should be marked with 8-0 polyglactin or 6-0 Plain gut for easier identification at closure. A modification of the limbal approach involves only a single-sided radial extension. Closure involves placing an absorbable suture (prefer 8-0, but 6-0 will also do) at each edge of conjunctival flap and approximating it to the adjacent intact limbal conjunctiva with interrupted sutures. Radial extensions can be left unsutured, or closed with a single stitch, but ensure no Tenon's has prolapsed.

Fornix incisions are usually the preferred technique by experienced surgeons due to the cosmetic benefit and quicker, more comfortable recovery for the patient. It is made approximately 8–10 mm in length, starting about 8 mm behind the limbus, nasally or temporally as required. Here the Tenon's must be grasped and incised separately to gain access to the episcleral space. Some prefer a more oblique orientation of the incision, the exact nature of which varies with surgeon preference, type of surgery, etc. After surgery, the incision can be closed with an absorbable suture usually single interrupted (some even choose continuous) or can be left unsutured with close approximation. Ensure that no Tenon's is prolapsing after closure.

Other types of incisions can be Swan type over the muscle insertion, between limbus and muscle (paralimbal) or two small incisions on either side of insertion of a muscle as devised in minimally invasive strabismus surgery (MISS).

EXPOSURE AND ISOLATION

A detailed discussion about each type of surgery in strabismus is beyond the scope of this chapter, but we have tried to outline the basic approaches in greater detail with certain salient points about specific procedures. It is hoped that this helps the beginner strabismus surgeon to begin to form a solid foundation on which to build upon with experience.

Rectus Muscles

Adequate exposure is a must for accurate and safe surgery. After gaining entry to the episcleral space, an opening is made in intermuscular septa to reach bare sclera. A squint hook is passed from one end of the muscle insertion (begin with tip directed away from the insertion and rotate it by slight pressure on the sclera to enter beneath the muscle) to the other. At all times remain anterior to the equator and in close contact with the globe to avoid disturbing oblique insertions, orbital fat, and vortex veins. For beginners, for LR, it is preferred to hook the muscle from the superior border to avoid IO fibers being included and for SR, it is preferred to hook from the nasal side to avoid SO. Slight traction and tilt on the hook exposes the intermuscular septae better, which should be meticulously dissected under visualization. A second muscle hook is inserted from the other side if there is doubt about the completeness of fibers being included. The space between the muscle and bare sclera should be free of all attachments, but avoid any excessive dissection to preserve anatomy and prevent bleeding and subsequent scarring. After complete muscle isolation on the hook, sharp dissection of the muscle capsule and intermuscular septum is done under direct visualization. Some prefer blunt cleaning of the capsule using cotton-tipped sterile buds. To ensure bloodless field, one should be careful from the start—ensure sharp dissection is not close to fleshy portion of rectus muscle, avoid anterior ciliary vessels at insertion, and apply pressure when muscle belly divided, with minimal cauterization, if at all.

A modified Swan incision (directly over the insertion) for SR in order to preserve the conjunctiva and Tenon's for a possible future antiglaucoma surgery can be considered in some patients. For IR isolation, it is important to be aware of the thick mass of fascia about 10 mm behind its insertion, the Lockwood ligament with the IO included. It is important for larger IR recessions (>4–5 mm), like in thyroid ophthalmopathy, where some prefer to dissect the intermuscular membrane well posterior to the Lockwood ligament in order to prevent lower lid retraction. Others use a suture passed through this tissue, to secure and attach the Lockwood ligament and lower lid retractors forward and avoid its undue recession so as to not affect the palpebral aperture size. Vortex veins lie about 10 mm behind IR insertion and must be avoided during any manipulation.

For ensuring all fibers are hooked, a heel-toe maneuver and a pole test can be performed. For *heel-toe* (angle of muscle hook is heel, end bulb is toe), the hook is tented up at its toe end, gently trying to rotate the same toward limbus. If this is easily achieved, it indicates complete muscle fibers having been hooked, but if the heel tends to move posteriorly, then some fibers are probably left out. The *pole test* is recommended as a final step to ensure that the entire rectus muscle has been hooked. The toe of a small hook (Steven's hook) is placed on bare sclera behind the muscle insertion. While maintaining slight pressure on the globe, the toe is moved around the muscle insertion, till it is located anterior to the insertion. If some fibers have not been hooked or the muscle split, the toe gets caught and one is unable to bring it anterior to insertion. This should prompt a delicate search for any missed muscle fibers.

Obliques

For SO, an incision parallel to the limbus (7–8 mm from it) is preferred, about 5–6 mm in length, near the insertion of the SR in either the superotemporal quadrant (preferred for insertion manipulation) or the superomedial quadrant (preferred for tendon part). Some prefer a superior limbal incision for better exposure and manipulation. During SO isolation, minimal disturbance of the surrounding fascia should be done to minimize scarring.

Tenon's capsule is divided separately, a large muscle hook passed beneath SR to rotate the eye inferiorly. The toe of the large muscle hook would be covered by fascia which should not be disturbed. Better exposure can be achieved if a separate small tissue retractor (like Barbie's retractor) is used to retract the upper eyelid and conjunctiva rather than rely on a lid speculum. Avoid the vortex veins which emerge on either side of the SR, a little behind the equator. The entire tendon insertion of the SO can be identified by passing a flat instrument like an iris repositor between it and the underlying sclera from anterior to posterior, visualized as a thin, white shiny membrane spreading out in a fan-shaped manner beneath the SR (after it is retracted nasally). Once the SO is identified, a small incision is made through Tenon's fascia directly over the tendon. The tendon can then be hooked with a small hook. The SO is one of the most common muscles with anatomical variations; this should always be anticipated during dissection.

Some prefer a nasal approach for certain surgeries on SO, like tucking, tendon expansion, or chicken suture.

The conjunctival incision, usually fornix, for IO is made just anterior to the mid-portion of the distal half of the muscle, followed by incision in the Tenon's capsule to reach the episcleral space. The belly of IO muscle is embedded in the posterior Tenon's capsule and must be shelled out taking care to avoid splitting the muscle. At the mid-portion also lies a vortex vein, in nearly all cases and should be protected. To improve exposure, LR and IR are identified and retracted if needed. As the eye ball is rotated superonasally, usually the posterior border of IO should be directly visualized. Important landmarks to ensure that IO has been identified are the simultaneous visualization of the posterior border of IO, vortex vein, and sclera. A hook is then used to lift the IO (first directed toward floor of orbit then drawn anteriorly) from the anterior end and dissect it posteriorly, making sure that no portion of the muscle is left behind (try to visualize the posterior edge from the under-side as the muscle is lifted) and ensure that the fat pad is not disturbed. The surgeon sharply dissects the IO muscle capsule while the assistant places the capsule under mild traction. Careful dissection is done of the fascia surrounding the muscle, including the intermuscular septum posterior to it while ensuring no fat prolapse occurs.

GENERAL SUTURING GUIDELINES

The next step after isolation is to secure the muscle by suturing. Some prefer to clear the Tenon's near the insertion by mild cautery before sutures are passed in order to clear the field and to prevent sutures being weakened by transmitted heat later.

For securing rectus muscles, a general technique can be used which aims to prevent any muscle slip within the capsule while simultaneously securing both ends and preventing central sag. For this purpose, we prefer a double armed, 6-0 polyglactin suture on a spatulated needle **(Figs. 4A and B)**. For recessions securing the muscle about 1 mm away from scleral insertion is the preferred site.

There are many variations and surgeon preferences for securing the muscle with sutures. Our preferred technique is described.

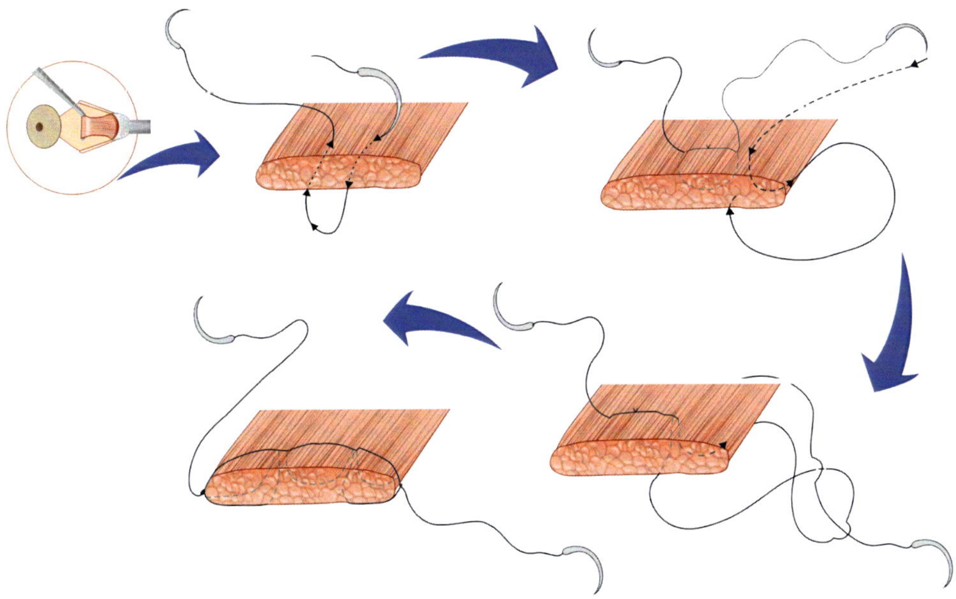

A

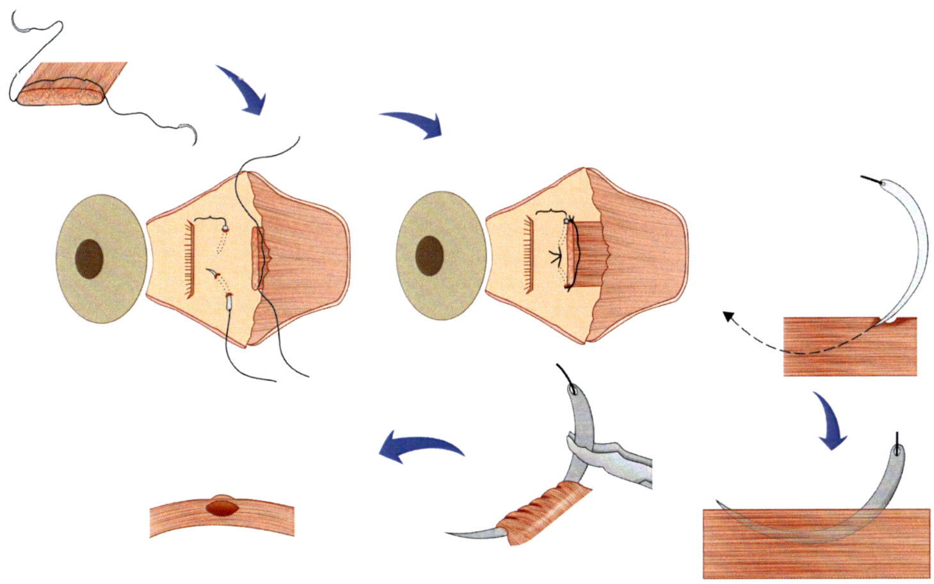

B

Figs. 4A and B: Steps for securing sutures through a rectus muscle and through scleral insertion. (A) Placement of sutures in muscle; (B) Placement of sutures attaching muscle to sclera.

The needle is passed through the center of the muscle to make a central knot (prevents sagging) which should not be over tightened. The ends are kept unequal to help in identification of muscle anatomy later, especially after disinsertion. On either side of the central stitch, most surgeons prefer a half-thickness pass or a transverse pass which comes out of the side of the muscle. It is not uncommon for the beginner surgeon to be superficial in this pass, hence some prefer a full thickness to prevent a potential muscle slip. A second, full-thickness pass is taken just behind the first one and the needle brought out half way between edge and the central suture bite. A "figure of 8" loop is made and the needle is brought out from the smaller outer loop in order to make a secure locking stitch. Similar passes and knots are made at other edge of muscle, ensuring that the muscle is not crumpled or bunched up due to tightness of the sutures and both ends are in a straight line to prevent muscle slant. This general technique can be used for most recessions and resections.

Muscle plication aims to preserve the blood supply, hence only the edges of muscle (about 15% from either end) should be manipulated. Here a separate single-ended 6-0 polyglactin for either end of the muscle is used. After visualization of the anterior ciliary arteries, the needle is entered in a transverse pass about 15% from the edge. A locking knot is tied and a second full thickness pass just behind the first one is taken to secure the edge well. Similarly the other edge of the muscle is also secured. After making a mattress loop on either edge of the scleral insertion site, the sutures are secured after either pulling muscle loop above the suture, or pushing it into the globe by using an iris retractor. This needs diligent assistance and experience on both the surgeon side and the assistant side. Knotting is done while the muscle loop is tight and fold of muscle is at the edge of insertion site.

The scleral pass of the needle should be aimed at about 0.2 mm depth and 1.5 mm in length. This is practically achieved by first ensuring a stable globe by using locking forceps or tissue holding forceps at the cut end of muscle stump near insertion. The area of scleral point entry is measured as per procedure and usually marked with tip of forceps or calipers, which temporarily causes point dehydration by compression of scleral fibers and the sclera appears darkened. It should be noted that it is the point of entry that is measured and not the exit location. Remember the muscle sits at the point of needle entry and the suture knots sit at the point of needle exit. The needle pass should be just visible beneath the superficial scleral fibers. This should be the case throughout the course of the needle in sclera and it should never be directed deep, but aimed to be just parallel. After the length of one needle pass, it is directed superficially to exit the sclera. Some prefer to partially make a "crossing-sword pass" which approaches, but does not intersect with the second needle's pass. Some others prefer to keep the scleral passes apart in order to ensure the muscle is stretched and not bunched up at new insertion. A simple traction is maintained on the sutures while knotting, which is usually enough to prevent any sag. In case of central laxity or sag noted, single interrupted stitch is usually enough.

RECTUS MUSCLE WEAKENING PROCEDURES

The aim here is to weaken the action of the muscle while in most cases minimizing any limitation of ductions. This can be achieved by recessions, retroequatorial myopexy (Faden), marginal myotomy (partial thickness cuts in muscle), tenotomy/myectomy or disinsertion (removal of muscle-tendon complex from scleral insertion), and lengthening (by sutures or silicone expanders) **(Fig. 5)**.

Recession

Principle

The insertion is moved closer to the origin of the muscle in the same plane, producing a slackening of muscle fibers and altering the torque vector. Recession beyond the equatorial/tangential point of the globe when the eye moves into the action of the muscle leads to mechanical limitation and can cause duction deficits and is hence avoided.

Method

Muscle is exposed and secured with 6-0 polyglactin sutures about 1 mm near insertion. Muscle is detached leaving a <1 mm stump (minimizes bleeding, makes measurement accurate, and does not leave cosmetic stump). Measure the intended recession needed by calipers and mark a point on sclera from either ends of the insertion. The detached tendon is re-inserted maintaining the original width of the muscle.

Some Aphorisms

- The MR does not have direct attachments to adjacent obliques, hence easier to become "lost."
- Large SR recessions may cause lid retraction, similar to the IR surgery.
- The effect of a combined bilateral recession or recess—resect procedure at one setting is usually more than that of a sequential one.
- IR recession should be conservatively done, as downgaze is more critical if compromised.

Variations: Usually Used for A/V Pattern Strabismus

- *Oblique/slanting insertion*: Amount of recession varied between one pole of new insertion and the other. Example: Inferior pole of MR insertion recessed more than superior pole to weaken muscle action more in downgaze.
- Insertion of horizontal recti can be raised or lowered one or half tendon width to weaken muscle more in up or downgaze. The shifting is done such that the muscle insertion remains concentric to the limbus.

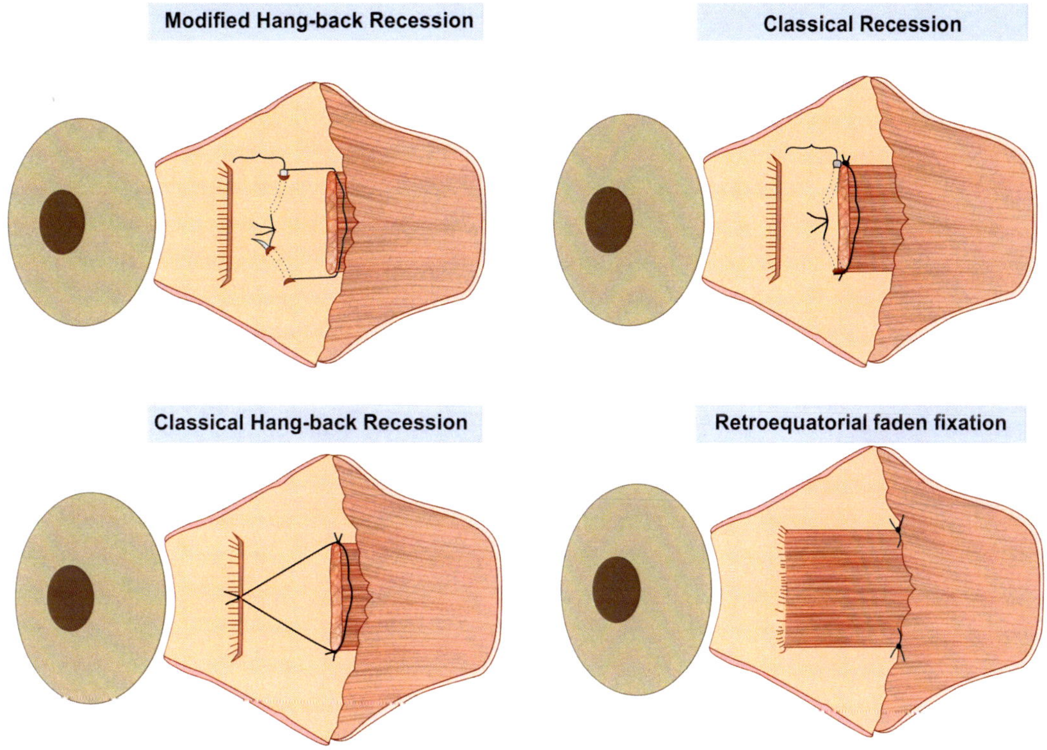

Fig. 5: Common muscle weakening procedures.

Other Variations in Recessions

Hang Back

Method for hang-back: The muscle is secured as before and disinserted. Locking forceps at insertion stump are used to stabilize the globe. The needles are passed in front of the sclera, just anterior to insertion and brought out close together. The muscle is pulled anteriorly up to the insertion before measuring, else unexpected larger recession effect might occur. Calipers are placed perpendicular to globe at the insertion site and measurement is taken on the suture length and demarcated by a locking artery or needle holder. Suture is tied over the needle holder and trimmed after which globe is allowed to rotate away from muscle, so that the muscle retracts and "hangs back on the suture."

Method for hemi hang-back: Here the procedure is almost entirely similar, however the scleral sutures are passed mid-way behind insertion and the intended amount of recession. This is used to avoid suturing deep posterior over sclera, especially with LR as it is closer to macula.

Indications for Larger Recessions (Supramaximal Recessions)

- *LR paralysis*: Recession of contracted, tight ipsilateral MR (to allow eye to abduct) and contralateral MR (to limit adduction and increase gaze comitance when LR is not innervated).
- *Duane retraction syndrome (DRS)*: Recess contralateral MR (to enlarge the field of binocular vision)
- *Dissociated vertical deviation (DVD)*: To prevent up-drift by supramaximal SR recessions
- *Infantile esotropia (ET) with larger deviations*: Supramaximal recessions of both medial rectus muscle.
- *Congenital nystagmus with marked face turn*: Recess MR in one and LR in other eye to use null area.
- ET associated with blind microphthalmic eye.

Retroequatorial Myopexy or Faden Operation

The aim is to cause a progressive weakening effect as the eye moves into the field of action of the operated rectus muscle without affecting primary position alignment much.

Principle

The muscle is attached to the globe far posterior to insertion, using sutures through edges or belly of muscle, causing the lever arm to shorten progressively as the muscle contracts, but without appreciable muscle slackness. Hence, the weakening increases as the eye moves into the field of action of the operated muscle. It has recently been theorized that it is not the lever arm which is affected much, rather the posterior fixation suture causes posterior displacement of pulley sleeve system during muscle contraction resulting in mechanical restriction of globe movement seen after surgery.

Method

Rectus muscle is detached from globe at insertion and one or more circumferentially placed mattress sutures (using nonabsorbable 5-0 Mersilene or 4-0 Dacron) are used to attach the muscle belly to the underlying sclera at the distance where the Faden stitch is planned. The scleral bites should be 3–4 mm on either side of the muscle with at least 80% of fibers in fixation. The muscle is then re-inserted at the original insertion. Many surgeons prefer to not detach the original insertion, if no added recession is planned.

If recession is planned with Faden operation, sutures are passed through the muscle at a point which is "Faden" distance less than recession (Example: for a 15 mm Faden and 4 mm recession, muscle is fixed at 11 mm distance). The sutures in sclera are placed at the same distance (15 mm) and recession of required amount is then performed (4 mm).

The distances behind insertion recommended for Faden operation are as follows:

- *MR*: 12–14 mm
- *LR*: 16–20 mm
- *SR*: 14–16 mm
- *IR*: 14–16 mm.

Some Aphorisms

- The difference between the Faden operation and that of supramaximal recession is that although the lever arm progressively shortens in both, only the latter results in increased muscle slackness.
- A reverse leash effect may be produced which leads to some progressive mechanical restriction as the eye moves further into the field of action of the operated muscle.
- An alternative to Faden is the "Pulley-suture" where instead of the posterior rectus muscle belly being sutured to sclera, it is sutured into the thick pulley overlying the orbital layer of the posterior muscle for a similar effect as traditional Faden.

Indications

Technically difficult and requiring good assistance, Faden operation is popular still for a variety of patients:

- Nonaccommodative convergence excess ET (MR)
- Nystagmus blockade syndrome (MR)
- DVD (SR)
- Paralytic strabismus (contralateral synergist)
- DRS type 1 (contralateral MR)
- Additional weakening effect over an already recessed muscle.

Z Myotomy

Principle

The muscle length is lengthened by means of transverse incisions along the belly of the muscle.

Method

The area of muscle to be cut is first crushed with straight artery forceps. Three transverse incisions are made through two-thirds of the muscle width at 5 mm intervals behind the muscle insertion, two on one side and the other on opposite, alternating. Avoid cautery as it may lead to excess adhesions leading to erroneous Faden effect.

It is usually used to augment an already maximally recessed muscle for greater weakening effect.

Free Tenotomy

Disinsertion of a rectus muscle without scleral reattachment is utilized when maximal weakening effect is needed.

Method

Simply cutting the muscle at insertion might lead to later reattachment, exerting some effect on the globe. Hence, the muscle is allowed to retract within the Tenon's capsule and the opening closed with sutures. This can be better ensured if simultaneous resection of part of muscle is done, so that forward migration is unlikely.

Recession with Fixation to Adjacent Periosteum over the Orbital Wall

Perhaps the most efficient way to maximally weaken a rectus muscle is to recess and transfer it to the adjacent periosteum. It is usually performed for the LR muscle in longstanding exotropia in third nerve palsy or in exotropic Duane retraction syndrome. It is also occasionally used on the IR in conditions such as congenital fibrosis of the EOMs where patient adopts a large chin up compensatory head posture.

Method

Limbal incision is preferred. LR is isolated, hooked, and secured using 5-0 Mersilene (nonabsorbable suture) as routine. The suture can be passed under direct visualization or through periorbital fat tissue to reach the periosteum without actually exposing the periosteum. For the latter, a sturdy needle (S-14 or S-24) is preferred bent at an acute angle for periosteal bite, along with a malleable retractor to protect the globe during suture retrieval.

Some Aphorisms

- A rectus muscle can still have some action on the globe, despite maximal recession or even tenotomy, this is due to secondary connections of the muscle to the globe through the Tenon's and surrounding tissues. Hence, periosteal fixation is needed for maximal weakening effect, but even this may not be total.

RECTUS MUSCLE STRENGTHENING PROCEDURES

The aim here is to improve the muscle action without causing undue limitation of movement or to augment a paralyzed muscle **(Fig. 6)**. Classical resection and plication are now the favored techniques. Transposition is preferred for chronic nerve palsies and disinnervations.

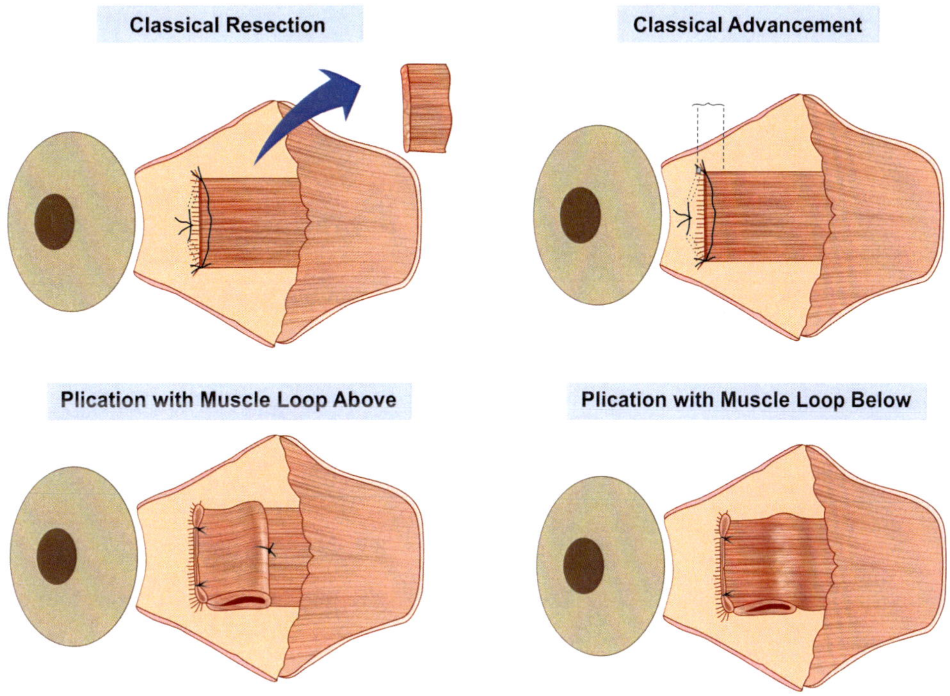

Fig. 6: Some muscle strengthening techniques.

Resection

Principle

The muscle is strengthened by shortening it while maintaining its action through the point of original insertion. Similar to recession, safe limits are defined to prevent mechanical restriction.

Method

After adequate exposure and isolation of muscle as per the required indication, muscle can either be secured with sutures at appropriate distance, the portion of muscle in front of the sutures is excised and the shortened muscle reattached to original insertion.

Few Aphorisms

- If the central tendon sags using the direct suture method, an additional central bite can be taken to prevent recession effect being added.
- Resection produces greater postoperative reaction such as conjunctival chemosis and redness than most other strabismus surgeries as direct muscle transection is done in a vascular area and sutures are close to limbus.
- Greater effect is obtained with simultaneous recession of ipsilateral antagonist.

Rectus Muscle Plication (Also Known as "Tuck")

Principle

Muscle is shortened and hence strengthened similar to resection, but no part is excised, rather it is folded in such a manner that the lever arm is shortened by a fixed amount. This can be achieved by double-breasting or cinching or simple suture fixation.

Method

Two double armed mattress sutures can be secured at either end of the muscle at appropriate distance from limbus as per the indication. The muscle loop is pulled up and brought close to insertion site, after which the mattress sutures are tightened. The loop is then sutured to keep it flat against the globe. Alternatively the two ends of the muscle can be secured by single-ended sutures as described in the suturing section.

Few Aphorisms

- The measurements are the same as resection.
- Plication needs diligent assistance, but has the potential advantage of being reversible, no possibility of muscle loss or slip, and less reaction postoperatively.
- Slight cosmetic disadvantages due to muscle bunching may occur in some cases.
- The benefit of preserving the anterior ciliary artery supply usually trumps the above-mentioned drawbacks.

Advancement

Alternative strengthening procedure where the muscle is isolated, detached, and re-inserted close to limbus, thereby "stretching" it, hence making it taut and more effective. Reverse of recession, but usually not preferred due to short insertion-limbus distance and the cosmetic blemish due to new insertion being visible. It is useful in consecutive squint, where recession has already been performed as well as in some paralytic strabismus.

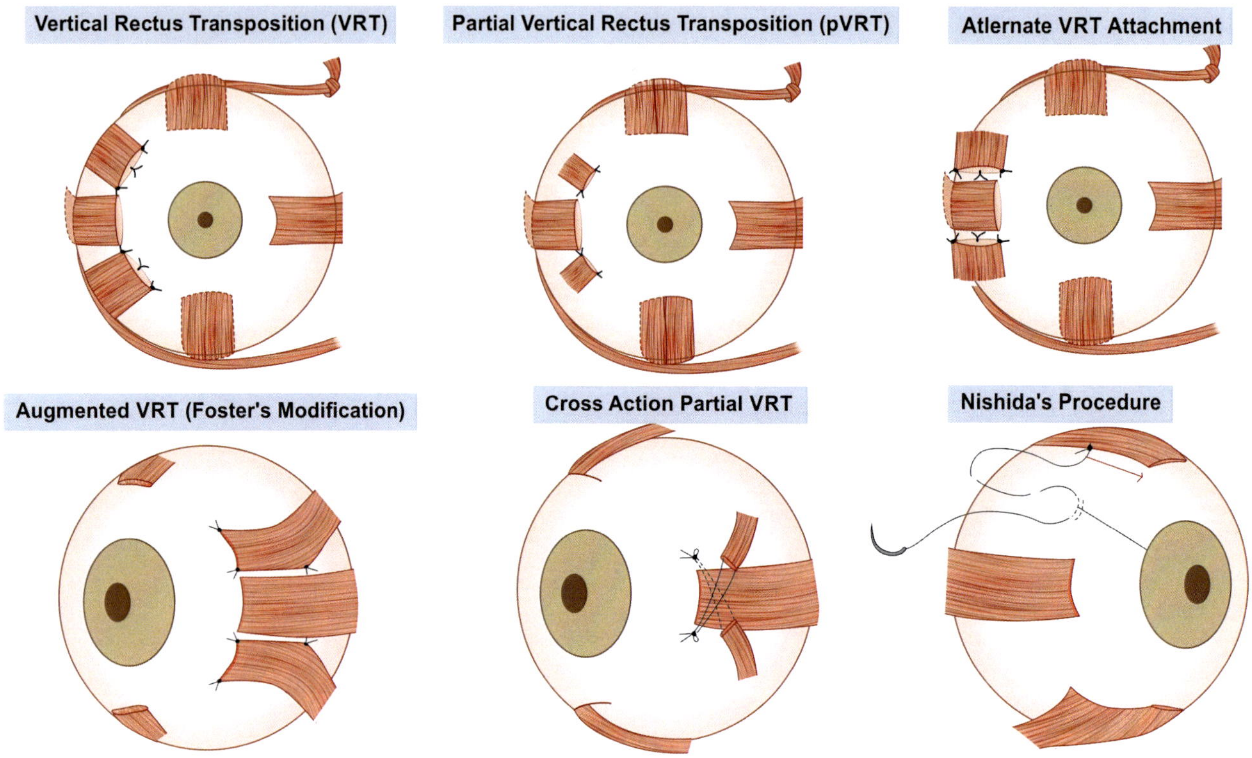

Fig. 7: Some transposition procedures.

Transposition

If the function of a muscle cannot be improved by a strengthening procedure, the adjacent muscles can be used to improve the action of the paralyzed muscle **(Fig. 7)**.

Principle

Utilization of adjacent muscles in place of a paralyzed or absent muscle by changing the vector of the adjacent muscles such that their line of action aids the affected muscle.

Procedure

Prerequisite before transposition is the absence of any restriction of the antagonist as tested by FDT. If the antagonist is tight, recession should be done and dissection to free adhesions should be completed. Then the adjacent muscles are exposed, isolated, and secured with partial or complete disinsertion and sutured to sclera adjacent to the paralyzed muscle, as per indication. Many types have been described; a short summary of the same is given in **Table 1.**

Aphorisms

- Though partial transposition is said to preserve the ciliary supply, there is still a possible risk of anterior segment ischemia and this should be kept in mind as well as patient to be counseled about. It is advisable to not transect more than two whole rectus insertions at a single operation.
- Rarely noted to have torsional effects, so those with good vision and fusion capability should be warned about the same.

OBLIQUE MUSCLE SURGERIES

Due to the unique nature of the oblique muscles, we describe their surgeries separately.

Inferior Oblique

Common indications for weakening include primary inferior oblique overaction (IOOA), SO palsy with IOOA, and DVD with IOOA.

Inferior Oblique Recession

Aim is to produce controlled weakening of all functions of the IO in a graded and reversible manner **(Table 2)**.

Method: After a fornix incision (preferred), the IO is isolated and secured. It is detached from the site of its insertion (some prefer to secure it with sutures; 6-0 polyglactin after detachment) and mild cautery applied to the proximal edge (some prefer use of hemostat). The muscle is then sutured to the sclera along its normal course, commonly the anterior muscle suture is secured 2–4 mm posterior to the temporal border of the IR insertion, just near the temporal edge. Graded recession has been described by many authors in different preferences.

Myectomy of the Inferior Oblique

Some surgeons believe that despite the multiple varieties of recession, the IO overactions can recur unless a large segment is removed (IO myectomy) **(Fig. 8)**.

Method: For myectomy, after the IO is hooked, it is clamped between two hemostatic forceps for 1–2 minutes. The muscle

TABLE 1: Transposition procedure.

S. No.	*Name*	*Affected muscle or disease*	*Transposed muscle*	*Special information*
1.	Hummelsheim	LR palsy	Lateral halves of SR and IR (vertical rectus transposition—VRT)	5-0 Mersilene used
2.	Jensen	LR palsy	Lateral halves of SR and IR are tied with upper and lower halves of LR	knots tied at equator
3.	O'Connor	LR palsy	Vertical recti to LR with LR cinching	LR cinch
4.	Callahan	Elevator palsy	Upper halves of MR and LR	Tied next to SR
5.	Knapp	Elevator palsy (SR)	Horizontal recti to SR	Complete dis-insertion and sutured next to SR
7.	Helveston	III N. Palsy (MR)	Preserved sclera used to transpose	LR recession done
			Vertical recti (medial halves) to MR	

(IR: inferior rectus; LR: lateral rectus; MR: medial rectus; SR: superior rectus)

TABLE 2: Inferior oblique recession.

S. No.	*Method*	*Position of insertion of the secured IO*	*Approximate amount of recession obtained*
1.	Fink (1962)	6 mm posterior and 6 mm inferior to lower border of LR	8 mm
2.	Park; Apt and Call (1978)	3 mm posterior and 2 mm temporal to the lateral pole of IR	10 mm
3.	Maximal recession	Reinsertion at scleral exit of the inferior temporal vortex vein	14 mm
4.	Modified Elliot and Nankin (recession-cum-anteropositioning)	Anterior end at lateral end of IR with the posterior end being 5 mm posterior along the lateral border of IR	Supramaximal weakening effect, weakening the effect severely in downgaze
5.	Stager's anterior and nasal transposition	IO inserted 2 mm nasal to the insertion of the IR	IOOA with absent SO, antielevation syndrome significant upshoot and downshoot in DRS
6.	Pure anteropositioning (Sharma)	IO inserted just at the inferior edge of the LR	Antero-positions of the IO without any practical effect on torsion, comparable to about 8 mm recession
7.	Total anteropositioning	Entire width of the IO is placed anterior to the IR	Weakens elevation in adduction almost completely, may cause antielevation syndrome
8.	Recession of the anterior fibers	Anterior half fibers separately hooked and split about 12–14 mm and recessed.	Selectively weakens extorsion, useful in torsional Kestenbaum

(DRS: Duane retraction syndrome; IO: inferior oblique; IOOA: inferior oblique overaction; IR: inferior rectus; LR: lateral rectus; SO: superior oblique)

is then cut with tenotomy scissors in between; cautery is sometimes added to prevent the highly vascular muscle from bleeding.

Denervation and Extirpation of the Inferior Oblique

Reserved for pronounced and recurrent IOOA but is infrequently used. The procedure involves transection of the neurovascular bundle combined with removal of a large portion of the IO muscle's distal segment. The nerve to the IO is a fusiform structure on the posterior border of the muscle. This can be hooked and stocked to identify a tight band which is then cauterized.

Some Aphorisms

- Good exposure and assistance is must for any procedure involving the IO.
- Important structures such as the macula (near IO insertion) and vortex vein proximity must be kept in mind and protected.
- Excessive dissection is avoided to prevent orbital fat prolapse and fat adherence syndrome.
- Unilateral recession and anterior transposition of the IO can cause hypotropia in primary position, hence used for unilateral hypertropia by many surgeons. But the limitation of elevation in abduction should be kept in mind causing antielevation syndrome.

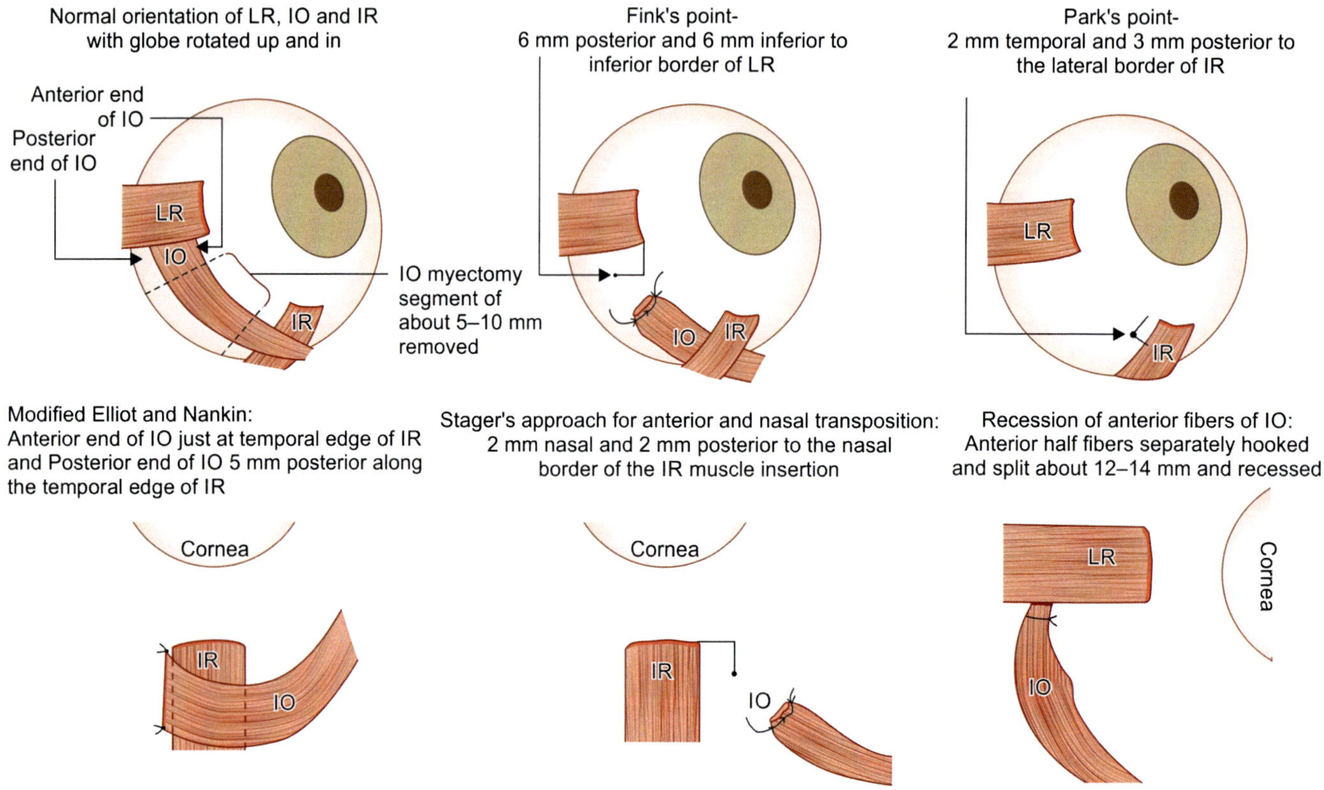

Fig. 8: Inferior oblique procedures.
(IO: inferior oblique; IR: inferior rectus; LR: lateral rectus)

Strengthening Procedures on Inferior Oblique

Strengthening procedures are rarely performed, although advancement has few indications such as abnormal head posture (AHP) in congenital nystagmus. However, as it lacks a good tendinous part, resection usually does not work. Some have tried double breasting or plication and found it to be successful.

Advancement in the form of selective strengthening of the anterior fibers (half or entire width) is done. These fibers are disinserted and advanced superiorly from its insertion toward the SR.

Superior Oblique

Strengthening Procedures on Superior Oblique

Principle: Strengthening the action of the SO is usually carried out using tucking procedures. When all fibers (anterior and posterior) are subjected to tucking, all three functions are increased (incyclotorsion, depression, and abduction). If only anterior fibers are tucked, the incyclotorsion action is enhanced, which is needed when excyclotorsion is the main problem.

Superior Oblique Tuck

Method: After adequate exposure as outlined above, the SO is hooked by placing a small hook on the sclera adjacent to the temporal border of the SR and anterior to the identified SO tendon. The small hook is moved posteriorly as it is held against the sclera. It is then turned superiorly and withdrawn anteriorly, this isolates the SO tendon. The small hook is then exchanged with a larger one and the surrounding attachments between the SR and SO are dissected bluntly.

The tendon can be held with a tendon tucker or a hook (with clamp) and measurement done as per indication. A nonabsorbable suture is passed at the marked part of the tendon (after double folding) and tied. The tucked portion is then allowed to retract back into sub-Tenon's space. Some prefer to suture the same temporally to avoid mechanical restriction.

Some Aphorisms

- Tissues during this procedure and in general for all SO surgeries should be handled with extreme care and minimal dissection to avoid iatrogenic Brown syndrome.
- After tuck, FDT is performed to ensure no tightness of SO (the inferior limbus should be able to cross the horizontal line joining the two canthi without undue force).
- A 4 + 4 mm double folding produces 8 mm tuck which is enough for a 3+ SO over-action (SOOA).
- Selective tuck of the anterior fibers can be done as part of torsional Kestenbaum.

Selective Strengthening of Superior Oblique Muscle (Harada-Ito Procedure and its Modifications)

Aim

Mainly used to strengthen intorsion.

Method

The anterior fibers are the ones which run nearly parallel to the globe and are responsible for intorsion. After isolation of the SO tendon on the temporal side, it is divided longitudinally using two small hooks to about 8–10 mm posterior to its insertion at sclera. The anterior 3 mm is separated from the rest. An anterior tenting of these fibers is achieved using nonabsorbable sutures. The suture is then anchored to the temporal end of the SR.

Harada-Ito plus procedure refers to the incorporation of a few fibers of the posterior part of the SO tendon, which corrects small amounts of hypertropia in addition to the excyclotropia countering effect.

Fell's modification of the Harada-Ito procedure is typically used in bilateral SO palsy, with minimal vertical deviation but significant extorsion. Here the anterior portion of the SO tendon is advanced, after its isolation as above, but using absorbable sutures to secure the anterior 3 mm of fibers. These fibers are then detached from sclera at insertion and advanced temporally. It is then secured to the sclera 8 mm posterior and 2 mm superior to the superior edge of the LR, such that the edge is perpendicular but flat to the superior border of LR.

Weakening Procedures on Superior Oblique

Tenotomy and Tenectomy

After direct identification of the SO, in tenotomy the tendon is disinserted after isolation (full tendon width) and left to retract **(Figs. 9A and B)**. Results are variable.

Tenectomy involves cutting a part of the SO between two hemostats after identification and hooking, nasal to SR. This causes generalized weakening of all functions. In both tenotomy and tenectomy, the tendon is completely transected.

Posterior Tenectomy of Posterior Tenectomy

Here, after hooking the SO, the anterior (1–2 mm width) fibers are spared and a wedge of posterior fibers are excised. This selectively weakens the depression and abduction in down gaze. This is useful for correction pattern strabismus without significant effect on torsion.

Recession of the Superior Oblique

After disinsertion, the tendon is inserted 4 mm nasal to the SR. Graded recession may be done by reinserting closer to SR for lesser effect as per indication. Sometimes the above procedure may cause limitation of depression in downgaze due to anterior placement of SO.

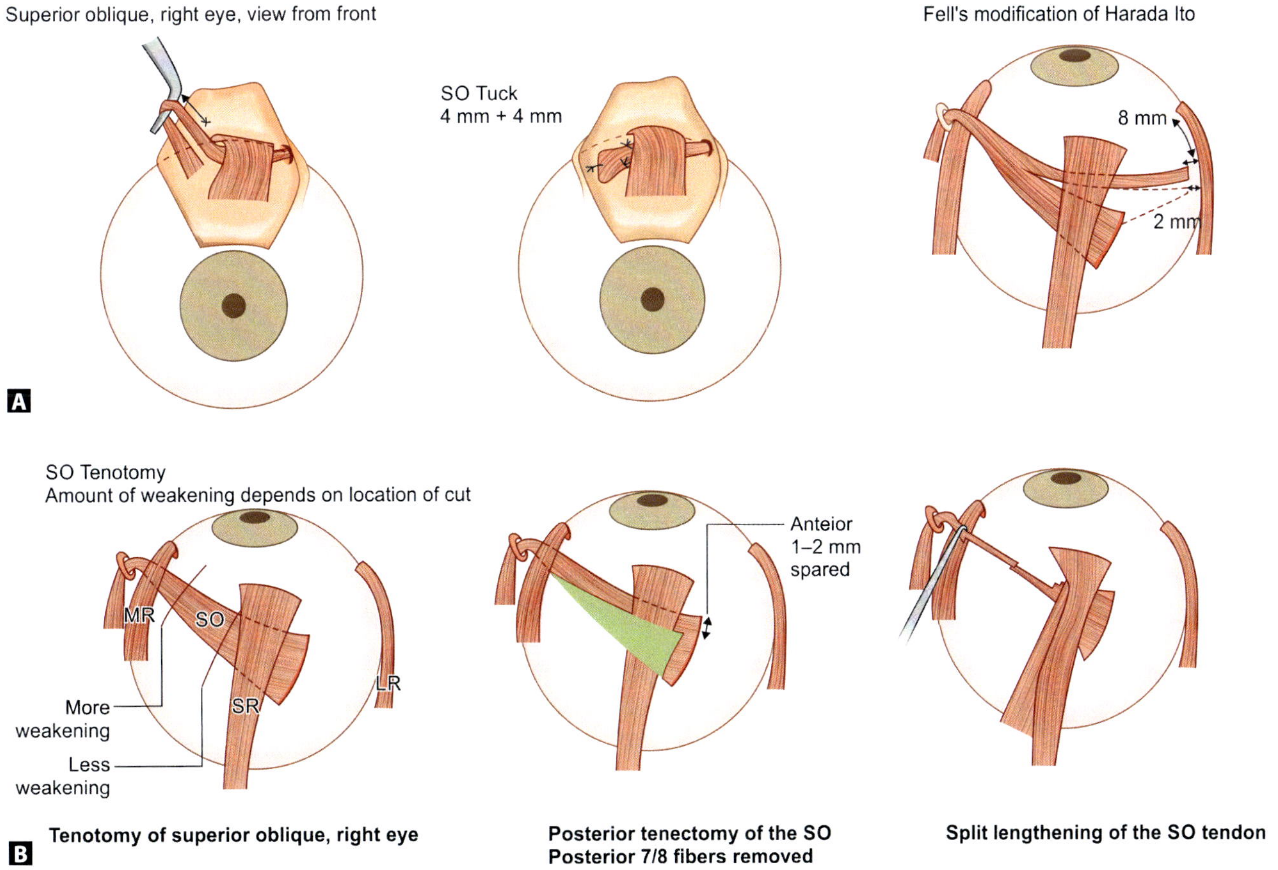

Figs. 9A and B: Superior oblique (SO) procedures. (A) Orientation from front; (B) Orientation from above.

Silicone Band Expander

Superior oblique is isolated nasal to the SR as described above (temporal approach preferred). Two double armed 5-0 Mersilene sutures are placed in the tendon 2 mm apart, the temporal one being 3–4 mm nasal to the nasal border of SR. The tendon is transected and the silicone band (same as used for scleral buckling surgery—2/2.5 mm wide with length varying 5–8 mm) is sutured between the cut ends of the tendon. Tenon's over the tendon and expander is closed with absorbable sutures.

Chicken Suture

Instead of a silicone band, a nonabsorbable suture can be used to separate and expand the cut ends of the SO tendon.

Few Aphorisms

- *Advantage of silicone band*: Fan-shaped insertion preserved, and graded weakening can be achieved.
- *Disadvantage of silicon band*: Possible undesirable adhesions and band exposure/extrusion.

Split Tendon Expansion of Superior Oblique

Similar to silicone band, splitting the tendon be used to lengthen the SO and hence weaken it. Here after isolation of the SO tendon, it is split up to 10 mm length. After the half widths are separated, they are joined together effectively making the length of the segment double.

ADJUSTABLE TECHNIQUES (FIGS. 10A AND B)

Aim

The adjustable addition to strabismus surgeries and its many variations hopes to achieve better postoperative alignment. Some believe it is more to ensure that the muscle does not remain where we certainly do not want it to be, rather than being exact in where we do want it to be. It is more useful in surgeries where variability in outcomes is higher, like incomitant strabismus, especially thyroid eye disease, reoperations, and those with sensory anomalies and diplopia.

Method

There are many approaches described, we summarize a couple here. Either limbal or fornix approach can be used, but limbal preferred.

Bow Type

Bow type can be used for routine recession as well as resection. After rectus muscle isolation and exposure, two

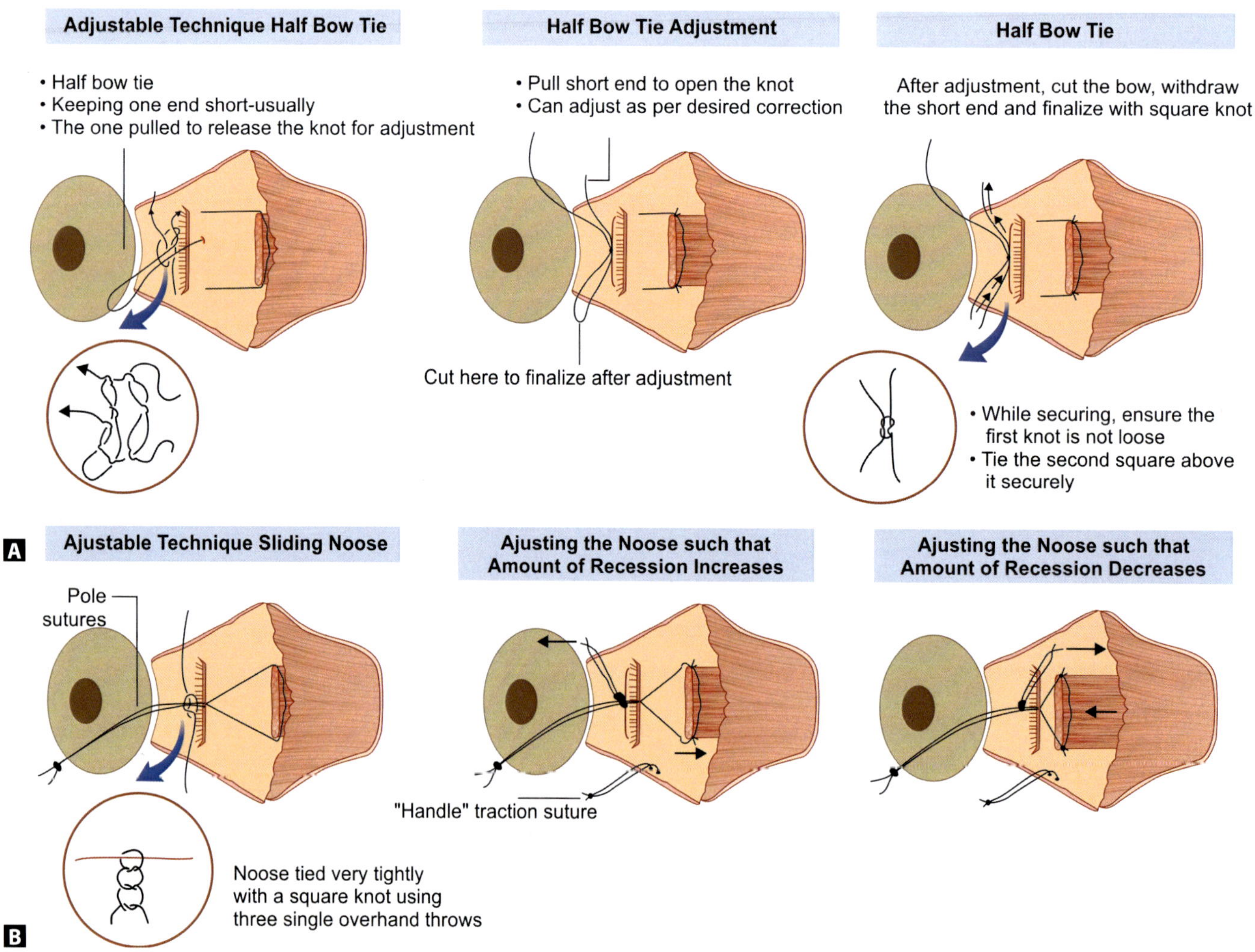

Figs. 10A and B: Adjustable suture techniques.

separate sutures are passed at each end of muscle. The sutures are brought either directly or through a short scleral tunnel to the muscle insertion, maintaining width of the insertion. The two ends are tied with each other in a bow tie knot technique. The half knot is opened at the time of adjustment, secured after due assessment. The ends are cut short enough for adjustment. The limbal conjunctiva sutured with a 5 mm bare sclera.

Sliding Noose (Or Cinch Knot)

After placement of muscle sutures into sclera, a second absorbable suture is tied around the two muscle sutures after they exit sclera. Adjustment is achieved by either sliding the noose anteriorly or posteriorly, as per assessment. After desired position is reached, the muscle sutures are tied securely over the cinch knot.

ADVANCES AND SPECIAL PROCEDURES

Minimally Invasive Strabismus Surgery

Initially propounded by Gobin and later made famous by Mojon, this is truly minimal access surgery, as the name implies.

Principle

Surgical access to the muscles using two small key-hole conjunctival incisions followed by dissection of the muscle from the surrounding tissue through the same openings followed by recession, plication, transposition, etc. (MISS has been adapted for a variety of strabismus surgeries over the years).

Aim

To achieve strabismus surgery with minimal disturbance of natural anatomy and for better healing, using key-hole conjunctival incision sites placed strategically close to the area of manipulation for the muscle in question. Other benefits being improved cosmesis, less irritation and reducing complications such as Dellen and Tenon's prolapse.

Method

- Limbal traction suture (Prolene 6-0) secured with artery forceps to move eye away from the field of action of the muscle in question.
- Edges of muscle visualized through the conjunctiva.
- Conjunctival incisions are made radial, parainsertional 1-2 mm in length which may range in number from 2 to 6 as per the case requirement. Start from insertion site visualized and travel backward along the length of the muscle.
- After incisions, a small hook is placed to ensure edges of the muscle are clearly identified.
- Using Westcott scissors, the episcleral tissue is gently dissected to better delineate the muscle edge. Dissection is continued over the muscle to join the two incisions in order to create a tunnel covered with overlying intact conjunctiva.
- Hook muscle completely after the above and dissect check ligaments as well as intermuscular septum about 6–7 mm posteriorly.
- *Recession in MISS*: After retracting conjunctiva over tendon, full thickness locking bites using single-ended 6-0 polyglactin are secured at each end of muscle insertion. The amount of recession required is measured and marked on sclera. Scleral sutures are preplaced using partial thickness bites which run parallel to muscle edge at both sides. After confirming secure placement of sutures, muscle is disinserted using Westcott scissors under the conjunctiva. Ensure that the sutures and overlying conjunctiva is not damaged. The muscle is secured at the intended distance by tightening the preplaced sutures which are then tied off.
- *Plication in MISS*: The conjunctival openings are similar as above, parallel along the edge of the muscle and the amount of plication is measured on calipers and marked. A forceps is used to grasp the muscle at the location and a single-ended 6-0 polyglactin is passed full thickness through conjunctiva, Tenon's, and muscle. It is brought out through the conjunctival opening, the loop of the suture between muscle and conjunctiva is grasped with forceps and drawn out of the incision. This is required to free the suture from the conjunctiva and Tenon's ensuring that it freely passes through muscle belly. Its end is brought out and tied to the needle end, securing the muscle with locking knot. The needle is then passed through sclera at the insertion site, partial thickness, parallel bites on each side of insertion. The muscle tendon is drawn forward using an iris spatula and can either be flattened above or below the muscle belly. Good assistance is needed, such that while tightening the muscle does not sag backward. Suture is tied off to achieve plication.
- Conjunctiva is stretched backward in order to make the scleral pass, this can be difficult in older people and resurgeries. In the very young, excess Tenon's may compromise visualization.
- Conjunctival opening is closed using self-buried knots (continuous inverted sutures) with 8-0 vicryl.

Some Aphorisms

- During incision step, the ciliary vessels on the muscle do not move, while conjunctival vessels do, this is helpful to localize the muscle before incisions are placed.
- To facilitate some surgical steps, it may be necessary to create tunnels between the key-hole incisions.
- The openings are kept as far away from the limbus as possible, such that they can be joined together to create a larger opening if needed. This is useful especially in the initial transition phase to this technique.

- The location of the incisions are planned such that they are completely covered by the lids except in upgaze or downgaze.
- Microscope visualization is preferred for this technique.

LOOP MYOPEXY

Yokoyama in 2001 proposed a surgical idea for heavy eye syndrome or myopic strabismus fixus convergens (having inferior shift of LR and nasal shift of SR). He suggested uniting the LR and SR to convert them into behaving like a muscle pulley, pushing the herniated eyeball back into the muscle cone.

Method

After conjunctival incision, isolate the LR and SR. A nonabsorbable suture (5-0 Ethibond) is passed through lateral half of SR and superior half of LR about 14–16 mm behind limbus and tied with locking knots. Scleral fixation is not necessary, but performed by some as a modification. Scleral fixation is risky in highly myopic eyes and inadvertent globe perforation during scleral pass should be avoided.

Another variation is to perform scleral fixation using 240 silicone retinal band with Watzke sleeve as a tethering aid instead of the sutures. Some perform MR recession if FDT shows restriction, while others prefer a staged approach.

NISHIDA'S PARTIAL TENDON TRANSPOSITION PROCEDURE

Nishida (2003) described a procedure for chronic LR palsy cases to strengthen abduction and at the same time not compromising primary and downgaze position with vessel sparing approach.

Method

Nonabsorbable (5-0 polyester braided or 6-0 polypropylene nonbraided) suture is inserted at the temporal edge (one-third width of muscle) of each vertical rectus muscle, about 8–10 mm posterior to insertion. The sutures should avoid the ciliary vessels during muscle bite. The scleral bites are then taken 10–12 mm behind limbus at the superotemporal or inferotemporal quadrant. This in effect transposes the vertical recti partially along the vector of LR without tenotomy or muscle splitting, thus preventing anterior segment ischemia.

In 2013, the same group modified this procedure to not even involve splitting. Here the lateral muscle belly margins of the SR and IR are directly sutured onto the sclera (superotemporal or inferonasal quadrant). Here the sutures transfer the lateral muscle bellies temporally creating additional muscle insertion as new points of action, similar to pulleys. The transposed bellies thus change the vector of vertical recti along LR, generating additional force at suturing point.

Y SPLIT AND MEDIAL TRANSPOSITION OF LATERAL RECTUS

Another procedure described for complete third nerve palsy is the Y split and medial transposition of LR. This has also been modified and used to treat the upshoot and downshoot observed in DRS along with ipsilateral recession of the LR to counter the cocontraction.

Method

A near complete conjunctival peritomy is done via limbal approach. LR is exposed, isolated, and split 15–22 mm posteriorly. Preferably two locking bites using nonabsorbable 6-0 polyester sutures are placed at the edge of each of the split muscle halves. Muscle halves are disinserted and the sutures are passed through the eye of Gass muscle hook. Using the Gass hook, the upper half is passed under the SR and SO tendon behind its insertion and the lower half is passed between the globe and both IR and IO. The upper and lower halves are then re-attached to the superior and inferior border of MR insertion, respectively. When combined with MR resection, this procedure gives greater correction (beyond 80 PD).

For DRS, a further recession of about 6–7 mm of the LR is performed to reduce the increased tension due to stretch obtained by the Y-split and also treats severe upshoot and downshoot due to co-contraction.

CROSS VERTICAL RECTUS TRANSPOSITION FULL WIDTH OR PARTIAL FOR DUANE'S RETRACTION SYNDROME: ABDUCTION DEFICIT

Vertical rectus transposition (VRT), earlier described by Hummelsheim for complete sixth nerve palsy, has also been utilized with various modifications for DRS.

Aim

The aim here is to change the vector of the vertical recti such that the affected loss of adduction or abduction is compensated, without compromising primary position and downgaze. This also improves binocular field as well as shifts the field toward the affected gaze.

Method

Full tendon, partial tendon, or a single muscle VRT have all been described for DRS. A newer modification involves partial splitting of both SR and IR with vessel sparing steps. The two halves are secured on nonabsorbable 5-0 polyester sutures and disinserted. Each half is brought beneath the LR and secured at the opposite corners of the LR insertion. In contrast to classical VRT and partial vertical rectus transposition (pVRT), here the new insertion is not along the spiral of Tillaux, rather one end is beneath the LR leading to an oblique orientation of the insertion. Various modifications with adjustable techniques have been described for the same as well.

Some Aphorisms

- The transposed muscles do not have active innervation in the field of gaze of the affected muscle, hence allows the weakening of the antagonist to have greater effect.
- *Other means of augmenting the VRT have been suggested*: Ipsilateral MR weakening; ipsilateral LR plication; transposed muscle resection; crossed adjustable approach, etc. A detailed view is beyond the scope of the present work, but has been summarized in the work by Doyle and Hunter (JAAPOS, 2019—see suggested reading).

TETHERING OR PERIOSTEAL (MECHANICAL) FIXATION OF THE GLOBE

Sometimes, despite supramaximal surgeries, the eyes cannot be aligned even in the primary position, especially for long-standing restrictive and postparalytic strabismus. In such cases, mechanical fixation of the globe in the primary position using the periosteal tissue for tethering is an alternative.

Method

An apically based periosteal flap is created from any of the orbital walls. A periosteal elevator is used to separate the flap from the orbital bone, using 5-0 Mersilene it is secured at the anterior edge. The flap is then sutured to sclera, anterior to the paralyzed rectus muscle insertion. Some prefer to utilize an additional titanium plate affixed to the orbital wall adjacent to the paralyzed muscle for extra stability. Here, the suture arises from the posterior aspect of the plate and is sutured to sclera in a similar manner as above. The globe is then rotated to the periosteal flap (or titanium plate) and fixed into place using nonabsorbable sutures.

Few Aphorisms

- The surgeon may not be able to visualize the actual site of suturing of the flap onto sclera, hence experienced judgment is advised.
- Initial overcorrection is preferred.

Supramaximal Recess–Resect Procedures

Recess and resect procedure larger than the conventional measurements on horizontal rectus muscle surgery has been tried for large angle horizontal strabismus. The strabismus is around 70–80 PD and is not amenable to correction with two muscle surgery. The normal alternative is engaging one muscle of the other eye also. Since in these large angle tropias, the fixing eye is the normal eye, the patient and relatives may be apprehensive and may not agree for surgery on the normal eye; and therefore super- or supramaximal recess–resect procedure can be tried. The procedure is more relevant in sensory exotropias (exotropia in long-standing loss of vision/deep amblyopia). Resection of 8.5 mm of MR and 12.5 recession of LR is done. The problem of incomitance and deficit abduction should be borne in mind.

TRANSPLANTATION

True muscle transplantation has been described for very large angle ET or exotropia. The aim is to overcome 70–80 PD or more of horizontal strabismus and 20–25 PD of vertical in patients having even larger degrees of deviation. "True" muscle transplantations consist of transplanting the resected portion of a muscle to the ipsilateral antagonist muscle to lengthen the muscle and enhance its weakness. Though this portion of muscle has no contractile force and remains as a fibrotic band, very similar to the silicone band used to weaken the SO muscle. The advantage is its replacement for supramaximal recessions and nonconcurrence of patient to touch the sound eye. But this procedure has not gained much popularity.

Mini-Tenotomy

Central or edge mini-tenotomy has been described as an adjunct procedure to achieve 2–4 PD of correction by additional weakening of rectus muscle. It can be performed under topical anesthesia (with added 2.5% phenylephrine for vasoconstriction), the insertion is grasped with toothed forceps through intact conjunctiva, after identifying the same by following ciliary vessels. After confirmation, central 2–3 mm of the tendon is cut using Westcott scissors through intact conjunctiva.

AMNIOTIC MEMBRANE TRANSPLANTATION

Amniotic membrane is useful to prevent recurrence of adhesions in patients with restrictive strabismus of long-standing duration caused by conjunctival scarring, fat adherence, or muscle contracture.

SUGGESTED READING

1. Coats DK, Olitsky SE. Strabismus Surgery and its Complications. Berlin/Heidelberg: Springer-Verlag; 2007.
2. Doyle JJ, Hunter DG. Transposition procedures in Duane retraction syndrome. J AAPOS. 2019;23(1):5-14.
3. Kushner BJ. Strabismus: Practical Pearls You Won't Find in Textbooks. Berlin: Springer; 2017.
4. Ludwig IH, Clark RA, Stager DR Sr. New strabismus surgical techniques. J AAPOS. 2013;17(1):79-88.
5. Sharma P. Strabismus Simplified. New Delhi: CBS Publishers & Distributors; 2013.
6. Wright KW, Strube YNJ. Color Atlas of Strabismus Surgery. New York: Springer-Verlag New York; 2015.

27

CHAPTER

Complications of Strabismus Surgery

Shivanand J Sheth, Syed Faraaz Hussain

INTRODUCTION

Surgical complications are an integral part of any surgical procedure. The only way to avoid complications is to avoid doing surgery. Surgical complications are directly related to the number of surgeries and therefore, statistically, less number of surgeries will result in less number of complications or denial of complications by a surgeon is another option. But our purpose does not fit to any of these categories. Our goal and desire is to obtain the best possible result without any complications. However, this ideal situation does not always prevails and we must be conversant with all types of complications and learn to avoid and treat them.

Normally, in strabismus surgery, three varieties of complications can occur. First, a complication not acceptable to the patient, e.g., over- or undercorrection of the alignment. Second, a known complication which occurs commonly in many patients and resolves with time. Third, an inadvertent serious complication which was not anticipated by the surgeon. It is imperative and prudent on part of the surgeon to explain in plain language, the types of complications which may occur. An "informed consent", in this regard, is the best insurance. We can also relate complications as mild and severe, which are enumerated in **Table 1**.

Another problem with the most common, so-called complication with strabismus surgery, is obvious under- or overcorrection. It becomes more relevant as this result of surgery cannot be hidden and therefore is the biggest area dissatisfaction. However you must explain to the patient preoperatively about the success of alignment; persistence of strabismus is the end result of an unsuccessful surgery. An ideal result from strabismus surgery should include the following:

- Minimum postoperative discomfort
- No conjunctival scarring
- Normal palpebral aperture
- Normal ductions and versions
- Normal visual acuity
- Most importantly, orthotropia.

But this perfect postoperative situation is seldom present. If above stated ideal result is not obtainable, then an "acceptable" result should be tried for. Intermittent exotropia, paresis of ocular muscles, or complex strabismus are some conditions where "perfect" result cannot be expected; and this should be explained clearly to the patient. Even in other less complex cases, an acceptable result could include small undercorrection or overcorrection, minimum vertical deviation, barely visible lid fissure anomaly, minimum conjunctival redness, no suture granuloma, and timely resolution of suture knots and inflammation, to name a few. Some early postoperative phenomena which are transient and should not be narrated to the patient as complications include transient suture reaction, subconjunctival hemorrhage, slight lid edema, conjunctival abrasions, and dellen formations. All these postoperative situations are not avoidable most of times, and in practice, should not be considered as complications per se, and the patient should be pacified accordingly.

Situations mentioned in **Table 1**, which persist after a stipulated time, can be labeled as complications and treated accordingly.

There could be complications unrelated to the strabismus surgery, that is, complications arising from general or local anesthesia, intra- or postoperatively **(Table 2)**.

TABLE 1: Strabismus surgery complications.

Mild	*Severe*
Dellen	Globe perforation
Chronic red eye	Orbital infection
Pyogenic granuloma	Endophthalmitis
Tenon's prolapse	Surgically-induced necrotizing scleritis
Epithelial inclusion cyst	Slipped muscle
Chemosis	Lost muscle
Suture granuloma	Retinal detachment
	Fat adherence syndrome
	Anterior segment ischemia

TABLE 2: Strabismus surgery complications by steps.

Preoperative	*Intraoperative*	*Postoperative*
• Non-cooperative patient • Incorrect assessment • Amount of deviation • Prior history • Inadequate amblyopia treatment • Inadequate refraction	• *Anesthesia related*: – Malignant hyperthermia – Cardiac arrest – Oculocardiac reflex and bradycardia – Allergy – Gastritis • *Intraoperative surgery related*: – Muscle hematoma – Inappropriate incision – Scleral perforation – Muscle-tendon rupture – Loose sutures – Orbital hemorrhage – Hyphema – Lost and/or slipped muscle – Muscle split in two (PITS) – Tenon's rupture with fat prolapse	• Endophthalmitis • Suture granuloma • Tenon's prolapse • Conjunctival cyst • Dellen • Anterior segment ischemia • Overcorrection and undercorrection • Orbital cellulitis • Adherence syndrome • Conjunctival scar • Iatrogenic Brown syndrome • Lid fissure anomalies

(PITS: pulled-in-two syndrome)

Strabismus surgery complications (minor and major) have a prevalence of about 1 in 400, with the most common serious complication being globe perforation (1:1,000), while retinal detachment and endophthalmitis are the least common. Anterior segment ischemia has been reported around 1 in 13,000.

Most preoperative issues can be prevented by diligent workup, having standard operating procedures and a "time-out" before induction of any patient.

ANESTHESIA RELATED

These being the few instances where the patient's life can be threatened, due care must to taken to prevent the same.

Cardiac issues must be ruled out in all cases under going strabismus surgery. Cardiac arrest, though an extremely rare complication, can occur and should be prevented by better preparation preoperatively, including a check by a general physician, as well as an anesthetist.

Malignant Hyperthermia

A true life-threatening emergency, occurring as an acute event due to extreme heat production by the body, usually triggered by inhalational agents (e.g., halothane) and muscle relaxants (e.g., succinylcholine) leading to sequence of events causing excess muscle contraction and anaerobic metabolism with cell death. More common in children, can occur sporadically, also supposed to have genetic and familial predisposition.

How to Identify?

Tachycardia is the earliest sign, with unstable blood pressure (BP) and tachypnea. Cyanosis, trismus, elevated CO_2 levels, electrolyte imbalance eventually lead to renal failure, cardiac arrest, and disseminated intravascular coagulation causing death.

Prevention

Intravenous (IV) dantrolene (muscle relaxant) preoperatively and before induction in predisposed individuals usually leads to uneventful anesthesia.

How to Treat?

Stop triggering agents and complete surgery. Hyperventilate with 100% O_2, along with IV dantrolene and efforts to reduce body temperature (IV iced saline, iced lavage of stomach, bladder and rectum, and iced blanket). To treat systemic complications as efficiently as possible (cardiac failure, renal failure, hyperkalemia, and metabolic acidosis).

Oculocardiac Reflex

Oculocardiac reflex (OCR) is another important life-threatening possibility, albeit extremely rare.

How to Identify?

Sinus bradycardia, ectopic beats, and sinus arrest noted during manipulation of EOMs, especially medial rectus (MR).

Prevention

Always perform squint surgery with anesthetist stand-by, even if topical or peribulbar route is used. On noting even the early signs, muscle should be released till heart rate stabilizes. Some prefer to give preoperative atropine intramuscular or even intraglossal (0.1 mg/kg), but this should be done with the coordination of anesthetist.

How to Treat?

Intravenous atropine (0.15 mg/kg) should be given, if OCR persists. In recalcitrant cases, one can give retrobulbar lignocaine block; which blocks the afferent arm of the reflex.

INTRAOPERATIVE (SURGERY RELATED)

Hemorrhage

This is one of the most common complications of most types of extraocular surgeries, including strabismus. Predispositions such as uncontrolled hypertension, antiplatelet medications, and blood dyscrasias should be kept in mind.

How to Identify?

Conjunctival hemorrhages are usually due to retrobulbar or peribulbar anesthesia. Any active bleeding is usually obvious on table, once the conjunctival incision is made. Conjunctival ecchymosis and chemosis is usually obvious, and in cases of orbital hemorrhage (usually due to blocks), sudden raised IOP and proptosis can be noted. Muscle hemorrhage can rarely become severe enough to cause muscle hematoma, but when it occurs it can jeopardize the muscle surgery. Such severe cases are usually due to an underlying arterial bleed, missed at the time of surgery.

Orbital hematoma, when a vortex vein has been cut, causes a large, anterior, and unsightly hematoma. It is rare, but can be severe, though usually well controlled with pressure.

Postoperative subconjunctival hemorrhage is nearly an ubiquitous phenomena and preoperative counseling usually benefits.

How to Prevent?

For most types of hemorrhages, careful planning before the procedure (prefer sub-Tenon's block to retrobulbar, etc.) and meticulous inspection before conjunctival incision is usually enough. As a dictum, any sharp tipped instruments, especially scissors should be used only under good visualization, with tips and entire shaft visible before blade closure. Topical vasoconstrictors are preferred by some, but can increase BP. Light cautery can be done at the expected steps of surgery which predisposes to hemorrhages (conjunctival incision and muscle disinsertion) or pressure is usually enough. History of any blood dyscrasias or use of blood-thinning drugs should be taken.

How to Treat?

For mild intraoperative cases, pressure and light cautery are usually enough. Some prefer swabstick soaked in 1:1,000 adrenaline with the knowledge of anesthetists. For severe hemorrhage (orbital or muscle which may compromise optic nerve), lateral canthotomy is performed.

Globe Perforation

Globe perforation is most common among the severe complications of strabismus surgery, but rarely leading to poor or very poor visual outcomes. Complex surgeries, needing deeper tissue dissection and passage of needles posteriorly (Faden, etc.) or those with thin sclera are at higher risk. Rarely, the type of needle if erroneously chosen with wider breadth or cutting type instead of spatulated, may lead to greater risk of globe perforation.

How to Identify?

It can go unrecognized in many cases on table. Many a times the surgeon gets the feel of a deeper pass of the needle and suspects perforation. A bead of vitreous at the needle tip or a small brown uveal tissue might be visible at the entry or exit site of needle. Rarely dark deoxygenated blood might be visible as a bead. Globe may become soft, even without visible loss of vitreous or blood.

How to Prevent?

Check needles, keep surgical field clear, and good exposure before needle pass. Ensure assistant and surgeon are both comfortable. Avoid suturing in areas with scleral thinning. Avoid excess pull on tissues, including muscle. Hang back or modifications may be preferable if surgical access difficult or thin sclera.

How to Treat?

In case of strong suspicion of perforation, remove suture and needle from the said site and place at alternative location before proceeding. If visible vitreous, excise it flush to globe surface and suture site with 6-0 polyglactin suture interrupted bites. Indirect ophthalmoscopy to be performed when suspected perforation, preferable dilate on table, and examine before closure of case. In case of noted retinal break, vitreoretinal opinion should be sought.

Slipped/Lost Muscle

There is a significant difference between a slipped muscle and the term lost muscle. A muscle is not actually "lost". During surgery, it has simply been lost from hold and retracted into the orbit and is lost from view and cannot be seen. This is a serious intraoperative complication.

In contrast, a "slipped" muscle occurs gradually during the postoperative period. The slipped muscle may remain attached to the sclera, albeit, further back than where it was attached; or it may slip back into its capsule while the capsule remains attached to the sclera.

The MR is most likely to be lost because it is not attached with other muscles by intermuscular fascia nor to the orbit. Loss of this muscle can occur intraoperatively, when extensive dissection of the intermuscular fascia has been done and the muscle has slipped from hold. In another situation, the sutures attaching the muscle to the sclera give way, and the muscle retracts back into the orbit. This can be seen in the immediate postoperative period. The inferior rectus (IR) is well in association with inferior oblique and Lockwood's ligament; the superior rectus with superior oblique, such that it is highly unlikely of these muscles getting lost in the orbit and out of view. The complication will be evident as the eye will not move in the direction of the lost muscle.

Prevention

- The sutures should be placed properly in the muscle tissue, taking precaution to incorporate full thickness of the muscle. As a rule, the sutures are placed 0.5–1.0 mm, behind the line of muscle disinsertion, not at the margin of cut end. This extra placement is adjusted in the final surgical numbers.
- Place the needle into the sclera at least 0.2–0.3 mm deep and creating a track of at least 1.5 mm long.
- The synthetic absorbable sutures should be well tied, with multiple knots (at least for MR).
- Do not dissect the intermuscular septum beyond the emergence of muscle from the posterior Tenon. This ensures that the muscle remains visible even if the suture knot has slipped and its attachment to sclera is lost.

Management

If the muscle is lost on table or seen on the postoperative day of dressing, the patient should be taken again in operating room and the exploration of muscle tried. A few drops of phenylephrine 5% should be instilled in the operative area to blanch the Tenon's capsule that will make the red muscle more conspicuous.

If the lost muscle is detected in late postoperative period, the best option is to get an MRI done and identify the position of the lost muscle. A careful and cautious retrievement of muscle should be tried and reattached to the intended site. No blind groping should be tried as this can cause further injury and orbital hemorrhage. If the attempt is futile, then a muscle transposition surgery is the option.

Muscle/Tendon Rupture

During the course of surgery, the muscle or tendon can rupture. This usually happens when excessive force is applied with the muscle hook or the muscle is stretched too much between two hooks.

The best prevention is to apprise the assistant beforehand regarding manipulation of muscle and keep him/her comfortable.

Posterior Chamber Hemorrhage

Posterior chamber hemorrhage is uncommon and usually iatrogenic; occurring because of scleral/retinal perforation. Caution regarding the suture bites has already been discussed.

■ POSTOPERATIVE

Chronic Red Eye

Redness after strabismus surgery is almost ubiquitous, but its persistence is the bothersome issue. If red eye remains or recurs weeks to months after surgery, patients are concerned, and rightfully so, especially about cosmesis. It is usually complained about by patients or guardians, especially if persistent. Diffuse conjunctival congestion, localized congestion over muscle insertion site or over suture site is usually noted.

How to Prevent?

It can be prevented by meticulous dissection with avoidance of orbital fat prolapse during posterior dissection. Removal of clots before conjunctival closure, burying knots, and prevention of Tenon's prolapse are all good practices to prevent persistence of red eye. Also care should be taken not to include the plica or caruncle in the conjunctival closure.

How to Treat?

Intense topical steroids for a month postoperatively can be given in those having predisposition to bleeding and fragile conjunctiva, like reoperations. Rarely, long-term topical steroids and lubricants are indicated. In persistent cases, depot subconjunctival steroids can be given to reduce inflammation and conjunctival bulk.

Anterior Segment Ischemia

It is defined as spectrum of changes secondary to compromise of the anterior segment circulation of eye, which can range from mild reversible symptoms to phthisis. Specific to strabismus surgery, the typical anterior segment ischemia described is usually noted after surgery on three recti muscles or more, and particularly if both vertical muscles are involved, where the anterior ciliary vessels from the muscular branches have been severed. Most patients recover within 2 weeks but some may take 3 months. Circulation is established from collaterals from deep circulation and never from recanalization of the anterior ciliary vessels. Mild ischemia is seen in many of patients even with two muscle surgery, but it is mild and not clinically significant.

Olver and Lee have graded anterior segment ischemia as follows:

- *Grade 1*: Reduced iris circulation
- *Grade 2*: With pupillary signs
- *Grade 3*: With uveitis
- *Grade 4*: With keratopathy.

Severe ischemia leads to blurring of vision and pain within 24 hours of the surgery. Pupils are dilated and conjunctival congestion present postoperatively. Conjunctival congestion is normal in postoperative period; pupillary dilatation may be due to preoperative peribulbur anesthesia used, which should normalize in couple of days. Persistent pupillary dilation with hazy vision, should herald anterior segment ischemia. Anterior chamber is deep with flare and circulating pigment. Vitreous shows haze and intraocular pressure (IOP) is reduced. Iris angiography shows poor arterial filling, especially adjacent to the operated rectus muscles. Delayed changes include cataract formation, iris atrophy and pupillary abnormalities, ciliary shut-down, and eventually can lead to phthisis bulbi, if very severe.

The first three grades of the disorder are not significant clinically, but the fourth grade is severe with corneal edema, deep folds, heavy flare with hypopyon, and sometimes cataract. Hypotony can result and patients with modern therapy can recover, but permanent damage from cataract, corneal scarring, and macular changes result.

How to Prevent?

The following points should be taken into consideration to avoid anterior segment ischemia:

- Vertical muscles are more susceptible to ischemia though they have two vessels but are not backed by long posterior ciliary arteries.
- Older and vascularly compromised patients are more prone.
- When more than three muscle surgery is necessary, it should be done after a gap of few years.
- Even then, a "tucking" procedure is advisable than resection.
- It is not practically possible to predict which patients will have clinically significant anterior segment ischemia, but patients with atherosclerosis, hypertension, and vascularly compromised patients and elderly persons are more prone for the disorder.

Treatment

In acute phase, pain is treated with 1% atropine topically to relieve ciliary spasm; administration of high dose of local and systemic steroids is the standard treatment. Local circulation can be improved by IV dextran 40 in a 5–10% dextrose saline solution. For first 2 days, 1 L per day followed by 500 mL for next 3 days. Serum electrolytes, sugars, and renal function must be monitored diligently. Long-term oral steroids with slow taper are usually required in severe cases, but most patients do show improvement without significant vision loss after prolonged course.

Adherence Syndrome

It is usually caused by abnormal attachments developing between structures in the orbit after strabismus surgery due to damage to muscle cone, Tenon's capsule, or the connective tissue network among the orbital fat leading to its prolapse followed by fibro-fatty scarring. It is mostly seen after surgery of inferior oblique, but trauma and lid surgeries can also be causative. A high degree of care and suspicion must be kept in mind in all such cases and one should be on the lookout for the fatty yellowish reflex noted on table. Postoperatively, patient usually presents with progressive hypotropia and limitation of elevation.

How to Prevent?

During inferior oblique surgery, the posterior edge of the muscle should be visualized when attempting dissection avoiding damage to the posterior Tenon's and orbital fat. Excessive bleeding to be avoided, use of minimal cautery and removal of blood clots before closure should be done.

How to Treat?

If noted during surgery, careful reposition with removal of excess fat can be attempted and the posterior Tenon's repaired. Postoperatively, especially in established cases, surgical exploration of inferior fornix with meticulous dissection, excision of orbital fat noted, repair of posterior Tenon's defect followed by recession of IR. Amniotic membrane grafting is usually advised. Corticosteroid irrigations, plastic sheets, mesh repair, and sleeves around muscles have all been attempted, but results in reoperations are relatively poor.

Infection

Infection as a whole, after strabismus surgery, is quite uncommon in the modern era.

Acute conjunctivitis, with discharge, can be easily avoided with preoperative topical antibiotics and use of povidone iodine preoperatively. If at all it occurs, it is mostly if the patient has not taken due aseptic precautions, and can be treated effectively. Two important infections can occur which are matter of concern, but are extremely rare.

1. Endophthalmitis is fortunately extremely rare (1 in 30,000) after strabismus surgery. It is recognized by the usual signs of conjunctival hyperemia, lid swelling and pain, anterior chamber reaction with or without hypopyon, and vitreous haze. Vision is seriously affected and continuously diminishes. With the first confirmatory signs, a vitreoretinal surgeon consultation should be done.
2. Orbital cellulitis is another dreaded, but again rare complication. Severe conjunctival congestion and chemosis, pain, proptosis, and limitation of ocular movements are the cardinal signs.

Prevention

Endophthalmitis usually occurs when there has been a perforation during surgery and the precautions have been already previously highlighted. Orbital cellulitis, in most part, is due to poor preoperative aseptic preparation and the infection has gone into the orbit during surgery. Postpone surgery if clinical evidence of conjunctivitis or blepharitis in immediate preoperative period is noted. Meticulous preoperative instillation povidone iodine (5%) in the conjunctival sac, along with sterility maintenance at all times is absolutely necessary. Steroid-antibiotic ointment at end of the procedure is usually advised. Topical antibiotics drops along with anti-inflammatory drops should be given for a week or two depending upon the local condition. Lubricating drops should also be given at least for two weeks till the sutures start dissolving.

Prolapse of Tenon's Capsule

Prolapse of the Tenon's fascia is an unsightly sight in postoperative period. It occurs where there has been incomplete closure of the conjunctival wound.

It usually shrinks with time and no intervention is required. Only in cases where it is extensive, then reposition and proper suturing of conjunctiva is required.

Chronic Suture Granuloma

It is again a rare postoperative complication occurring in <0.5% of cases. A red, raised, and hard protruding mass at the site of muscle insertion. Occurs a week after surgery and though not painful, but may produce some discomfort. It consists of chronic inflammatory cells and it takes some weeks to disappear. It usually subsides with the absorption of sutures, but slight protuberance can remain.

Treatment consists of topical steroids for 2–3 weeks. If it does not subside, then it can be surgically removed, once the absorption period of sutures has completed. With the modern day polyglactic or polyglycolic acid sutures, which are inert, this complication is very rare.

Dellen

A dellen is a local depression in the cornea near the limbus. It is caused by localized dehydration of the cornea and "shrinkage" of stroma at that point. It is differentiated from ulcer or cornea melt, that it has an intact epithelium, although there is pooling of fluorescein dye at that point. It is not alarming and does not interfere with the result of strabismus surgery. It is most commonly seen with limbal conjunctival incisions.

Treatment consists of patching the eye for a few days; the cornea gets hydrated and the dellen disappears. Alternatively, lubricant drops may be used till the dellen disappears.

Postoperative Brown Syndrome

Iatrogenic Brown syndrome results when the superior oblique tendon is tucked or shortened by resection, thus limiting its excursion in upgaze during adduction. The superior oblique muscle has unique anatomy, with the muscle, trochlea, and the reflected tendon working independently. This means that the superior oblique tendon has an excursion potential of 16 mm from extreme downgaze to extreme upgaze. When a tuck is done or the tendon is resected, the amount of available tendon is reduced, that is, the amount of tendon from trochlea to the insertion is shortened and the full elevation in adduction cannot be achieved and Brown syndrome results.

Prevention

The best way to prevent postoperative Brown syndrome is to avoid surgery to shorten the superior oblique tendon. Normally, in cases of congenital superior oblique palsy, enough redundant tendon is available and shortening procedure does not create Brown syndrome, but in acquired disorders, the surgery should be avoided and inferior oblique surgery should be the choice.

Treatment

Usually small discrepancy of limitation of elevation in adduction can be overlooked if there is no gross problem to the patient. In any case, few weeks' time should be given postoperatively, during which the condition subsides spontaneously. If not, then resurgery to reverse tuck or recession procedure should be thought of.

POSTOPERATIVE CARE

Planning of postoperative care begins during the surgery.

Eye and Personal Care

- Avoid antibiotic eye drops during the surgery and keep the cornea moist to prevent damage to cornea. Suture conjunctiva or approximate edges well enough to prevent Tenon's or bare sclera exposure. Keep knots small or buried. Wash clots before closure. Pad well or counsel accordingly if left open (depending upon type of surgery).
- In all cases, as a precaution, antibiotic and anti-inflammatory drops, usually combined, should be given for first one week 4–5 times-a-day. In selected cases, if warranted, these drops can be continued for further one week along with lubricating drops.
- Discharge from the hospital to be coordinated with anesthetist, including schedule for suture adjustment.
- Before discharge, check for evidence of slipped muscle or any significant infection.
- Corrective glasses as preoperatively should be continued unless having prisms or needing adjustment later.
- Occlusion, if to be continued, should be started 2 weeks postoperatively, after all conjunctival hyperemia and inflammation has subsided.
- Children can return to school in about 7–10 days, but should avoid swimming, sports, and heavy exercise for 2 weeks.
- Adults can return to routine indoor work in a week as per comfort level, but to take due care for asepsis and avoid heavy exercise. Work involving dirty surroundings or exposure to environmental hazards should be avoided for 2 weeks.

SUGGESTED READING

1. Agrawal S. Strabismus for every Ophthalmologist. New Delhi, India: Springer. 2019.
2. David C, Skott O. Strabismus Surgery and its Complications. USA: Springer; 2007.
3. Del Monte MA, Archer SM. Atlas of Pediatric Ophthalmology and Strabismus Surgery. Mischigan, USA: Churchill Livingstone; 1993.

4. Helveston EM. (2005). Surgical Management of Strabismus, 5th edition. [online] Available from: https://www.aao.org/assets/86858597-4bc8-4e9b-a94f-8960daf40cb0/636343503861030000/strabismus-surgical-management-of-strabismus-ehelveston-pdf?inline=1. [Last accessed October, 2021].
5. James R, Wilson ME, Saunders RA, Trivedi RH. Pediatric Ophthalmology: Current Thought and a Practical Guide. Germany: Springer; 2009.
6. Kushner, Burton J. Strabismus: Practical Pearls You Won't Find in Textbooks. USA: Springer; 2017.
7. Leuder GT. Pediatric Practice Ophthalmology. St Louis, USA: McGraw Hill; 2011.
8. Mein J, Trimble R. Diagnosis and Management of Ocular Motility Disorders, 2nd edition. London: Blackwell Ltd.; 1995.
9. Prieto-Diaz J, Souza-Diaz CR. Strabismus, 4th edition. Boston: Butterworth & Heinemann; 2000.
10. Robison HD, Nelson LB, Olitsky SE. Harley's Pediatric Ophthalmology, 6th edition. Philadelphia, PA: Lippincott Williams & Wilkins; 2005.
11. Sharma PI. Strabismus Simplified. New Delhi, India: CBS Publishers; 2013.
12. Taylor D, Hoyt CS. Pediatric ophthalmology and strabismus. London: Elsevier Saunders; 2005.
13. Wright KW, Strube YNJ. Colour Atlas of Strabismus Surgery, 4th edition. USA: Springer; 2015.

28

CHAPTER

Nonsurgical Management of Strabismus

Rohit Saxena, Monika Yadav

INTRODUCTION

Nonsurgical treatment forms a very important component of managing various forms of strabismus. While some forms of strabismus may be completely corrected by using nonsurgical interventions, even those requiring surgery usually need some form of nonsurgical management pre- or post-surgery to ensure long-term stability or improve binocular outcomes.

Subnormal visual acuity (VA) can either be a cause of strabismus or a result of it and therefore a major component of nonsurgical management is improvement of VA prior to doing any surgical intervention. Moreover certain neuromuscular anomalies can be adequately controlled by nonsurgical means. This chapter shall discuss components of nonsurgical treatment of strabismus and amblyopia.

OPTICAL TREATMENT

Optical treatment includes use of optical modalities such as spectacles including use of bifocals and prisms for correction of refractive error and for the deviation.

Refractive Correction

Subnormal VA in one or both eyes can result in impaired fusion thereby contributing to strabismus. Providing appropriate refractive correction improves the quality of image on the fovea thereby promoting fusion and also helps in restoring proper balance between convergence and accommodation. Hence, a good baseline refraction under appropriate cycloplegia is essential. Cycloplegic agent of choice depends upon the age of the patient. Atropine is the preferred cycloplegic agent in children up to 7–8 years of age, especially those with dark irides. The ointment form is better compared to drops as it remains in the eye longer and is unlikely to travel down the nasolacrimal duct and get systemically absorbed in significant quantities. **Table 1** enlists cycloplegic drugs used along with its dosages and tonus allowances.

In cases of esotropia, the full refractive error measured under age-appropriate cycloplegia should be prescribed. Initially when hypermetropia is corrected for the first time, some children may experience blurring of distance vision as they are unable to relax accommodation while wearing their glasses. This acceptance of glasses can be improved by ensuring immediate use of the prescribed spectacles before the effect of the cycloplegia wears off. However, if the child continues to resist the spectacles, repeat of cycloplegia can be given for 3–4 days so that the accommodation can be relaxed and the child starts to see a clear image with the spectacles. This will remove the stimulus for accommodation as the cycloplegia wears off. Also, it is essential to explain to the patient or parents, in the case of children, that it is important to wear glasses all the time despite patient having clear vision

TABLE 1 : Cycloplegic drugs used in ophthalmology.

Name of drug	*Percentage*	*Age till which indicated*	*Dosage*	*Duration after which retinoscopy to be done*	*Period of post mydriatic test*	*Duration of action*	*Tonus allowance*
Atropine sulfate	1% ointment	< 5 years	tds × 3 days	4th day	After 3 weeks	2–3 weeks	1D
Homatropine hydrobromide	2% drops	5–8 years	One drop every 10 min × 6 times	After 90 min of instillation of first drop	After 3 days	2–3 days	0.5 D
Cyclopentolate hydrochloride	1% drops	8 years and above	1 drop every 15 min × 3 times	After 90 min of instillation of first drop	After 6–18 hours	6–18 hours	0.75 D

without glasses particularly in conditions of accommodative esotropia. The distance vision should be carefully monitored as in a young child, distance vision clarity is extremely important otherwise the child shall refrain from wearing corrective glasses or be at a risk of developing amblyopia.

However, in certain cases, either under correction or overcorrection of refractive error is needed. In cases of exodeviation, slight under correction of hypermetropic refractive error or overcorrection of myopic refractive error can help to control the exodeviation. However, this is usually not tolerated in the long-term and the patient can develop asthenopic symptoms.

Bifocal spectacles are prescribed in patients having high accommodative-convergence over accommodation (AC/A) ratio and consequent esodeviation which is more at near than distance. Important point to note is that the use of bifocals must ensure that the esodeviation is completely countered at near with its use. Minimal lens power needed to overcome near deviation should be used. This is obtained by adding plus lenses starting from 1 and gradually increasing power by +0.5 and simultaneously measuring the deviation.

Also, bifocals are prescribed on the basis of measurements made during the initial examination as no further change in deviation has been noted following use of bifocals on follow-up.

Design of bifocals is equally important. Executive-type bifocals are preferred and the separation line between the near and distance fixation should bisect the pupil as the patient looks straight. It is therefore important to give written instruction to the optician to make pupil bisecting bifocal glasses. Progressive lenses are not preferred as it is not possible to ensure that the maximum power of the near add is used every time the child looks at a near object. Regular use of bifocals may cause fusional amplitudes to develop spontaneously in many patients, after which the bifocals may be reduced step by step and eventually discontinued.

Attempts of weaning off bifocal glasses can be done by the age of 7–8 years. Surgical treatment may be considered in the form of bilateral MR recession if a patient still continues to require bifocals to maintain fusion during the early teenage years or if fusional control of the near deviation is no longer possible.

In patients with myopia and high AC/A ratio, the patient might become dependent on bifocals after the myopia is corrected as now the patient has to use accommodative effort to see clearly at near, which he was not used to doing until his refractive error was uncorrected.

Indications of Prism Therapy

Box 1 enlists various indications for prisms in the management of strabismus.

BOX 1: Indications for prisms in the management of strabismus.

- They are used in patients with small concomitant deviations to optically eliminate the deviation
- In patients with symptomatic phorias to eliminate asthenopia
- To correct residual deviations following strabismus surgeries
- In incomitant strabismus to relieve the diplopia
- To improve fusional vergences in convergence and divergence insufficiency
- In cases of nystagmus to treat the head posture as well as improve the visual acuity by prescribing prisms with base away from null point
- For cosmetic reasons in patients where surgery is not indicated

Prism Adaptation Test

This test has been used to calculate the target angle in patients with esotropia. After fully correcting the refractive error, base out prisms are prescribed to patients for residual esotropia. Patients are reviewed after 2 weeks, if further increase in deviation is noted, prism power is increased till a stable prism adapted angle is achieved, for which the surgery is ultimately undertaken. A multicenter prospective and randomized study showed that the success rate of patients for whom target angle was taken as stable prism adapted angle was higher (89%) vis-à-vis those operated for conventional angle (79%).

Also in cases of long-standing strabismus, where a "pseudo fovea" comes into existence, chances of postoperative diplopia can be predicted and ascertained, by placing an appropriate prism to neutralize the deviation and then enquire about the presence of diplopia. If there is no complain of diplopia, the surgeon can go ahead safely; but if diplopia is complained, then the patient should be warned of transient diplopia, so that there is no postoperative panic.

PHARMACOLOGICAL TREATMENT

Miotics

Miotics are helpful in patients with high AC/A ratio as they induce accommodation without requiring any central accommodative effort thereby reducing the associated convergence. Depth of focus is also increased due to the attendant miosis. 0.03% solution of echothiophate iodide is used, starting with once-daily (OD) dosing. Dose is titrated to achieve the desired effect. A study found 0.03% solution of ecothiopate iodide as effective as 0.125% solution in controlling accommodative esotropia.

The use of miotics is beneficial only if some degree of binocularity can be achieved, hence minor reduction in deviation does not justify their use.

Miotics can be used both diagnostically for differentiating accommodative and non-accommodative strabismus and therapeutically in patients with high AC/A ratio and those non-compliant to medications, postoperatively to enhance fusion in cases of consecutive esotropia and to treat amblyopia along with atropine.

Ecothiopate iodide tends to lower down the levels of cholinesterase, thereby prolonging the effect of succinyl choline, hence caution should be exercised in patients planned for surgery under general anesthesia.

Most common ocular reactions to miotics include transient blurring of vision, generalized darkening of the field of vision, and development of iris cysts. The incidence of iris cysts ranges from 20 to 50% of all children treated with miotics, these cysts tend to develop near pupillary margin and may appear from 2 to 40 weeks after the beginning of therapy. However, they tend to regress spontaneously after discontinuation of therapy.

Currently bifocals are clearly preferred over miotics in the management of accommodative esotropia with high AC/A ratio due to the side effects and lack of availability, but can rarely be used in children who do not tolerate glasses.

Atropine

Atropine is an anticholinergic agent that acts on muscarinic receptors in the ciliary body causing paralysis of accommodation with subsequent loss of accommodative convergence. Atropine sulfate 1% ointment is used as a cycloplegic agent for refraction in children <5 years of age. Guibor advocated the use of atropine in children with esotropia for a duration of at least 6 months before surgery. The underlying mechanism was suppression of the accommodative-convergence mechanism. However, this treatment modality is not much in vogue. At present, the role of atropine is for cycloplegia prior to refraction in children and for the treatment of amblyopia which shall be discussed ahead.

Botulinum Toxin

Botulinum toxin type A is a US Food and Drug Administration (FDA)-approved drug for use in both adult strabismus and blepharospasm. Botulinum toxin acts by inhibiting the extracellular release of Ach at the neuromuscular junction thus causing chemical denervation of the target muscle where it is injected. This action is temporary and the effect usually lasts for about 3 months with type A botulinum toxin. Botulinum toxin in strabismus mainly acts by weakening the contraction of a particular muscle in order to straighten the eye. The needle is inserted into the target muscle under the guidance of electromyography (EMG) and the toxin is injected into the muscle.

Box 2 enlists various indications for use of botulinum toxin in strabismus.

ORTHOPTIC EXERCISES

The goal of orthoptic treatment is to improve binocular vision, and convert manifest squint into latent squint. It does so by combating suppression, helps to convert anomalous retinal correspondence (ARC) to normal retinal correspondence (NRC), and also improves fusional amplitudes. Amblyopia if present should always be treated before starting the orthoptic exercises. This is then followed by antisuppression therapy, diplopia training, and finally improvement of fusional amplitudes.

Antisuppression Training

Suppression is a binocular phenomenon used to combat diplopia through active central inhibition of disparate and confusing images originating from the retina of the deviated eye. However, development of suppression acts as an obstacle to the development of binocular vision.

The primary aim of antisuppression exercises is to make the patient aware of the diplopia in heterophoria as well as hetrotropias. Diplopia training can be done by making the patient aware of the physiological diplopia wherein the patient is asked to be aware of the diplopia of the distant object while he is focusing on a near target or the patient is asked to be aware of the diplopia of a near object while he is focusing on a distant object.

Another method is using red filter where the red filter is placed in front of the dominant eye of the patient and the patient is either asked to trace a drawing with a red pencil or select red beads for a necklace. Patients can also be made aware of diplopia using prisms in which a vertical prism of strength enough to shift the image outside the scotoma is placed in front of one eye and the patient is asked to appreciate the diplopia. Gradually, the strength of the prism is reduced so the patient can appreciate the diplopia even without prisms.

Suppression can be treated by rapidly moving the visual target on the synoptophore in front of the suppressed eye across the suppression scotoma (macular massage) or slowly moving the target from the periphery toward the scotoma and then slowly crossing the object to the other side (crossing technique) so as to gradually reduce the scotoma

BOX 2: Indications of botulinum toxin in strabismus.

- *Infantile esotropia:* It helps in initial rehabilitation of patients in very young kids up to 18 months of age thus postponing the surgery. Here the Botox is injected bilaterally into the medial rectus helping with the ocular alignment up to 10 prism diopters in 70 to 75 percent patients
- *Acquired esotropia in children:* Many such cases achieve peripheral fusion with Botulinum toxin injection
- In sixth nerve palsy, the toxin is injected into the medial rectus to straighten the eyes
- In sensory strabismus it is primarily used to prevent muscle contracture
- Acute onset esotropia in older children
- Small angle esotropia in older children and adults
- In large angle deviations higher doses of the toxin can be injected in the muscle, although it is associated with greater complication rates such as ptosis

and the patient can superimpose. Tibbs binocular trainer and cheiroscope can also be used for diplopia training exercises.

Fusion Training

Fusion training is used to improve the convergence as well as divergence amplitudes depending on the requirement and is very useful in the management of phorias. It can be done using:

- *Synoptophore*: After placing the fusion slides, the arms of the synoptophore are placed at an angle where the patient is able to fuse and then the arms are either gradually converged (for convergence amplitudes) or they are diverged (for improving the divergence amplitudes) till patient has diplopia. Gradually with this exercise, the fusional amplitudes of the patient improve.
- *Prisms*: Here the prisms are placed in front of the eyes base out (for improving convergence amplitudes) and base in (for improving divergence amplitudes) at a strength where the patient can fuse the target object. The strength of the prisms is gradually increased so as to improve the fusional amplitudes.

Convergence Insufficiency

Orthoptic exercises are most effective and form the primary line of treatment for convergence insufficiency. Suppression if present should be treated first before starting the convergence exercises.

Initially, the NRC is improved using advancement exercises where the patient is asked to place the tip of a pencil in front of nose at a point where he can see a single image. At this time he should be able to appreciate physiological diplopia with the distant objects appearing double. This ensures that the patient is doing the exercise binocularly. Patient is then asked to slowly advance the pencil toward the nose and as soon as he sees a double image he is asked to fuse and again advance the pencil. Jump exercises where the patient is asked repeatedly to shift focus between objects placed at 6 m and 33 cm can also be used. The near target is then brought closer up to 5 cm.

Diplopia training can also be done by asking the patient to focus at a near target while being aware of the physiologic diplopia of a distant object. The near target is then removed and the patient is asked to maintain the convergence for increasing periods while diplopia is maintained at distance. This exercise develops voluntary convergence.

Fusional amplitudes for convergence can then be improved using the synoptophore, base out prisms, convergence card, or stereogram in uncrossed position.

Occlusion

Apart from amblyopia management, it has been advised in the treatment of intermittent exotropia. Occluding the dominant eye for 4–6 hours a day in a patient of intermittent exotropia has been given to decrease the angle of deviation and reports show some benefit in patients with small angle intermittent exotropia where they may become exophoric. However, a randomized trial did not find any advantage of occlusion over no treatment.

MANAGEMENT OF AMBLYOPIA

Management of amblyopia has been fully discussed in Chapter 5. But since treatment of amblyopia forms an integral part of nonsurgical management of strabismus, only a passing note is given here **(Box 3)**. Universally amblyopia is defined as a unilateral or bilateral diminution of best-corrected visual acuity (BCVA) due to ocular misalignment or form sense deprivation. According to Snellen's acuity chart, it is defined as the difference of two Snellen's lines between two eyes or BCVA less than 6/12 in both eyes.

Refractive Correction

Proper assessment and correction of refractive error is the first step in the management of patients with amblyopia. Refraction with the use of age-appropriate cycloplegia should be done and a prescription for glasses should be given. It is very important to check for compliance as children with anisometropic amblyopia with small refractive error in the better eye are often reluctant to wear glasses.

Occlusion

The principle of occlusion of the sound eye is that the amblyopic eye is forced to take part in the visual system actively and secondly, it also stops the inhibitory stimuli to the amblyopic eye. Before starting the occlusion therapy, it is important to correctly document baseline VA and do a proper refractive correction of the patient. A period of 4–6 weeks of refractive adaptation should be given before occlusion is started. The earlier the occlusion therapy begins, the better the results though occlusion therapy can be successful even in older age. On follow-up it is important to check the vision of the sound eye as there is always the risk of "occlusion amblyopia".

Penalization

The principle of penalization is to blur the image of the better eye so that the patient prefers to use the amblyopic eye. Atropine use was firstly advocated for this in 1903 by Worth. The use of miotic in amblyopic eyes and atropine in the better eye has also been described. According to these authors,

BOX 3: Modalities for amblyopia treatment.

- Refractive correction
- Occlusion
- Penalization
- Pharmacological treatment- levodopa- carbidopa, citicoline
- CAM treatment
- Dichoptic treatment

these drugs will cause the patient to prefer the amblyopic eye for near fixation while the sound eye continues to fixate at distance.

Systemic Medications

Certain systemic medications like levodopa and citicholine have been used as an adjunct in the treatment of amblyopia.

Other modalities of treatment include CAM treatment, dichoptic training, pleoptics, and surgical intervention for underlying amblyogenic factors including strabismus and refractive errors.

Of these modalities, pleoptics need a special mention as it serves as a modality for treating visual morbidity resulting from eccentric fixation development in dense amblyopia.

Pleoptics

It is a modality of treatment of amblyopia in patients with eccentric fixation. Patients with eccentric fixation do not assume central fixation on covering the fellow eye. Such patients can fixate on the object non-foveolarly as demonstrated by Bangerter in 1955. Bangerter classified fixation patterns in amblyopia into 3 types:

1. Central fixation
2. Eccentric fixation (non-foveolar fixation)
3. No fixation

Eccentric fixation areas could be either para-foveolar, parafoveal or peripheral eccentric. Furthermore, it was found that non-foveolar fixation could occur in vertical eccentricity as well. It was nasal to the fovea in patients with esotropia and temporal to the fovea in patients with exotropia. Eccentric fixation is a cause for concern because it offers less visual quality as compared to foveal fixation and patients with this condition would not tend to go back to the foveal fixation pattern due to long-standing deviation and deep amblyopia. Eccentric fixation could be either steady or wandering, the latter is considered a good prognostic sign while managing it.

Diagnosis of eccentric fixation can be made grossly by holding a small light source in front of the patient's head in midline and covering the fellow eye. If eccentric fixation is present, the patient will make no or very small redressal movement. Haidinger's brushes or Maxwell's spot can be used to detect subtle forms of eccentric fixation.

Haidinger's brushes are yellowish brush-like shapes that seem to radiate from point of fixation when polarized preferably blue light is viewed. In the case of central fixation, the center of the brush coincides with the fixation target, with eccentric fixation brushes appear peripheral to the fixation point. Maxwell spot contains a dark spot in the blue region of the visible spectrum which represents the macula. Position of this dark spot relative to that of the fixation mark is a sensitive index of the retinal area used for fixation.

Clinically visuoscope, as devised by Cuppers is used to check fixation. It contains a star, the center of which coincides with the fovea in cases of central fixation, but not in cases of eccentric fixation. Pleoptics is used to manage cases of amblyopia with eccentric fixation.

Two methods are used; Bangerter's method and Cupper's method.

Bangerter's Method

The area on the retina used for eccentric fixation is dazzled with bright flashes of light while protecting the fovea with a disc projecting onto it. This is followed by intermittent stimulation of the macula by light. The procedure is carried out under direct visualization of the fundus and continued till central scotoma vanishes and fixation becomes central.

Cupper's Method

The principle is to establish the physiological superiority of fovea over the retinal periphery. The fovea is protected by a black mark and the retinal periphery including the area used for eccentric fixation is dazzled with bright light. This produces negative after-images with a central clear spot corresponding to the fovea. This treatment is complemented with exercise using Haidinger's brushes or after-images which are visualized only by the fovea of the patient.

Pleoptics treatment method was found to be effective mainly in older and cooperative children and a lot of time and effort were required before noticeable results were evident. Although pleoptics is no longer clinically practiced so frequently, partly due to a decrease in eccentric fixation and deep amblyopia cases as the development of amblyopia is now picked up at an early age and treated, it is important to remember the principles of the same. It could be a helpful modality in patients who lose their better eye due to some reason, and their amblyopic eye does not recover by itself.

ROLE OF PRISMS

Ophthalmology study is completely based on optical devices. Prism is also an optical device, which is extensively used in ophthalmology. Ophthalmic prisms are a transparent, triangular, refracting medium which contains a base and an apex. The apical angle determines the power of a prism.

Optical Principle of Prisms

Refraction through a prism obeys Snell's law of refraction **(Fig. 1)**. The light ray deviates towards the base and the image is displaced towards the apex. Hence, the eye perceives the image to be formed towards the apex and makes a refixation movement towards it when the prism is placed in front of the eye. The net change in the direction of the light ray is called the angle of deviation which depends on:

1. Refractive index of the material used to make the prism
2. Refracting angle (α) of the prism
3. Angle of incidence of the light ray.

The power of the prism also depends on its position in front of the eye which results due to differences in the angle of incidence. There are two defined positions, prentice position and position of minimum deviation **(Fig. 2)**. In the prentice position, the surface of the prism is at 90 degrees to the ray of light such that all deviation takes place at the other surface. The angle of minimum deviation is when the angle of incidence equals the angle of emergence. Since the angle of deviation in prentice position is more than the angle of minimum deviation, the power of any prism in the prentice position is greater than its power in the position of minimum deviation.

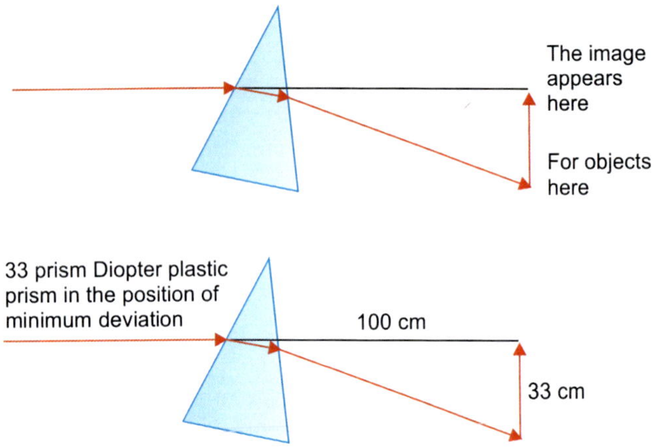

Fig. 1: Optics of prism.

Power of a prism is calculated by the amount of deviation of light rays at a fixed distance. Thus, 1 prism diopter (PD) power is deviation of rays by 1 centimeter at a distance of 1 meter.

Types of Prisms

Prisms are made of glass, acrylic, or fluorite. In ophthalmology, usually plastic (acrylic) prisms are used. They can be used as loose prisms, in a trial frame, in a prism bar or attached to lens as Fresnel prisms.

Fresnel Prisms

These consist of a plastic sheet of parallel tiny prisms of identical refracting angles **(Fig. 3)**. It is based on the principle, that the power of an optical system does not depend on the thickness of the individual elements or their separation. Thus, the overall prismatic effect is the same as that of a single large prism. They can be incorporated into the patient's glasses and allow prismatic correction up to 40 PD. Certain problems can occur like a decrease in visual acuity, contrast sensitivity and chromatic aberration. However, by matching the refractive index of the spectacle lens material and the prism, these issues can be reduced.

Prisms can be used both diagnostically and therapeutically in strabismus. They can either be trial set prisms, loose prisms, prism bars, or Fresnel prisms. Prisms in the trial set

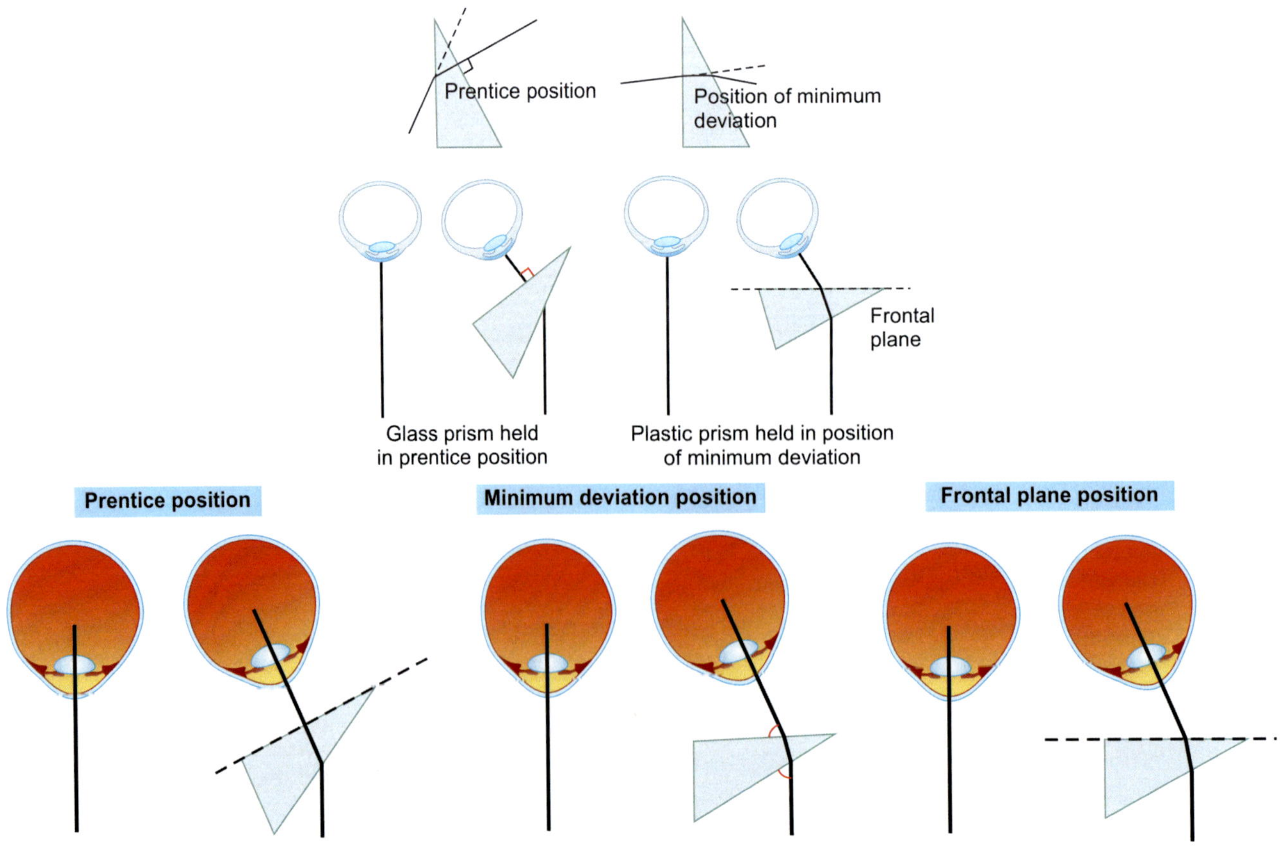

Fig. 2: Position of prisms.

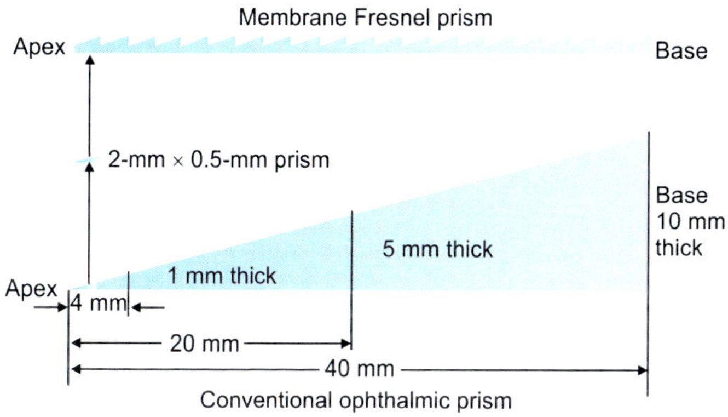

Fig. 3: Fresnel prisms.

range from ½ PD to 12 PD, loose prisms range from 5 PD to 60 PD while prism bars range from 1 PD to 40 PD. Fresnel prisms range from 1 PD to 40 PD.

Therapeutic Uses of Prisms

Orthoptic Exercises

Orthoptic exercises have been an established part of therapy for heterophoria, intermittent strabismus, convergence insufficiency, and accommodative problems for many years. Fusional amplitudes can be developed by placing prisms of increasing power in front of the eye and asking patient to attempt fusion.

Prisms in Treatment of Phorias and Tropias

Prisms are more commonly used for the treatment of heterophorias than tropias. They can be used both for esophoria as well as exophoria with their apex pointing towards the direction of deviation. Accurate cycloplegic refraction followed by prescription of appropriate glasses should be done first and then the minimum power of prism that eliminates symptoms should be prescribed. In small amounts of exophoria, optical correction or orthoptic exercises may benefit; but large degrees of exophoria require surgical intervention or alleviation of problems temporarily with prisms.

Patients with intermittent exotropia with asthenopia and diplopia can benefit with base-in prisms. Small constant deviations may also benefit with prisms to overcome diplopia.

Prisms for Abnormal Head Posture/Nystagmus

Use of 'yoked' prisms has shown to benefit in nystagmus. Prescribing bilateral yoked prisms with base in the same direction of head turn, i.e., with right head turn, base-out prism in right eye and base-in prism in left eye, will keep the eyes in null position and decrease the head turn.

Prisms to Relieve Diplopia

Prisms are used to relieve diplopia and increase the field of binocular single vision in patients with incomitant strabismus like acquired third, fourth, or sixth cranial nerve palsies as well as in acute acquired comitant esotropia, decompensated heterophoria, and convergence insufficiency. These prisms also stimulate the unaffected antagonistic muscle in paralytic strabismus, thereby preventing its secondary contracture.

Convergence Insufficiency

In these cases, the deviation is greater at near than at distance fixation. This occurs mostly due to low AC/A ratio or decreased fusional vergence. Though orthoptic exercises are the first line of management, in cases where they fail, use of base-in prisms decreases the symptoms significantly especially in the presbyopic age.

CONCLUSION

Nonsurgical management of strabismus forms an important component of strabismus treatment. Bulk of it aims at improving VA, thereby improving fixation behavior, along with developing fusional controls prior to undertaking any definitive surgical treatment.

SUGGESTED READING

1. Bangerter A. The purpose of pleoptics. Ophthalmologica. 1969; 158:334.
2. Campos EC, Schiavi C, Benedetti P, Bolzani R, Porciatti V. Effect of citicoline on visual acuity in amblyopia: Preliminary results. Graefe's Arch Clin Exp Ophthalmol. 1995;233(5):307-12.
3. Efficacy of prism adaptation in the surgical management of acquired esotropia. Prism Adaptation Study Research Group. Arch Opthalmol. 1990;108(9):1248-56.
4. Elkington AR, Frank HJ, Greaney MJ. Clinical Optics, 3rd edition. Oxford: Blackwell; 1984, Ch 4 Prisms.
5. Flanders M, Sarkis N. Fresnel membrane prisms: clinical experience. Can J Ophthalmol. 1999;34(6):335-40.
6. Linksz A. Theory of pleoptics. Int Ophthalmol Clin. 1961;1:747.
7. Ludwig IH, Parks MM, Jetson PP. Long-term results of bifocal therapy for accommodative esotropia. J Pediatr Ophthalmol Strabismus. 1989;26(6):264-70.
8. Noorden GK von, Morris J, Edelman P. Efficacy of bifocals in the treatment of accommodative esotropia. Am J Ophthalmol. 1978;85(6):830-4.
9. Pediatric Eye Disease Investigator Group. A randomized trial of atropine regimens for treatment of moderate amblyopia in children. Ophthalmology. 2004;111(11):2076-85.
10. Repka MX, Wallace DK, Beck RW, Kraker RT, Birch EE, Cotter SA, et al. Two-year follow-up of a 6-month randomized trial of atropine vs patching for treatment of moderate amblyopia in children. Arch Ophthalmol. 2005;123(2):149-57.
11. Scheiman MM, Hertle RW, Beck RW, Edwards AR, Birch E, Cotter SA, et al. Randomized trial of treatment of amblyopia in children aged 7 to 17 years. Arch Ophthalmol. 2005;123(4): 437-47.
12. Scheiman MM, Hertle RW, Kraker RT, Beck RW, Birch EE, Felius J, et al. Patching vs atropine to treat amblyopia in children aged 7 to 12 years: A randomized trial. Arch Ophthalmol. 2008; 126(12):1634-42.
13. Sofi IA, Gupta SK, Bharti A, Tantry TG. Efficiency of the occlusion therapy with and without levodopa-carbidopa in amblyopic children-A tertiary care centre experience. Int J Health Sci (Qassim). 2016;10(2):249-57.
14. Thompson JT, Guyton DL. Ophthalmic prisms: measurement errors and how to minimize them. Ophthalmology. 1983;90(3): 204-10.
15. Véronneau-Troutman S. Fresnel prisms and their effects on visual acuity and binocularity. Trans Am Ophthalmol Soc. 1978;76: 610-53.

29

CHAPTER

Nystagmus in Children

Dhikshitha Balaji, Jordan Murray, Fatema Ghasia

INTRODUCTION

Nystagmus is an involuntary, rhythmic, and rapid eye oscillation of one or both eyes. The etiology is variable; it can be due to vestibular tone imbalance, "leakiness" of the neural integrator, or abnormality of the slow, smooth eye-movement subsystem. It can result in reduced visual acuity due to excessive motion of images on the retina, sometimes with oscillopsia. It can also cause decreased depth perception, balance, and coordination. Nystagmus can be classified into two major types. Jerk nystagmus which is characterized by a pathologic slow phase drifting in one direction with a corrective fast phase "jerking" in the opposite direction and pendular nystagmus, which is less common, consists of slow phases with "pendular" oscillations to either side. Nystagmus can also be manifest, meaning always present, or latent, occurring when one eye is covered. In addition, nystagmus can be classified by the direction of the fast phase (horizontal, vertical, or torsional) as well as whether it is conjugate (the amplitude and direction of nystagmus are the same in both eyes) or disconjugate (the amplitude and direction vary between the eyes). Other clinical characteristics include the waveform, amplitude, and frequency of nystagmus. The types of nystagmus and eye oscillations have been characterized in a National Eye Institute Sponsored Workshop and Classification of Eye Movement Abnormalities and Strabismus (CEMAS) **(Box 1)**.

Nystagmus is commonly encountered in pediatric patients. Pediatric nystagmus can be contrasted with adult-onset nystagmus both clinically and in etiology. In children, the most common nystagmus is infantile nystagmus syndrome (INS) or fusion maldevelopment nystagmus syndrome (FMNS), formerly called latent nystagmus. In both adults and children, acquired nystagmus may be associated with neurological lesions of the vestibular and ocular motor pathways in the brainstem and/or cerebellum. Nystagmus is frequently seen in patients with retinal disorders. In fact, 76% of patients with inherited retinal dystrophies reported nystagmus, one of the most constant clinical features noticed by parents.

BOX 1: Eye movement disorders as classified by National Eye Institute Sponsored Workshop: Classification of Eye Movement Abnormalities and Strabismus.

- *Physiologic nystagmus*:
  - Vestibular nystagmus
  - Optokinetic nystagmus
- *Physiologic fixational movements*:
  - Microtremor
  - Slow drifts
  - Microsaccades
- *Pathologic nystagmus*:
  - Fusion maldevelopment nystagmus
  - Infantile nystagmus syndrome
  - Spasmus nutans syndrome
  - Vestibular nystagmus (central or peripheral imbalance and central instability)
  - Gaze-holding deficiency nystagmus (endgaze, rebound, and gaze instability nystagmus)
  - Vision loss (prechiasmal, chiasmal, and postchiasmal)
  - Other pendular nystagmus and nystagmus associated with disease of central myelin-multiple sclerosis, pendular nystagmus associated with tremor of palate, and pendular vergence nystagmus associated with Whipple's disease
  - Ocular bobbing
  - Lid nystagmus
- *Saccadic intrusions and oscillations*:
  - Square wave jerk and oscillations
  - Square wave pulses
  - Saccadic pulses
  - Induced convergence retraction
  - Dissociated ocular oscillations
  - Hypermetric saccades
  - Macrosaccadic oscillations
  - Ocular flutter
  - Flutter dysmetria
  - Opsoclonus
  - Psychogenic flutter
  - Superior oblique myokymia

Accurate diagnosis of nystagmus type often requires ocular motility recordings; however clinical history and examination are also important. The history should cover onset, pre- and perinatal complications, family history, growth, and development milestones. Patients with congenital or fusion maldevelopment nystagmus almost never have oscillopsia. They may present with abnormal head position. However, acquired nystagmus in children and adults frequently presents with oscillopsia, blurred vision, and double vision, if there is coexisting strabismus. Optical coherence tomography (OCT), particularly with a hand-held spectral domain OCT, is clinically useful to produce reliable retinal measurements and identify the cause of nystagmus by differentiating albinism, PAX6 mutations, achromatopsia, or atypical foveal hypoplasia. Hand-held OCT for infants and young children has been shown to be comparable to adult OCT and could be used to predict visual acuity in preverbal children, facilitating focused examinations, and earlier diagnosis. Furthermore, through OCT, clinicians will be able to document stages of foveal development and cone photoreceptor degeneration, which can aid in diagnosis and prediction of prognosis for patients with infantile nystagmus. For suspected retinal disorders such as achromatopsia or Leber congenital amaurosis (LCA), retinal electrophysiologic testing like electroretinography (ERG), OCT, and molecular genetic testing may yield higher diagnoses than an MRI scan. Neuroimaging may be useful if there are coexistent optic nerve abnormalities or atrophy, or if the diagnosis of INS is ambiguous. Finally, nystagmus can be distinguished from other abnormal involuntary eye movements because of its slow speeds and rhythmicity. Diagnoses to rule out include saccadic intrusions such as opsoclonus or ocular flutter, ocular bobbing, and oculogyric crises.

In the following chapter, we will cover important characteristics of the most common types of nystagmus in children.

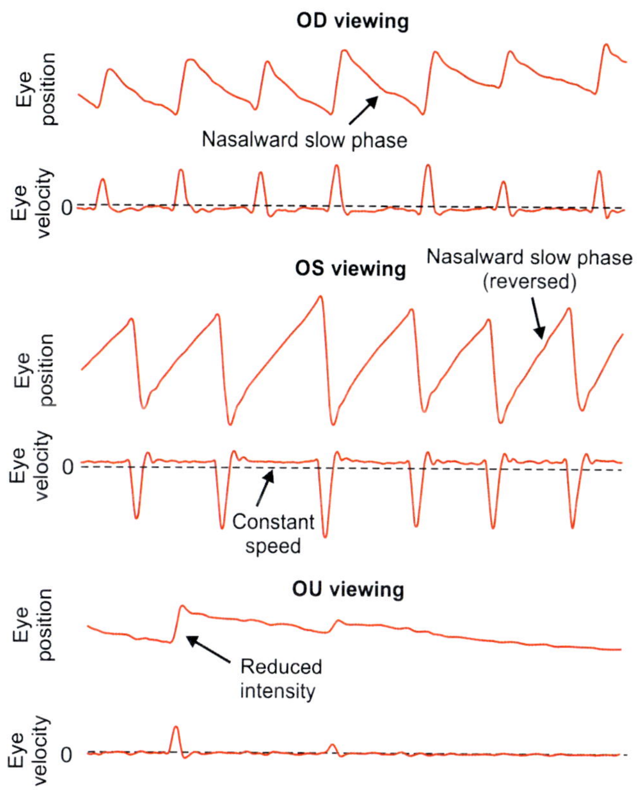

Fig. 1: Eye position and velocity in fusion maldevelopment nystagmus syndrome (FMNS). Eye positions and velocities versus time for a patient with FMN under OD (top), OS (middle), and OU (bottom) viewing conditions. FMN can be identified by linear or decelerating slow phases that are nasalward with respect to the viewing eye, resulting in a reversal in direction between OD and OS monocular viewing. FMN was formerly called latent nystagmus because its reduced intensity during binocular viewing gave the impression that the condition would be evident only on covering one eye.

TYPES OF NYSTAGMUS

Fusion Maldevelopment Nystagmus Syndrome (Latent Nystagmus)

Fusion maldevelopment nystagmus syndrome is a jerk nystagmus of both eyes that becomes apparent or markedly enhanced when one eye is covered. The uncovered eye drifts in a pathologic nasally directed slow phase movement and then corrected with a temporally directed fast phase. The covered eye also moves in the same direction, but may vary in amplitude. If FMNS is present with both eyes viewing, it is called manifest latent nystagmus. Manifest latent nystagmus occurs in as many as 50% of patients with infantile strabismus, while true latent nystagmus is rare.

Fusion maldevelopment nystagmus syndrome develops due to disruption of binocularity in infancy. Congenital esotropia impeding binocular vision early in infancy is the leading cause, but any disorder than disturbs development of binocular fusion can cause FMNS. It is strongly associated with presence of strabismus and dissociated vertical deviation (DVD). Regarding diagnosis with eye movement recordings, the slow phases in FMNS are typically in decreasing exponential or linear velocity form. This is in contrast to congenital nystagmus, which shows increasing exponential velocity form. **Figure 1** depicts the features of FMNS including reversal in the direction of quick phase per the viewing eye, increased intensity during monocular viewing condition and the constant velocity of the slow phases.

Clinical Pearls

- Depending on the viewing eye, FMNS exhibits reversal of direction of nystagmus. For example, there is right-beating nystagmus when the right eye is viewing and left-beating nystagmus when the left eye is viewing.
- Fogging technique is helpful to measure monocular visual acuity. Complete occlusion during testing can result in underestimation of acuity due to appearance of latent nystagmus under monocular viewing conditions. Fogging can be applied with a +5.00 D lens placed over the viewing eye.

Infantile Nystagmus Syndrome

Causes of Infantile Nystagmus Syndrome

Infantile nystagmus syndrome, formerly called congenital nystagmus, is a bilateral, conjugate, horizontal-torsional, and pendular or jerk nystagmus. It is present at birth or in early infancy, at an estimated prevalence of 2.4 in 1,000, and persists throughout life. INS can be idiopathic or correlated with albinism, retinal disease, visual deprivation early in life, congenital aniridia, underdeveloped optic nerves, or congenital cataract.

Infantile nystagmus syndrome should be differentiated from acquired nystagmus, which appears later in life. Age at onset and waveform characteristics of the nystagmus should be considered to make this distinction. Eye movement recordings can measure waveforms, such as through electrooculography, scleral search coil, and video eye-tracking **(Fig. 2)**. Over the first year of life, INS waveforms evolve. They begin triangular, then become pendular, and finally jerk at around 1 year of age. On attempted visual fixation, INS nystagmus increases. However, it decreases with convergence **(Fig. 3)** or eyelid closure. If the nystagmus is asymmetrical or unilateral, neurological disease should be suspected.

Patients with idiopathic INS do not have known lesions; rather they are hypothesized to develop nystagmus after failure of sensorimotor integration in infancy due to abnormal postnatal visual experience. Of children with idiopathic INS, about 25% have a mutation in the *FRMD7* gene. When patients with a *FRMD7* mutation underwent retinal image studies using OCT, they were found to have significantly shallower foveal pits, abnormal optic nerve head morphology with decreased optic disk area, decreased retinal nerve fiber layer thickness, and decreased cup area and depth. This suggests that abnormal afferent system development is associated with FRMD7 mutations.

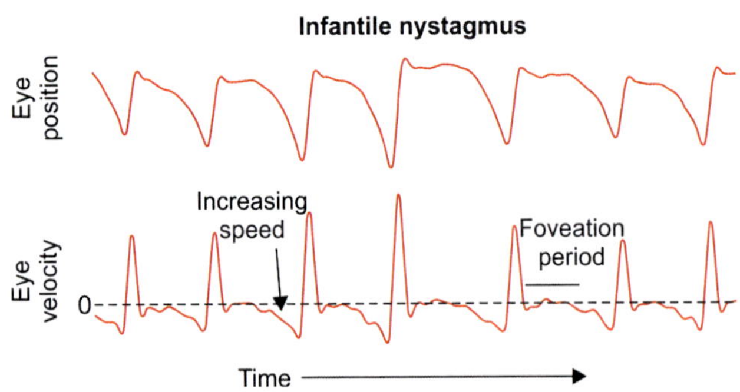

Fig. 2: Eye position and velocity in infantile nystagmus. It highlights the key-differentiating feature seen in patients with infantile nystagmus syndrome (INS) compared to fusion maldevelopment nystagmus syndrome (FMNS). INS patients increasing eye velocity in contrast to FMNS subjects with linear or decelerating slow phase velocities. The foveation periods are defined as brief periods of time when the eye is still and is pointed at the target of interest. During these periods, the eye velocity is at a minimum and visual acuity is at the best.

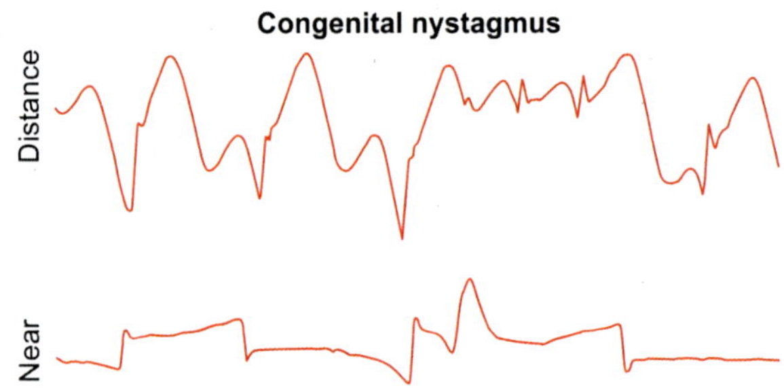

Fig. 3: Change in nystagmus intensity with vergence. It highlights the reduction of nystagmus intensity (frequency × amplitude) with convergence in a patient with idiopathic infantile nystagmus syndrome.

Because the disease is genetically heterogeneous, involving genes of retinal and brain development, and also associated with other conditions, identifying the underlying cause of INS can be difficult. A novel diagnostic next-generation sequencing gene panel can be used to provide genetic diagnoses, particularly for genes *FRMD7*, *CACNA1F*, *TYR*, *CRYBA1*, and *TYRP1*. High- and low-frequency head oscillations can be seen in patients with INS. These are abnormal oscillations that do not influence foveation periods and are not used as a compensatory mechanism to improve vision in INS patients.

Infantile nystagmus syndrome can be associated with sensory anomalies including albinism, achiasma, isolated foveal hypoplasia, congenital retinal dystrophies, and rod-cone dystrophies. Here we will focus on albinism and retinal dystrophies, particularly LCA and achromatopsia.

Albinism has a particularly strong association with INS, with almost 90% of patients with albinism also having nystagmus. The lack of pigmentation of retinal pigment epithelium (RPE) and melanin leads to foveal hypoplasia and subsequent abnormal routing of optic nerves. Normal foveal development begins at fetal week 25 and finishes 15–45 months after birth. In albinism, PAX6 mutations, or in isolation, this developmental process is disturbed, leading to foveal hypoplasia. It is possible to document the degree of foveal hypoplasia, representing different stages of arrested development, by using OCT as a diagnostic aid and prognostic indicator. A grading system has been proposed, in which grade 1 foveal hypoplasia is due to partial displacement of the inner retinal layers resulting in a rudimentary pit. This process fails in grades 2, 3, and 4. In grades 1 and 2, lengthening of the outer segment is a sign of cone photoreceptor specialization, a process that fails in grade 3 and 4. In grades 1, 2, and 3, there is successful migration of cone photoreceptors represented by outer nuclear layer widening. In grade 4, that developmental process completely fails to occur. **Figures 4A to F** depict fundus photos and OCT images from a child with albinism. Histologically, there are decreased melanosomes, causing ocular symptoms, or decreased melanin in melanosomes, causing oculocutaneous symptoms. Additionally, rods are abnormally present in

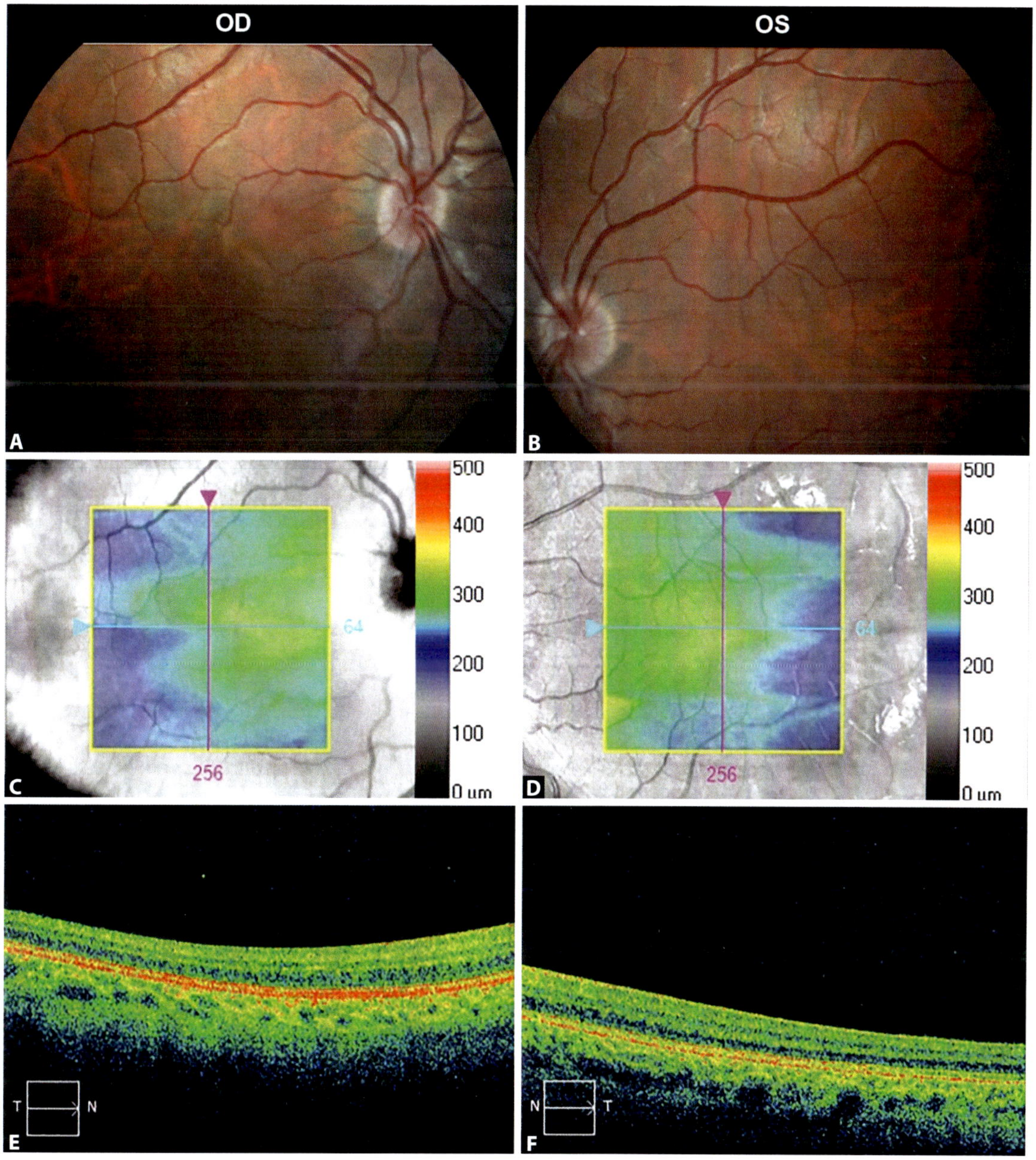

Figs. 4A to F: Fundus pictures and optical coherence tomography (OCT) images showing foveal hypoplasia in albinism. Fundus photos depict foveal hypoplasia with lack of foveal pigment and absent foveal reflex in both eyes. The Cirrus OCT images of the macula at the expected fovea demonstrating lack of normal retinal doming and depression of the retina at the expected fovea.

the fovea, where typically only cones are present. Ocular involvement of albinism varies in individuals, but typically results in decreased visual acuity, photophobia, nystagmus, iris transillumination, and a blond-appearing fundus. ERG is normal in albinism, and may even show extremely large responses due to light scatter.

Another cause of infantile nystagmus is retinal dystrophies. Major conditions of retinal dystrophy associated with early-onset nystagmus include LCA and achromatopsia, congenital stationary night blindness, Bardet-Biedl syndrome, Joubert syndrome, and Alström syndrome. All are causes of nystagmus due to deficits of rod and cone systems. Color blindness, low vision, increased sensitivity to bright lights, and nystagmus represent cone dysfunction. On the other hand, night vision issues and reduced peripheral visual fields indicate problems with the rods.

Leber congenital amaurosis is an autosomal recessive and heterogeneous condition that produces large-amplitude, low-frequency nystagmus, or roving eye movements. Nystagmus can also be upbeating and asymmetric, though this is less common. Infants should be examined for bilateral staphylomatous macular lesions. In a subset of patients with LCA, developmental delay, hearing loss, epilepsy, cerebellar abnormalities, and hypotonia has been observed. Optic disks eventually become pale as retinal pigmentary abnormalities become evident.

Achromatopsia is another autosomal recessive and heterogeneous condition that presents with lower-amplitude and higher-frequency nystagmus. Children are typically light-averse (photodysphoria), have decreased visual acuity, and may not be able to distinguish colors. Children also sometimes present with short stature, small hands and feet, premature puberty, minimal dysmorphism, and unilateral parental isodisomy of chromosome 14.

Full-field ERG is useful to observe retinal cod-cone function and is the clinical gold standard in the identification of hereditary retinal disorders. A handheld, noninvasive ERG recording system can also be used as a feasible, fast, and effective alternative in children to minimize discomfort and risk. For achromatopsia, glasses or contact lenses allow wavelengths of low luminous light to be transmitted to the retina while absorbing short wavelength light.

Treatments for Infantile Nystagmus Syndrome

Surgical: Surgical treatments for INS vary depending on intensity of nystagmus, abnormal head position, and whether strabismus is also present.

Surgery to improve abnormal head position: The Kestenbaum procedure **(Table 1)** is used to move and broaden the null zone, improving visual function and creating better foveations for a broader horizontal range. This procedure can be used to improve head position in patients with INS with coexisting strabismus. 40% and 60% augmented Kestenbaum procedure can be performed for moderate (30°) and severe (45°) head positioning. In concordant cases, meaning surgery to correct head position would also correct the strabismus, an augmented Kestenbaum procedure can be performed on the fixating eye. In a Kestenbaum procedure, both eyes are turned parallel in the direction of the abnormal head posture by combined recess and resect surgery on each eye. However, there are also discordant cases, in which a surgical correction on the fixating eye for head position would make strabismus worse. One option to address discordant cases is to reduce the surgical dose in the fixating eye while maintaining maximal surgery in the fellow eye. Surgery to correct head positioning has a high success rate, with 95% of patients resolving symptoms at 1–3 weeks. By 2 years, 82% still had successful head positioning. Long-term follow-up at 10 years showed that only 21% of patients required another operation. Surgical planning for these results consisted of an augmented

TABLE 1: Kestenbaum procedure: The suggested surgical amounts. It shows the suggested surgical amounts for the Kestenbaum and augmented Kestenbaum procedures as described by Buckley and Bruce Shields in the "Atlas of Ophthalmic Surgery".

	Head turn to the right—eyes gaze left	
	Right eye—esotropic	
	Lateral rectus recession	*Medial rectus recession*
Classic (5,6,7,8) (5 + 8 = 6 + 7)	8	5
Augmented (+ 40%)	11	7
Augmented (+ 60%)	13	8
	Left eye—exotropic	
	Medial rectus resection	*Lateral rectus recession*
Classic (5,6,7,8) (5 + 8 = 6 + 7)	6	7
Augmented (+ 40%)	8.5	10
Augmented (+ 60%)	9.5	11
	Head turn to the left—eyes gaze right	
	Right eye—exotropic	
	Lateral rectus recession	*Medial rectus resection*
Classic (5,6,7,8) (5 + 8 = 6 + 7)	7	6
Augmented (+ 40%)	10	8.5
Augmented (+ 60%)	11	9.5
	Left eye—esotropic	
	Medial rectus recession	*Lateral rectus resection*
Classic (5,6,7,8) (5 + 8 = 6 +7)	5	8
Augmented (+ 40%)	7	11
Augmented (+ 60%)	8	13

Kestenbaum procedure for patients with horizontal face turn without strabismus. Patients with coexisting horizontal face turn and strabismus were treated with decreased dose of surgery in the fellow eye. For discordant strabismus, surgical dosage was decreased in the fixated eye while a full 60% augmentation was done in the nonfixating eye.

Tetonomy with reattachment: Tenotomy and reattachment of the four rectus muscles or tenotomy on two rectus muscles with large recessions of the other two rectus muscles for face turns <20 can be employed. Tenotomies are thought to reduce foveation time and improve real-world functioning. The proposed mechanism is that afferent proprioceptive receptors increase firing rate due to the tetonomy, causing the feedback loop to the brain to relax muscle tension. However, the isolated four-muscle tetonomy remains controversial and is indicated in <10% of cases.

Four muscle recession: Recess-resect procedures of four vertical rectus muscles may also be considered for patients with vertical null zone. Bilateral vertical extraocular muscle surgery of the combined vertical recti and oblique muscles in children with horizontal INS has also been shown to improve or resolve chin-down or chin-up vertical head posture. For four muscles recession, medial rectus muscles are recessed less than the lateral rectus muscles. However, four muscles recession may produce hypometric saccades and decrease the efficacy of the surgery.

Medical: One-time surgical treatment is typically favored over lifelong medical treatment. However, gabapentin, memantine, and topical brinzolamide have shown possible benefit in children with INS. Drug therapy largely focuses on augmenting the inhibitory neurotransmitter system or inhibiting the excitatory neurotransmitter system. For example, clonazepam can be used to treat downbeat nystagmus while baclofen has been successful in treating acquired periodic alternating nystagmus. Contact lenses have also been used to treat INS, the mechanism potentially related to increasing afferent feedback from the inner eyelids and conjunctiva and base out prisms can be prescribed to patients with suppression of nystagmus with convergence.

Clinical Pearls

- Structural eye abnormalities should be ruled out due to frequent association of INS with afferent visual pathway abnormalities.
- Foveal hypoplasia can be identified with OCT.
- *FRMD7* gene mutations have been associated with X-linked INS.

Spasmus Nutans

Spasmus nutans is a triad of nystagmus, head nodding, and torticollis, beginning in infancy and usually disappearing in childhood. The nystagmus is disconjugate, asymmetric, and high frequency, and can be horizontal, vertical, or torsional. The nystagmus can increase in frequency with convergence. The head nodding is an adaptive mechanism that may improve visual acuity by suppressing the nystagmus. Head nodding in spasmus nutans differs from that in INS, which are pathologic tremors that do not improve visual acuity. Interestingly, while the pathologic neurologic pathways for both spasmus nutans and INS are speculative, spasmus nutans has greater environmental associations such as nonwhite ethnicity, low home luminance, gestational age, and low socioeconomic status.

The age of onset is typically between 6 and 12 months of age, and sometimes noticed when the baby is feeding. Amblyopia is frequently associated with spasmus nutans, especially when the nystagmus is asymmetric, as well as strabismus. In diagnosis, suprasellar tumors, which present similarly, should be ruled out through neuroimaging and monitoring of visual, neurologic, and endocrine function. Identical eye movements have also been seen in children with Down syndrome, third ventricular tumors, optic nerve, chiasmal, or parachiasmal gliomas, and some in fetal alcohol syndrome. Therefore, the distinction cannot be made solely through eye and head movement recordings and consultation with a pediatric neurologist as well as CT or MRI of the head is indicated. Also, retinal dystrophies may also simulate spasmus nutans; electroretinograms can be used to distinguish the two. If there are no associated central nervous system (CNS) abnormalities, spasmus nutans typically resolves on clinical observation by 2 years but subclinical nystagmus is usually still evident on eye movement recordings until 5–12 years of age. Good visual acuity can be predicted for children with spasmus nutans, who may develop both visual acuity and stereovision during phases of compensatory head nodding.

Clinical Pearls

Retinal dystrophies should be suspected in patients in whom nystagmus does not resolve by 2 years of age and who have no CNS abnormalities.

Neurologic Nystagmus

Though all nystagmus is neurologic in origin, neurologic nystagmus refers nystagmus that results from intracranial lesions or systemic neurologic disease. Neurologic disease should be suspected, especially if the nystagmus is asymmetrical or unilateral. Common concurrent neurologic symptoms include vertigo, nausea, headaches, relative afferent pupillary defect, papilledema, optic atrophy, and visual loss. Neurodegenerative diseases may also produce horizontal nystagmus before other clinical signs appear.

Acquired Neurologic Nystagmus

Neurologic nystagmus is typically acquired and can present with coexisting strabismus. Exodeviations and particularly pattern strabismus can be associated with neurologic disorders. Ocular cranial nerve palsies can also cause strabismus along with nystagmus, as diseases affecting these nerves result in motility disturbance and weakness of corresponding muscles. For example, a sixth nerve palsy necessitates an aggressive workup in a child and presents with other cranial nerve involvement, nystagmus, papilledema, and strabismus.

Nystagmus due to Brain Tumor

Of children presenting with brain tumors to ophthalmologists, 24% had nystagmus. Because the visual system of a child is still developing, including visual fields, foveal maturation, and occipital cortex development, brain tumors put children at risk of vision loss or other morbidities such as strabismus and nystagmus. A clinical examination of various eye movements can be helpful to distinguish central and peripheral oculomotor and vestibular disorders. For example, a saccadic smooth pursuit would indicate a central oculomotor disturbance. Hypermetric saccades can be seen in cerebellar impairments while hypometric saccades are more common in brainstem lesions or neurodegenerative disorders.

Patients with nystagmus should be examined in the primary position, gazing straight ahead. Fixation nystagmus typically increases with fixation and is caused by a central disorder, typically of the brainstem or cerebellum. Horizontal-torsional spontaneous nystagmus is suppressed by fixation, suggesting that brainstem and cerebellum functioning is intact. Rather, this type of nystagmus points to peripheral vestibular disorder. Nystagmus that is purely horizontal, vertical, or torsional usually is a result of central disease.

For children presenting with asymmetric nystagmus, spasmus nutans, retinal diseases, optic nerve hypoplasia, and intracranial masses should be considered. If the patient has normal visual acuity and ocular examination and lack of head titubation, spasmus nutans is less likely than underlying retinal disease, neurological disorder, or optic pathway glioma (OPG). In children with OPGs, nystagmus can be explained through subclinical damage to ganglion cell axons that control gaze holding or from compressive damage of visuomotor centers in the midbrain that control gaze holding. Asymmetric nystagmus typically resolves after treatment of OPG, though visual prognosis is moderate to poor. Monocular nystagmus can be a presenting sign of an OPG, so its presence should raise suspicion of a tumor with prompt imaging.

While central positional nystagmus (CPN) is usually caused by peripheral vestibular disorder, it has also been reported in association with several lesions in the posterior fossa, including infarction, hemorrhage, tumor, or demyelinating disease. CPN due to a central lesion presents as an apogeotropic nystagmus during supine roll test or as downbeat nystagmus in prone or straight head-handing position. It is either vertical or purely torsional and persistent. The nystagmus results from erroneous processing of signals, which do not properly estimate the rotational velocity of the head and gravity direction.

Vertical Nystagmus

Vertical nystagmus can also be ascribed to neurologic causes. It is rarely present and can be classified as upbeating or downbeating. Both forms can be affected by head position and convergence. The pathophysiology is not completely understood, but upbeat nystagmus may be due to pontine or medullary lesions that result in primary hypoactivity of the excitatory superior vestibular nucleus-ventral tegmental tract (SVN-VTT) pathway, while downbeat nystagmus results from floccular damage to the same pathway. In both cases, there seems to be no major primary involvement of the excitatory downward vestibular pathway. A second hypothesis is that gravity may influence vertical spontaneous nystagmus, as it facilitates the downward vestibular system while restraining the upward system. Consequently, an additional and physiologically stronger excitatory SVN-VTT pathway may have developed in order to counteract gravity. Because the upward pathway must be permanently active to maintain primary eye position, a lesion affecting excitatory branches or inhibitory branches could result in upbeating or downbeating nystagmus. Rarely, vertical nystagmus is familial and visual acuity is typically good.

Upbeating nystagmus in infancy is usually associated with anterior visual pathway disease. A complete ophthalmologic examination should be performed to identify any structural abnormalities, including optic nerve pathologies. If ocular examination is unremarkable, an ERG to evaluate retinal dystrophies should be considered.

Congenital downbeating nystagmus is rare in infancy, but typically occurs with positive family history. The major clinical characteristics as described by CEMAS are a conjugate, upward drift of the eye followed by a downward fast face with a gravity-dependent component, and a horizontal gaze-evoked nystagmus component. Downbeating nystagmus resolves in most cases by 2 years of age. In older children, acquired forms of downbeating nystagmus call for neuroimaging to evaluate for abnormalities in the craniocervical junction, such as Arnold–Chiari malformations. Other pathophysiologic hypotheses include deficient cerebellar inhibition of the brainstem, imbalance of vestibular pathways, gravity-dependent anomaly of normal upward drift, or impaired vertical smooth pursuit. Both horizontal nystagmus and downbeating nystagmus can co-occur, resulting in a nystagmus with an oblique slow phase in Arnold–Chiari malformation. In this case, downbeat nystagmus can occur from compression of a herniated cerebellum against the caudal brainstem. Other eye movement disorders in patients with Arnold–Chiari malformations are esotropia secondary to divergence insufficiency, seesaw nystagmus, skew deviation, periodic alternating nystagmus, and shifted null position of the horizontal gaze-evoked nystagmus. The goals of eye muscle surgery for patients with downbeating nystagmus is to move the upgaze eccentric null position closer to the primary position by moving both eyes down and treating coexisting strabismus.

Horizontal Gaze-evoked Nystagmus

Gaze-evoked nystagmus is a horizontal nystagmus that typically occurs with cerebellar and brainstem lesions, reflecting a loss of the common neural integrator. In gaze-evoked nystagmus, drifts move the eyes away from the target and a null position where drifts are absent **(Figs. 5A and B)**. There is failure to maintain eccentric gaze position because of defective gaze-holding mechanisms due to dysfunction of vestibulocerebellar structures.

Nystagmus due to Demyelinating Syndromes

Finally, demyelinating syndromes of the cerebellum or tracts between cerebellum and brainstem, though very rare in children, can also lead to nystagmus. For example, the most common causes of acquired pendular nystagmus are disorders of central myelin, particularly multiple sclerosis (MS). About 40–76% of MS patients experience eye movement disorders and acquired pendular nystagmus is a classic source of oscillopsia.

Opsoclonus and Ocular Flutter

Ocular flutter is a series of intermittent bursts of conjugate saccades occurring strictly in the horizontal plane without an intersaccadic interval. It is a rare symptom that occurs in the context of many diseases including cancerous malignancies, paraneoplastic or autoimmune diseases, drug intoxication, head trauma, or postviral infection. Its true prevalence may be obscured by self-limiting cases.

Opsoclonus and ocular flutter are on a continuum, sharing pathogenesis, and localizing significance. Opsoclonus is an ocular dyskinesia with sudden, involuntary, arrhythmic, and chaotic conjugate saccadic ocular movements without an intersaccadic interval. In contrast to ocular flutter, opsoclonus eye movements are multidirectional and can be in any plane **(Figs. 6A to C)**. Symptoms include oscillopsia and visual blurring. It is present during fixation, smooth pursuit, convergence, and persists during sleep and eyelid closure. It has been observed transiently in healthy term and preterm neonates. However, as many as 50% of children with opsoclonus have tumors of neural crest origin, such as neuroblastoma. Of those patients with neuroblastoma, 2–3% are affected by opsoclonus-myoclonus ataxia syndrome, in which generalized myoclonus and ataxia coexist. It has also been associated with parainfectious, metabolic, and toxic etiologies, particularly viral encephalitis. The syndrome is mainly hypothesized to be caused by immunological cross-reactivity between the tumor and normal cerebellar neurons. The antineuronal antibodies associated with opsoclonus include anti-Ri, anti-Hu, and anti-Yo. Testing of these antibodies is not regularly done because the majority of patients with opsoclonus are seronegative. Instead, whole body imaging is recommended to identify the tumor.

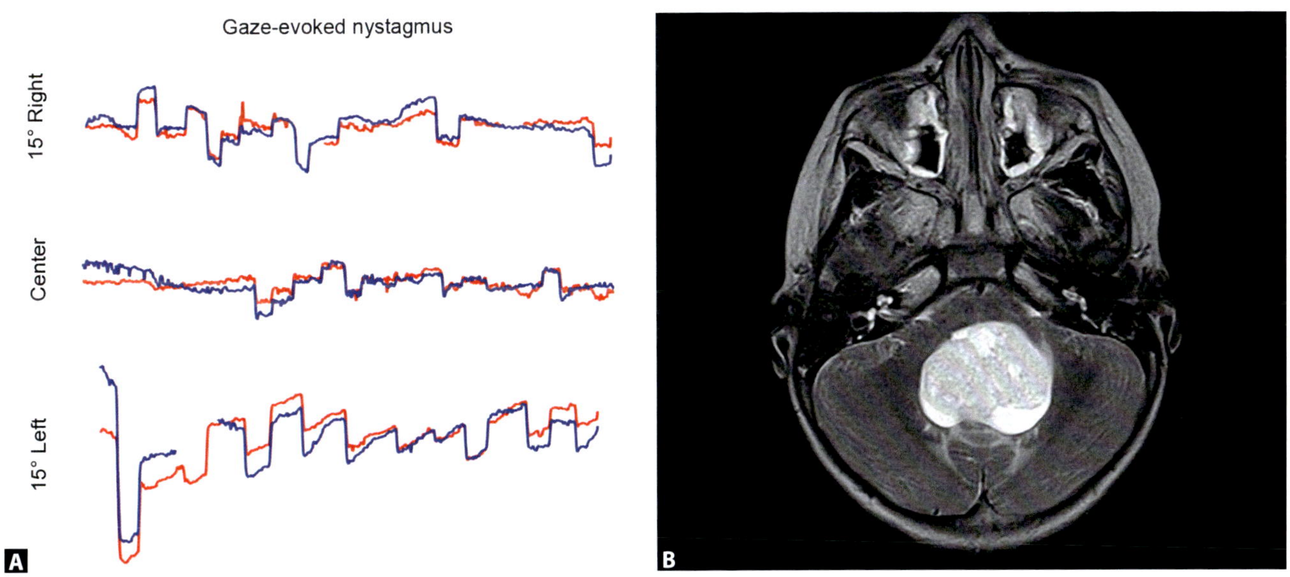

Figs. 5A and B: (A) Horizontal eye position traces for asymmetric gaze-evoked nystagmus in a child with pilocytic astrocytoma. OS (blue) and OD (red) horizontal eye position traces (up corresponds to rightward eye movements) for a patient with gaze-evoked nystagmus as a dot displayed at 15° to the right (top), centrally (middle), and 15° to the left (bottom) was fixated upon with both eyes. In the last case, the gaze direction evokes a periodic oscillation with quick phases and rightward linear slow phases that is not evident when fixating centrally or to the right; (B) MRI showing the brainstem/cerebellar tumor. There is a large heterogeneously enhancing multilobulated mass centered within and expanding the fourth ventricle, appear to arise from the superior aspect of the cerebellar vermis. The enhancing portion of the mass measures 4 × 5 × 5.5 cm.

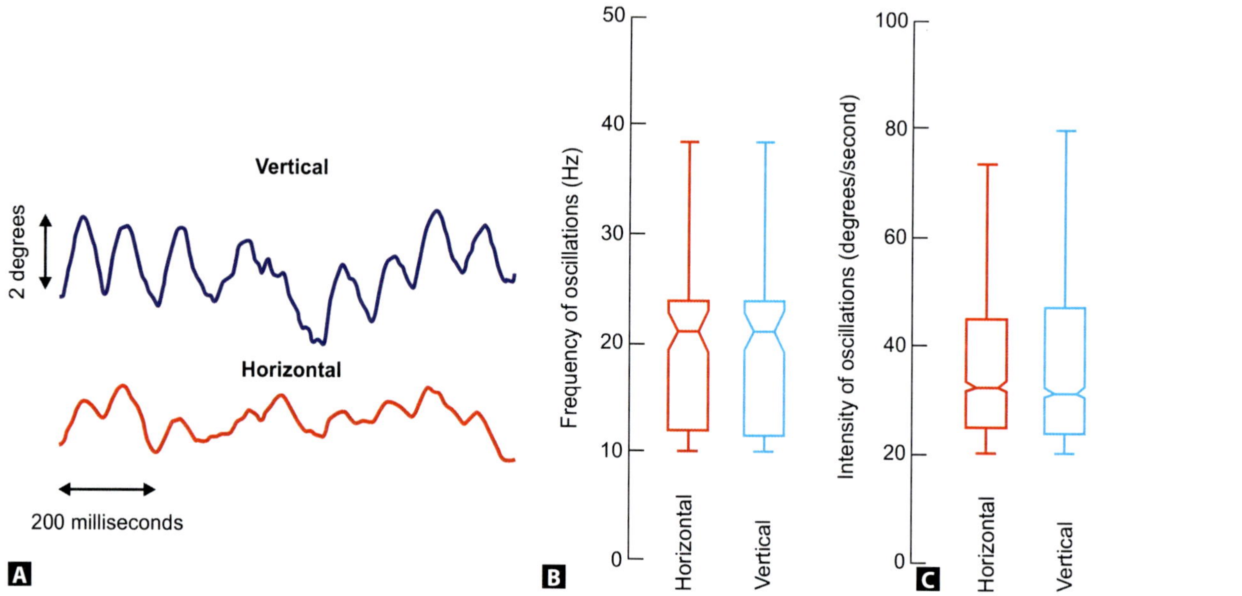

Figs. 6A to C: Eye movements for micro-opsoclonus. (A) This panel depicts example of micro-opsoclonus. Blue lines depict vertical eye movements, while red lines are horizontal eye movements. Eye positions are plotted on Y-axis, and corresponding time is plotted on X-axis; (B) Box and whisker plots summarize the frequency of microsaccadic oscillations from all four patients. Red box and whisker plot depict horizontal oscillation frequency, while blue illustrates the frequencies of vertical oscillations. Notch represents 95% confidence interval, horizontal line in the center of the notch is median frequency, and length of the box is interquartile interval, while whiskers depict the range; (C) This panel depicts box and whisker plots summarizing the intensity (peak to trough velocity difference) of micro-opsoclonus. Blue box and whisker plot depict vertical oscillations, while red is horizontal.

Symptoms include gross motor delay with decreased muscle tone as well as sleep and speech difficulties. Management options include treatment with corticosteroids, intravenous immunoglobulins, tumor surgery, or chemotherapy. Clonazepam may be utilized in patients that did not respond to immune suppressants. Adrenocorticotropic hormone (ACTH) may be superior to corticosteroid treatments, according to recent studies. Interestingly, nearly 100% of patients with opsoclonus-myoclonus syndrome survive, while 75% of Horner's syndrome patients and 11% of orbital metastasis patients survive. Even with successful treatment, children often have long-term neurologic sequelae.

Voluntary Nystagmus

Voluntary nystagmus is a benign, pendular, conjugate, high frequency, and low amplitude movement of the eyes initiated and terminated on command. It appears similarly to ocular flutter, but the movement is not sustained beyond 20–30 seconds. The inability to sustain the movement is the key feature that differentiates voluntary nystagmus from other pathologic forms of flutter. It can be initiated during convergence and may be associated with mild widening of palpebral fissures with facial grimaces. It can also be familial with various generations showing similar parameters of nystagmus such as duration, amplitude, and frequency.

NYSTAGMUS BLOCKAGE SYNDROME

Definition

It is a motor adaptation in a case of nystagmus to increase vision when the patient has to focus on a visually demanding task. There is an inverse relationship between the amount of esotropia and amplitude of nystagmus.

Clinical Findings

The patient is orthotropic with manifest nystagmus when inattentive, but there is esotropia with minimal nystagmus when attentive. The fixing eye is preferred to be adducted so that the face turn is in the direction of the fixing eye. There is an absence of nystagmus when the fixating eye is in adduction with the appearance of a manifest jerky nystagmus as the fixating eye moves into primary position and abduction.

These patients can become esotropic with time due to sustained convergence and secondary changes in the medial rectus muscles.

Diagnosis is assisted by the presence of pupillary constriction during esotropia.

This entity must be differentiated from

- *Infantile esotropia with manifest-latent nystagmus:* Nystagmus will be present even in the presence of esotropia.
- *Bilateral sixth nerve paralysis:* Absence of nystagmus and presence of true abduction deficits.
- *Infantile esotropia with crossed fixation:* There is no nystagmus as fixation is maintained in the primary position or in abduction. Second, an esotropia caused by adduction of both eyes, which is frequently seen with the nystagmus blockage syndrome (NBS), does not occur in alternating esotropia with crossed fixation where the fixating eye, as a rule, is in the primary position and only the non-fixating eye is adducted. Third, patients with

crossed fixation are alternators; amblyopia does not occur with alternating strabismus but is seen with the NBS.

Management

Patient is prescribed appropriate refractive correction with alternate occlusion.

Surgical management involves bimedial recession with posterior fixation sutures. The correction should be planned for the manifest angle of esotropia at the time of visual demand.

SUMMARY

Nystagmus type	*Pathogenesis*	*Symptoms*	*Diagnosis*	*Treatment*	*Prognosis*
Fusion maldevelopment nystagmus syndrome	Any disorder that disturbs development of binocular fusion, particularly congenital esotropia	• Nystagmus that becomes apparent or enhanced when one eye is covered • Strongly associated with strabismus and dissociated vertical divergence • *Nystagmus blockage syndrome*: Head turn such that viewing eye is in adducting position	Eye movement recordings of fast and slow phases	• Combination of medical, optical, and surgical treatments to improve visual acuity and binocular function • Surgical therapy can be performed to correct abnormal head posture and strabismus, with the possibility of improving visual acuity	FMNS patients typically have impaired stereopsis despite strabismus and amblyopia therapies
Infantile nystagmus syndrome	• Idiopathic • Correlated with albinism, retinal disease, visual deprivation early in life, congenital iris absence, underdeveloped optic nerves, or congenital cataract • *FRMD7* gene mutation	• Nystagmus increases on attempted fixation, but decreases with convergence or eyelid closure • High- and low-frequency head oscillations	• Gene sequencing panel • Eye movement recordings for waveforms	• *Surgeries*: Kestenbaum procedure to improve abnormal head position, tetonomy with reattachment, and four muscles recession • *Medically*: Gabapentin, memantine and topical brinzolamide • Others base out prism to induce convergence and dampen nystagmus and contact lenses	Depends on underlying cause, but generally waveforms decrease in amplitude and frequency until 6–8 years of age and remain stable afterwards unless associated with progressive disease
Spasmus nutans	• Rare, idiopathic • Environmental associations such as nonwhite ethnicity, low home luminance, gestational age, and low socioeconomic status	• Nystagmus is disconjugate, asymmetric, high frequency; can be horizontal, vertical, or torsional • Nystagmus can increase in frequency with convergence • Head nodding	Triad of nystagmus, head nodding, and torticollis	Observation once CNS abnormalities are ruled out	• Typically begins in infancy and resolves on clinical observation by 2 years, but subclinical nystagmus persists until 5–12 years • Good visual acuity is predicted, as children may develop both visual acuity and stereovision during phases of compensatory head nodding

Contd...

Contd...

Nystagmus type	*Pathogenesis*	*Symptoms*	*Diagnosis*	*Treatment*	*Prognosis*
Neurologic nystagmus	• Acquired with neurologic disorders or ocular cranial nerve palsies • Vertical nystagmus can be upbeat or downbeat • Upbeat nystagmus is possibly due to pontine or medullary lesions involving SVN-VTT pathway or anterior visual pathway disease • Downbeat nystagmus is possibly due to floccular damage involving SVN-VTT pathway • Horizontal nystagmus can be gaze evoked and associate with brain tumor • Associated with demyelinating disease	• Vertigo, nausea, headaches, relative afferent pupillary defect, papilledema, optic atrophy, and visual loss • Brain tumor • Upbeating or downbeating nystagmus • Horizontal gaze-evoked nystagmus	• Ophthalmologic and neurologic examination to identify structural abnormalities including nerve pathologies • ERG to evaluate retinal dystrophies	• Treatment of underlying neurologic cause • Eye muscle surgery to move eyes closer to primary position	Depends on underlying cause
Opsoclonus	• Can be observed transiently in healthy term and preterm neonates • Tumors of neural crest origin in children • Parainfectious, metabolic, and toxic etiologies • Immunological cross-reactivity between the tumor and normal cerebellar neurons	• Eye movements are multidirectional and can be in any plane • Oscillopsia and visual blurring • Present during fixation, smooth pursuit, convergence, and persists during sleep and eyelid closure	Whole body imaging to identify potential tumor	Can include corticosteroids, intravenous immunoglobulins, tumor surgery, and chemotherapy	Even with successful treatment, children often have long-term neurologic sequelae
Ocular flutter	Rare symptom that occurs in the context of many diseases including cancerous malignancies, paraneoplastic or autoimmune diseases, drug intoxication, head trauma, or postviral infection	Intermittent bursts of conjugate saccades occurring strictly in the horizontal plane without an intersaccadic interval	Eye movement recordings	Treatment of underlying cause	Usually self-limiting
Voluntary nystagmus	Thought to be familial	Pendular, conjugate, high frequency, low amplitude movement of the eyes on command	The inability to sustain the movement is the key feature that differentiates voluntary nystagmus from other pathologic forms of flutter	Does not require treatment	*Benign*: Initiated and terminated on command

(CNS: central nervous system; ERG: electroretinography; FMNS: fusion maldevelopment nystagmus syndrome; SVN-VTT: superior vestibular nucleus-ventral tegmental tract)

D

G

H

M

T